Medical Terminology Systems

Systems

A Body Systems Approach

SIXTH EDITION

Barbara A. Gylys (GĬL-Ĭs), MEd, CMA-A (AAMA)
Professor Emerita
College of Health and Human Services
Coordinator of Medical Assisting Technology
University of Toledo
Toledo, Ohio

Mary Ellen Wedding, MEd, MT(ASCP), CMA, (AAMA) AAPC
Professor of Health Professions
College of Health Science and Human Services
University of Toledo
Toledo, Ohio

F.A. Davis Company • Philadelphia

What's INSIDE...▶

MEDICAL TERMINOLOGY SYSTEMS
A Body Systems Approach, 6th Edition

CLEAR, CONCISE PRESENTATION
using the classic word-building and body systems approach to learning.

CHAPTER OUTLINES
to orient students to each chapter's content

KEY TERMS
highlighted in the beginning of each chapter

ABBREVIATIONS
for common terms

HOW DOES WORD BUILDING WORK?
It begins with the basics

- ■ **Introduces word elements**
  - • Roots
  - • Combining forms
  - • Suffixes
  - • Prefixes

- ■ **Reviews each element one by one**

- ■ **Applies the principles of word building to each body system**
  - • Learn the parts from which words are built
  - • Decipher words based on knowledge of word parts

- ■ **Uses mnemonic devices and interactive activities** (in the book and on the CD) to make word building fun and increase retention

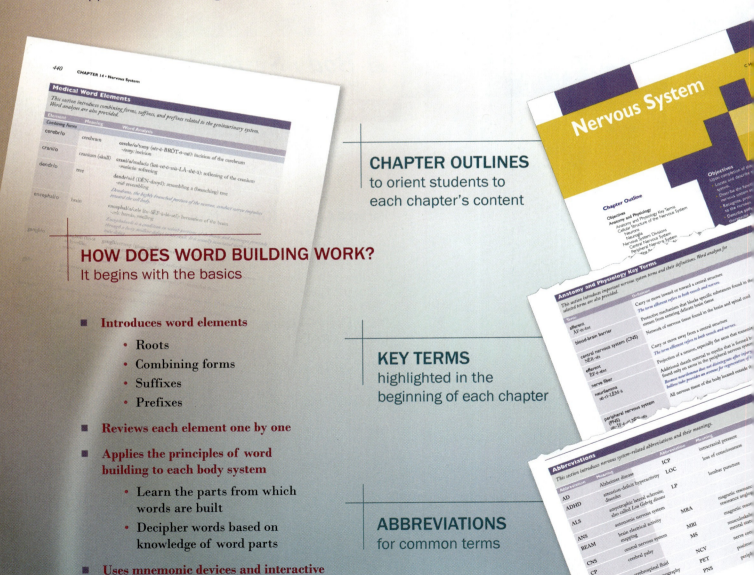

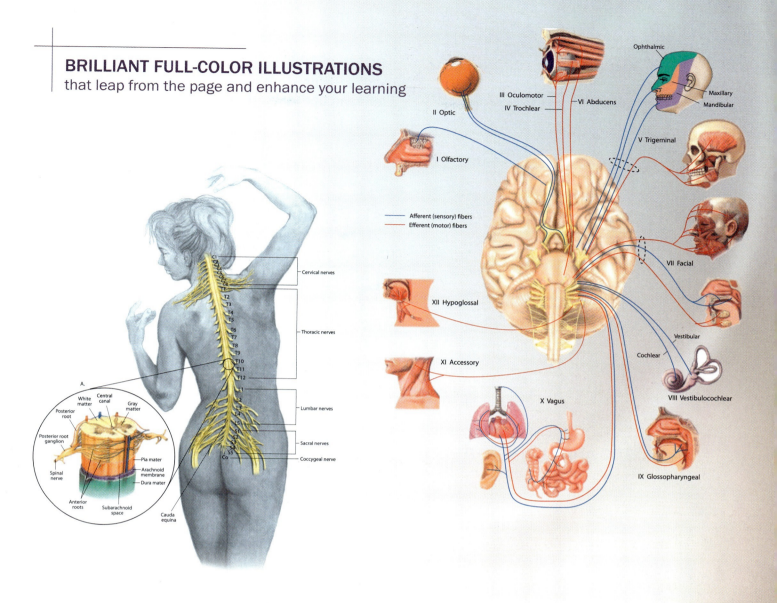

BRILLIANT FULL-COLOR ILLUSTRATIONS
that leap from the page and enhance your learning

Ophthalmic

II Optic

III Oculomotor
IV Trochlear
VI Abducens

Maxillary
Mandibular

I Olfactory

V Trigeminal

Afferent (sensory) fibers
Efferent (motor) fibers

VII Facial

XII Hypoglossal

XI Accessory

Vestibular

Cochlear

X Vagus

VIII Vestibulocochlear

IX Glossopharyngeal

Cervical nerves

Thoracic nerves

Lumbar nerves

Sacral nerves

Coccygeal nerve

A.

White matter
Central canal
Gray matter

Posterior root

Posterior root ganglion

Spinal nerve

Anterior roots

Subarachnoid space

Pia mater
Arachnoid membrane
Dura mater

Cauda equina

C1
C2
C3
C4
C5
C6
C7
C8
T1
T2
T3
T4
T5
T6
T7
T8
T9
T10
T11
T12
L1
L2
L3
L4
L5
S1
S2
S3
S4
S5
Co

ANATOMY
that's detailed and precise

(3) Dendrites

(1) Cell body

(6) Schwann cell

Schwann cell nucleus

(7) Neurilemma

(4) Axon

(2) Nucleus

(4) Axon

(5) Myelin sheath

(8) Node of Ranvier

(10) Axon terminal

(10) Axon terminal

Mitochondrion

Synaptic bulb

(11) Neurotransmitter

(9) Synapse

Dendrite of receiving neuron

Receptor sites

A.

B.

...A Unique Blend
OF WORDS AND ART

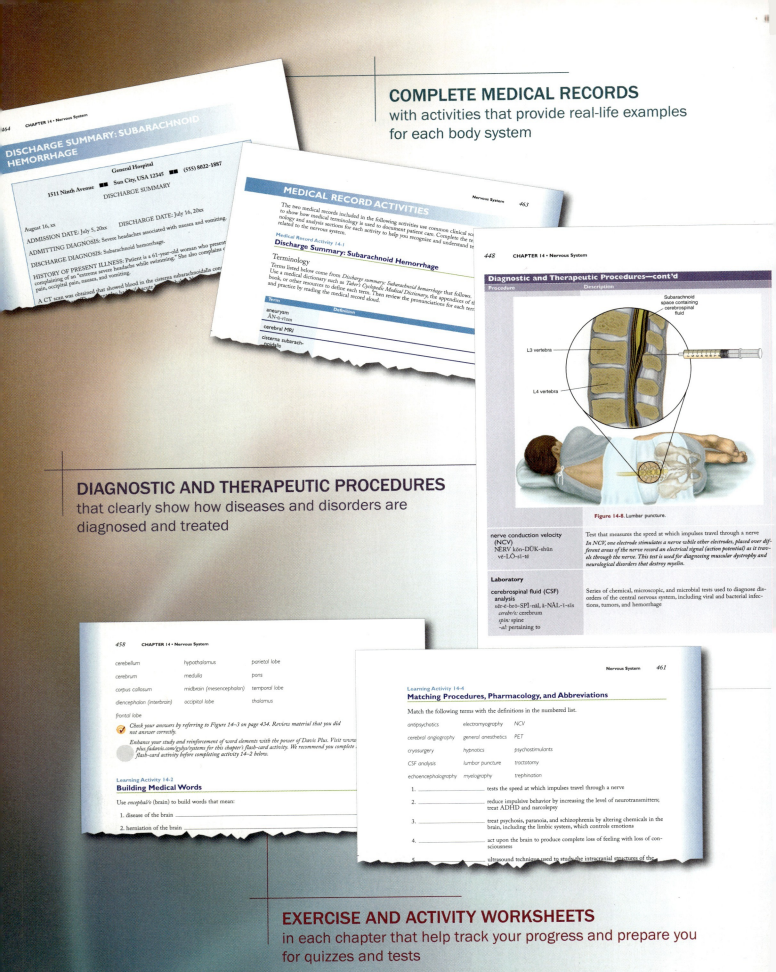

COMPLETE MEDICAL RECORDS

with activities that provide real-life examples for each body system

---

DISCHARGE SUMMARY: SUBARACHNOID HEMORRHAGE

General Hospital

1511 Ninth Avenue ■■ Sun City, USA 12345 ■■ (555) 8022-1887

DISCHARGE SUMMARY

August 16, xx

ADMISSION DATE: July 5, 20xx   DISCHARGE DATE: July 16, 20xx

ADMITTING DIAGNOSIS: Severe headaches associated with nausea and vomiting.

DISCHARGE DIAGNOSIS: Subarachnoid hemorrhage.

HISTORY OF PRESENT ILLNESS: Patient is a 61-year-old woman who present complaining of an "extreme severe headache while swimming." She also complains of pain, occipital pain, nausea, and vomiting.

A CT scan was obtained that showed blood in the cisterna subarachnoidalis con

---

MEDICAL RECORD ACTIVITIES

The two medical records included in the following activities use common clinical sce to show how medical terminology is used to document patient care. Complete the te nology and analysis sections for each activity to help you recognize and understand te related to the nervous system.

Medical Record Activity 14-1

Discharge Summary: Subarachnoid Hemorrhage

Terminology

Terms listed below come from *Discharge summary: Subarachnoid hemorrhage* that follows. Use a medical dictionary such as *Taber's Cyclopedic Medical Dictionary* to define each term. book, or other resources to define each term. Then review the pronunciations for each term and practice by reading the medical record aloud.

Term	Definition
aneurysm ĂN-ū-rĭzm	
cerebral MRI	
cisterna subarach- noidalis	

DIAGNOSTIC AND THERAPEUTIC PROCEDURES

that clearly show how diseases and disorders are diagnosed and treated

---

Diagnostic and Therapeutic Procedures—cont'd

Procedure	Description

Subarachnoid space containing cerebrospinal fluid

L3 vertebra

L4 vertebra

Figure 14-8. Lumbar puncture.

nerve conduction velocity (NCV) NĔRV kŏn-DŬK-shŭn vē-LŎ-sĭ-tē	Test that measures the speed at which impulses travel through a nerve *In NCV, one electrode stimulates a nerve while other electrodes, placed over different areas of the nerve record an electrical signal (action potential) as it travels through the nerve. This test is used for diagnosing muscular dystrophy and neurological disorders that destroy myelin.*

Laboratory

cerebrospinal fluid (CSF) analysis sĕr-ē-brō-SPĪ-năl, ă-NĂL-ĭ-sĭs *cerebr/o:* cerebrum *spin:* spine *-al:* pertaining to	Series of chemical, microscopic, and microbial tests used to diagnose disorders of the central nervous system, including viral and bacterial infections, tumors, and hemorrhage

---

cerebellum	hypothalamus	parietal lobe
cerebrum	medulla	pons
corpus callosum	midbrain (mesencephalon)	temporal lobe
diencephalon (interbrain)	occipital lobe	thalamus
frontal lobe		

✓ *Check your answers by referring to Figure 14–3 on page 434. Review material that you did not answer correctly.*

Enhance your study and reinforcement of word elements with the power of Davis Plus. Visit www. plus.fadavis.com/gylys/systems for this chapter's flash-card activity. We recommend you complete flash-card activity before completing activity 14–2 below.

Learning Activity 14-2

Building Medical Words

Use *encephal/o* (brain) to build words that mean:

1. disease of the brain _____

2. herniation of the brain _____

Learning Activity 14-4

Matching Procedures, Pharmacology, and Abbreviations

Match the following terms with the definitions in the numbered list.

antipsychotics	electromyography	NCV
cerebral angiography	general anesthetics	PET
cryosurgery	hypnotics	psychostimulants
CSF analysis	lumbar puncture	tractotomy
echoencephalography	myelography	trephination

1. _____ tests the speed at which impulses travel through a nerve

2. _____ reduce impulsive behavior by increasing the level of neurotransmitters; treat ADHD and narcolepsy

3. _____ treat psychosis, paranoia, and schizophrenia by altering chemicals in the brain, including the limbic system, which controls emotions

4. _____ act upon the brain to produce complete loss of feeling with loss of consciousness

5. _____ ultrasound technique used to study the intracranial structures of the

---

EXERCISE AND ACTIVITY WORKSHEETS

in each chapter that help track your progress and prepare you for quizzes and tests

COMPLETE LEARNING AND TEACHING EXPERIENCE!

The full **Medical Terminology Systems** package includes the text, Term*Plus* CD-ROM, and Audio CD.

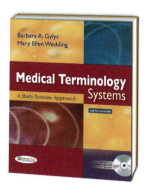 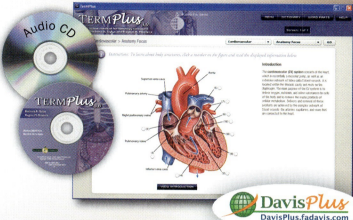

- **Audio CD**
  - Listen-and-learn activities for more than 300 terms

- **Term*Plus* 3.0 CD-ROM**
  - Competency based, self-paced
  - Mac & PC compatible
  - Interactive exercises, such as anatomy labeling, crossword puzzles, word drag-and-drop, and word scrambles

- **Student Resources Online at Davis*Plus***
  (No fee—No password—No registration)
  - Audio pronunciations—Downloadable to an iPod or MP3 player for study on the go
  - Flash Card and Medical Record Activities
  - Word Search Activities
  - Animations—almost 20 in all

- **Instructor Resources Available Upon Adoption Online at Davis*Plus* and on CD-ROM**
  - 25 PowerPoint Slideshows
  - Wimba Electronic Test Bank—Nearly 1,250 multiple-choice, true/false, short answer, and matching items
  - Interactive Teaching Tool—A wealth of activities for each body system—52 in all
  - Searchable image bank with approximately 150 images
  - Activity Pack including a Resource Kit for uploading to Blackboard or other learning management systems

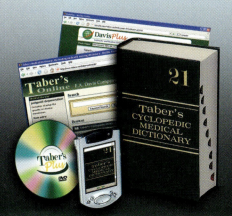

TABER'S CYCLOPEDIC MEDICAL DICTIONARY, 21ST EDITION

Edited by Donald Venes, MD, MSJ

Taber's brings meanings to life! To thrive in the ever-changing world of healthcare, you need a respected, trusted, and cutting-edge cyclopedic resource. In hand, online, or on your mobile device—anywhere and everywhere—turn to Taber's 21 and the Taber's*Plus* DVD.

www.fadavis.com

F. A. Davis Company
1915 Arch Street
Philadelphia, PA 19103
www.fadavis.com

Printed in the United States of America

Last digit indicates print number: 10 9 8 7 6 5 4 3 2 1

Senior Acquisitions Editor: Andy McPhee
Manager of Content Development: George W. Lang
Developmental Editor: Brenna H. Mayer
Art and Design Manager: Carolyn O'Brien

As new scientific information becomes available through basic and clinical research, recommended treatments and drug therapies undergo changes. The author(s) and publisher have done everything possible to make this book accurate, up to date, and in accord with accepted standards at the time of publication. The author(s), editors, and publisher are not responsible for errors or omissions or for consequences from application of the book, and make no warranty, expressed or implied, in regard to the contents of the book. Any practice described in this book should be applied by the reader in accordance with professional standards of care used in regard to the unique circumstances that may apply in each situation. The reader is advised always to check product information (package inserts) for changes and new information regarding dose and contraindications before administering any drug. Caution is especially urged when using new or infrequently ordered drugs.

Library of Congress Cataloging-in-Publication Data
Gylys, Barbara A.
  Medical terminology systems : a body systems approach / Barbara A. Gylys, Mary Ellen Wedding. — 6th ed.
      p. cm.
  Includes index.
  ISBN 978-0-8036-2090-2
  1. Medicine—Terminology. I. Wedding, Mary Ellen. II. Title.
  [DNLM: 1. Terminology as Topic—problems and Exercises. W 15 G997ma 2009]
  R123.G94 2009
  610. 1'4—dc22   2009006473

This Book is Dedicated with Love

to my best friend, colleague, and husband, Julius A. Gylys, and *to my children,*
Regina Maria and Julius Anthony, and *to my grandchildren, Andrew Masters,*
Julia Masters, Caitlin Masters, Anthony Mychal Bishop-Gylys,
and Matthew James Bishop-Gylys **B.A.G.**

to my loving grandchildren, Andrew Arthur Kurtz, Katherine
Louise Kurtz, Daniel Keith Wedding II, Carol Ann Estelle Wedding,
Jonathan Michael Kurtz, Donald Keith Wedding III,
Emily Michelle Wedding, Katelyn Christine Wedding,
and David Michael wedding **M.E.W.**

Acknowledgments

The authors would like to acknowledge the valuable contributions of F. A. Davis's editorial and production team who were responsible for this project:

- **Andy McPhee, Senior Acquisitions Editor,** who provided the overall design and layout for the sixth edition. His vision and guidance focused the authors at the onset of the project, and his support throughout this endeavor provided cohesiveness.
- **Brenna H. Mayer, Developmental Editor,** whose careful and conscientious edits and suggestions for the manuscript are evident throughout the entire work. Her enthusiasm and untiring assistance and support during this project are deeply appreciated and the authors extend their sincerest gratitude.

In addition, we wish to acknowledge the many, exceptionally dedicated publishing partners that helped in this publication:

- Stephanie A. Casey, Administrative Assistant
- Yvonne N. Gillam, Associate Developmental Editor
- Kate Margeson, Illustrations Coordinator
- Frank J. Musick, Developmental Editor, Electronic Publishing
- Bob Butler, Production Manager
- Carolyn O'Brien, Art and Design Manager
- David Orzechowski, Managing Editor
- Kirk Pedrick, Electronic Product Development Manager, Electronic Publishing
- Elizabeth Y. Stepchin, Developmental Associate.

We also extend our sincerest appreciation to Neil K. Kelly, Executive Director of Sales, Sally J. Daluge, Senior Regional Manager, and their staff of sales representatives whose continued efforts have undoubtedly contributed to the success of this textbook.

Joanne Leming
Director
Allied Health Programs
Nevada Career Institute
Las Vegas, Nevada

Marti Lewis, EdD, RN, CMA-AC (AAMA)
Former Dean (retired)
Mathematics, Engineering, Science, and Health
Olympic College
Bremerton, Washington

Susan Perreira, MS, CMA, RMA
Associate Professor and Coordinator
Medical Assisting Program
Capital Community College
Hartford, Connecticut

Marilyn Reeder, MS, CMA (AAMA), CNA, CHUC
Instructor
Health Sciences and Medicine
GASC Technology Center
Flint, Michigan

Amy Semenchuk, RN, BSN
Department Chair
Health Occupations
Rockford Business College
Rockford, Illinois

Carol Tamparo, PhD, CMA (AAMA)
Former Dean
Health Sciences & Business (retired)
Lake Washington Technical College
Tacoma, Washington

Claire Travis, BA, MA (Educ), MBA, CPHQ
Director
Allied Health
Salter School
Worcester, Massachusetts

LaTanya Young, RMA (AMT), PA-C, MMSc, MPH
Assistant Professor and Coordinator
Medical Assisting Program
Clayton State University
Morrow, Georgia

Preface

The sixth edition of *Medical Terminology Systems: A Body Systems Approach* continues to live up to its well-established track record of presenting medical word-building principles based on competency-based curricula. The popular, basic features of the previous edition have been enhanced and expanded.

Systems is designed with the educational foundation of a textbook-workbook that complements all teaching formats, including traditional lecture, distance learning, and independent or self-paced study. The purpose of the book is to help students learn medical terminology so they can effectively communicate with other members of the health care team. A variety of pedagogical features help them develop a solid foundation in medical terminology to broaden their medical vocabulary. Although the study of medical terminology demands hard work and discipline, various self-paced activities offer interest and variety to the learning process. A variety of activities and resources are available to adopters of the textbook on DavisPlus at *www.davisplus.fadavis.com.*

All changes in the sixth edition are structured to help in the learning process and improve retention of medical terms. Many new, visually impressive, full-color illustrations have been added to this edition. The art work throughout the book is specifically designed to present accurate and aesthetically pleasing representations of anatomical structures, disease conditions, and medical procedures. Illustrations augment course content in new and interesting ways and help make difficult concepts clear.

The sixth edition continues to present eponyms without showing the possessive form, such as *Bowman capsule, Cushing syndrome,* and *Parkinson disease.* Medical dictionaries as well as the American Association for Medical Transcription and the American Medical Association support these changes. The sixth edition contains a summary of medical abbreviations and their meanings. New to this edition is a summary of common symbols as well as an updated list of "do-not-use" abbreviations. The summaries are found in Appendix B, Common Abbreviations and Symbols.

Each body systems chapter continues to incorporate the most current technological changes in medicine. Educators and practitioners in various health care disciplines have offered many helpful suggestions for this edition, which have been incorporated. A newly developed list of key anatomy and physiology terms, complete with pronunciations and definitions, sets a solid base for the chapter.

Also new to this edition is a body connections section for each body systems chapter. This table identifies the interrelationship among the body systems and helps put each of them into a clear perspective for the student. Diagnostic and therapeutic procedures have also been expanded. Finally, pharmacology information has been edited to include drugs most commonly used in medical treatment. This section continues to provide generic and trade names, along with their therapeutic actions.

Here is a brief summary of chapters:

- **Chapter 1** explains the techniques of medical word-building using basic word elements.
- **Chapter 2** categorizes major surgical, diagnostic, symptomatic, and grammatical suffixes.
- **Chapter 3** presents major prefixes of position, number and measurement, direction, and other parameters.
- **Chapter 4** introduces anatomical, physiological, and pathological terms. It also presents combining forms denoting cellular and body structure, body position and direction, regions of the body, and additional combining forms related to diagnostic methods, and pathology. General diagnostic and therapeutic terms are described and provide a solid foundation for specific terms addressed in the body system chapters that follow.
- **Chapters 5 through 15** are organized according to specific body systems and may be taught in any sequence. These chapters include key anatomical and physiological terms; basic anatomy and physiology; a body connections table; combining forms, suffixes, and prefixes; pathology; diagnostic, symptomatic, and related terms; diagnostic and therapeutic procedures; pharmacology; abbreviations; learning activities; and medical record activities. All activities allow self-assessment and evaluation of competency.
- **Appendix A: Answer Key** contains answers to each learning activity to validate proficiency and provide immediate feedback for student assessment. Although the answer key for the terminology section of each medical record is not included in this appendix, it is available to adopters in the Activity Pack.
- **Appendix B: Common Abbreviations and Symbols** includes an updated, comprehensive list of medical abbreviations and their meanings and a new summary of common symbols as well as an updated list of "do-not-use" abbreviations.

- **Appendix C: Glossary of Medical Word Elements** contains alphabetical lists of medical word elements and their meanings. This appendix presents two methods for word-element indexing—first by medical word element, then by English term.
- **Appendix D: Index of Genetic Disorders** lists genetic disorders presented in the textbook.
- **Appendix E: Index of Diagnostic Imaging Procedures** lists radiographic and other diagnostic imaging procedures presented in the textbook.
- **Appendix F: Index of Pharmacology** lists medications presented in the textbook.
- **Appendix G: Index of Oncological Disorders** lists oncological disorders presented in the textbook.

Instructor's Resource Disk

The Instructor's Resource Disk (IRD) features many new, innovative instructional aids designed to make teaching medical terminology easier and more effective. The supplemental teaching aids can be used in various educational settings—traditional classroom, distance learning, or independent or self-paced studies. The IRD consists of an Activity Pack, three PowerPoint presentations, a searchable image bank, an Interactive Teaching Tool (ITT), animations, and a Wimba computerized test bank, a powerful, user-friendly test-generation program.

Activity Pack

The Activity Pack has been expanded to meet today's instructional needs and now includes:

- *Suggested Course Outlines.* Course outlines are provided to help you plan the best method of covering material presented in the textbook. A newly designed course outline is provided for textbooks packaged with Term *Plus,* the completely revised and updated interactive software. Now it will be easy to correlate instructional software with textbook chapters.
- *Student and Instructor-Directed Activities.* These comprehensive teaching aids have been updated and new ones have been added for this edition. They offer an assortment of activities for each body-system chapter. Activities can be used as course requirements or as supplemental material. In addition, activities can be assigned as individual or collaborative projects. For group projects, Peer Evaluation Forms have been provided.
- *Community and Internet Resources.* This section provides an expanded list of resources, including technical journals, community organizations, and Internet sites to complement course content.
- *Supplemental Medical Record Activities.* The supplemental medical record activities have been updated and include student activities that complement and expand information presented in the body system chapters. As in the textbook, these activities use common clinical scenarios to show how medical terminology is used to document patient care. Medical terms, their pronunciations, and a medical record analysis are provided for each record, along with an answer key. In addition, each medical record highlights a specific body system and correlates it with a medical specialty. Medical records can be used for various activities, including oral reports, medical coding, medical transcribing, or individual assignments.
- *Crossword Puzzles.* These fun, educational activities are included for each body system chapter. They are designed to reinforce material covered in the chapter and can be used individually or in groups. They can also be used for extra credit or "just for fun." An answer key is included for each puzzle.
- *Pronunciations and Answer Keys.* We've continued to provide a special answer key for the medical record research activities in the textbook. This key should prove helpful as you present course material and grade assignments.
- *Master Transparencies.* The transparency pages offer large, clear, black-and-white anatomical illustrations perfect for making overhead transparencies and are provided for each body system.

PowerPoint Presentations

This edition of *Systems* contains three powerful PowerPoint presentations for your use. *Lecture Notes* provides an outline-based presentation for each body system chapter. It consists of a chapter overview, main functions of the body system, and selected pathology, vocabulary, and procedures. Full-color illustrations from the book are included. *MedTerm Workout* is an interactive presentation in which terms drop into view at a click of the mouse. Students can be prompted to say the term aloud, define the term, or provide other feedback before moving to the next term. *Name That Part* is a unique interactive PowerPoint presentation that alows you to guide students in identifying specific parts of a body system. No other medical terminology book offers this innovative ancillary, and we hope you find it useful in your classroom.

Image Bank

New to this edition is an Adobe Flash-based image bank that contains all illustrations from the textbook. It is fully searchable and allows users to zoom in and out and display a JPG image of an illustration that can be copied into a Microsoft Word document or PowerPoint presentation.

Interactive Teaching Tool

The Interactive Teaching Tool (ITT) is a newly incorporated instructional ancillary for use in the classroom. The tool is an Adobe Flash application of images from the book, followed by questions and answers relevant to the illustration. You can zoom in and out of images and test students' knowledge as you lead discussion of the content.

Animations

We've also developed five new animations to help students better visualize complex concepts. For instance, one animation explores the pathology of gastroesophageal reflux diseases, or GERD. Another shows the various stages of pregnancy and delivery. We think these innovative tools will help students better understand important processes and procedures and the medical terms that go along with them.

Electronic Test Bank

This edition offers a powerful Wimba test-generating program that allows you to create custom-made or randomly generated tests in a printable format from a test bank of more than 1,240 multiple-choice test items as well as numerous true-false and matching questions. The program requires Windows 95, Windows 98, or Windows NT and is available for Macintosh on request.

Audio CD

Some versions of *Systems* are packaged with an audio CD recording. The CD provides exercises designed to strengthen spelling, pronunciation, and understanding of selected medical terms. The audio CD can also be used in beginning transcription and medical secretarial courses. Transcription skills are be developed by typing each word as it is pronounced. After the words are typed, spelling can be corrected by referring to the textbook or a medical dictionary.

Term *Plus*

Term *Plus* is a powerful, interactive CD-ROM program offered with some texts, depending on which version has been selected. Term *Plus* is a competency-based, self-paced, multimedia program that includes graphics, audio, and a dictionary culled from *Taber's Cyclopedic Medical Dictionary*, 20th ed. Help menus provide navigational support. The software comes with numerous interactive learning activities, including:

- Anatomy Focus
- Tag the Elements (Drag-and-Drop)
- Spotlight the Elements
- Concentration
- Build Medical Words
- Programmed Learning
- Medical Vocabulary
- Chart Notes
- Spelling
- Crossword Puzzles
- Word Scramble

All activities can be graded and the results printed or e-mailed to an instructor. That makes the CD-ROM especially valuable as a distance-learning tool because it provides evidence of student drill and practice in various learning activities.

Taber's Cyclopedic Medical Dictionary

The world-famous *Taber's Cyclopedic Medical Dictionary* is the recommended companion reference for this book. Virtually all terms in *Systems* may be found in *Taber's*. In addition, *Taber's* contains etymologies for nearly all main entries presented in this textbook.

We hope you enjoy this new edition as much as we enjoyed preparing it. We think you will find this the best edition ever.

Barbara A. Gylys
Mary Ellen Wedding

Contents at a Glance

Contents

CHAPTER **5**   **Integumentary System**   *71*

Basic Elements of a Medical Word

Chapter Outline

Objectives

Upon completion of this chapter, you will be able to:

- Identify the four word elements used to build medical words.
- Divide medical words into their component parts.
- Apply the basic rules to define and build medical words.
- Locate the pronunciation guidelines chart and interpret pronunciation marks.
- Pronounce medical terms presented in this chapter.
- Demonstrate your knowledge of this chapter by completing the learning activities.

Medical Word Elements

The language of medicine is a specialized vocabulary used by health care practitioners. Many current medical word elements originated as early as the 1st century B.C., when Hippocrates practiced medicine. With advancements in medicine, new terms have evolved to reflect these innovations. For example, radiographic terms, such as *magnetic resonance imaging* (MRI) and *ultrasound* (US), are now used to describe current diagnostic procedures.

A medical word consists of some or all of the following elements: word root, combining form, suffix, and prefix. How you combine these elements, and whether all or some of them are present in a medical term, determines the meaning of a word. The purpose of this chapter is to help you identify these elements in order to construct medical terms correctly.

Word Roots

A **word root** is the foundation of a medical term and contains its primary meaning. All medical terms have at least one word root. Most word roots are derived from Greek or Latin language. Thus, two different roots may have the same meaning. For example, the Greek word *dermatos* and the Latin word *cutane* both refer to the skin. As a general rule, Greek roots are used to build words that describe a disease, condition, treatment, or diagnosis. Latin roots are used to build words that describe anatomical structures. Consequently, the Greek root *dermat* is used primarily in terms that describe a disease, condition, treatment, or diagnosis of the skin; the Latin root *cutane* is used primarily to describe an anatomical structure. (See Table 1-1.)

Table 1-1	**Examples of Word Roots**		
This table lists examples of word roots as well as their phonetic pronunciations. Begin learning the pronunciations as you review the information below.			
English Term	**Greek or Latin Term***	**Word Root**	**Word Analysis**
skin	dermatos (Gr)	dermat	**dermat**/itis (dĕr-mă-TĪ-tĭs): inflammation of the skin
			A term that describes a skin disease
	cutis (L)	cutane	**cutane**/ous (sŭb-kū-TĀ-nē-ŭs): pertaining to the skin
			A term that describes an anatomical structure
kidney	nephros (Gr)	nephr	**nephr**/oma (nĕ-FRŌ-mă): tumor of the kidney
			A term that describes a kidney disease
	renes (L)	ren	**ren**/al (RĒ-năl): pertains to the kidney
			A term that describes an anatomical structure
mouth	stomatos (Gr)	stomat	**stomat**/itis (stō-mă-TĪ-tĭs): inflammation of the mouth
			A term that describes any inflammatory condition of the mouth
	oris (L)	or	**or**/al (OR-ăl): pertaining to the mouth
			A term that describes an anatomical structure

*It is not important to know the origin of a medical word. This information is provided here to help avoid confusion and illustrate that there may be two different word roots for a single term.

Combining Forms

A **combining form** is created when a word root is combined with a vowel. The vowel, known as a *combining vowel*, is usually an *o*, but sometimes it is an *i*. The combining vowel has no meaning of its own, but enables two word elements to be connected. Like the word root, the combining form is the basic foundation to which other word elements are added to build a complete medical word. In this text, a combining form will be listed as *word root/vowel* (such as *gastr/o*), as illustrated in Table 1-2.

Suffixes

A **suffix** is a word element placed at the end of a word that changes the meaning of the word. In the terms tonsill/*itis*, and tonsill/*ectomy*, the suffixes are –*itis* (inflammation) and –*ectomy* (excision, removal). Changing the suffix changes the meaning of the word. In medical terminology, a suffix usually describes a pathology (disease or abnormality), symptom, surgical or diagnostic procedure, or part of speech. Many suffixes are derived from Greek or Latin words. (See Table 1-3.)

Table 1-2   Examples of Combining Forms

This table illustrates how word roots and vowels create combining forms. Learning combining forms rather than word roots makes pronunciation a little easier because of the terminal vowel. For example, in the table below, the word roots gastr *and* nephr *are difficult to pronounce, whereas their combining forms* gastr/o *and* nephr/o *are easier to pronounce.*

Word Root	+	Vowel	=	Combining Form	Meaning
erythr/	+	o	=	erythr/o	red
gastr/	+	o	=	gastr/o	stomach
hepat/	+	o	=	hepat/o	liver
immun/	+	o	=	immun/o	immune, immunity, safe
nephr/	+	o	=	nephr/o	kidney
oste/	+	o	=	oste/o	bone

Table 1-3   Examples of Suffixes

This table lists examples of pathological suffixes as well as their phonetic pronunciations. Begin learning the pronunciations as you review the information below.

Combining Form	+	Suffix	=	Medical Word	Meaning
	+	**-itis** (inflammation)	=	**gastritis** găs-TRĪ-tĭs	inflammation of the stomach
gastr/o (stomach)	+	**-megaly** (enlargement)	=	**gastromegaly** găs-trō-MĔG-ă-lē	enlargement of the stomach
	+	**-oma** (tumor)	=	**gastroma** găs-TRŌ-mă	tumor of the stomach
	+	**-itis** (inflammation)	=	**hepatitis** hĕp-ă-TĪ-tĭs	inflammation of the liver
hepat/o (liver)	+	**-megaly** (enlargement)	=	**hepatomegaly** hĕp-ă-tō-MĔG-ă-lē	enlargement of the liver
	+	**-oma** (tumor)	=	**hepatoma** hĕp-ă-TŌ-mă	tumor of the liver

Prefixes

A **prefix** is a word element attached to the beginning of a word or word root. However, not all medical terms have a prefix. Adding or changing a prefix changes the meaning of the word. The prefix usually indicates a number, time, position, direction, or negation. Many of the same prefixes used in medical terminology are also used in the English language. (See Table 1-4.)

Basic Guidelines

Defining and building medical words are crucial skills in mastering medical terminology. Following the basic guidelines for each will help you develop these skills.

Defining Medical Words

Here are three basic steps for defining medical words using *gastroenteritis* as an example.

1. Define the suffix, or last part of the word. In this case, the suffix *-itis, which means inflammation.*
2. Define the first part of the word (which may be a word root, combining form, or prefix). In this case, the combining form *gastr/o means stomach.*
3. Define the middle parts of the word. In this case, the word root *enter* means *intestine.* When you analyze *gastroenteritis* following the three previous rules, the meaning is:

1. inflammation (of)
2. stomach (and)
3. intestine.

Thus, the meaning of *gastroenteritis* is *inflammation (of) stomach (and) intestine.* Table 1-5 on page 4 further illustrates this process.

Table 1-4	**Examples of Prefixes**

This table lists examples of prefixes as well as their phonetic pronunciations. Begin learning the pronunciations as you review the information below.

Prefix	+	Word Root	+	Suffix	=	Medical Word	Meaning
an- (without, not)	+	**esthes** (feeling)	+	**-ia** (condition)	=	**anesthesia** ăn-ĕs-THĒ-zē-ă	condition of not feeling
hyper- (excessive, above normal)	+	**therm** (heat)	+	**-ia** (condition)	=	**hyperthermia** hī-pĕr-THĔR-mē-ă	condition of excessive heat
intra- (in, within)	+	**muscul** (muscle)	+	**-ar** (pertaining to)	=	**intramuscular** ĭn-tră-MŬS-kū-lăr	pertaining to within the muscle
para- (near, beside; beyond)	+	**nas** (nose)	+	**-al** (pertaining to)	=	**paranasal** păr-ă-NĀ-săl	pertaining to (area) near the nose
poly- many, much	+	**ur** (urine)	+	**-ia** (condition)	=	**polyuria** pŏl-ē-Ū-rē-ă	condition of much urine

---

Table 1-5	**Defining Gastroenteritis**

This table illustrates three steps of defining a medical word using the example gastroenteritis.

Combining Form	Middle	Suffix
gastr/o	**enter/**	**-itis**
stomach	intestine	inflammation
(step 2)	(step 3)	(step 1)

Building Medical Words

There are three basic rules for building medical words.

Rule #1

A word root links a suffix that begins with a vowel.

Rule #2

A combining form (root + *o*) links a suffix that begins with a consonant.

Rule #3

A combining form links a root to another root to form a compound word. This rule holds true even if the next root begins with a vowel, as in *osteoarthritis*. Keep in mind that the rules for linking multiple roots to each other are slightly different from the rules for linking roots and combining forms to suffixes.

Rule 1

Word Root	+	Suffix	=	Medical Word	Meaning
hepat	+	**-itis**	=	**hepatitis**	inflammation of the liver
liver		inflammation		hĕp-ă-TĪ-tĭs	

Rule 2

Combining Form	+	Suffix	=	Medical Word	Meaning
hepat/o	+	**-cyte**	=	**hepatocyte**	liver cell
liver		cell		HĔP-ă-tō-sīt	

Rule 3

Combining Form	+	Word Root	+	Suffix	=	Medical Word	Meaning
oste/o	+	**chondr**	+	**-itis**	=	**osteochondritis**	inflammation of bone and cartilage
(bone)		cartilage		inflammation		ŏs-tē-ō-kŏn-DRĪ-tĭs	
		arthr	+	**-itis**	=	**osteoarthritis**	inflammation of bone and joint
		joint		inflammation		ŏs-tē-ō-ăr-THRĪ-tĭs	

 It is Time to review medical word elements by completing Learning Activity 1–1. and 1–2.

Pronunciation Guidelines

Although pronunciations of medical words usually follows the same rules that govern pronunciations of English words, some medical words may be difficult to pronounce when first encountered.

Therefore, selected terms in this book include phonetic pronunciation. Also, pronunciation guidelines can be found on the inside front cover of this book and at the end of selected tables. Use them whenever you need help with pronunciation of medical words.

It is Time to review pronunciations, analysis of word elements, and defining medical terms by completing Learning Activities 1-3, 1-4, and 1-5.

LEARNING ACTIVITIES

The following activities provide a review of the basic medical word elements introduced in this chapter. Complete each activity and review your answers to evaluate your understanding of this chapter.

Learning Activity 1-1

Understanding Medical Word Elements

Fill in the following blanks to complete the sentences correctly.

1. The four elements used to form words are _____.

2. A root is the main part or foundation of a word. In the words *arthritis, arthroma,* and *arthroscope,* the root is _____.

Identify the following statements as true or false. If false, rewrite the statement correctly on the line provided.

3. A combining vowel is usually an e.	True	False
4. A word root links a suffix that begins with a consonant.	True	False
5. A combining form links multiple roots to each other.	True	False
6. A combining form links a suffix that begins with a consonant.	True	False
7. To define a medical word, first define the prefix.	True	False
8. In the term *intramuscular, intra* is the prefix.	True	False

Underline the word root in each of following combining forms.

9. splen/o (spleen)

10. hyster/o (uterus)

11. enter/o (intestine)

12. neur/o (nerve)

13. ot/o (ear)

14. dermat/o (skin)

15. hydr/o (water)

✓ *Check your answers in Appendix A. Review material that you did not answer correctly.*

Correct Answers _____ × 6.67 = _____ % Score

Learning Activity 1-2

Identifying Word Roots and Combining Forms

Underline the word roots in the following medical words.

Medical Word	Meaning
1. nephritis	inflammation of the kidneys
2. arthrodesis	fixation of a joint
3. dermatitis	inflammation of the skin
4. dentist	specialist in teeth
5. gastrectomy	excision of the stomach
6. chondritis	inflammation of cartilage
7. hepatoma	tumor of the liver
8. muscular	pertaining to muscles
9. gastria	condition of the stomach
10. osteoma	tumor of the bone

Underline the combining forms below.

11. nephr	kidney
12. hepat/o	liver
13. arthr	joint
14. oste/o/arthr	bone, joint
15. cholangi/o	bile vessel

 Check your answers in Appendix A. Review material that you did not answer correctly.

Correct Answers _____ × 6.67 = _____ % Score

Learning Activity 1-3

Understanding Pronunciations

Review the pronunciation guidelines (located inside the front cover of this book) and then underline the correct answer in each of the following statements.

1. The diacritical mark ¯ is called a (breve, macron).

2. The diacritical mark ˘ is called a (breve, macron).

3. The ¯ indicates the (short, long) sound of vowels.

4. The ˘ indicates the (short, long) sound of vowels.

5. The combination *ch* is sometimes pronounced like *(k, chiy)*. Examples are *cholesterol, cholemia.*

6. When *pn* is at the beginning of a word, it is pronounced only with the sound of *(p, n)*. Examples are *pneumonia, pneumotoxin.*

7. When *pn* is in middle of a word, the *p (is, is not)* pronounced. Examples are *orthopnea, hyperpnea.*

8. When *i* is at the end of a word, it is pronounced like *(eye, ee)*. Examples are *bronchi, fungi, nuclei.*

9. For *ae* and *oe*, only the (first, second) vowel is pronounced. Examples are *bursae, pleurae.*

10. When *e* and *es* form the final letter or letters of a word, they are commonly pronounced as (combined, separate) syllables. Examples are *syncope, systole, nares.*

✓ *Check your answers in Appendix A. Review material that you did not answer correctly.*

Correct Answers _____ × 10 = _____ % Score

Learning Activity 1-4

Identifying Suffixes and Prefixes

Pronounce the following medical terms. Then analyze each term and write the suffix in the right-hand column. The first suffix is completed for you.

Term	Suffix
1. thoracotomy thōr-ă-KŎT-ō-mē	-tomy
2. gastroscope GĂS-trō-skōp	
3. tonsillitis tŏn-sĭl-Ī-tĭs	
4. gastroma GĂS-trō-mă	
5. tonsillectomy tŏn-sĭl-ĔK-tō-mē	

Pronunciation Help	Long Sound	ā — rate	ē — rebirth	ī — isle	ō — over	ū — unite
	Short Sound	ă — alone	ĕ — ever	ĭ — it	ŏ — not	ŭ — cut

Pronounce the following medical terms. Then analyze each term and write the element that is a prefix in the right-hand column. The first prefix is completed for you.

Term	Prefix
6. anesthesia ăn-ĕs-THĒ-zē-ă	an-
7. hyperthermia hī-pĕr-THĔR-mē-ă	
8. intramuscular ĭn-tră-MŬS-kū-lăr	
9. paranasal păr-ă-NĀ-săl	
10. polyuria pŏl-ē-Ū-rē-ă	

✓ *Check your answers in Appendix A. Review material that you did not answer correctly.*

Correct Answers _____ × 10 = _____ % Score

Defining Medical Words

The three basic steps for defining medical words are:

1. Define the last part of the word, or **suffix**.

2. Define the first part of the word, or **prefix, word root,** or **combining form.**

3. Define the **middle** of the word.

First pronounce the term aloud. Then apply the above three steps to define the terms in the following table. If you are not certain of a definition, refer to Appendix C, Part 1, of this textbook, which provides an alphabetical list of word elements and their meanings.

Term	Definition
1. gastritis găs-TRĬ-tĭs	_____
2. nephritis nĕf-RĪ-tĭs	_____
3. gastrectomy găs-TRĔK-tō-mē	_____
4. osteoma ŏs-tē-Ō-mă	_____
5. hepatoma hĕp-ă-TŌ-mă	_____
6. hepatitis hĕp-ă-TĪ-tĭs	_____

Refer to the section "Building Medical Words" on page 5 to complete this activity. Write the number for the rule that applies to each listed term as well as a short summary of the rule. Use the abbreviation WR to designate *word root*, CF to designate *combining form*. The first one is completed for you.

Term	Rule	Summary of the Rule
7. arthr/itis ăr-THRĪ-tĭs	*I*	*A WR links a suffix that begins with a vowel.*
8. scler/osis sklĕ-RŌ-sĭs	____	_____
9. arthr/o/centesis ăr-thrō-sĕn-TĒ-sĭs	____	_____
10. colon/o/scope kō-LŎN-ō-skōp	____	_____
11. chondr/itis kŏn-DRĪ-tĭs	____	_____
12. chondr/oma kŏn-DRŌ-mă	____	_____
13. oste/o/chondr/itis ŏs-tē-ō-kŏn-DRĪ-tĭs	____	_____
14. muscul/ar MŬS-kū-lăr	____	_____
15. oste/o/arthr/itis ŏs-tē-ō-ăr-THRĪ-tĭs	____	_____

Check your answers in Appendix A. Review material that you did not answer correctly.

Correct Answers _____ × 6.67 = _____ % Score

Suffixes

Chapter Outline

Objectives

Upon completion of this chapter, you will be able to:

- Define and provide examples of surgical, diagnostic, pathological, and related suffixes.
- Determine how to link combining forms and word roots to various types of suffixes.
- Identify adjective, noun, and diminutive suffixes.
- Locate and apply guidelines for pluralizing terms.
- Pronounce medical terms presented in this chapter.
- Demonstrate your knowledge of the chapter by completing the learning activities.

Suffix Linking

In medical words, a suffix is added to the end of a word root or combining form to change its meaning. For example, the combining form *gastr/o* means *stomach*. The suffix *-megaly* means *enlargement*, and *-itis* means *inflammation*. *Gastr/o/megaly* is an enlargement of the stomach; *gastr/itis* is an inflammation of the stomach. Whenever you change the suffix, you change the meaning of the word. Suffixes are also used to denote singular and plural forms of a word as well as a part of speech. The following tables provide additional examples to reinforce the rules you learned in Chapter 1. (See Tables 2–1 and 2–2.)

Words that contain more than one word root are known as compound words. Multiple word roots within a compound word are always changed to combining forms so that the roots are joined together with a combining vowel, regardless of whether the second word root begins with a vowel or a consonant. Notice that a combining vowel is used in the Table 2–2 between **gastr** and **enter,** even though the second word root, **enter,** begins with a vowel.

Keep in mind the rule for linking multiple roots is slightly different from the rules for linking word roots to suffixes. Recall from Chapter 1 that suffixes that begin with a vowel are linked with a word root; suffixes that begin with a consonant are linked with a combining form.

Table 2-1 Word Roots and Combining Forms with Suffixes

This table provides examples of word roots used to link a suffix that begins with a vowel. It also lists combining forms (root + o) used to link a suffix that begins with a consonant.

Element	+	Suffix	=	Medical Word	Meaning
Word Roots					
gastr (stomach)	+	**-itis** (inflammation)	=	**gastritis** găs-TRĪ-tĭs	inflammation of the stomach
hemat (blood)	+	**-emesis** (vomiting)	=	**hematemesis** hĕm-ăt-ĔM-ĕ-sĭs	vomiting of blood
arthr (joint)	+	**-itis** (inflammation)	=	**arthritis** ăr-THRĪ-tĭs	inflammation of a joint
Combining Forms					
gastr/o (stomach)	+	**-dynia** (pain)	=	**gastrodynia** găs-trō-DĬN-ē-ă	pain in the stomach
hemat/o (blood)	+	**-logy** (study of)	=	**hematology** hē-mă-TŎL-ō-jē	study of blood
arthr/o (joint)	+	**-centesis** (surgical puncture)	=	**arthrocentesis** ăr-thrō-sĕn-TĒ-sĭs	surgical puncture of a joint

Table 2-2 Compound Words with Suffixes

This table shows examples of medical terms with more than one word root, and also suffixes linked together with word roots when the suffix begins with a vowel.

Combining Form	+	Word Root	+	Suffix	=	Medical Word	Meaning
gastr/o (stomach)	+	**enter** (intestine)	+	**-itis** (inflammation)	=	**gastroenteritis** găs-trō-ĕn-tĕr-Ī-tĭs	inflammation of stomach and intestine
oste/o (bone)	+	**arthr** (joint)	+	**-itis** (inflammation)	=	**osteoarthritis** ŏs-tē-ō-ō-ăr-THRĪ-tĭs	inflammation of bone and joint
encephal/o (brain)	+	**mening** (meninges)	+	**-itis** (inflammation)	=	**encephalomeningitis** ĕn-sĕf-ă-lō-mĕn-ĭn-JĪ-tĭs	inflammation of brain and meninges

Surgical, Diagnostic, Pathological, and Related Suffixes

Surgical suffixes describe a type of invasive procedure performed on a body part. (See Table 2–3.) Diagnostic suffixes denote a procedure or test performed to identify the cause and nature of an illness. Pathological suffixes describe an abnormal condition or disease. (See Table 2–4.)

Suffix Types

An effective method in mastering medical terminology is to learn the major types of suffixes in categories. By grouping the surgical, diagnostic, pathological, related, as well as grammatical suffixes, they will be easier to remember.

Table 2-3	Common Surgical Suffixes	
	This table lists commonly used surgical suffixes along with their meanings and word analyses.	
Suffix	**Meaning**	**Word Analysis**
-centesis	surgical puncture	arthr/o/**centesis** (ăr-thrō-sĕn-TĒ-sĭs): puncture of a joint space with a needle and the withdrawal of fluid *arthr/o:* joint *Arthrocentesis may also be performed to obtain samples of synovial fluid for diagnostic purposes, instill medications, and remove fluid from joints to relieve pain.*
-clasis	to break; surgical fracture	oste/o/**clasis** (ŏs-tē-ŌK-lă-sĭs): surgical fracture of a bone to correct a deformity *oste/o:* bone
-desis	binding, fixation (of a bone or joint)	arthr/o/**desis** (ăr-thrō-DĒ-sĭs): binding together of a joint *arthr/o:* joint *Arthrodesis is a surgical procedure to fuse bones across the joint space in a degenerated, unstable joint.*
-ectomy	excision, removal	append/**ectomy** (ăp-ĕn-DĔK-tō-mē): excision of the appendix *append:* appendix
-lysis	separation; destruction; loosening	thromb/o/**lysis** (thrŏm-BŎL-ĭ-sĭs): destruction of a blood clot *thromb/o:* blood clot *Drug therapy is usually used to dissolve a blood clot.*
-pexy	fixation (of an organ)	mast/o/**pexy** (MĂS-tō-pĕks-ē): fixation of the breast(s) *mast/o:* breast *Mastopexy, an elective surgery, is performed to affix sagging breasts in a more elevated position, commonly improving their shape.*
-plasty	surgical repair	rhin/o/**plasty** (RĪ-nō-plăs-tē): surgical repair of the nose *rhin/o:* nose *Plastic surgery to change the size or shape of the nose.*
-rrhaphy	suture	my/o/**rrhaphy** (mī-OR-ă-fē): suture of a muscle *my/o:* muscle
-stomy	forming an opening (mouth)	trache/o/**stomy** (trā-kē-ŎS-tō-mē): forming an opening into the trachea *trache/o:* trachea (windpipe) *A tracheostomy is an artificial opening performed to bypass an obstructed upper airway.*

(continued)

Table 2-3	Surgical Suffixes—cont'd		
-tome	instrument to cut	oste/o/**tome** (ŎS-tē-ō-tōm): instrument to cut bone *oste/o:* bone *An osteotome is a surgical chisel used to cut through bone.*	
-tomy	incision	trache/o/**tomy** (trā-kē-ŎT-ō-mē): incision (through the neck) into the trachea *trache/o:* trachea (windpipe) *Tracheotomy is performed to gain access to an airway below a blockage.*	
-tripsy	crushing	lith/o/**tripsy** (LĬTH-ō-trĭp-sē): crushing a stone *lith/o:* stone, calculus *Lithotripsy is a surgical procedure for eliminating a stone in the kidney, ureter, bladder, or gallbladder.*	

 It is time to review surgical suffixes by completing Learning Activities 2–1, 2–2, and 2–3.

Table 2-4	Diagnostic, Pathological, and Related Suffixes

This table lists commonly used diagnostic, pathological, and related suffixes along with their meanings and word analyses.

Suffix	Meaning	Word Analysis
Diagnostic		
-gram	record, writing	electr/o/cardi/o/**gram** (ē-lĕk-trō-KĂR-dē-ō-grăm): record of the electrical activity of the heart *electr/o:* electricity *cardi/o:* heart
-graph	instrument for recording	cardi/o/**graph** (KĂR-dē-ŏ-grăf): instrument for recording electrical activity of the heart *cardi/o:* heart
-graphy	process of recording	angi/o/**graphy** (ăn-jē-ŎG-ră-fē): process of recording blood vessels *angi/o:* vessel (usually blood or lymph) *Angiography is the radiographic imaging of blood vessels afte injection of a contrast medium.*
-meter	instrument for measuring	pelv/i/**meter*** (pĕl-VĬM-ĕ-tĕr): instrument for measuring the pelvis *pelv/i:* pelvis
-metry	act of measuring	pelv/i/**metry*** (pĕl-VĬM-ĕ-trē): act or process of measuring the dimension of the pelvis *pelv/i:* pelvis
-scope	instrument for examining	endo/**scope** (ĔN-dō-skōp): instrument for examining within *endo-:* in, within *An endoscope is a flexible or rigid instrument consisting of a tube and optical system for observing the inside of a hollow organ or cavity.*
-scopy	visual examination	endo/**scopy** (ĕn-DŎS-kō-pē): visual examination within *endo-:* in, within *Endoscopy is performed to visualize a body cavity or canal using a specialized lighted instrument called an endoscope.*

Table 2-4	Diagnostic, Pathological, and Related Suffixes—cont'd	
Suffix	**Meaning**	**Word Analysis**
Pathological and Related		
-algia	pain	neur/**algia** (nū-RĂL-jē-ă): pain of a nerve *neur: nerve* *The pain of neuralgia usually occurs along the path of a nerve.*
-dynia		ot/o/**dynia** (ō-tō-DĬN-ē-ă): pain in the ear; earache *ot/o: ear*
-cele	hernia, swelling	hepat/o/**cele** (hĕ-PĂT-ō-sēl): hernia of the liver *hepat/o: liver*
-ectasis	dilation, expansion	bronchi/**ectasis** (brŏng-kē-ĔK-tă-sĭs): dilation or expansion of one or more bronchi *bronchi: bronchus (plural, bronchi)* *Bronchiectasis is associated with various lung conditions and is commonly accompanied by chronic infection.*
-edema	swelling	lymph/**edema** (lĭmf-ĕ-DĒ-mă): swelling and accumulation of tissue fluid *lymph: lymph* *Lymphedema may be caused by a blockage of the lymph vessels.*
-emesis	vomiting	hyper/**emesis** (hī-pĕr-ĔM-ĕ-sĭs): excessive vomiting *hyper-: excessive, above normal*
-emia	blood condition	an/**emia** (ă-NĒ-mē-ă): blood condition caused by a decrease in red blood cells (erythrocytes) *an-: without, not*
-gen	forming, producing, origin	carcin/o/**gen** (kăr-SĬN-ō-jĕn): forming, producing, or origin of cancer *carcin/o: cancer* *A carcinogen is a substance or agent, such as cigarettes, that causes the development or increases the incidence of cancer.*
-genesis		carcin/o/**genesis** (kăr-sĭ-nō-JĔN-ĕ-sĭs): forming or producing cancer *carcin/o: cancer* *Carcinogenesis is the transformation of normal cells into cancer cells, commonly as a result of chemical, viral, or radioactive damage to genes.*
-iasis	abnormal condition (pro-duced by something specific)	chol/e/lith/**iasis*** (kō-lē-lĭ-THĪ-ă-sĭs): abnormal condition of gallstones *chol/e: bile, gall* *lith: stone, calculus* *Cholelithasis is the presence or formation of gallstones in the gallbladder or common bile duct.*
-itis	inflammation	gastr/**itis** (găs-TRĪ-tĭs): inflammation of the stomach *gastr: stomach*
-lith	stone, calculus	chol/e/**lith*** (KŌ-lē-lĭth): gallstone *chol/e: bile, gall*
-malacia	softening	chondr/o/**malacia** (kŏn-drō-măl-Ā-shē-ă): softening of the articular cartilage, usually involving the patella *chondr/o: cartilage*

(continued)

Table 2-4	Diagnostic, Pathological, and Related Suffixes—cont'd

Suffix	Meaning	Word Analysis
-megaly	enlargement	cardi/o/**megaly** (kăr-dē-ō-MĔG-ă-lē): enlargement of the heart *cardi/o:* heart
-oma	tumor	neur/**oma** (nū-RŌ-mă): tumor composed of nerve tissue *neur:* nerve *A neuroma is a benign tumor composed chiefly of neurons and nerve fibers, usually arising from a nerve tissue. It may also be a swelling of a nerve that usually results from compression.*
-osis	abnormal condition; increase (used primarily with blood cells)	cyan/**osis** (sī-ă-NŌ-sĭs): dark blue or purple discoloration of the skin and mucous membrane *cyan:* blue *Cyanosis indicates a deficiency of oxygen in the blood.*
-pathy	disease	my/o/**pathy** (mī-ŎP-ă-thē): disease of muscle *my/o:* muscle
-penia	decrease, deficiency	erythr/o/**penia** (ĕ-rĭth-rō-PĒ-nē-ă): decrease in red blood cells *erythr/o:* red
-phagia	eating, swallowing	dys/**phagia** (dĭs-FĀ-jē-ă): inability or difficulty in swallowing *dys-:* bad; painful; difficult
-phasia	speech	a/**phasia** (ă-FĀ-zē-ă): absence or impairment of speech *a-:* without, not
-phobia	fear	hem/o/**phobia** (hē-mō-FŌ-bē-ă): fear of blood *hem/o:* blood
-plasia	formation, growth	dys/**plasia** (dĭs-PLĀ-zē-ă): abnormal formation or growth of cells, tissues, or organs *dys-:* bad; painful; difficult *Dysplasia is a general term for abnormal formation of an anatomic structure.*
-plasm		neo/**plasm** (NĒ-ō-plăzm): new formation or growth of tissue *neo-:* new *A neoplasm is an abnormal formation of new tissue, such as a tumor or growth.*
-plegia	paralysis	hemi/**plegia** (hĕm-ē-PLĒ-jē-ă): paralysis of one side of the body *hemi-:* one half *Hemiplegia affects the right or left side of the body and is usually caused by a brain injury or stroke.*
-ptosis	prolapse, downward displacement	blephar/o/**ptosis** (blĕf-ă-rō-TŌ-sĭs): drooping of the upper eyelid *blephar/o:* eyelid
-rrhage	bursting forth (of)	hem/o/**rrhage** (HĔM-ĕ-rĭj): bursting forth (of) blood *hem/o:* blood *Hemorrhage refers to a loss of a large amount of blood within a short period, either externally or internally.*
-rrhagia		men/o/**rrhagia** (mĕn-ō-RĀ-jē-ă): profuse discharge of blood during menstruation *men/o:* menses, menstruation

Table 2-4	Diagnostic, Pathological, and Related Suffixes—cont'd	
Suffix	**Meaning**	**Word Analysis**
-rrhea	discharge, flow	dia/**rrhea** (dī-ă-RĒ-ă): abnormally frequent discharge or flow of fluid fecal matter from the bowel *dia–:* through, across
-rrhexis	rupture	arteri/o/**rrhexis** (ăr-tē-rē-ō-RĔK-sĭs): rupture of an artery *arteri/o:* artery
-sclerosis	abnormal condition of hardening	arteri/o/**sclerosis** (ăr-tē-rē-ō-sklĕ-RŌ-sĭs): abnormal condition of hardening of an artery *arteri/o:* artery
-spasm	involuntary contraction, twitching	blephar/o/**spasm** (BLĔF-ă-rō-spăsm): twitching of the eyelid *blephar/o:* eyelid
-stenosis	narrowing, stricture	arteri/o/**stenosis** (ăr-tē-rē-ō-stĕ-NŌ-sĭs): abnormal narrowing of an artery *arteri/o:* artery
-toxic	poison	hepat/o/**toxic** (HĔP-ă-tō-tŏk-sĭk): poisonous to the liver *hepat/o:* liver
-trophy	nourishment, development	dys/**trophy** (DĬS-trō-fē): bad nourishment *dys–:* bad; painful; difficult *Dystrophy is an abnormal condition caused by improper nutrition or altered metabolism.*

*The *i* in *pelv/i/meter* and *pelv/i/metry* and the *e* in *chol/e/lithiasis* and *chol/e/lith* are exceptions to the rule of using the connecting vowel *o*.

 It is time to review diagnostic, pathological, and related suffixes by completing Learning Activities 2–4 and 2–5.

Grammatical Suffixes

Grammatical suffixes are attached to word roots to form parts of speech, such as adjectives and nouns, or singular or plural forms of medical words. They are also used to denote a diminutive form, or smaller version, of a word—for example, *tubule,* which means a small tube. Many of these same suffixes are used in the English language. (See Table 2–5.)

Table 2-5	Adjective, Noun, and Diminutive Suffixes	
This table lists adjective, noun, and diminutive suffixes along with their meanings and word analyses.		
Suffix	**Meaning**	**Word Analysis**
Adjective		
-ac	pertaining to	cardi/**ac** (KĂR-dē-ăk): pertaining to the heart *cardi:* heart
-al		neur/**al** (NŪ-răl): pertaining to a nerve *neur:* nerve
-ar		muscul/**ar** (MŬS-kū-lăr): pertaining to muscle *muscul:* muscle

(continued)

Table 2-5	Adjective, Noun, and Diminutive Suffixes—cont'd	
Suffix	**Meaning**	**Word Analysis**
-ary		pulmon/**ary** (PŬL-mō-nĕr-ē): pertaining to the lungs *pulmon:* lung
-eal		esophag/**eal** (ē-sŏf-ă-JĒ-ăl): pertaining to the esophagus *esophag:* esophagus
-ic		thorac/**ic** (thō-RĂS-ĭk): pertaining to the chest *thorac:* chest
-ical*		path/o/log/**ical** (păth-ō-LŎJ-ĭ-kăl): pertaining to the study of disease *path/o:* disease *log:* study of
-ile		pen/**ile** (PĒ-nīl): pertaining to the penis *pen:* penis
-ior		poster/**ior** (pŏs-TĒ-rē-or): pertaining to the back of the body *poster:* back (of body), behind, posterior
-ous**		cutane/**ous** (kū-TĀ-nē-ŭs): pertaining to the skin *cutane:* skin
-tic		acous/**tic** (ă-KOOS-tĭk): pertaining to hearing *acous:* hearing
Noun		
-esis	condition	di/ur/**esis** (dī-ū-RĒ-sĭs): abnormal secretion of large amounts of urine *di-:* double *ur:* urine
-ia		pneumon/**ia** (nū-MŌ-nē-ă): infection of the lung usually caused by bacteria, viruses, or diseases *pneumon:* air; lung
-ism		hyper/thyroid/**ism** (hī-pĕr-THĪ-royd-ĭzm): condition characterized by overactivity of the thyroid gland *hyper-:* excessive, above normal *thyroid:* thyroid gland
-iatry	medicine; treatment	pod/**iatry** (pō-DĪ-ă-trē): specialty concerned with treatment and prevention of conditions of the feet *pod:* foot
-ician	specialist	obstetr/**ician** (ŏb-stĕ-TRĬSH-ăn): physician who specializes in the branch of medicine concerned with pregnancy and childbirth *obstetr:* midwife
-ist		hemat/o/log/**ist** (hē-mă-TŎL-ō-jĭst): physician who specializes in the treatment of disorders of blood and blood-forming tissues *hemat/o:* blood *log:* study of
-y	condition; process	neur/o/path/**y** (nū-RŎP-ă-thē): disease condition of the nerves *neur/o:* nerve *path:* disease

Table 2-5	Adjective, Noun, and Diminutive Suffixes—cont'd	
Suffix	**Meaning**	**Word Analysis**
Diminutive		
-icle	small, minute	ventr/**icle** (VĔN-trĭ-kl): small cavity, as of the brain or heart *ventr:* belly, belly side
-ole		arteri/**ole** (ăr-TĒ-rē-ōl): the smallest of the arteries; minute artery *arteri:* artery
		Arteries narrow to form arterioles (small arteries), which branch into capillaries (the smallest blood vessels).
-ule		ven/**ule** (VĔN-ūl): small vein continuous with a capillary *ven:* vein

*The suffix *-ical* is a combination of *-ic* and *-al.* **The suffix *-ous* also means *composed of or producing.*

 It is time to review grammatical suffixes by completing Learning Activity 2–6.

Plural Suffixes

Many medical words have Greek or Latin origins and follow the rules of these languages in building singular and plural forms. Once you learn these rules, you will find that they are easy to apply. You will also find that some English endings have also been adopted for commonly used medical terms. When a word changes from a singular to a plural form, the suffix of the word is the part that changes. A summary of the rules for changing a singular word into its plural form is located on the inside back cover of this textbook. Use it to complete Learning Activity 2–7 and whenever you need help forming plural words.

 It is time to review the rules for forming plural words by completing Learning Activity 2–7.

LEARNING ACTIVITIES

The following activities provide review of the suffixes introduced in this chapter. Complete each activity and review your answers to evaluate your understanding of the chapter.

Learning Activity 2-1
Building Surgical Words

Use the meanings in the right column to complete the surgical words in the left column. The first one is completed for you. Note: The word roots are underlined in the left column.

Incomplete Word   Meaning

1. episi/o/t o m y _____   incision of the perineum

2. col _____   excision (of all or part)* of the colon

3. arthr/o/_____   surgical puncture of a joint (to remove fluid)

4. splen_____   excision of the spleen

5. col/o/_____   forming an opening (mouth) into the colon

6. oste/o/_____   instrument to cut bone

7. tympan/o/_____   incision of the tympanic membrane

8. trache/o/_____   forming an opening (mouth) into the trachea

9. mast_____   excision of a breast

10. lith/o/_____   incision to remove a stone or calculus

11. hemorrhoid_____   excision of hemorrhoids

Build a surgical word that means

12. forming an opening (mouth) into the colon: _____

13. excision of the colon: _____

14. instrument to cut bone: _____

15. surgical puncture of a joint: _____

16. incision to remove a stone: _____

17. excision of a breast: _____

18. incision of the tympanic membrane: _____

19. forming an opening (mouth) into the trachea: _____

20. excision of the spleen:_____

✔   *Check your answers in Appendix A. Review any material that you did not answer correctly.*

Correct Answers _____ × 5 = _____ % Score

_____

*Information in parentheses is used to clarify the meaning of the word but not to build the medical term.
Note: If you are not satisfied with your level of comprehension in Learning Activity 2–1, review it and complete the exercise again.

Learning Activity 2-2

Building More Surgical Words

Use the meanings in the right column to complete the surgical words in the left column. The word roots are underlined in the left column.

Incomplete Word

Meaning

1. arthr/o/ _____
2. rhin/o/ _____
3. ten/o/ _____
4. my/o/ _____
5. mast/o/ _____
6. cyst/o/ _____
7. oste/o/ _____
8. lith/o/ _____
9. enter/o/ _____
10. neur/o/ _____

fixation or binding of a joint
surgical repair of the nose
surgical repair of tendons
suture of a muscle
fixation of a (pendulous)* breast
suture of the bladder
surgical fracture of a bone
crushing of a stone
separation of intestinal (adhesions)
crushing a nerve

Build a surgical word that means

11. surgical repair of the nose: _____
12. fixation of a joint: _____
13. suture of a muscle: _____
14. fixation of a (pendulous) breast: _____
15. suture of the bladder: _____
16. repair of tendons: _____
17. surgical fracture of a bone: _____
18. crushing stones: _____
19. separation of intestinal (adhesions): _____
20. crushing a nerve: _____

Check your answers in Appendix A. Review any material that you did not answer correctly.

Correct Answers _____ ✕ 5 = _____ % Score

---

*Information in parentheses is used to clarify the meaning of the word but not to build the medical term.

Learning Activity 2-3

Selecting a Surgical Suffix

Use the suffixes listed below to build surgical words in the right column that reflect the meanings in the left column.

-centesis	-ectomy	-plasty	-tome
-clasis	-lysis	-rrhaphy	-tomy
-desis	-pexy	-stomy	-tripsy

1. crushing of a stone: lith/o/ _____
2. puncture of a joint (to remove fluid)*:   arthr/o/ _____
3. excision of the spleen: splen/ _____
4. forming an opening (mouth) into the colon: col/o/ _____
5. instrument to cut skin: derma/ _____
6. forming an opening (mouth) into the trachea: trache/o/ _____
7. incision to remove a stone or calculus: lith/ _____ / _____
8. excision of a breast: mast/ _____
9. excision of hemorrhoids: hemorrhoid/ _____
10. incision of the trachea: trache/ _____ / _____
11. fixation of a breast: mast/ _____ / _____
12. excision of the colon: col/ _____
13. suture of the stomach (wall):   gastr/ _____ / _____
14. fixation of the uterus: hyster/ _____ / _____
15. surgical repair of the nose: rhin/ _____ / _____
16. fixation or binding of a joint: arthr/ _____ / _____
17. to break or surgically fracture a bone: oste/ _____ / _____
18. loosening of nerve (tissue):   neur/ _____ / _____
19. suture of muscle: my/o/ _____
20. incision of the tympanic membrane: tympan/ _____ / _____

✔ *Check your answers in Appendix A. Review any material that you did not answer correctly.*

Correct Answers _____ × 5 = _____ % Score

---

*Information in parentheses is used to clarify the meaning of the word but not to build the medical term.

Learning Activity 2-4

Selecting Diagnostic, Pathological, and Related Suffixes

Use the suffixes in this list to build diagnostic, pathological, and related words in the right column that reflect the meanings in the left column.

-algia	*-graph*	*-metry*	*-penia*	*-rrhage*
-cele	*-iasis*	*-oma*	*-phagia*	*-rrhea*
-ectasis	*-malacia*	*-osis*	*-phasia*	*-rrhexis*
-emia	*-megaly*	*-pathy*	*-plegia*	*-spasm*
-genesis				

1. tumor of the liver: hepat/ _____

2. pain (along the course) of a nerve: neur/ _____

3. dilation of a bronchus: bronchi/ _____

4. producing or forming cancer: carcin/o/ _____

5. abnormal condition of the skin: dermat/ _____

6. enlargement of the kidney: nephr/o/ _____

7. discharge or flow from the ear: ot/_____ / _____

8. rupture of the uterus: hyster/_____ / _____

9. spasm or twitching of the eyelid: blephar/_____ / _____

10. herniation of the bladder: cyst/_____ / _____

11. bursting forth (of) blood: hem/o/ _____

12. abnormal condition of a stone or calculus: lith/ _____

13. paralysis affecting one side (of the body):   hemi/ _____

14. disease of muscle (tissue):   my/_____ / _____

15. difficult or painful swallowing or eating: dys/ _____

16. softening of the bones: oste/_____ / _____

17. without (or absence of) speech: a/ _____

18. white blood condition: leuk/ _____

19. deficiency in red (blood) cells: erythr/_____ / _____

20. measuring the pelvis: pelv/i/ _____

   ✓ *Check your answers in Appendix A. Review any material that you did not answer correctly.*

Correct Answers _____ × 5 = _____ **% Score**

Learning Activity 2-5

Building Pathological and Related Words

Use the meanings in the right column to complete the pathological and related words in the left column.

Incomplete Word	Meaning
1. bronchi _____	dilation of a bronchus
2. chole _____	gallstone
3. carcin/o/ _____	forming or producing cancer
4. oste/ __ /_____	softening of bone
5. hepat/ __ / _____	enlargement of the liver
6. cholelith _____	abnormal condition of gallstones
7. hepat/ __ / _____	herniation of the liver
8. neur/o/ _____	disease of the nerves
9. dermat _____	abnormal condition of the skin
10. hemi _____	paralysis of one half of the body
11. dys _____	difficult swallowing
12. a _____	without (or absence of) speech
13. cephal _____	pain in the head; headache
14. blephar/ __ / _____	twitching of the eyelid
15. hyper _____	excessive formation (of an organ or tissue)

✅ *Check your answers in Appendix A. Review any material that you did not answer correctly.*

Correct Answers _____ × 6.67 = _____ % Score

Learning Activity 2-6

Selecting Adjective, Noun, and Diminutive Suffixes

Use the adjective suffixes in the following list to create a medical term. The first one is completed for you. Note: When in doubt about the validity of a word, refer to a medical dictionary.

-ac	-ary	-ic	-tic
-al	-eal	-ous	-tix

Element	Medical Term	Meaning
1. thorac/	*thoracic*	pertaining to the chest
2. gastr/		pertaining to the stomach
3. bacteri/		pertaining to bacteria
4. aqua/		pertaining to water
5. axill/		pertaining to the armpit
6. cardi/		pertaining to the heart
7. spin/		pertaining to the spine
8. membran/		pertaining to a membrane

Use the noun suffixes in the following list to create a medical term.

-er	-ism	-iatry
-ia	-ist	
-is	-y	

Element	Medical Term	Meaning
9. intern/		specialist in internal medicine
10. leuk/em/		condition of "white" blood
11. sigmoid/o/scop/		visual examination of the sigmoid colon
12. alcohol/		condition of (excessive) alcohol
13. pod/		treatment of the feet
14. allerg/		specialist in treating allergic disorders
15. man/		condition of madness

Use the diminutive suffixes in the following list to create a medical term.

-icle	-ole	-ula	-ule

Element	Medical Term	Meaning
16. arteri/		minute artery
17. ventr/		small cavity
18. ven/		small vein

✔ *Check your answers in Appendix A. Review any material that you did not answer correctly.*

Correct Answers _____ × 5.6 = _____ % Score

Learning Activity 2-7

Forming Plural Words

Review the guidelines for plural suffixes (located inside the back cover of this book). Then write the plural form for each of the following singular terms and briefly state the rule that applies. The first one is completed for you.

Singular	Plural	Rule
1. diagnosis	*diagnoses*	*Drop the is and add es.*
2. fornix		
3. vertebra		
4. keratosis		
5. bronchus		
6. spermatozoon		
7. septum		
8. coccus		
9. ganglion		
10. prognosis		
11. thrombus		
12. appendix		
13. bacterium		
14. testis		
15. nevus		

Check your answers in Appendix A. Review any material that you did not answer correctly.

Correct Answers _____ × 6.67 = _____ % Score

DavisPlus.fadavis.com

Enhance your study and reinforcement of suffixes with the power of DavisPlus. Visit www. davisplus.fadavis.com/gylys/systems *for the flash-card activity related to suffixes. We recommend you complete the flash-card activity before moving on to Chapter 3.*

Prefixes

Chapter Outline

Objectives

Upon completion of this chapter, you will be able to:

- Explain the use of prefixes in medical terminology.
- Explain how a prefix changes the meaning of a medical word.
- Identify prefixes of position, number and measurement, and direction.
- Demonstrate your knowledge of this chapter by completing the learning activities.

Prefix Linking

Most medical words contain a root or combining form with a suffix. Some of them also contain prefixes. A prefix is a word element located at the beginning of a word. Substituting one prefix for another alters the meaning of the word. For example, in the term *macro/cyte*, *macro-* is a prefix meaning *large*; *-cyte* is a suffix meaning cell. A *macrocyte* is a large cell. By changing the prefix *macro-* to *micro-* (small), the meaning of the word changes. A *microcyte** is a small cell. See Table 3–1 for three other examples of how a prefix changes the meaning of a word.

Prefix Types

Learning the major types of prefixes, such as prefixes of position, number and measurement, and direction, as well as some others, will help you master medical terminology.

Prefixes of Position, Number, Measurement, and Direction

Prefixes are used in medical terms to denote position, number and measurement, and direction. Prefixes of position describe a place or location. (See Table 3–2.) Prefixes of number and measurement describe an amount, size, or degree of involvement. (See Table 3–3.) Prefixes of direction indicate a pathway or route. (See Table 3–4.)

Other Common Prefixes

Many other common prefixes may also be used to change the meaning of a word. See Table 3–5 for a list of some other common prefixes.

Table 3-1	**Changing Prefixes and Meanings**

In this table, each word has the same root, nat *(birth) and suffix,* -al *(pertaining to). By substituting different prefixes, new words with different meanings are formed.*

Prefix	+	Word Root	+	Suffix	=	Medical Word	Meaning
pre- (before)	+				=	**prenatal** prē-NĀ-tăl	pertaining to (the period) before birth
peri (around)	+	**nat** (birth	+	**-al** (pertaining to)	=	**perinatal** pĕr-ĭ-NĀ-tăl	pertaining to (the period) around birth
post (after)	+				=	**postnatal** pōst-NĀ-tăl	pertaining to (the period) after birth

Table 3-2	**Prefixes of Position**

This table lists commonly used prefixes of position along with their meanings and word analyses.

Prefix	Meaning	Word Analysis
epi-	above, upon	**epi**/gastr/ic (ĕp-ĭ-GĂS-trĭk): pertaining to above the stomach *gastr:* stomach *–ic:* pertaining to
hypo-	under, below, deficient	**hypo**/derm/ic (hī-pō-DĔR-mĭk): pertaining to under the skin *derm:* skin *–ic:* pertaining to *Hypodermic injections are given under the skin.*
infra-	under, below	**infra**/cost/al (ĭn-fră-KŎS-tăl): below the ribs *cost:* ribs *–al:* pertaining to

*The suffix *-cyte* can also be broken down as a root *cyt* which a noun ending e (cyt/e).

Table 3-2	**Prefixes of Position—cont'd**	
Prefix	**Meaning**	**Word Analysis**
sub-		**sub**/nas/al (sŭb-NĀ-săl): under the nose *nas:* nose *-al:* pertaining to,
inter-	between	**inter**/cost/al (ĭn-tĕr-KŎS-tăl): between the ribs *cost:* ribs *-al:* pertaining to
post-	after, behind	**post**/nat/al (pōst-NĀ-tăl): pertaining to (the period) after birth *nat:* birth *-al:* pertaining to
pre-	before, in front of	**pre**/nat/al (prē-NĀ-tăl): pertaining to (the period) before birth *nat:* birth *-al:* pertaining to
pro-		**pro**/gnosis (prŏg-NŌ-sĭs): knowing before *-gnosis:* knowing *Prognosis is the prediction of the course and end of a disease and the estimated chance of recovery.*
retro-	backward, behind	**retro**/version (rĕt-rō-VĔR-shŭn): turning backwards *-version:* turning *Retroversion refers to tipping backward of an organ (such as the uterus) from its normal position.*

Table 3-3	**Prefixes of Number and Measurement**	

This table lists commonly used prefixes of number and measurement along with their meanings and word analyses.

Prefix	**Meaning**	**Word Analysis**
bi-	two	**bi**/later/al (bī-LĂT-ĕr-ăl): pertaining to two sides *later:* side *-al:* pertaining to
dipl-	double	**dipl**/opia (dĭp-LŌ-pē-ă): double vision *-opia:* vision
diplo-		**diplo**/bacteri/al (dĭp-lō-băk-TĒR-ē-ăl): bacteria linked together in pairs *bacteri:* bacteria *-al:* pertaining to *Diplobacteria reproduce in such a manner that they are joined together in pairs.*
hemi-	one half	**hemi**/plegia (hĕm-ē-PLĒ-jē-ă): paralysis of one half of the body *-plegia:* paralysis
hyper-	excessive, above normal	**hyper**/calc/emia (hī-pĕr-kăl-SĒ-mē-ă): excessive calcium in the blood *calc:* calcium *-emia:* blood condition

(continued)

Table 3-3	Prefixes of Number and Measurement—cont'd	
Prefix	**Meaning**	**Word Analysis**
macro-	large	**macro**/cyte (MĂK-rō-sīt): large cell *–cyte:* cell
micro-	small	**micro**/scope (MĪ-krō-skōp): instrument for examining small (objects) *–scope:* instrument for examining *The microscope is an optical instrument that greatly magnifies minute objects.*
mono-	one	**mono**/therapy (MŎN-ō-thĕr-a-pē): one treatment *–therapy:* treatment *An example of monotherapy is treatment using only a single drug or a single treatment modality.*
uni-		**uni**/nucle/ar (ū-nĭ-NŪ-klē-ăr): pertaining to one nucleus *nucle:* nucleus *–ar:* pertaining to
multi-	many, much	**multi**/gravida (mŭl-tĭ-GRĂV-ĭ-dă): woman who has been pregnant more than once *–gravida:* pregnant woman
poly-		**poly**/phobia (pŏl-ē-FŌ-bē-ă): fear of many things *–phobia:* fear
primi-	first	**primi**/gravida (prī-mĭ-GRĂV-ĭ-dă): woman during her first pregnancy *–gravida:* pregnant woman
quadri-	four	**quadri**/plegia (kwŏd-rĭ-PLĒ-jē-ă): paralysis of four limbs *–plegia:* paralysis
tri-	three	**tri**/ceps (TRĪ-cĕps): three heads *–ceps:* head *Triceps describes a muscle arising by three heads with a single insertion, as the triceps brachii of the posterior arm shown in Figure 10–1.*

Table 3-4	Prefixes of Direction	
This table lists commonly used prefixes of direction as well as their meanings and word analyses.		
Prefix	**Meaning**	**Word Analysis**
ab-	from, away from	**ab**/duction (ăb-DŬK-shŭn): movement of a limb away from (an axis of) the body *–duction:* act of leading, bringing, conducting
ad-	toward	**ad**/duction (ă-DŬK-shŭn): movement of a limb toward (an axis of) the body *–duction:* act of leading, bringing, conducting
circum-	around	**circum**/ren/al (sĕr-kŭm-RĒ-năl): pertaining to around the kidney *ren:* kidney *–al:* pertaining to

Table 3-4	Prefixes of Directions—cont'd	
Prefix	**Meaning**	**Word Analysis**
peri-		**peri**/odont/al (pĕr-ē-ō-DŎN-tăl): pertaining to around a tooth *odont:* teeth *-al:* pertaining to
dia-	through, across	**dia**/rrhea (dī-ă-RĒ-ă): flow through *-rrhea:* discharge, flow *Diarrhea is a condition of abnormally frequent discharge or flow of fluid fecal matter from the bowel.*
trans-		**trans**/vagin/al (trăns-VĂJ-ĭn-ăl): pertaining to across or through the vagina *vagin:* vagina *-al:* pertaining to
ecto-	outside, outward	**ecto**/gen/ous (ĕk-TŎJ-ĕ-nŭs): forming outside the body or structure *gen:* forming, producing, origin *-ous:* pertaining to, *An ectogenous infection is one that originates outside of the body.*
exo-		**exo**/tropia (ĕks-ō-TRŌ-pē-ă): turning outward (of one or both eyes) *-tropia:* turning
extra-		**extra**/crani/al (ĕks-tră-KRĀ-nē-ăl): outside the skull *crani:* cranium (skull) *-al:* pertaining to
endo-	in, within	**endo**/crine (ĔN-dō-krĭn): secrete within *-crine:* secrete *Endocrine describes a gland that secretes directly into the bloodstream.*
intra-		**intra**/muscul/ar (ĭn-tră-MŬS-kū-lăr): within the muscle *muscul:* muscle *-ar:* pertaining to
para-*	near, beside; beyond	**para**/nas/al (păr-ă-NĀ-săl): beside the nose *nas:* nose *-al:* pertaining to
super-	upper, above	**super**/ior (soo-PĒ-rē-or): pertaining to the upper part of a structure *-ior:* pertaining to
supra-	above; excessive; superior	**supra**/ren/al (soo-pră-RĒ-năl): pertaining to above the kidney *ren:* kidney *-al:* pertaining to
ultra-	excess, beyond	**ultra**/son/ic (ŭl-tră-SŎN-ĭk): pertaining to sound beyond (that which can be heard by the human ear) *son:* sound *-ic:* pertaining to

*Para- may also be used as a suffix meaning *to bear (offspring).*

Table 3-5	**Other Common Prefixes**

This table lists other commonly used prefixes along with their meanings and word analyses.

Prefix	Meaning	Word Analysis
a-*	without, not	**a**/mast/ia (ă-MĂS-tē-ă): without a breast *mast:* breast *–ia:* condition *Amastia may be the result of a congenital defect, an endocrine disorder, or mastectomy.*
an-**		**an**/esthesia (ăn-ĕs-THĒ-zē-ă): without feeling *–esthesia:* feeling *Anesthesia may be a partial or complete loss of sensation with or without loss of consciosness.*
anti-	against	**anti**/bacteri/al (ăn-tĭ-băk-TĒR-ē-ăl): against bacteria *bacteri:* bacteria *–al:* pertaining to *Antibacterials are substances that kill bacteria or inhibit their growth or replication.*
contra-		**contra**/ception (kŏn-tră-SĔP-shŭn): against conception or impregnation *–ception:* conceiving *Contraceptive techniques prevent pregnancy by means of medication, a device, or a method that blocks or alters one or more of the processes of reproduction.*
brady-	slow	**brady**/cardia (brăd-ē-KĂR-dē-ă): slow heart rate *–cardia:* heart
dys-	bad; painful; difficult	**dys**/tocia (dĭs-TŌ-sē-ă): difficult childbirth *–tocia:* childbirth, labor
eu-	good, normal	**eu**/pnea (ūp-NĒ-ă): normal breathing *–pnea:* breathing
hetero-	different	**hetero**/graft (HĔT-ĕ-rō-grăft): different transplant *–graft:* transplantation *A heterograft, also called a xenograft, is a transplant of tissue from another species that is used as a temporary graft in certain cases, as in treating a severely burned patient when tissue from the patient or from a tissue bank is not available.*

*The prefix *a-* is usually used before a consonant.
** The prefix *an-* is usually used before a vowel.

Table 3-5   Other Common Prefixes—cont'd

Prefix	Meaning	Word Analysis
homo-	same	**homo**/graft (HŌ-mō-grăft): same transplant *-graft:* transplantation *A homograft, also called an allograft, is a transplant of tissue obtained from a member of the patient's own species. Commonly transplanted organs include bone, kidney, lung, and heart. Recipients take immunosuppressive drugs to prevent tissue rejection.*
homeo-		**homeo**/plasia (hō-mē-ō-PLĀ-zē-ă): formation of new tissue similar to that already existing in a part *-plasia:* formation, growth
mal-	bad	**mal**/nutrition (măl-nŭ-TRĬ-shŭn): bad nutrition *Malnutrition refers to any disorder resulting from an inadequate or excessive intake of food.*
pan-	all	**pan**/arthr/itis (păn-ăr-THRĪ-tĭs): inflammation of all (or many) joints *arthr:* joint *-itis:* inflammation
pseudo-	false	**pseudo**/cyesis (soo-dō-sī-Ē-sĭs): false pregnancy *-cyesis:* pregnancy *Pseudocyesis is a condition in which a woman believes she is pregnant when she is not and begins to develop all the physical characteristics associated with pregnancy.*
syn-*	union, together, joined	**syn**/dactyl/ism (sĭn-DĂK-tĭl-ĭzm): condition of joined fingers or toes *dactyl:* fingers; toes *-ism:* condition *Syndactylism varies in degree of severity from incomplete webbing of the skin of two digits to complete union of digits and fusion of the bones and nails.*
tachy-	rapid	**tachy**/pnea (tăk-ĭp-NĒ-ă): rapid breathing *-pnea:* breathing

*** The prefix *syn-* appears as *sym-* before *b, p, ph,* or *m.*

 It is time to review prefixes by completing Learning Activities 3–1, 3–2, and 3–3.

LEARNING ACTIVITIES

The following activities provide review of the prefixes introduced in this chapter. Complete each activity and review your answers to evaluate your understanding of the chapter. You can also enhance your learning of prefixes with the power of *DavisPlus*. Visit *www.davisplus.fadavis.com/ gylys/systems* for this chapter's flash-card activity. We recommend you do so before completing the learning activities that follow.

Learning Activity 3-1
Identifying and Defining Prefixes

Place a slash after each of the following prefixes and then define the prefix. The first one is completed for you.

Word   Definition of Prefix

1. inter/dental   *between*
2. hypodermic   _____
3. epidermis   _____
4. retroversion   _____
5. sublingual   _____
6. transvaginal   _____
7. infracostal   _____
8. postnatal   _____
9. quadriplegia   _____
10. hypercalcemia   _____
11. primigravida   _____
12. microscope   _____
13. triceps   _____
14. polydipsia   _____
15. abduction   _____
16. anesthesia   _____
17. macrocyte   _____
18. intramuscular   _____
19. suprapelvic   _____
20. diarrhea   _____
21. circumduction   _____
22. adduction   _____
23. periodontal   _____
24. bradycardia   _____
25. tachypnea   _____
26. dystocia

27. e u p n e a   _____

28. h e t e r o g r a f t   _____

29. m a l n u t r i t i o n   _____

30. p s e u d o c y e s i s   _____

✔ *Check your answers in Appendix A. Review any material that you did not answer correctly.*

Correct Answers _____ ✕ 3.34 = _____ % Score

Learning Activity 3-2

Matching Prefixes of Position, Number and Measurement, and Direction

Match the following terms with the definitions in the numbered list.

diarrhea	*macrocyte*	*pseudocyesis*
ectogenous	*periodontal*	*quadriplegia*
hemiplegia	*polyphobia*	*retroversion*
hypodermic	*postoperative*	*subnasal*
intercostal	*prenatal*	*suprarenal*

1. _____ tipping back of an organ
2. _____ pertaining to under the skin
3. _____ before birth
4. _____ pertaining to under the nose
5. _____ after surgery
6. _____ pertaining to between the ribs
7. _____ false pregnancy
8. _____ pertaining to around the teeth
9. _____ flow through (watery bowel movement)
10. _____ pertaining to an origin outside (the body or structure)
11. _____ above the kidney
12. _____ paralysis of one half (of the body)
13. _____ paralysis of four (limbs)
14. _____ (abnormally) large blood cell
15. _____ many fears

✔ *Check your answers in Appendix A. Review any material that you did not answer correctly.*

Correct Answers _____ ✕ 6.67 = _____ % Score

Learning Activity 3-3

Matching Other Prefixes

Match the following terms with the definitions in the numbered list.

amastia	dyspepsia	homograft
anesthesia	dystocia	malnutrition
antibacterial	eupnea	panarthritis
bradycardia	heterograft	syndactylism
contraception	homeoplasia	tachycardia

1. _____ difficult digestion
2. _____ tissue transplant from a different species
3. _____ inflammation of many joints
4. _____ against bacteria
5. _____ slow heartbeat
6. _____ poor or bad nutrition
7. _____ without a breast
8. _____ without sensation
9. _____ good or normal breathing
10. _____ condition of fused fingers and toes
11. _____ rapid heartbeat
12. _____ against conception
13. _____ tissue transplant from the same species
14. _____ difficult childbirth
15. _____ formation of the same tissue

✔ *Check your answers in Appendix A. Review any material that you did not answer correctly.*

Correct Answers _____ ✕ 6.67 = _____ % Score

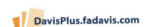
DavisPlus.fadavis.com

Enhance your study and reinforcement of prefixes with the power of DavisPlus. Visit
www.davisplus.fadavis.com/gylys/systems for the flash-card activity related to prefixes.
We recommend you complete the flash-card activity before moving on to Chapter 4.

Body Structure

CHAPTER

4

Chapter Outline

Objectives

Upon completion of this chapter, you will be able to:

- List the levels of organization of the body.
- Define and identify the three planes of the body.
- Identify the cavities, quadrants, and regions of the body.
- List and identify the terms related to direction, position, and planes of the body.
- Recognize, pronounce, spell, and build words related to body structure and identify common abbreviations.
- Describe diagnostic and therapeutic procedures and other terms associated with body structure.
- Demonstrate your knowledge of this chapter by completing the learning and medical record activities.

Introduction

This chapter provides the basic foundation for understanding the body system chapters that follow. It presents the basic structural and functional organization of the body—from the cellular level to the organism level. It also presents terms used to describe planes of the body, body cavities, quadrants and regions of the abdominal cavity, and divisions of the spinal column. These terms are an essential part of medical terminology and are used in all body systems. General concepts of **pathology** and terminology associated with the disease process are also provided. Finally, this chapter presents and describes terms associated with diagnostic and therapeutic procedures.

Body Structure Key Terms

This section introduces important terms associated with body structure, along with their definitions and pronunciations. Word analyses are also provided for selected terms.

Term	Definition
chromatin KRŌ-mă-tĭn	Structural component of the nucleus, composed of nucleic acids and proteins *Chromatin condenses to form chromosomes during cell division.*
chromosome KRŌ-mō-sōm	Threadlike structures within the nucleus composed of a deoxyribonucleic acid (DNA) molecule that carries hereditary information encoded in genes *Each sperm and each egg has 23 unpaired chromosomes. After fertilization, each cell of the embryo then has 46 chromosomes (23 pairs). In each pair of chromosomes, one chromosome is inherited from the father and the other from the mother.*
cytoplasm SĪ-tō-plăzm *cyt/o:* cell *-plasm:* formation, growth	Jellylike substance found within the cell membrane composed of proteins, salts, water, dissolved gases, and nutrients *All cellular structures, including the nucleus and organelles, are embedded in cytoplasm.*
deoxyribonucleic acid (DNA) dē-ok-sē-rē-bō-noo-KLĒ-ĭk ĂS-ĭd	Molecule that holds genetic information capable of replicating and producing an exact copy whenever the cell divides
diaphragm DĪ-ă-frăm	Muscular wall that divides the thoracic cavity from the abdominopelvic cavity *Alternating contraction and relaxation of the diaphragm is essential to the breathing process.*
metabolism mĕ-TĂB-ō-lĭzm	Sum of all physical and chemical changes that take place in a cell or an organism *Metabolism includes the building up (anabolism) and breaking down (catabolism) of body constituents.*
organelle or-găn-ĔL	Cellular structure that provides a specialized function, such as the nucleus (reproduction), ribosomes (protein synthesis), Golgi apparatus (removal of material from the cell), and lysosomes (digestion) *The membranes of many organelles act as sites of chemical reactions.*
pathology pă-THŎL-ō-jē *path/o:* disease *-logy:* study of	Study of the nature of diseases, their causes, development, and consequences. *Pathology as a branch of medicine includes the use of laboratory methods rather than clinical examination of signs and symptoms to study the causes, nature, and development of diseases.*

Body Structure Key Terms—cont'd

Term	Definition
peristalsis pĕr-ĭ-STĂL-sĭs	Rhythmic contraction and relaxation of the walls of a tubular organ to propel its contents onward

Pronunciation Help	Long Sound	ā—rate	ē—rebirth	ī—isle	ō—over	ū—unite
	Short Sound	ă—alone	ĕ—ever	ĭ—it	ŏ—not	ŭ—cut

Levels of Organization

The body is made up of several levels of structure and function. Each of these levels builds on the previous level, and contributes to the structure and function of the entire organism. (See Figure 4–1.) The levels of organization from least to most complex are:

- cell
- tissue
- organ
- system
- organism.

Cell

The study of the body at the cellular level is called *cytology.* The cell is the structural and functional unit of life. Body cells perform all activities associated with life, including utilizing food, eliminating waste, and reproducing. Cells consist of a cell membrane that encloses cytoplasm and a nucleus.

Cell Membrane and Cytoplasm

The cell membrane acts as a barrier that encloses the entire cell. It controls the transport of many substances to and from the cell. Within the cell membrane is a jellylike matrix of proteins, salts, water, dissolved gases, and nutrients called cytoplasm. Inside the cytoplasm are various structures called organelles that provide specialized functions for the cell. The largest cell organelle is the nucleus.

Nucleus

The nucleus is responsible for metabolism, growth, and reproduction. It also carries the genetic blueprint of the organism. This blueprint is found in a complex molecule called deoxyribonucleic acid (DNA) that is organized into threadlike structures called chromatin. When the cell is ready to divide, chromatin forms chromosomes, which carry thousands of genes that make up our genetic blueprint. In the human, there are about 31,000 genes that determine unique human characteristics. Genes pass biological information from one generation to the next. This biological information includes such traits as hair color, body structure, and metabolic activity. In the human, all cells except sperm cells and egg cells contain 23 pairs, or 46 chromosomes.

Tissue

Groups of cells that perform a specialized activity are called *tissues.* The study of tissues is called *histology.* Between the cells that make up tissues are varying amounts and types of nonliving, intercellular substances that provide pathways for cellular interaction. More than 200 cell types compose four major tissues of the body:

- **Epithelial tissue** covers surfaces of organs, lines cavities and canals, forms tubes and ducts, provides the secreting portions of glands, and makes up the epidermis of the skin. It is composed of cells arranged in a continuous sheet consisting of one or more layers.
- **Connective tissue** supports and connects other tissues and organs. It is made up of diverse cell types, including fibroblasts, fat cells, and blood.
- **Muscle tissue** provides the contractile tissue of the body, which is responsible for movement.
- **Nervous tissue** transmits electrical impulses as it relays information throughout the entire body.

Organ

Organs are body structures that perform specialized functions. They are composed of at least two or more tissue types. For example, the stomach is made up of connective tissue, muscle tissue, epithelial tissue, and nervous tissue. Muscle and connective tissue form the wall of the stomach. Epithelial and connective tissue cover the inner and outer surfaces of the stomach. Nervous tissue

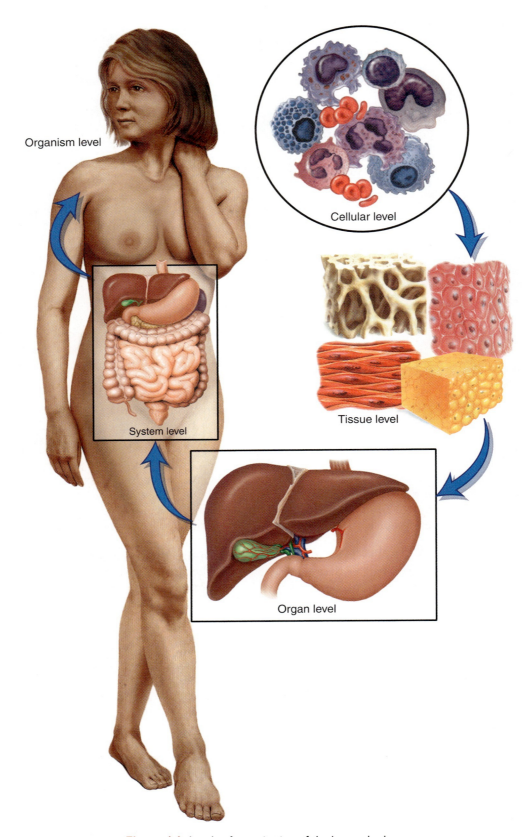

Organism level

Cellular level

Tissue level

System level

Organ level

Figure 4-1. Levels of organization of the human body.

penetrates the epithelial lining of the stomach and its muscular wall to stimulate the release chemicals for digestion and contraction for **peristalsis.**

System

A body system is composed of varying numbers of organs and accessory structures that have similar or related functions. For example, organs of the gastrointestinal system include the esophagus, stomach, small intestine, and bowel. Some of its accessory structures include the liver, gallbladder, and pancreas. The purpose of this system is to digest food, remove and use its nutrients, and expel waste products. Other body systems include the reproductive, respiratory, urinary, and cardiovascular systems.

Organism

The highest level of organization is the organism. An organism is a complete living entity capable of independent existence. All complex organisms, including humans, are made up of several body systems that work together to sustain life.

Anatomical Position

The **anatomical position** is a body posture used to locate anatomical parts in relation to each other. In this position, the body is erect and the eyes are looking forward. The upper limbs hang to the sides, with the palms facing forward. The lower limbs are parallel, with toes pointing straight ahead. No matter how the body is actually positioned—standing or lying down, facing forward or backward—or how the limbs are actually placed, the positions and relationships of a structure are always described as if the body were in the anatomical position.

Planes of the Body

To identify the different sections of the body, anatomists use an imaginary flat surface called a *plane.* The most commonly used planes are **midsagittal** (median), **coronal** (frontal), and **transverse** (horizontal). (See Table 4–1.) The section is named for the plane along which it is cut. Thus, a cut along a transverse plane produces a transverse, or horizontal, section. (See Figure 4–2.)

Prior to the development of modern imaging techniques, standard x-ray images showed only a single plane, and many body abnormalities were difficult, if not impossible, to see. Current imaging procedures, such as magnetic resonance imaging

Table 4-1	**Planes of the Body**	

This table lists planes of the body and their anatomical divisions.

Plane	Anatomical Division
Midsagittal (median)	Right and left halves
Coronal (frontal)	Anterior (ventral) and posterior (dorsal) aspects
Transverse (horizontal)	Superior (upper) and inferior (lower) aspects

(MRI) and computed tomography (CT), produce three-dimensional images on more than one plane. Thus, structural abnormalities and body masses that were previously not found using a standard single plane x-ray are now detected with scanning devices that show images taken in several body planes.

Body Cavities

Medical professionals locate structures or abnormalities by referring to the body cavity in which they are found. (See Figure 4–3.) The body has two major cavities:

- dorsal (posterior), including the cranial and spinal cavities
- ventral (anterior), including the thoracic and abdominopelvic cavities. (See Table 4–2.)

Abdominopelvic Divisions

The abdominopelvic area of the body lies beneath the **diaphragm.** It holds the organs of digestion (abdominal area) and the organs of reproduction and excretion (pelvic area). Two anatomical methods are used to divide this area of the body for medical purposes:

- quadrants
- regions.

Quadrants

Quadrants are four divisions of the lower torso used to show topographical location. They provide a means of locating specific sites for descriptive and diagnostic purposes. (See Table 4–3.) The

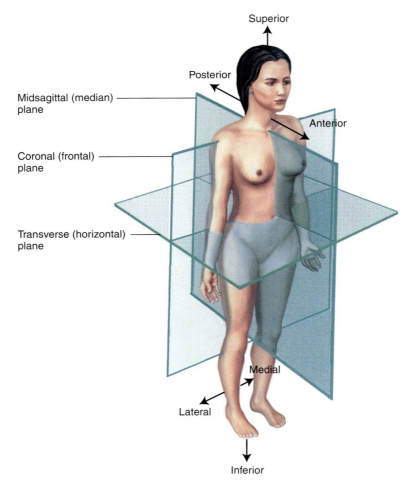

Figure 4-2. Body planes. Note that the body is in the anatomical position.

divisions of quadrants are used in clinical examinations and medical reports. Pain, lesions, abrasions, punctures, and burns are commonly described as located in a specific quadrant. Incision sites are also identified by using body quadrants as the method of location. An imaginary cross passing through the navel identifies the four quadrants. (See Figure 4–4A.)

Regions

Whereas the quadrants of the body are used primarily to identify topographical sites, the **abdominopelvic regions** are used mainly to identify the location of underlying body structures and visceral organs. (See Table 4–4.) For example, the stomach is located in the left hypochondriac and epigastric region; the appendix is located in the hypogastric region. (See Figure 4–4B.)

Spine

The spine is divided into sections corresponding to the vertebrae located in the spinal column. These divisions are:

- cervical (neck)
- thoracic (chest)
- lumbar (loin)
- sacral (lower back)
- coccyx (tailbone)

Directional Terms

Directional terms are used to show the position of a structure in relation to another structure. For example, the kidneys are superior to the urinary bladder. The directional phrase *superior to* denotes *above*. This example indicates that the kidneys are located above the urinary bladder. (See Table 4–5.)

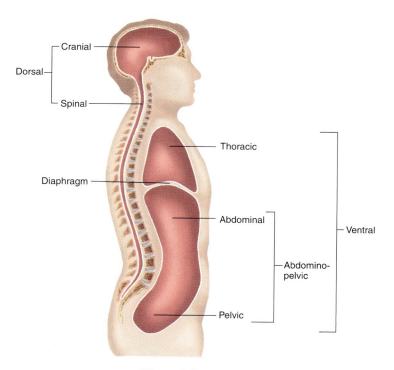

Figure 4-3. Body cavities.

Table 4-2	**Body Cavities**

This table lists the body cavities and some of the major organs found within them. The thoracic cavity is separated from the abdominopelvic cavity by a muscular wall called the diaphragm.

Cavity	Major Organ(s) in the Cavity
Dorsal	
Cranial	Brain
Spinal	Spinal cord
Ventral	
Thoracic	Heart, lungs, and associated structures
Abdominopelvic	Digestive, excretory, and reproductive organs and structures

Table 4-3	**Body Quadrants**

This table lists the quadrants of the body, their corresponding abbreviations, and their major structures.

Quadrant	Abbreviation	Major Structures
Right upper	RUQ	Right lobe of liver, gallbladder, part of pancreas, part of small and large intestines
Left upper	LUQ	Left lobe of liver, stomach, spleen, part of pancreas, part of small and large intestines
Right lower	RLQ	Part of small and large intestines, appendix, right ovary, right fallopian tube, right ureter
Left lower	LLQ	Part of small and large intestines, left ovary, left fallopian tube, left ureter

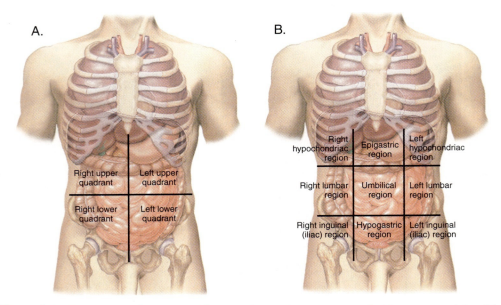

Figure 4-4. Quadrants and regions. (A) Four quadrants of the abdomen. (B) Nine regions of the abdomen.

Table 4-4	**Abdominopelvic Regions**

This table lists the names of the abdominopelvic regions and their location.

Region	Location
Left hypochondriac	Upper left region beneath the ribs
Epigastric	Region above the stomach
Right hypochondriac	Upper right region beneath the ribs
Left lumbar	Left middle lateral region
Umbilical	Region of the navel
Right lumbar	Right middle lateral region
Left inguinal (iliac)	Left lower lateral region
Hypogastric	Lower middle region beneath the navel
Right inguinal (iliac)	Right lower lateral region

⊕ *It is time to review the planes of the body and quadrants and regions of the abdominopelvic area by completing Learning Activities 4–1 and 4–2.*

Table 4-5	**Directional Terms**

This table lists directional terms along with their definitions. In this list, opposing terms are presented consecutively to aid memorization.

Term	Definition
Abduction	Movement away from the midsagittal (median) plane of the body or one of its parts
Adduction	Movement toward the midsagittal (median) plane of the body

Table 4-5	Directional Terms—cont'd	
	Term	**Definition**
	Medial	Pertaining to the midline of the body or structure
	Lateral	Pertaining to a side
	Superior (cephalad)	Toward the head or upper portion of a structure
	Inferior (caudal)	Away from the head, or toward the tail or lower part of a structure
	Proximal	Nearer to the center (trunk of the body) or to the point of attachment to the body
	Distal	Further from the center (trunk of the body) or from the point of attachment to the body
	Anterior (ventral)	Front of the body
	Posterior (dorsal)	Back of the body
	Parietal	Pertaining to the outer wall of the body cavity
	Visceral	Pertaining to the viscera, or internal organs, especially the abdominal organs
	Prone	Lying on the abdomen, face down
	Supine	Lying horizontally on the back, face up
	Inversion	Turning inward or inside out
	Eversion	Turning outward
	Palmar	Pertaining to the palm of the hand
	Plantar	Pertaining to the sole of the foot
	Superficial	Toward the surface of the body (external)
	Deep	Away from the surface of the body (internal)

 It is time to review body cavity, spine, and directional terms by completing Learning Activity 4–3.

Medical Word Elements

This section introduces combining forms, suffixes, and prefixes related to body structure. Word analyses are also provided.

Element	Meaning	Word Analysis
Combining Forms		
Cellular Structure		
cyt/o	cell	**cyt/o**/logist (sī-TŎL-ō-jĭst): specialist in study of cells –*logist:* specialist in the study of *Cytologists study the formation, structure, and function of cells.*
hist/o	tissue	**hist/o**/logy (hĭs-TŎL-ō-jē): study of tissues –*logy:* study of *Histology is the branch of science that investigates the microscopic structures and functions of tissues.*
kary/o	nucleus	**kary/o**/lysis (kăr-ē-ŎL-ĭ-sĭs): destruction of the nucleus –*lysis:* separation; destruction; loosening *Karyolysis results in death of the cell.*
nucle/o		**nucle/ar** (NŪ-klē-ăr): pertaining to the nucleus –*ar:* pertaining to

(continued)

Medical Word Elements—cont'd

Element	Meaning	Word Analysis
Position and Direction		
anter/o	anterior, front	**anter**/ior (ăn-TĔR-ē-or): pertaining to the front *-ior:* pertaining to
caud/o	tail	**caud**/ad (KAW-dăd): toward the tail *-ad:* toward *Caudad is opposite of craniad.*
crani/o	cranium (skull)	**crani**/al (KRĀ-nē-ăl): pertaining to the cranium *-al:* pertaining to
dist/o	far, farthest	**dist**/al (DĬS-tăl): pertaining to the farthest (point of attachment) *-al:* pertaining to *Distal refers to the point furthest from the center (trunk) of the body or from the point of attachment to the body. Thus, the fingers are distal to the wrist.*
dors/o	back (of body)	**dors**/al (DOR-săl): pertaining to the back (of the body) *-al:* pertaining to
infer/o	lower, below	**infer**/ior (ĭn-FĒR-rē-or): pertaining to a lower (structure or surface) *-ior:* pertaining to *The inferior surface is the undersurface of a structure or organ, or a place below a structure or organ.*
later/o	side, to one side	**later**/al (LĂT-ĕr-ăl): pertaining to a side *-al:* pertaining to
medi/o	middle	**medi**/ad (MĒ-dē-ăd): toward the middle *-ad:* toward
poster/o	back (of body), behind, posterior	**poster**/ior (pōs-TĔR-ē-or): pertaining to the back (of the body) *-ior:* pertaining to
proxim/o	near, nearest	**proxim**/al (PRŎK-sĭm-ăl): pertaining to the nearest (point of attachment) *-al: pertaining to* *Proximal refers to the point closest to the center (trunk) of the body or to the point of attachment to the body. Thus, the elbow is proximal to the wrist.*
ventr/o	belly, belly side	**ventr/al** (VĔN-trăl): pertaining to the belly side (front of the body) *-al: pertaining to*
Regions of the Body		
abdomin/o	abdomen	**abdomin**/al (ăb-DŎM-ĭ-năl): pertaining to the abdomen *-al: pertaining to*
cervic/o	neck; cervix uteri (neck of uterus)	**cervic**/al (SĔR-vĭ-kăl): pertaining to the neck *-al: pertaining to*

Medical Word Elements—cont'd

Element	Meaning	Word Analysis
crani/o	cranium (skull)	**crani**/al (KRĀ-nē-ăl): pertaining to the cranium *-al: pertaining to*

gastr/o	stomach	hypo/**gastr**/ic (hī-pō-GĂS-trĭk): pertaining to (the area) below the stomach
		  hypo-: under, below
		  -ic: pertaining to

ili/o	ilium (lateral, flaring portion of hip bone)	**ili**/al (ĬL-ē-ăl): pertaining to the ilium *-al:* pertaining to
inguin/o	groin	**inguin**/al (ĬNG-gwĭ-năl): pertaining to the groin *-al:* pertaining to *The groin is the depression located between the thigh and trunk.*
lumb/o	loins (lower back)	**lumb**/ar (LŬM-băr): pertaining to the loins (lower back) *-ar:* pertaining to

pelv/i
 	
pelv/o
	pelvis	**pelv/i**/meter* (pĕl-VĬM-ĕ-tĕr): instrument for measuring the pelvis
		  -meter: instrument for measuring
		pelv/ic (PĔL-vĭk): pertaining to the pelvis
		  -ic: pertaining to

spin/o	spine	**spin**/al (SPĪ-năl): pertaining to the spine *-al:* pertaining to
thorac/o	chest	**thorac**/ic (thō-RĂS-ĭk): pertaining to the chest *-ic:* pertaining to
umbilic/o	umbilicus, navel	**umbilic**/al (ŭm-BĬL-ĭ-kăl): pertaining to the navel *-al:* pertaining to
Color		
albin/o	white	**albin**/ism (ĂL-bĭn-ĭzm): condition of whiteness *-ism:* condition *Albinism is characterized by a partial or total lack of pigment in the skin, hair, and eyes.*
leuk/o		**leuk**/o/cyte (LOO-kō-sīt): white cell *-cyte:* cell *A leukocyte is a white blood cell.*
chlor/o	green	**chlor**/opia (klō-RŌ-pē-ă): green vision *-opia:* vision *Chloropia is a disorder in which viewed objects appear green. It is associated with a toxic reaction to digitalis.*

chrom/o	color	hetero/**chrom**/ic (hĕt-ĕr-ō-KRŌ-mĭk): pertaining to different colors
		  hetero-: different
		  -ic: pertaining to
		Heterochromia is associated with the iris or sections of the iris of the eyes. Thus, the individual with heterochromia may have one brown iris and one blue iris.

(continued)

Medical Word Elements—cont'd

Element	Meaning	Word Analysis
cirrh/o	yellow	**cirrh**/osis (sĭr-RŌ-sĭs): abnormal yellowing *-osis:* abnormal condition; increase (used primarily with blood cells) *In cirrhosis, the skin, sclera of the eyes, and mucous membranes take on a yellow color. Cirrhosis of the liver is usually associated with alcoholism or chronic hepatitis.*
jaund/o		**jaund**/ice (JAWN-dĭs): yellowing *-ice:* noun ending *Jaundice is caused by an abnormal increase of bilirubin (a yellow compound formed when red blood cells are destroyed) in the blood.*
xanth/o		**xanth**/o/cyte (ZĂN-thō-sīt): yellow cell *-cyte:* cell
cyan/o	blue	**cyan**/o/tic (sī-ăn-ŎT-ĭk): pertaining to blueness *-tic:* pertaining to *Cyanosis is associated with lack of oxygen in the blood.*
erythr/o	red	**erythr**/o/cyte (ĕ-RĬTH-rō-sīt): red cell *-cyte:* cell *An erythrocyte is a red blood cell.*
melan/o	black	**melan**/oma (mĕl-ă-NŌ-mă): black tumor *-oma:* tumor *Melanoma is a malignancy that arises from melanocytes.*

poli/o	gray; gray matter (of brain or spinal cord)	**poli**/o/myel/itis (pōl-ē-ō-mī-ĕl-Ī-tĭs): inflammation of the gray matter of the spinal cord
		  myel: bone marrow; spinal cord
		  -itis: inflammation

Other		

acr/o	extremity	**acr**/o/cyan/osis (ăk-rō-sī-ă-NŌ-sĭs): abnormal condition in which the extremities are blue
		  cyan: blue
		  -osis: abnormal condition; increase (used primarily with blood cells)

eti/o	cause	**eti**/o/logy (ē-tē-ŎL-ō-jē): study of the causes of disease *-logy:* study of

idi/o	unknown, peculiar	**idi**/o/path/ic (ĭd-ē-ō-PĂTH-ĭk): pertaining to an unknown (cause of) disease
		  path: disease
		  -ic: pertaining to

morph/o	form, shape, structure	**morph**/o/logy (mor-FŎL-ō-jē): study of form, shape, or structure *-logy:* study of
path/o	disease	**path**/o/logist (pă-THŎL-ō-jĭst): specialist in the study of disease *-logist:* specialist in the study of *Pathologists examine tissues, cells, and body fluids for evidence of disease.*

Medical Word Elements—cont'd

Element	Meaning	Word Analysis
radi/o	radiation, x-ray; radius (lower arm bone on thumb side)	**radi/o**/logist (rā-dē-ŎL-ŏ-jĭst): specialist in the study of radiation *-logist:* specialist in the study of *Radiologists are physicians who employ imaging techniques for diagnosing and treating disease.*
somat/o	body	**somat**/ic (sō-MĂT-ĭk): pertaining to the body *-ic:* pertaining to
son/o	sound	**son/o**/graphy (sō-NŎG-ră-fē): process of recording sound; also called *ultrasonography* *-graphy:* process of recording *Sonography employs ultrasound (inaudible sound) to produce images. It is a painless, noninvasive imaging technique that does not use x-rays.*
viscer/o	internal organs	**viscer**/al (VĬS-ĕr-ăl): pertaining to internal organs *-al:* pertaining to
xer/o	dry	**xer**/osis (zē-RŌ-sĭs): abnormal condition of dryness *-osis:* abnormal condition; increase (used primarily with blood cells) *Xerosis refers to abnormal dryness of the skin, mucous membranes, or conjunctiva.*
Suffixes		
-genesis	forming, producing, origin	path/o/**genesis** (păth-ō-JĔN-ĕ-sĭs): origin of disease *path/o:* disease *Pathogenesis refers to the origin or cause of an illness or abnormal condition.*
-gnosis	knowing	pro/**gnosis** (prŏg-NŌ-sĭs): knowing before *pro-:* before, in front of *Prognosis is the prediction of the course and end of a disease and the estimated chance of recovery.*
-gram	record, writing	arteri/o/**gram** (ăr-TĒ-rē-ō-grăm): record of an artery *An arteriogram is an x-ray film of an artery taken after injection of a radiopaque contrast medium.*
-graph	instrument for recording	radi/o/**graph** (RĀ-dē-ō-grăf): instrument for recording x-rays *radi/o:* radiation, x-rays; radius (lower arm bone on thumb side)
-graphy	process of recording	arthr/o/**graphy** (ăr-THRŎG-ră-fē): process of recording a joint *arthr/o:* joint *Arthrography is an x-ray examination of a joint, such as the knee, shoulder, or elbow, usually with the use of a contrast medium.*
-logist	specialist in the study of	dermat/o/**logist** (dĕr-mă-TŎL-ō-jĭst): specialist in the study of the skin *dermat/o:* skin
-logy	study of	hemat/o/**logy** (hē-mă-TŎL-ō-jē): study of blood *hemat/o:* blood
-meter	instrument for measuring	therm/o/**meter** (thĕr-MŎM-ĕ-tĕr): instrument for measuring heat *therm/o:* heat

(continued)

Medical Word Elements—cont'd

Element	Meaning	Word Analysis
-metry	act of measuring	ventricul/o/**metry** (věn-trĭk-ū-LŎM-ĕ-trē): act of measuring the ventricles *ventricul/o:* ventricle (of heart or brain)
-pathy	disease	gastr/o/**pathy** (găs-TRŎP-ă-thē): disease of the stomach *gastr/o:* stomach
Prefixes		
ab-	from, away from	**ab**/duction (ăb-DŬK-shŭn): act of bringing away from (midline of the body) *-duction:* act of leading, bringing, conducting *Abduction is the movement of a limb or body part away from the midline of the body.*
ad-	toward	**ad**/duction (ă-DŬK-shŭn): act of bringing toward (midline of the body) *-duction:* act of leading, bringing, conducting *Adduction is the movement of a limb toward the midline of the body.*
hetero-	different	**hetero**/morph/ous (hĕt-ĕr-ō-MOR-fŭs): different form or shape *morph:* form, shape, structure *-ous:* pertaining to *Heteromorphous refers to any deviation from a normal type or shape.*
homeo-	same, alike	**homeo**/plasia (hō-mē-ō-PLĀ-zē-ă): formation of same (tissue) *-plasia:* formation, growth *Homeoplasia is the formation of new tissue similar to that already existing in a part.*
infra-	below, under	**infra**/cost/al (ĭn-fră-KŎS-tăl): pertaining to (the area) below the ribs *cost:* ribs *-al:* pertaining to
peri-	around	**peri**/cardi/al (pĕr-ĭ-KĂR-dē-ăl): pertaining to (the area) around the heart *cardi:* heart *-al:* pertaining to
super-	upper, above	**super**/ior (soo-PĒ-rē-or): pertaining to the upper (area) *-ior:* pertaining to
trans-	across, through	**trans**/abdomin/al (trăns-ăb-DŎM-ĭ-năl): pertaining to (a direction) across or through the abdomen *abdomin:* abdomen *-al:* pertaining to
ultra-	excess, beyond	**ultra**/son/ic (ŭl-tră-SŎN-ĭk): pertaining to beyond (audible) sound *son:* sound *-ic:* pertaining to *Ultrasound includes sound frequencies too high to be perceived by the human ear.*

*The *i* in *pelv/i/meter* is an exception to the rule of using the connecting vowel *o.*

 It is time to review medical word elements by completing Learning Activity 4–4.

Pathology

All body cells require oxygen and nutrients for survival. They also need a stable internal environment that provides a narrow range of temperature, water, acidity, and salt concentration. This stable internal environment is called *homeostasis.* When homeostasis is disrupted and cells, tissues, organs, or systems are unable to function effectively, the condition is called *disease.* From a clinical point of view, disease is a **pathological** or **morbid** condition that presents a group of signs, symptoms, and clinical findings. **Signs** are objective indicators that are observable. A palpable mass and tissue redness are examples of signs. A **symptom** is subjective and is experienced only by the patient. Dizziness, pain, and malaise are examples of symptoms. Clinical findings are the results of radiologic, laboratory, and other medical procedures performed on the patient or his specimens.

Etiology is the study of the cause or origin of a disease or disorder. Some possible causes of diseases include:

- metabolic (such as diabetes)
- infectious (such as measles and mumps)
- congenital (such as cleft lip)
- hereditary (such as hemophilia)
- environmental (such as burns and trauma)
- neoplastic (such as cancer)

Establishing the cause and nature of a disease is called *diagnosis (Dx).* Determining a diagnosis helps in the selection of a treatment. A *prognosis* is the prediction of the course of a disease and its probable outcome. Any disease whose cause is unknown is said to be *idiopathic.*

A variety of diagnostic procedures are used to identify diseases and determine their extent or involvement. Diagnostic tests can be simple, such as listening to chest sounds with a stethoscope, or complex, such as a biopsy. Many of the diagnostic tests listed in this text can be categorized as surgical, clinical, endoscopic, laboratory, and radiological. Some tests include more than one testing modality.

Diagnostic, Symptomatic, and Related Terms

This section introduces diagnostic, symptomatic, and related terms and their meanings. Word analyses for selected terms are also provided.

Term	Definition
adhesion ăd-HĒ-zhŭn	Abnormal fibrous band that holds or binds together tissues that are normally separated *Adhesions may occur within body cavities as a result of surgery.*
analyte ĂN-ă-līt	Substance analyzed or tested, generally by means of laboratory methods *In a glucose tolerance test, glucose is the analyte.*
contrast medium KŎN-trăst MĔD-ē-ŭm	Substance injected into the body, introduced via catheter, or swallowed to facilitate radiographic images of internal structures that otherwise are difficult to visualize on x-ray films
dehiscence dĕ-HĬS-ĕns	Bursting open of a wound, especially a surgical abdominal wound
febrile FĔ-brĭl	Feverish; pertaining to a fever
homeostasis hō-mē-ō-STĀ-sĭs *homeo-:* same, alike *-stasis:* standing still	Relative constancy or balance in the internal environment of the body, maintained by processes of feedback and adjustment in response to external or internal changes *In homeostasis, such properties as temperature, acidity, and the concentrations of nutrients and wastes remain relatively constant.*

(continued)

Diagnostic, Symptomatic, and Related Terms—cont'd

Term	Definition
inflammation ĭn-flă-MĀ-shŭn	Body defense against injury, infection, or allergy that is marked by redness, swelling, heat, pain and, sometimes, loss of function *Inflammation is one mechanism used by the body to protect against invasion by foreign organisms and to repair injured tissue.*
morbid MOR-bĭd	Diseased; pertaining to a disease
nuclear medicine NŪ-klē-ăr	Branch of medicine concerned with the use of radioactive substances for diagnosis, treatment, and research
radiology rā-dē-ŎL-ō-jē *radi/o:* radiation, x-ray; radius (lower arm bone on thumb side) *-logy:* study of	Medical specialty concerned with the use of electromagnetic radiation, ultrasound, and imaging techniques for diagnosis and treatment of disease and injury (See Figure 4-5.)
interventional ĭn-tĕr-VĔN-shŭn-ăl	Radiological practice that employs fluoroscopy, CT, and ultrasound in nonsurgical treatment of various disorders *Examples of interventional radiology include balloon angioplasty and cardiac catheterization.*
therapeutic thĕr-ă-PŪ-tĭk *therapeut:* treatment *-ic:* pertaining to	Use of ionizing radiation in the treatment of cancer; also called *radiation oncology*

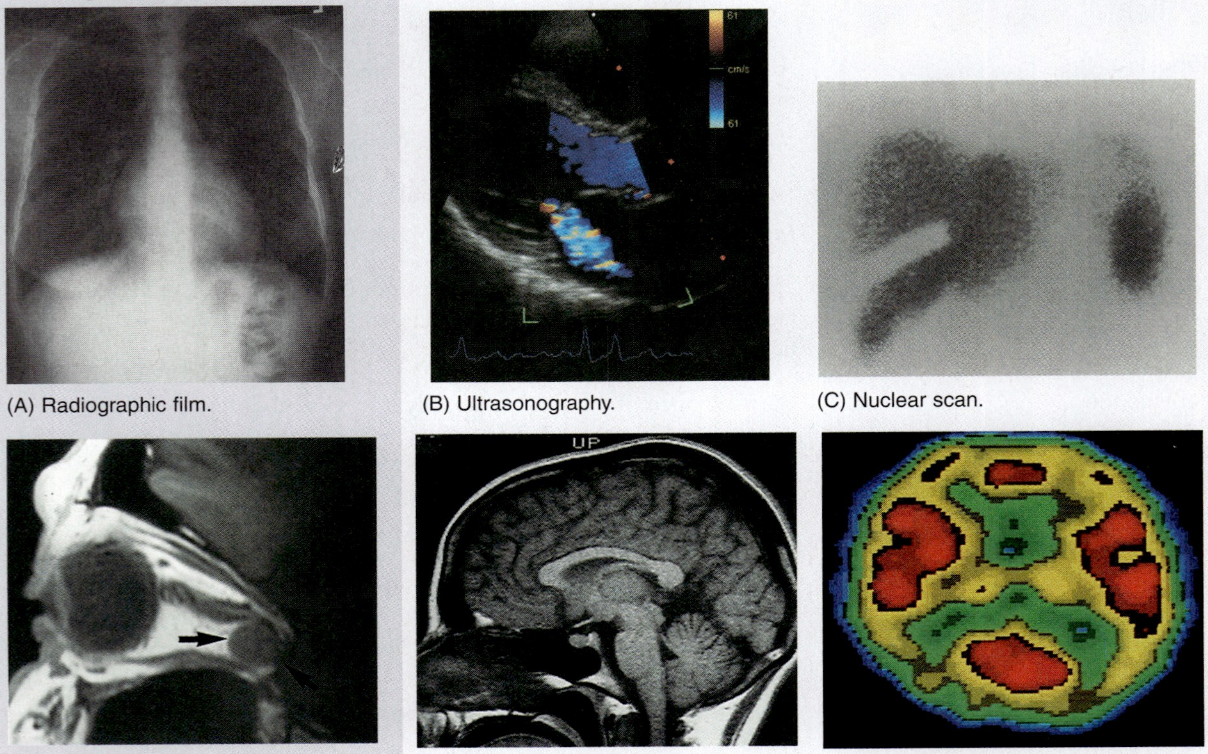

(A) Radiographic film.

(B) Ultrasonography.

(C) Nuclear scan.

(D) CT scan.

(E) MRI scan.

(F) PET scan of brain.

Figure 4-5. Medical imaging.

Diagnostic, Symptomatic, and Related Terms—cont'd

Term	Definition
radionuclides rā-dē-ō-NŪ-klīdz	Substances that emit radiation spontaneously; also called *tracers* *The quantity and duration of radioactive material used in these tests are safe for humans and should not have harmful effects.*
radiopharmaceutical rā-dē-ō-fărm-ă-SŪ-tĭ-kăl	Radionuclide attached to a protein, sugar, or other substance used to visualize an organ or area of the body that will be scanned
scan SKĂN	Term used to describe a computerized image by modality (such as CT, MRI, and nuclear imaging) or by structure (such as thyroid and bone)
sepsis SĔP-sĭs	Pathological state, usually febrile, resulting from the presence of microorganisms or their products in the bloodstream
suppurative SŬP-ū-ră-tĭv	Producing or associated with generation of pus

Diagnostic and Therapeutic Procedures

This section introduces procedures used to diagnose and treat a variety of disorders. Specific examples of these procedures are found in the body systems chapters. Descriptions are provided as well as pronunciations and word analyses for selected terms.

Procedure	Description
Diagnostic Procedures	
Endoscopic	
endoscopy ĕn-DŎS-kō-pē *endo-:* in, within *-scopy:* visual examination	Visual examination of a body cavity or canal using a specialized lighted instrument called an *endoscope* *Endoscopy is used for biopsy, surgery, aspirating fluids, and coagulating bleeding areas. The endoscope is usually named for the organ, cavity, or canal being examined, such as gastroscope and sigmoidoscope. (See Figure 4-6.) A camera and video recorder are commonly used during the procedure to provide a permanent record.*

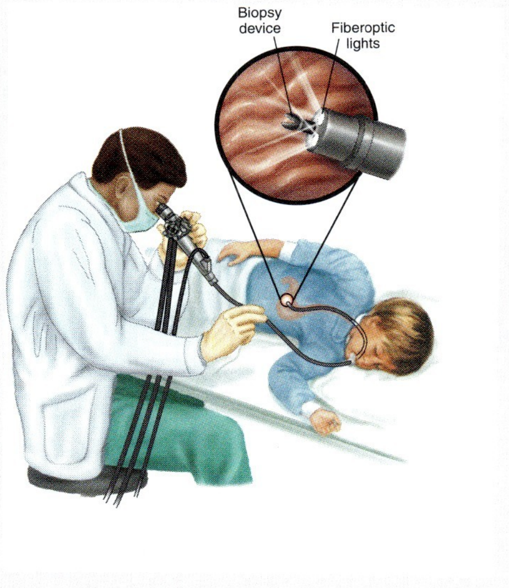

Figure 4-6. Endoscopy (gastroscopy).

(continued)

Diagnostic and Therapeutic Procedures—cont'd

Procedure	Description
laparoscopy lăp-ăr-ŎS-kō-pē *lapar/o:* abdomen *-scopy:* visual examination	Visual examination of the organs of the pelvis and abdomen through very small incisions in the abdominal wall
thoracoscopy thor-ă-KŎS-kă-pē *thorac/o:* chest *-scopy:* visual examination	Examination of the lungs, pleura, and pleural space with a scope inserted through a small incision between the ribs *Thoracoscopy is an endoscopic procedure usually performed for lung biopsy, repairing perforations in the lungs, and diagnosing pleural disease.*
Laboratory	
complete blood count (CBC)	Common blood test that enumerates red blood cells, white blood cells, and platelets; measures hemoglobin (the oxygen-carrying molecule in red blood cells); estimates red cell volume; and sorts white blood cells into five subtypes with their percentages *CBC can be performed using a manual or automated method.*
urinalysis (UA) ū-rĭ-NĂL-ĭ-sĭs	Common urine screening test that evaluates the physical, chemical, and microscopic properties of urine *Immediate UA can be performed with a dipstick test or the urine specimen can be sent to the laboratory for a full analysis.*
Radiographic	
computed tomography (CT) kŏm-PŪ-tĕd tō-MŎG-ră-fē *tom/o:* to cut *-graphy:* process of recording	Imaging technique achieved by rotating an x-ray emitter around the area to be scanned and measuring the intensity of transmitted rays from different angles; formerly called *computerized axial tomography* *In a CT scan, the computer generates a detailed cross-sectional image that appears as a slice. (See Figure 4-5D.) Tumor masses, bone displacement, and accumulations of fluid may be detected. This technique may be used with or without a contrast medium.*
Doppler DŎP-lĕr	Ultrasound technique used to detect and measure blood-flow velocity and direction through the cardiac chambers, valves, and peripheral vessels by reflecting sound waves off moving blood cells *Doppler ultrasound is used to identify irregularities in blood flow cause by blood clots, venous insufficiency, and arterial blockage.*
fluoroscopy floo-or-ŎS-kō-pē *fluor/o:* luminous, fluorescent *-scopy:* visual examination	Radiographic technique in which x-rays are directed through the body to a fluorescent screen that displays continuous motion images of internal structures *Fluoroscopy is used to view the motion of organs, such as the digestive tract, heart, and joints, or to aid in the placement of catheters or other devices.*

Diagnostic and Therapeutic Procedures—cont'd

Procedure	Description
magnetic resonance imaging (MRI) măg-NĔT-ĭk RĔZ-ĕn-ăns ĬM-ăj-ĭng	Noninvasive imaging technique that uses radiowaves and a strong magnetic field rather than an x-ray beam to produce multiplanar cross-sectional images (See Figure 4-5E.) *MRI is used to diagnose a growing number of diseases because it provides superior soft tissue contrast, allows multiple plane views, and avoids the hazards of ionizing radiation. MRI commonly proves superior to CT scan for most central nervous system images, particularly those of the brainstem and spinal cord as well as the musculoskeletal and pelvic areas. The procedure usually does not require a contrast medium.*
nuclear scan NŪ-klē-ăr	Diagnostic technique that uses a radioactive material (radiopharmaceutical) called a *tracer* that is introduced into the body (inhaled, ingested, or injected) and a specialized camera to produce images of organs and structures (See Figure 4-5C.) *A nuclear scan is the reverse of a conventional radiograph. Rather than being directed into the body, radiation comes from inside the body and is then detected by a specialized camera to produce an image.*
positron emission tomography (PET) PŎZ-ĭ-trŏn ē-MĬSH-ŭn tō-MŎG-ră-fē	Scanning technique using computed tomography to record the positrons (positive charged particles) emitted from a radiopharmaceutical, that produces a cross-sectional image of metabolic activity in body tissues to determine the presence of disease (See Figure 4-5F.) *PET is particularly useful in scanning the brain and nervous system to diagnose disorders that involve abnormal tissue metabolism, such as schizophrenia, brain tumors, epilepsy, stroke, and Alzheimer disease as well as cardiac and pulmonary disorders.*
radiography rā-dē-ŎG-ră-fē *radi/o:* radiation, x-ray, radius (lower arm bone on thumb side) *-graphy:* process of recording	Imaging technique that uses x-rays passed through the body or area and captured on a film; also called *x-ray* (See Figure 4-5A.) *On the radiograph, dense material, such as bone, appears white, and softer material, such as the stomach and liver, appears in shades of gray.*
single photon emission computed tomography (SPECT) FŌ-tŏn ē-MĬ-shŭn tō-MŎG-ră-fē *tom/o:* to cut *-graphy:* process of recording	Radiological technique that integrates computed tomography (CT) and a radioactive material (tracer) injected into the bloodstream to visualize blood flow to tissues and organs *SPECT differs from a PET scan in that the tracer remains in the blood stream rather than being absorbed by surrounding tissue. It is especially useful to visualize blood flow through arteries and veins in the brain.*
tomography tō-MŎG-ră-fē *tom/o:* to cut *-graphy:* process of recording	Radiographic technique that produces an image representing a detailed cross-section, or *slice,* of an area, tissue, or organ at a predetermined depth *Types of tomography include computed tomography (CT), positron emission tomography (PET), and single photon emission computed tomography (SPECT).*

(continued)

Diagnostic and Therapeutic Procedures—cont'd

Procedure	Description

ultrasonography (US)
ŭl-tră-sōn-ŎG-ră-fē
  ultra-: excess, beyond
  son/o: sound
  -graphy: process of recording
	Imaging procedure using high-frequency sound waves (ultrasound) that display the reflected "echoes" on a monitor; also called *ultrasound, sonography, echo,* and e*chography* (See Figure 4-5B.)
	US, unlike most other imaging methods, creates real-time moving images to view organs and functions of organs in motion. A computer analyzes the reflected echoes and converts them into an image on a video monitor. Because this procedure does not use ionizing radiation (x-ray), it is used for visualizing fetuses as well as the neck, abdomen, pelvis, brain, and heart.

Surgical

biopsy (bx) BĪ-ŏp-sē	Representative tissue sample removed from a body site for microscopic examination, usually to establish a diagnosis
frozen section (FS)	Ultra-thin slice of tissue cut from a frozen specimen for immediate pathological examination *FS is used primarily in oncological cases while the patient is still in the operating room. The evaluation by the pathologist helps determine if and how aggressively the surgeon will treat the patient.*
needle	Removal of a small tissue sample for examination using a hollow needle, usually attached to a syringe
punch	Removal of a small core of tissue using a hollow instrument (punch) *An anesthetic and suturing are usually required for a punch bx, and minimal scarring is expected.*
shave	Removal of tissue using a surgical blade to shave elevated lesions

Therapeutic Procedures

Surgical

ablation ăb-LĀ-shŭn	Removal of a part, pathway, or function by surgery, chemical destruction, electrocautery, freezing, or radio frequency (RF)
anastomosis ă-năs-tō-MŌ-sĭs	Surgical joining of two ducts, vessels, or bowel segments to allow flow from one to another (See Figure 4-7.)

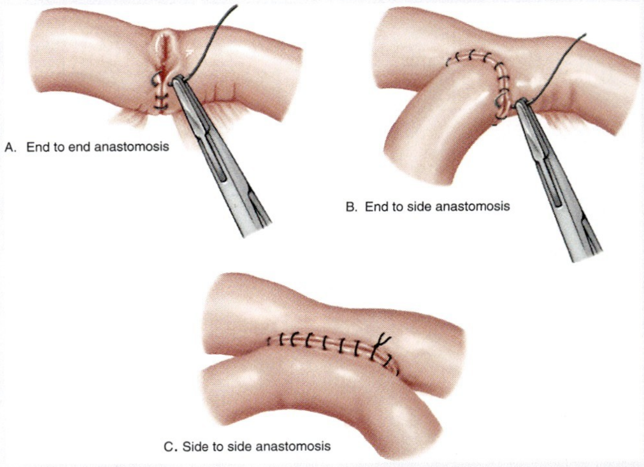

A. End to end anastomosis

B. End to side anastomosis

C. Side to side anastomosis

Figure 4-7. Anastomoses.

Diagnostic and Therapeutic Procedures—cont'd

Procedure	Description
cauterize KAW-tĕr-īz	Destroy tissue by electricity, freezing, heat, or corrosive chemicals
curettage kū-rĕ-TĂZH	Scraping of a body cavity with a spoon-shaped instrument called a *curette* (curet)
incision and drainage (I&D) ĭn-SĬZH-ŭn, DRĂN-ĭj	Incision made to allow the free flow or withdrawal of fluids from a wound or cavity
laser surgery LĀ-zĕr SŬR-jĕr-ē	Surgical technique employing a device that emits intense heat and power at close range to cut, burn, vaporize, or destroy tissues
radical dissection RĂD-ĭ-kăl dī-SĔK-shŭn	Surgical removal of tissue in an extensive area surrounding the surgical site in an attempt to excise all tissue that may be malignant and decrease the chance of recurrence *An example of a radical dissection procedure is radical mastectomy, in which the entire breast, surrounding lymph nodes, and sometimes adjacent muscles are removed.*
resection rē-SĔK-shŭn	Partial excision of a bone, organ, or other structure

 It is time to review diagnostic and therapeutic terms and procedures by completing Learning Activity 4–5.

Abbreviations

This section introduces body structure abbreviations and their meanings.

Abbreviation	Meaning	Abbreviation	Meaning
ant	anterior	**MRI**	magnetic resonance imaging
AP	anteroposterior	**PET**	positron emission tomography
Bx, bx	biopsy	**post**	posterior
CBC	complete blood count	**RF**	rheumatoid factor; radio frequency
CT	computed tomography	**RLQ**	right lower quadrant
DNA	deoxyribonucleic acid	**RUQ**	right upper quadrant
DSA	digital subtraction angiography	**sono**	sonogram
Dx	diagnosis	**SPECT**	single photon emission computed tomography
FS	frozen section	**Sx**	symptom
I&D	incision and drainage	**Tx**	treatment
LAT, lat	lateral	**UA**	urinalysis
LLQ	left lower quadrant	**U&L, U/L**	upper and lower
LUQ	left upper quadrant	**US**	ultrasound ultrasonography

LEARNING ACTIVITIES

The following activities provide a review of the body structure terms introduced in this chapter. Complete each activity and review your answers to evaluate your understanding of the chapter.

Learning Activity 4-1
Identifying Body Planes

Label the following illustration using the terms below.

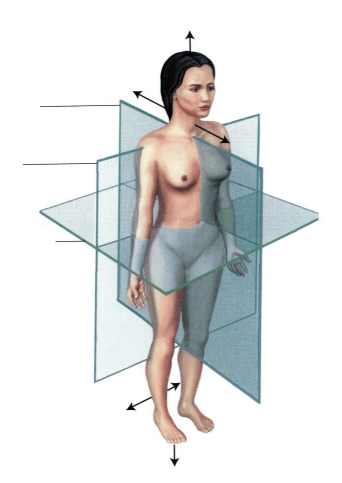

anterior	*lateral*	*posterior*
coronal (frontal) plane	*medial*	*superior*
inferior	*midsagittal (median) plane*	*transverse (horizontal) plane*

 Check your answers by referring to Figure 4–2 on page 44. Review material that you did not answer correctly.

Identifying Abdominopelvic Divisions

Label the quadrants on Figure A and regions on Figure B using the terms below.

A.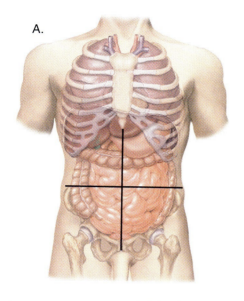
B.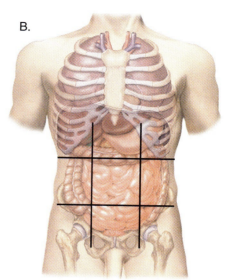

epigastric region	left lumbar region	right lower quadrant
hypogastric region	left upper quadrant	right lumbar region
left hypochondriac region	right hypochondriac region	right upper quadrant
left iliac region	right iliac region	umbilical region
left lower quadrant		

 Check your answers by referring to Figure 4–4A and 4–4B on page 46. Review material that you did not answer correctly.

Learning Activity 4-3

Matching Body Cavity, Spine, and Directional Terms

Match each term on the left with its meaning on the right.

1. _____ abdominopelvic
2. _____ adduction
3. _____ cervical

4. _____ coccyx
5. _____ deep
6. _____ eversion
7. _____ inferior (caudal)
8. _____ inversion
9. _____ lumbar

10. _____ plantar
11. _____ posterior (dorsal)
12. _____ prone
13. _____ proximal

14. _____ superficial
15. _____ thoracic

a. pertaining to the sole of the foot

b. tail bone

c. ventral cavity that contains heart, lungs, and associated structures

d. toward the surface of the body (external)

e. lying horizontal with face downward

f. turning outward

g. nearer to the center (trunk of the body)

h. ventral cavity that contains digestive, reproductive, and excretory structures

i. turning inward or inside out

j. part of the spine known as the neck

k. movement toward the median plane

l. away from the head; toward the tail or lower part of a structure

m. away from the surface of the body (internal)

n. part of the spine known as the *loin*

o. near the back of the body

✔ *Check your answers in Appendix A. Review any material that you did not answer correctly.*

Correct Answers _____ × 6.67 = _____ % Score

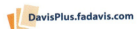
DavisPlus.fadavis.com

Enhance your study and reinforcement of word elements with the power of DavisPlus. Visit www. davisplus.fadavis.com/gylys/systems *for this chapter's flash-card activity. We recommend you complete the flash-card activity before completing Activities 4–4 and 4–5 below.*

Matching Word Elements

Match the following word elements with the definitions in the numbered list.

Combining	Forms	Suffixes	Prefixes
caud/o	kary/o	-genesis	ad-
dist/o	leuk/o	-gnosis	infra-
dors/o	morph/o	-graphy	ultra-
eti/o	poli/o		
hist/o	somat/o		
idi/o	viscer/o		
jaund/o	xer/o		

1. _____ nucleus
2. _____ far, farthest
3. _____ process of recording
4. _____ knowing
5. _____ white
6. _____ internal organs
7. _____ yellow
8. _____ tissue
9. _____ forming, producing, origin
10. _____ below, under
11. _____ excess, beyond
12. _____ tail
13. _____ back (of body)
14. _____ gray
15. _____ cause
16. _____ form, shape, structure
17. _____ dry
18. _____ unknown, peculiar
19. _____ toward
20. _____ body

Check your answers in Appendix A. Review any material that you did not answer correctly.

Correct Answers _____ × 5 = _____ % Score

Learning Activity 4-5

Matching Diagnostic and Therapeutic Terms and Procedures

Match the following terms with the definitions in the numbered list.

ablation	fluoroscopy	radionuclide
cauterize	morbid	resection
Doppler	nuclear scan	suppurative
endoscopy	punch biopsy	thoracoscopy
febrile	radiology	ultrasonography

1. _____ specialty concerned with the use of electromagnetic radiation, ultrasound, and imaging techniques

2. _____ measurement of blood flow in a vessel by reflecting sound waves off moving blood cells

3. _____ imaging technique that employs high-frequency sound waves

4. _____ visual examination of the lungs, pleura, and pleural space with a scope inserted through a small incision between the ribs

5. _____ excision of a core sample of tissue for examination

6. _____ visual examination of a cavity or canal using a special lighted instrument

7. _____ use of a radioactive material and scanning device to determine, size, shape, location, and function of various organs and structures

8. _____ radiographic technique that directs x-rays to a fluorescent screen and displays "live" images on a monitor

9. _____ disease, or pertaining to disease

10. _____ substance that emits radiation spontaneously; also called *tracer*

11. _____ feverish; pertaining to a fever

12. _____ partial excision of a bone, organ, or other structure

13. _____ producing or associated with generation of pus

14. _____ destruction of tissue by electricity, freezing, heat, or corrosive chemicals

15. _____ removal of a part, pathway, or function by surgery, chemical destruction, electrocautery, freezing, or radiofrequency (RF)

✔ *Check your answers in Appendix A. Review any material that you did not answer correctly.*

Correct Answers _____ × 6.67 = _____ % Score

MEDICAL RECORD ACTIVITIES

The two medical records included in the following activities use common clinical scenarios to show how medical terminology is used to document patient care. Complete the terminology and analysis sections for each activity to help you recognize and understand terms related to body structure.

Medical Record Activity 4-1
Radiological Consultation Letter: Cervical and Lumbar Spine

Terminology

Terms listed below come from the *Radiological Consultation Letter: Cervical and Lumbar Spine* that follows. Use a medical dictionary such as *Taber's Cyclopedic Medical Dictionary*, the appendices of this book, or other resources to define each term. Then review the pronunciations for each term and practice by reading the medical record aloud.

Term	Definition
AP	
atlantoaxial ăt-lăn-tō-ĂK-sē-ăl	
cervical SĔR-vĭ-kăl	
lateral LĂT-ĕr-ăl	
lumbar LŬM-băr	
lumbosacral junction lŭm-bō-SĀ-krăl	
odontoid ō-DŎN-toyd	
sacral SĀ-krăl	
scoliosis skō-lĕ-Ō-sĭs	
spasm SPĂZM	
spina bifida occulta SPĪ-nă BĬF-ĭ-dă ŏ-KŬL-tă	
vertebral bodies VĔR-tĕ-brăl	

Listen and Learn Online! *will help you master the pronunciation of selected medical words from this medical record activity. Visit* www.davisplus.com/gylys/systems *to find instructions on completing the* Listen and Learn Online! *exercise for this section and to practice pronunciations.*

PATHOLOGY REPORT: RADIOLOGICAL CONSULTATION LETTER: CERVICAL AND LUMBAR SPINE

Physician Center

2422 Rodeo Drive ■■ **Sun City, USA 12345** ■■ **(555) 333-2427**

May 3, 20xx

John Roberts, MD
1115 Forest Ave
Sun City, USA 12345

Dear Doctor Roberts:

Thank you for referring Chester Bowen to our office. Mr. Bowen presents with neck and lower back pain of more than 2 years' duration. Radiographic examination of June 14, 20xx reveals the following: AP, lateral, and odontoid views of the cervical spine demonstrate some reversal of normal cervical curvature, as seen on lateral projection. There is some right lateral scoliosis of the cervical spine. The vertebral bodies, however, appear to be well maintained in height; the intervertebral spaces are well maintained. The odontoid is visualized and appears to be intact. The atlantoaxial joint appears symmetrical.

Impression: Films of the cervical spine demonstrate some reversal of normal cervical curvature and a minimal scoliosis, possibly secondary to muscle spasm, without evidence of recent bony disease or injury. AP and lateral films of the lumbar spine, with spots of the lumbosacral junction, demonstrate an apparent minimal spina bifida occulta of the first sacral segment. The vertebral bodies, however, are well maintained in height; the intervertebral spaces appear well maintained.

Pathological Diagnosis: Right lateral scoliosis with some reversal of normal cervical curvature.

If you have any further questions, please feel free to contact me.

Sincerely yours,

Adrian Jones, MD
Adrian Jones, MD

aj:bg

Analysis

Review the medical record *Radiological Consultation Letter: Cervical and lumbar spine* to answer the following questions.

1. What was the presenting problem?

_____

2. What were the three views of the radiological examination of June 14, 20xx?

_____

3. Was there evidence of recent bony disease or injury?

_____

4. Which cervical vertebrae form the atlantoaxial joint?

_____

5. Was the odontoid fractured?

_____

6. What did the AP and lateral films of the lumbar spine demonstrate?

_____

Medical Record Activity 4-2

Radiology Report: Injury of Left Wrist, Elbow, and Humerus

Terminology

Terms listed below come from the *Radiology Report: Injury of Left Wrist, Elbow, and Humerus* that follows. Use a medical dictionary such as *Taber's Cyclopedic Medical Dictionary*, the appendices of this book, or other resources to define each term. Then review the pronunciations for each term and practice by reading the medical record aloud.

Term	Definition
anterior	
AP	
distal DĬS-tăl	
dorsal DOR-săl	
epicondyle ĕp-ĭ-KŎN-dīl	
humerus HŪ-mĕr-ŭs	
lucency LOO-sĕnt-sē	
medial MĒ-dē-ăl	

Term	Definition
mm	
posterior	
radius RĂ-dē-ŭs	
ulna ŬL-nă	
ventral-lateral VĔN-trăl-LĂT-ĕr-ăl	

 Listen and Learn Online! *will help you master the pronunciation of selected medical words from this medical record activity. Visit* www.davisplus.com/gylys/systems *to find instructions on completing the Listen and Learn Online! exercise for this section and to practice pronunciations.*

RADIOLOGY REPORT : INJURY OF LEFT WRIST, ELBOW, AND HUMERUS

General Hospital

1511 Ninth Avenue ■■ **Sun City, USA 12345** ■■ **(555) 802-1887**

RADIOLOGY REPORT

Date: June 5, 20xx   Patient: Hill, Joan
Physician: Adrian Jones, MD   DOB: 5/25/19xx
Examination: Left wrist, left elbow, and left humerus   X-ray No: 43201

LEFT WRIST: Images obtained with the patient's arm taped to an arm board. There are fractures through the distal shafts of the radius and ulna. The radial fracture fragments show approximately 8-mm overlap with dorsal displacement of the distal radial fracture fragment. The distal ulnar shaft fracture shows ventral-lateral angulation at the fracture apex. There is no overriding at this fracture. No additional fracture is seen. Soft-tissue deformity is present, correlating with the fracture sites.

LEFT ELBOW AND LEFT HUMERUS: Single view of the left elbow was obtained in the lateral projection. AP view of the humerus was obtained to include a portion of the elbow. A third radiograph was obtained but is not currently available for review. There is lucency through the distal humerus on the AP view along its medial aspect. It would be difficult to exclude fracture just above the medial epicondyle. On the lateral view, there is elevation of the anterior and posterior fat pad. These findings are of some concern. Repeat elbow study is recommended.

Jason Skinner, MD
Jason Skinner, MD

JS: bg

D: 6-05-20xx
T: 6-05-20xx

Analysis

Review the medical record *Radiology Report: Injury of Left Wrist, Elbow, and Humerus* to answer the following questions.

1. Where are the fractures located?

_____

2. What caused the soft-tissue deformity?

_____

3. Did the radiologist take any side views of the left elbow?

_____

4. In the AP view of the humerus, what structure was also visualized?

_____

5. What findings are cause for concern to the radiologist?

_____

Integumentary System

CHAPTER

5

Chapter Outline

Objectives

Upon completion of this chapter, you will be able to:

- Locate the major organs of the integumentary system and describe their structure and function.
- Describe the functional relationship between the integumentary system and other body systems.
- Pronounce, spell, and build words related to the integumentary system.
- Describe pathological conditions, diagnostic and therapeutic procedures, and other terms related to the integumentary system.
- Explain pharmacology associated with the treatment of skin disorders.
- Demonstrate your knowledge of this chapter by completing the learning and medical record activities.

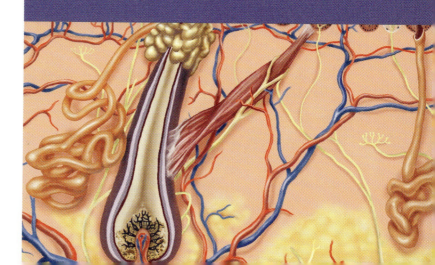

Anatomy and Physiology

The skin, also called *integument*, is the largest organ in the body. Together with its accessory organs (hair, nails, and glands), the skin makes up the **integumentary system.** Its elaborate system of distinct tissues includes glands that produce several types of secretions, nerves that transmit impulses, and blood vessels that help regulate body temperature. The skin covers and protects all outer surfaces of the body and performs many vital functions, including the sense of touch. (See Figure 5–1.)

Skin

The skin protects underlying structures from injury and provides sensory information to the brain. Beneath the skin's surface is an intricate network of nerve fibers that register sensations of temperature, pain, and pressure. Other important functions of the skin include protecting the body against ultraviolet rays, regulating body temperature, and preventing dehydration. The skin also acts as a reservoir for food and water. It also **synthesizes** vitamin D when exposed to sunlight. The skin consists of two distinct layers: the epidermis and the dermis. A subcutaneous layer of tissue binds the skin to underlying structures.

Epidermis

The outer layer, the (1) **epidermis,** is relatively thin over most areas but is thickest on the palms of the hands and the soles of the feet. Although the epidermis is composed of several sublayers called *strata*, the (2) **stratum corneum** and the (3) **basal layer**, which is the deepest layer, are of greatest importance.

The stratum corneum is composed of dead flat cells that lack a blood supply and sensory receptors. Its thickness is correlated with normal wear of the area it covers. The basal layer is the only layer of the epidermis that is composed of living cells

Anatomy and Physiology Key Terms

This section introduces important terms, along with their definitions and pronunciations. Word analyses for selected terms are also provided.

Term	Definition
androgen ĂN-drō-jĕn	Generic term for an agent (usually a hormone, such as testosterone and androsterone) that stimulates development of male characteristics
ductule DŬK-tūl *duct:* to lead; carry *-ule:* small, minute	Very small duct
homeostasis hō-mē-ō-STĀ-sĭs *homeo-:* same, alike *-stasis:* standing still	State in which the regulatory mechanisms of the body maintain an internal environment within tolerable levels, despite changes in the external environment *The regulatory mechanisms of the body control temperature, acidity, and the concentration of salt, food, and waste products.*
scrotum SKRŌ-tŭm	Pouch of skin in the male that contains the testicles
synthesis SĬN-thĕs-ĭs	Formation of a complex substance by the union of simpler compounds or elements *Skin synthesizes vitamin D (needed by bones for calcium absorption).*
synthesize SĬN-thĕ-sīz	To produce by **synthesis**

Pronunciation Help	Long Sound	ā—rate	ē—rebirth	ī—isle	ō—over	ū—unite
	Short Sound	ă—alone	ĕ—ever	ĭ—it	ŏ—not	ŭ—cut

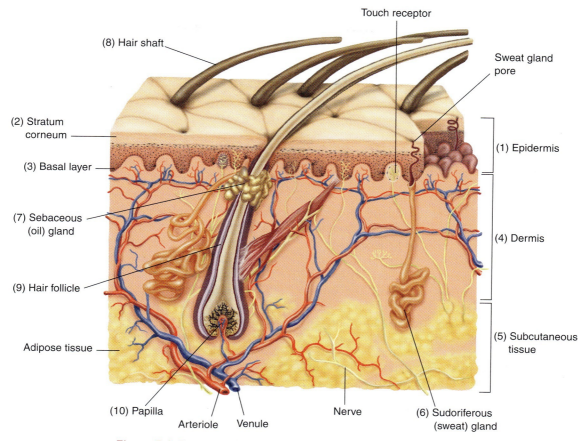

Touch receptor

(8) Hair shaft

Sweat gland pore

(2) Stratum corneum

(1) Epidermis

(3) Basal layer

(7) Sebaceous (oil) gland

(4) Dermis

(9) Hair follicle

(5) Subcutaneous tissue

Adipose tissue

(10) Papilla

Arteriole   Venule

Nerve

(6) Sudoriferous (sweat) gland

Figure 5-1. Structure of the skin and subcutaneous tissue.

where new cells are formed. As these cells move toward the stratum corneum to replace the cells that have been sloughed off, they die and become filled with a hard protein material called *keratin.* The relatively waterproof characteristic of keratin prevents body fluids from evaporating and moisture from entering the body. The entire process by which a cell forms in the basal layer, rises to the surface, becomes keratinized, and sloughs off takes about 1 month.

In the basal layer, special cells called *melanocytes* produce a black pigment called *melanin.* Melanin provides a protective barrier from the damaging effects of the sun's ultraviolet radiation, which can cause skin cancer. Moderate sun exposure increases the rate of melanin production and results in a suntan. However, overexposure results in sunburn due to melanin's inability to absorb sufficient ultraviolet rays to prevent the burn.

Differences in skin color are attributed to the amount of melanin in each cell. Dark-skinned people produce large amounts of melanin and are less likely to have wrinkles or skin cancer.

Production of melanocytes is genetically regulated and, thus, inherited. Local accumulations of melanin are seen in pigmented moles and freckles. An absence of pigment in the skin, eyes, and hair is most likely due to an inherited inability to produce melanin. An individual who cannot produce melanin has a marked deficiency of pigment in the eyes, hair, and skin and is known as an *albino.*

Dermis

The second layer of the skin, the (4) **dermis,** also called *corium,* lies directly beneath the epidermis. It is composed of living tissue and contains numerous capillaries, lymphatic vessels, and nerve endings. Hair follicles, **sebaceous** (oil) glands, and **sudoriferous** (sweat) glands are also located in the dermis.

The (5) **subcutaneous layer,** also called *hypodermis,* binds the dermis to underlying structures. It is composed primarily of loose connective tissue and **adipose** (fat) tissue interlaced with blood vessels. The subcutaneous layer stores fats, insulates and cushions the body, and regulates temperature.

The amount of fat in the subcutaneous layer varies with the region of the body and sex, age, and nutritional state.

Accessory Organs of the Skin

The accessory organs of the skin consist of integumentary glands, hair, and nails. The glands play an important role in defending the body against disease and maintaining homeostasis, whereas the hair and nails have more limited functional roles.

Glands

Two important glands located in the dermis produce secretions: the (6) **sudoriferous (sweat) glands** produce sweat and the (7) **sebaceous (oil) glands** produce oil. These two glands are **exocrine glands** because they secrete substances through ducts to an outer surface of the body rather than directly into the bloodstream.

The sudoriferous glands secrete perspiration, or sweat, onto the surface of the skin through pores. Pores are most plentiful on the palms, soles, forehead, and **axillae** (armpits). The main functions of the sudoriferous glands are to cool the body by evaporation, excrete waste products, and moisten surface cells.

The sebaceous glands are filled with cells, the centers of which contain fatty droplets. As these cells disintegrate, they yield an oily secretion called *sebum.* The acidic nature of sebum helps destroy harmful organisms on the skin, thus preventing infection. When ductules of the sebaceous glands become blocked, acne may result. Congested sebum causes formation of pimples or whiteheads. If the sebum is dark, it forms blackheads. Sex hormones, particularly androgens, regulate production and secretion of sebum. During adolescence, secretions increase; as the person ages, secretions diminish. The loss of sebum, which lubricates the skin, may be one of the reasons for the formation of wrinkles that accompany old age. Sebaceous glands are present over the entire body except on the soles of the feet and the palms of the hands. They are especially prevalent on the scalp and face; around such openings as the nose, mouth, external ear, and anus; and on the upper back and scrotum.

Hair

Hair is found on nearly all parts of the body except for the lips, nipples, palms of the hands, soles of the feet, and parts of the external genitalia. The visible part of the hair is the (8) **hair shaft**; the part that is embedded in the dermis is the hair root. The root, together with its coverings, forms the (9) **hair follicle.** At the bottom of the follicle is a loop of capillaries enclosed in a covering called the (10) **papilla.** The cluster of epithelial cells lying over the papilla reproduces and is responsible for the eventual formation of the hair shaft. As long as these cells remain alive, hair will regenerate even if it is cut, plucked, or otherwise removed. **Alopecia** (baldness) occurs when the hairs of the scalp are not replaced because of death of the papillae (singular, *papilla*).

Like skin color, hair color is related to the amount of pigment produced by epidermal melanocytes. Melanocytes are found at the base of the hair follicle. Melanin ranges in color from yellow to reddish brown to black. Varying amounts of melanin produce hair ranging in color from blond to brunette to black; the more abundant the melanin, the darker the hair. Heredity and aging affect melanin levels. A decrease or an absence of melanin causes loss of hair color.

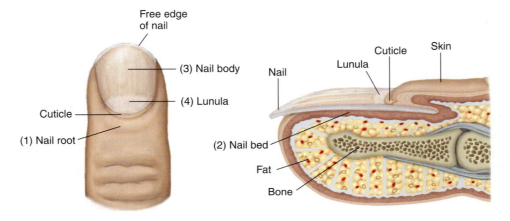

Figure 5-2. Structure of a fingernail.

Connecting Body Systems–Integumentary System

The main function of the skin is to protect the entire body, including all of its organs, from the external environment. Specific functional relationships between the skin and other body systems are summarized below.

Blood, lymph, and immune
- Skin is the first line of defense against the invasion of pathogens in the body.

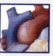

Cardiovascular
- Cutaneous blood vessels dilate and constrict to help regulate body temperature.

Digestive
- Skin absorbs vitamin D (produced when skin is exposed to sunlight) needed for intestinal absorption of calcium.
- Excess calories are stored as subcutaneous fat.

Endocrine
- Subcutaneous layer of the skin stores adipose tissue when insulin secretions cause excess carbohydrate intake to fat storage.

Female Reproductive
- Subcutaneous receptors provide pleasurable sensations associated with sexual behavior.
- Skin stretches to accommodate the growing fetus during pregnancy.

Genitourinary
- Receptors in the skin respond to sexual stimuli.
- Skin provides an alternative route for excreting salts and nitrogenous wastes in the form of perspiration.

Musculoskeletal
- Skin synthesizes vitamin D needed for absorption of calcium essential for muscle contraction.
- Skin also synthesizes vitamin D needed for growth, repair, and maintenance of bones.

Nervous
- Cutaneous receptors detect stimuli related to touch, pain, pressure, and temperature.

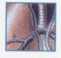

Respiratory
- Skin temperature may influence respiratory rate. As temperature increases, respiratory rate may also increase.
- Hairs of the nasal cavity filter particles from inspired air before it reaches the lower respiratory tract.

 It is time to review anatomy by completing Learning Activity 5–1.

Nails

Nails protect the tips of the fingers and toes from bruises and injuries. (See Figure 5–2.) Each nail is formed in the (1) **nail root** and is composed of keratinized stratified squamous epithelial cells producing a very tough covering. As the nail grows, it stays attached and slides forward over the layer of epithelium called the (2) **nail bed.**

This epithelial layer is continuous with the epithelium of the skin. Most of the (3) **nail body** appears pink because of the underlying vascular tissue. The half-moon–shaped area at the base of the nail, the (4) **lunula**, is the region where new growth occurs. The lunula has a whitish appearance because the vascular tissue underneath does not show through.

Medical Word Elements

This section introduces combining forms, suffixes, and prefixes related to the integumentary system. Word analyses are also provided.

Element	Meaning	Word Analysis
Combining Forms		
adip/o	fat	**adip**/osis (ăd-ĭ-PŌ-sĭs): abnormal condition of fat *-osis:* abnormal condition; increase (used primarily with blood cells) *Adiposis is an abnormal accumulation of fatty tissue in the body.*
lip/o		**lip/o**/cele (LĬP-ō-sēl): hernia containing fat *-cele:* hernia, swelling
steat/o	skin	**steat**/itis (stē-ă-TĪ-tĭs): inflammation of fatty (adipose) tissue *-itis:* inflammation
cutane/o		sub/**cutane**/ous (sŭb-kū-TĀ-nē-ŭs): pertaining to beneath the skin *sub-:* under, below *-ous:* pertaining to
dermat/o		**dermat/o**/plasty (DĔR-mă-tō-plăs-tē): surgical repair of the skin *-plasty:* surgical repair
derm/o		hypo/**derm**/ic (hī-pō-DĔR-mĭk): pertaining to under the skin *hypo-:* under, below *-ic:* pertaining to *A hypodermic injection is one in which the needle is inserted under the skin.*
hidr/o	sweat	**hidr**/aden/itis (hī-drăd-ĕ-NĪ-tĭs): inflammation of the sweat glands *aden:* gland *-itis:* inflammation *Do not confuse* hidr/o *(sweat) with* hydr/o *(water).*
sudor/o		**sudor**/esis (soo-dō-RĒ-sĭs): profuse sweating *-esis:* condition
ichthy/o	dry, scaly	**ichthy**/osis (ĭk-thē-Ō-sĭs): abnormal condition of dry or scaly skin *-osis:* abnormal condition; increase (used primarily with blood cells) *Ichthyosis can be any of several dermatological conditions in which the skin is dry and hardened (hyperkeratotic), resembling fish scales. A mild form of ichthyosis, called* winter itch, *is commonly seen on the legs of older patients, especially during the winter months.*
kerat/o	horny tissue; hard; cornea	**kerat**/osis (kĕr-ă-TŌ-sĭs): abnormal condition of horny tissue *-osis:* abnormal condition; increase (used primarily with blood cells) *Keratosis is a thickened area of the epidermis or any horny growth on the skin, such as a callus or wart.*
melan/o	black	**melan**/oma (mĕl-ă-NŌ-mă): black tumor *-oma:* tumor
myc/o	fungus (plural, *fungi)*	dermat/o/**myc**/osis (dĕr-mă-tō-mī-KŌ-sĭs): fungal infection of the skin *dermat/o:* skin *-osis:* abnormal condition; increase (used primarily with blood cells) *Melanoma is a malignant tumor of melanocytes that commonly begins in a darkly pigmented mole and can metastasize widely.*

Medical Word Elements—cont'd

Element	Meaning	Word Analysis
onych/o	nail	**onych/o**/malacia (ŏn-ĭ-kō-mă-LĀ-shē-ă): softening of the nails *-malacia:* softening
ungu/o		**ungu**/al (ŬNG-gwăl): pertaining to the nails *-al:* pertaining to
pil/o	hair	**pil/o**/nid/al (pī-lō-NĬ-dăl): pertaining to hair in a nest *nid:* nest *-al:* pertaining to *A pilonidal cyst commonly develops in the skin at the base of the spine. It develops as a growth of hair in a dermoid cyst.*
trich/o		**trich/o**/pathy (trĭk-ŎP-ă-thē): disease involving the hair *-pathy:* disease
scler/o	hardening; sclera (white of eye)	**scler/o**/derma (sklĕ-rō-DĔR-mă): hardening of the skin *-derma:* skin *Scleroderma is an autoimmune disorder that causes the skin and internal organs to become progressively hardened due to deposits of collagen. It may occur as a localized form or as a systemic disease.*
seb/o	sebum, sebaceous	**seb/o**/rrhea (sĕb-ō-RĒ-ă): discharge of sebum *-rrhea:* discharge, flow *Seborrhea is an excessive secretion of sebum from the sebaceous glands.*
squam/o	scale	**squam**/ous (SKWĀ-mŭs): pertaining to scales (or covered with scales) *-ous:* pertaining to
xen/o	foreign, strange	**xen/o**/graft (ZĔN-ō-grăft): skin transplantation from a foreign donor (usually a pig) for a human; also called *heterograft.* *Xenografts are used as a temporary graft to protect the patient against infection and fluid loss.* *-graft:* transplantation
xer/o	dry	**xer/o**/derma (zē-rō-DĔR-mă): dry skin *-derma:* skin *Xeroderma is a chronic skin condition characterized by dryness and roughness and is a mild form of ichthyosis.*
Suffixes		
-cyte	cell	lip/o/**cyte** (LĬP-ō-sīt): fat cell *lip/o:* fat
-derma	skin	py/o/**derma** (pī-ō-DĔR-mă): pus in the skin *py/o:* pus *Pyoderma is an acute, inflammatory, purulent bacterial dermatitis. It may be primary, such as impetigo, or secondary to a previous skin condition.*
-logist	specialist in the study of	dermat/o/**logist** (dĕr-mă-TŎL-ō-jĭst): specialist in treatment of skin disorders *dermat/o:* skin
-logy	study of	dermat/o/**logy** (dĕr-mă-TŎL-ō-jē): study of the skin (and its diseases) *dermat/o:* skin

(continued)

Medical Word Elements—cont'd

Element	Meaning	Word Analysis
-therapy	treatment	cry/o/**therapy** (krī-ō-THĔR-ă-pē): use of cold in the treatment (of disease) *cry/o:* cold *Cryotherapy is used to destroy tissue by freezing with liquid nitrogen. Cutaneous warts and actinic keratosis are common skin disorders that respond well to cryotherapy treatment.*

Prefixes

Element	Meaning	Word Analysis
an-	without, not	**an**/hidr/osis (ăn-hĭ-DRŌ-sĭs): abnormal condition of absence of sweat *hidr:* sweat *-osis:* abnormal condition; increase (used primarily with blood cells)
dia-	through, across	**dia**/phoresis (dī-ă-fă-RĒ-sĭs): excessive or profuse sweating; also called *sudoresis* or *hyperhidrosis* *-phoresis:* carrying; transmission
epi-	above, upon	**epi**/derm/is (ĕp-ĭ-DĔR-mĭs): above the skin *derm:* skin *-is:* noun ending *Epidermis is the outermost layer of the skin.*
homo-	same	**homo**/graft (HŌ-mō-grăft): transplantation of tissue between individuals of the same species; also called *allograft* *-graft:* transplantation
hyper-	excessive, above normal	**hyper**/hidr/osis (hī-pĕr-hī-DRŌ-sĭs): excessive or profuse sweating; also called *diaphoresis* or *sudoresis* *hidr:* sweat *-osis:* abnormal condition; increase (used primarily with blood cells)
sub-	under, below	**sub**/ungu/al (sŭb-ŬNG-gwăl): pertaining to beneath the nail of a finger or toe *ungu:* nail *-al:* pertaining to

 It is time to review medical word elements by completing Larning Activity 5–2. For audio pronunciations of the above-listed key terms, you can visit www.davisplus.fadavis.com/gylys/systems to download this chapter's Listen and Learn exercises or use the book's audio CD (if included).

Pathology

General appearance and condition of the skin are clinically important because they may provide clues to body conditions or dysfunctions. Pale skin may indicate shock; red, flushed, very warm skin may indicate fever and infection. A rash may indicate allergies or local infections. Even chewed fingernails may be a clue to emotional problems. For diagnosis, treatment, and management of skin disorders, the medical services of a specialist may be warranted. **Dermatology** is the medical specialty concerned with diseases that directly affect the skin and systemic diseases that manifest their effects on the skin. The physician who specializes in diagnosis and treatment of skin diseases is known as a **dermatologist.**

Skin Lesions

Lesions are areas of tissue that have been pathologically altered by injury, wound, or infection. Lesions may affect tissue over an area of a definite size (**localized**) or may be widely spread throughout the body (**systemic**). Evaluation of skin lesions, injuries, or changes to tissue helps establish the diagnosis of skin disorders. Lesions are described as primary or secondary. **Primary skin lesions** are the initial reaction to **pathologically**

altered tissue and may be flat or elevated. **Secondary skin lesions** are changes that take place in the primary lesion due to infection, scratching, trauma, or various stages of a disease. Lesions are also described by their appearance, color, location, and size as measured in centimeters. Some of the major primary and secondary skin lesions are described and illustrated in Figure 5–3.

Burns

Burns are tissue injuries caused by contact with thermal, chemical, electrical, or radioactive agents. Although burns generally occur on the skin, they can also affect the respiratory and digestive tract linings. Burns that have a local effect are not as serious as those that have a systemic effect.

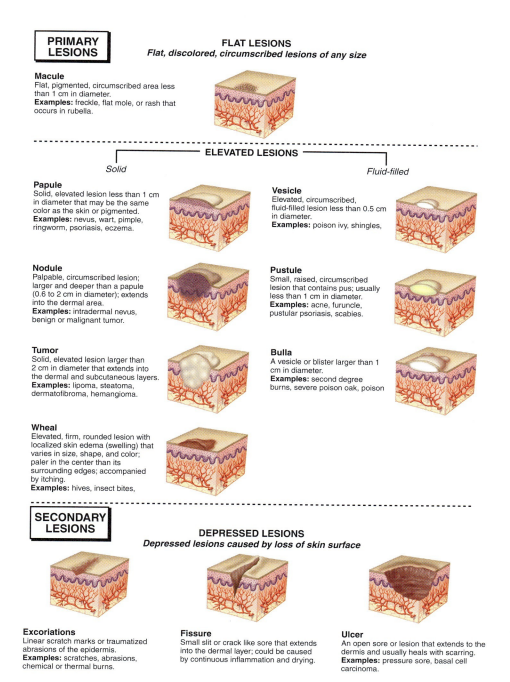

Figure 5-3. Primary and secondary lesions.

 It is time to review skin lesions by completing Learning Activity 5–3.

Systemic effects are life threatening and may include dehydration, shock, and infection.

Burns are usually classified as first-, second-, or third-degree burns. The extent of injury and degree of severity determine a burn's classification. **First-degree (superficial) burns** are the least serious type of burn because they injure only the top layers of the skin, the epidermis. These burns are most often caused by brief contact with either dry or moist heat (**thermal burn**), spending too much time in the sun (**sunburn**), or exposure to chemicals. Injury is restricted to local effects, such as skin redness (**erythema**) and acute sensitivity to sensory stimuli (**hyperesthesia**), such as touch, heat, or cold. Generally, blisters do not form and the burn heals without scar formation. **Second-degree (partial-thickness) burns** are deep burns that damage both the epidermis and part of the dermis. These burns may be caused by contact with flames, hot liquids, or chemicals. Symptoms mimic those of first-degree burns, but fluid-filled blisters (**vesicles** or **bullae**) form and the burn may heal with little or no scarring. See Figure 5–4.)

In **third-degree (full-thickness) burns**, the epidermis and dermis are destroyed and some of the underlying connective tissue is damaged, leaving the skin waxy and charred with insensitivity to touch. The underlying bones, muscles, and tendons may also be damaged. These burns may be caused by corrosive chemicals, flames, electricity, or extremely hot objects; immersion of the body in extremely hot water, or clothing that catches fire. Because of the extensiveness of tissue destruction,

ulcerating wounds develop and the body attempts to heal itself by forming scar tissue. Skin grafting (**dermatoplasty**) is commonly required to protect the underlying tissue and assist in recovery.

A formula for estimating the percentage of adult body surface area affected by burns is to apply the Rule of Nines. This method assigns values of 9% or 18% of surface areas to specific regions. The formula is modified in infants and children because of the proportionately larger head size. (See Figure 5–5.) To determine treatment, it is important to know the amount of the burned surface area because IV fluids for hydration are required to replace fluids lost from tissue damage.

Oncology

Neoplasms are abnormal growths of new tissue that are classified as benign or malignant. **Benign neoplasms** are noncancerous growths composed of the same type of cells as the tissue in which they are growing. They harm the individual only insofar as they place pressure on surrounding structures. If the benign neoplasm remains small and places no pressure on adjacent structures, it commonly is not removed. When it becomes excessively large, causes pain, or places pressure on other organs or structures, excision is necessary. **Malignant neoplasms** are composed of cells that are invasive and spread to remote regions of the body. These cells show altered function, altered appearance, and uncontrolled growth. They invade surrounding tissue and, ultimately, some of the malignant cells from the

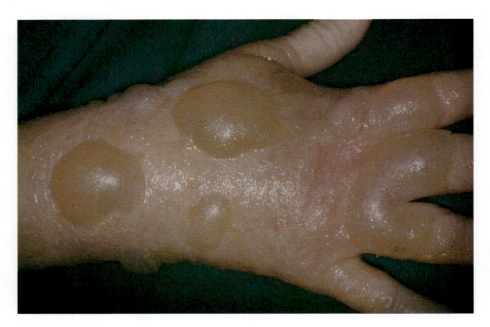

Figure 5-4. Second-degree burn of the hand. From Goldsmith, Lazarus, & Tharp: *Adult and Pediatric Dermatology: A Color Guide to Diagnosis and Treatment.* FA Davis, Philadelphia, 1997, p 318, with permission.

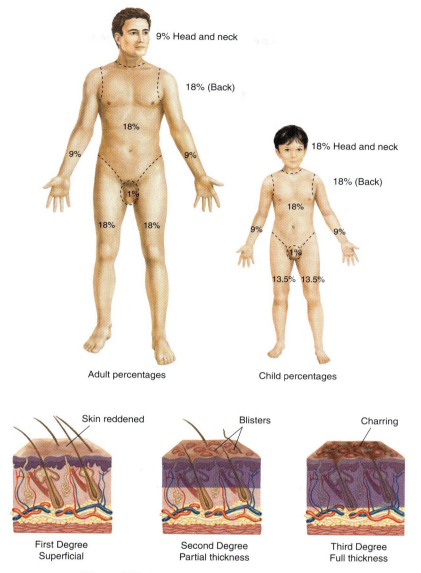

Figure 5-5. Rule of Nines and burn classification.

primary tumor may enter blood and lymph vessels and travel to remote regions of the body to form secondary tumor sites, a process called *metastasis*. The presence of a malignant growth (tumor), is the disease called *cancer*. The ability to invade surrounding tissues and spread to remote regions of the body is a distinguishing feature of cancer. If left untreated, cancer is usually progressive and generally fatal.

Cancer (CA) treatment includes surgery, chemotherapy, immunotherapy, and radiation therapy. **Immunotherapy,** also called *biotherapy,* is a recent treatment that stimulates the body's own immune defenses to fight tumor cells. To provide the most effective treatment, the physician may prescribe one of the above treatments or use a combination of them (**combined modality treatment**).

Grading and Staging Systems

Pathologists grade and stage tumors for **diagnostic** and **therapeutic** purposes. A **tumor** grading system is used to evaluate the appearance and maturity of malignant cells in a tumor. Pathologists commonly describe tumors by four grades of severity based on the microscopic appearance of their cells. (See Table 5–1.) A patient with a grade I tumor has the best **prognosis**; one with grade IV tumor has the poorest prognosis.

The tumor, node, metastasis (TNM) system of staging is used to identify the invasiveness of the malignant tumor. It also helps the **oncologist**

Table 5-1	Tumor Grading	

The table below defines the four tumor grades and their characteristics.

Grading	Tumor Characteristics
Grade I Tumor cells well differentiated	• Close resemblance to tissue of origin, thus, retaining some specialized functions
Grade II Tumor cells moderately differentiated	• Less resemblance to tissue of origin • More variation in size and shape of tumor cells • Increased mitoses
Grade III Tumor cells poorly to very poorly differentiated	• Only remotely resembles tissue of origin • Marked variation in shape and size of tumor cells • Greatly increased mitoses
Grade IV Tumor cells very poorly differentiated	• Little or no resemblance to tissue of origin • Extreme variation in size and shape of tumor cells

determine the most effective method of treatment. The TNM system stages tumors according to three basic criteria:

- **T**—size and invasiveness of the primary tumor
- **N**—nodal involvement
- **M**—spreading of the primary tumor to remote regions of the body (**metastasis**).

Numbers are used to indicate size or spread of the tumor. The higher the number, the greater the extent or spread of the malignancy. For example, T2 designates a small tumor; M0 designates no evidence of metastasis. (See Table 5–2.)

Basal Cell Carcinoma

Basal cell carcinoma, the most common type of skin cancer, is a malignancy of the basal layer of the epidermis, or hair follicles. This type of cancer is commonly caused by overexposure to sunlight. (See Figure 5–6.) These tumors are locally invasive but rarely metastasize. Basal cell carcinoma is most prevalent in blond, fair-skinned men and is the most common malignant tumor affecting white people. Although these tumors grow slowly, they commonly ulcerate as they increase in size and develop crusting that is firm to the touch. Metastases are uncommon with this type of cancer; however, the disease can invade the tissue sufficiently to destroy an ear, nose, or eyelid. Depending on the location, size, and depth of the lesion, treatment may include curettage and electrodesiccation, chemotherapy, surgical excision, irradiation, or chemosurgery.

Squamous Cell Carcinoma

Squamous cell carcinoma arises from skin that undergoes pathological hardening (**keratinizing**) of epidermal cells. It is an invasive tumor with potential for metastasis and occurs most commonly in fair-skinned white men over age 60. Repeated overexposure to the sun's ultraviolet rays greatly increases the risk of squamous cell carcinoma. Other predisposing factors associated with this type of cancer include radiation therapy, chronic skin irritation and inflammation, exposure to cancer causing agents (**carcinogens**), including tar and oil, hereditary diseases (such as **xeroderma pigmentosum** and **albinism**), and the presence of premalignant lesions (such as **actinic keratosis** or **Bowen disease**).

There are two types of squamous cell carcinoma: those that are confined to the original site (**in situ**) and those that penetrate the surrounding tissue (**invasive**). Treatment may consist of surgical excision; curettage and electrodesiccation, which provide good cosmetic results for smaller lesions; radiation therapy, usually for older or debilitated patients; and chemotherapy, depending on the location, size, shape, degree of invasion, and condition of underlying tissue. A combination of these treatment methods may be required for a deeply invasive tumor.

Malignant Melanoma

Malignant melanoma is a neoplasm composed of abnormal melanocytes that commonly begin in a darkly pigmented mole. Although malignant melanoma is relatively rare, the incidence is rising more rapidly than any other malignancy.

Table 5-2 — TNM System of Staging

*The table below outlines the tumor, node, metastasis (TNM) system of staging, including designations, stages, and degrees of tissue involvement.**

Designation	Stage	Tissue involvement
Tumor		
T0		No evidence of tumor
Tis	Stage I	Carcinoma in situ indicates the tumor is in a defined location and shows no invasion into surrounding tissues
T1, T2, T3, T4	Stage II	Primary tumor size and extent of local invasion, where T1 is small with minimal invasion and T4 is large with extensive local invasion into surrounding organs and tissues
Node		
N0		Regional lymph nodes show no abnormalities
N1, N2, N3, N4	Stage III	Degree of lymph node involvement and spread to regional lymph nodes, where N1 is less involvement with minimal spreading and N4 is more involvement with extensive spreading
Metastasis		
M0		No evidence of metastasis
M1	Stage IV	Indicates metastasis

*The designations Tx, Nx, and Mx indicate that the tumor, node, or metastasis cannot be assessed clinically.

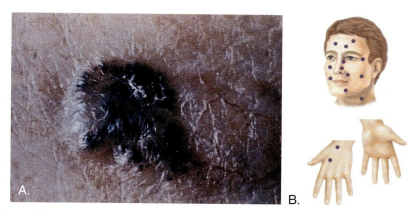

Figure 5-6. (A) Basal cell carcinoma (late stage). (B) common sites of basal cell carcinoma.

It is the most lethal of the skin cancers and can metastasize extensively to the liver, lungs, or brain.

Several factors may influence the development of melanoma, but persons at greatest risk have fair complexions, blue eyes, red or blonde hair, and freckles. Excessive exposure to sunlight and severe sunburn during childhood are believed to increase the risk of melanoma in later life. Avoiding the sun and using sunscreen have proved effective in preventing the disease.

Melanomas are diagnosed by **biopsy** along with histological examination. Treatment requires surgery to remove the primary cancer, along with adjuvant therapies to reduce the risk of metastasis. The extent of surgery depends on the size and location of the primary tumor and is determined by staging the disease.

It is time to review burn and oncology terms by completing Learning Activity 5–4.

Diagnostic, Symptomatic, and Related Terms

This section introduces diagnostic, symptomatic, and related terms and their meanings. Word analyses for selected terms are also provided.

Term	Definition
abscess ĂB-sĕs	Localized collection of pus at the site of an infection (characteristically a *staphylococcal* infection) *When a localized abscess originates in a hair follicle, it is called a* **furuncle***, or boil. A cluster of furuncles in the subcutaneous tissue results in the formation of a* **carbuncle***. (See Figure 5-7.)* **Figure 5-7.** Dome-shaped abscess that has formed a furuncle in hair follicles of the neck. Large furuncles with connecting channels to the skin surface form a carbuncle.
acne ĂK-nē	Inflammatory disease of the sebaceous glands and hair follicles of the skin with characteristic lesions that include blackheads (comedos), inflammatory papules, pustules, nodules, and cysts; usually associated with seborrhea; also called *acne vulgaris* *Acne results from thickening of the follicular opening, increased sebum production, and the presence of bacteria. It is associated with an inflammatory response. The face, neck, and shoulders are common sites for this condition.*
alopecia ăl-ō-PĒ-shē-ă	Partial or complete loss of hair resulting from normal aging, an endocrine disorder, a drug reaction, anticancer medication, or a skin disease; commonly called *baldness*
Bowen disease BŌ-ĕn	Form of intraepidermal carcinoma (squamous cell) characterized by red-brown scaly or crusted lesions that resemble a patch of psoriasis or dermatitis; also called *Bowen precancerous dermatosis* *Treatment for Bowen disease includes curettage and electrodesiccation.*
cellulitis sĕl-ū-LĪ-tĭs	Diffuse (widespread), acute infection of the skin and subcutaneous tissue *Cellulitis is characterized by a light glossy appearance of the skin, localized heat, redness, pain, swelling, and, occasionally, fever, malaise, and chills.*
chloasma klō-ĂZ-mă	Pigmentary skin discoloration usually occurring in yellowish brown patches or spots
comedo KŎM-ē-dō	Typical small skin lesion of acne vulgaris caused by accumulation of keratin, bacteria, and dried sebum plugging an excretory duct of the skin *The closed form of comedo, called a* whitehead, *consists of a papule from which the contents are not easily expressed.*

Diagnostic, Symptomatic, and Related Terms—cont'd

Term	Definition
dermatomycosis děr-mă-tō-mī-KŌ-sĭs *dermat/o:* skin *myc:* fungus *-osis:* abnormal condition; increase (used primarily with blood cells)	Infection of the skin caused by fungi *A common type of dermatomycosis is called* **ringworm.**
ecchymosis ĕk-ĭ-MŌ-sĭs	Skin discoloration consisting of a large, irregularly formed hemorrhagic area with colors changing from blue-black to greenish brown or yellow; commonly called a *bruise* (See Figure 5-8.) **Figure 5-8.** Ecchymosis.
eczema ĔK-zĕ-mă	Chronic skin inflammation characterized by erythema, papules, vesicles, pustules, scales, crusts, scabs, and, possibly, itching *Symptoms of eczema may occur alone or in combination.*
erythema ĕr-ĭ-THĒ-mă	Redness of the skin caused by swelling of the capillaries *An example of erythema is a mild sunburn or nervous blushing.*
eschar ĔS-kăr	Damaged tissue following a severe burn
impetigo ĭm-pĕ-TĪ-gō	Bacterial skin infection characterized by isolated pustules that become crusted and rupture
keratosis kĕr-ă-TŌ-sĭs *kerat:* horny tissue, hard; cornea *-osis:* abnormal condition; increase (used primarily with blood cells)	Thickened area of the epidermis or any horny growth on the skin (such as a callus or wart)
lentigo lĕn-TĪ-gō	Small brown macules, especially on the face and arms, brought on by sun exposure, usually in a middle-aged or older person *These pigmented lesions of the skin are benign and no treatment is necessary unless cosmetic repair is desired.*
pallor PĂL-or	Unnatural paleness or absence of color in the skin

(continued)

Diagnostic, Symptomatic, and Related Terms—cont'd

Term	Definition
pediculosis pĕ-dĭk-ū-LŌ-sĭs *pedicul:* lice *-osis:* abnormal condition; increase (used primarily with blood cells)	Infestation with lice, transmitted by personal contact or common use of brushes, combs, or headgear
petechia pĕ-TĒ-kē-ă	Minute, pinpoint hemorrhage under the skin *A petechia is a smaller version of an ecchymosis.*
pressure ulcer ŬL-sĕr	Skin ulceration caused by prolonged pressure from lying in one position that prevents blood flow to the tissues, usually in bedridden patients; also known as *decubitus ulcer* *Pressure ulcers are most commonly found in skin overlying a bony projection, such as the hip, ankle, heel, shoulder, and elbow.*
pruritus proo-RĪ-tŭs	Intense itching
psoriasis sō-RĪ-ă-sĭs	Chronic skin disease characterized by circumscribed red patches covered by thick, dry, silvery, adherent scales caused by excessive development of the basal layer of the epidermis (See Figure 5-9.) *New psoriasis lesions tend to appear at sites of trauma. They may be found in any location but commonly on the scalp, knees, elbows, umbilicus, and genitalia. Treatment includes topical application of various medications, keratolytics, phototherapy, and ultraviolet light therapy in an attempt to slow hyperkeratosis.* 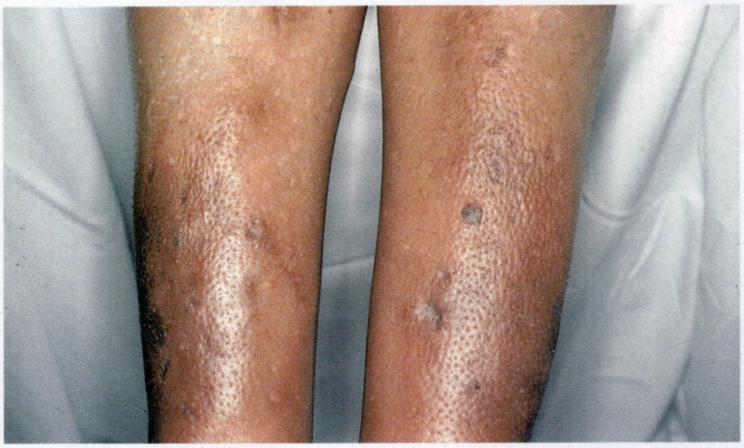
purpura PŬR-pŭ-ră	Any of several bleeding disorders characterized by hemorrhage into the tissues, particularly beneath the skin or mucous membranes, producing ecchymoses or petechiae *Hemorrhage into the skin shows red darkening into purple and then brownish yellow and finally disappearing in 2 to 3 weeks. Areas of discoloration do not disappear under pressure.*

Figure 5-9. Psoriasis. From Goldsmith, Lazarus, & Tharp: *Adult and Pediatric Dermatology: A Color Guide to Diagnosis and Treatment.* FA Davis, Philadelphia, 1997, p 381, with permission.

Term	Definition
scabies SKĀ-bēz	Contagious skin disease transmitted by the itch mite, commonly through sexual contact *Scabies manifests as papules, vesicles, pustules, and burrows and causes intense itching commonly resulting in secondary infections. The axillae, genitalia, inner aspect of the thighs, and areas between the fingers are most commonly affected.*
tinea TĬN-ē-ăh	Fungal skin infection whose name commonly indicates the body part affected; also called *ringworm* *Examples include tinea barbae (beard), tinea corporis (body), tinea pedis (athlete's foot), tinea versicolor (skin), tinea cruris (jock itch).*
urticaria ŭr-tĭ-KĂR-ē-ă	Allergic reaction of the skin characterized by the eruption of pale red, elevated patches called *wheals* or *hives* (See Figure 5-10)

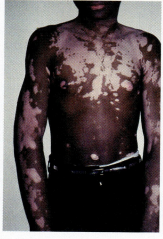

Figure 5-10. Urticaria. From Goldsmith, Lazarus, & Tharp: *Adult and Pediatric Dermatology: A Color Guide to Diagnosis and Treatment.* FA Davis, Philadelphia, 1997, p 381, with permission.

Term	Definition
verruca vĕr-ROO-kă	Epidermal growth caused by a virus; also known as warts. Types include plantar warts, juvenile warts, and venereal warts *Verrucae may be removed by cryosurgery, electrocautery, or acids; however, they may regrow if the virus remains in the skin.*
vitiligo vĭt-ĭl-Ī-gō	Localized loss of skin pigmentation characterized by milk-white patches (See Figure 5-11.)

Figure 5-11. Vitiligo. From Goldsmith, Lazarus, & Tharp: *Adult and Pediatric Dermatology: A Color Guide to Diagnosis and Treatment.* FA Davis, Philadelphia, 1997, p 121, with permission.

(continued)

Diagnostic and Therapeutic Procedures

This section introduces procedures used to diagnose and treat skin disorders. Descriptions are provided as well as pronunciations and word analyses for selected terms.

Procedure	Description
Diagnostic Procedures	
Clinical	

skin test (ST)	Any test in which a suspected allergen or sensitizer is applied to or injected into the skin to determine the patient's sensitivity to it *Most commonly used skin tests are the intradermal, patch, and scratch tests used for allergy testing. The intensity of the response is determined by the wheal-and-flare reaction after the suspected allergen is applied. Positive and negative controls are used to verify normal skin reactivity (See Figure 5-12.)* A. **Figure 5-12.** Skin tests. (A) Intradermal allergy test reactions. (B) Scratch (prick) skin test kit for allergy testing. B.
intradermal ĭn-tră-dĕr-măl	Skin test that identifies suspected allergens by subcutaneously injecting small amounts of extracts of the suspected allergens and observing the skin for a subsequent reaction *Intradermal skin tests are used to determine immunity to diphtheria (Schick test) or tuberculosis (Mantoux test).*
patch	Skin test that identifies suspected allergens by topical application of the substance to be tested (such as food, pollen, and animal fur), usually on the forearm, and observing for a subsequent reaction *After the patch is removed, a lack of noticeable reaction indicates a negative result; skin reddening or swelling indicates a positive result.*
scratch (prick)	Skin test that identifies suspected allergens by placing a small quantity of the suspected allergen on a lightly scratched area of the skin *Redness or swelling at the scratch sites within 10 minutes indicates an allergy to the substance, or a positive test result. If no reaction occurs, the test result is negative.*

Diagnostic and Therapeutic Procedures—cont'd

Procedure	Description
Surgical	
biopsy BĪ-ŏp-sē	Representative tissue sample removed from a body site for microscopic examination *Skin biopsies are used to establish or confirm a diagnosis, estimate prognosis, or follow the course of disease. Any lesion suspected of malignancy is removed and sent to the pathology laboratory for evaluation.*
needle	Removal of a small tissue sample for examination using a hollow needle, usually attached to a syringe
punch	Removal of a small core of tissue using a hollow punch
shave	Removal of surgical blade is used to remove elevated lesions
frozen section (FS)	Ultrathin slice of tissue from a frozen specimen for immediate pathological examination *FS is commonly used for rapid diagnosis of malignancy after the patient has been anesthetized to determine treatment options.*
Therapeutic Procedures	
chemical peel	Chemical removal of the outer layers of skin to treat acne scarring and general keratoses; also called *chemabrasion* *Chemical peels are also commonly used for cosmetic purposes to remove fine wrinkles on the face.*
debridement dā-brēd-MŎN	Removal of necrotized tissue from a wound by surgical excision, enzymes, or chemical agents *Debridement is used to promote healing and prevent infection.*
dermabrasion DĔRM-ă-brā-zhŭn	Rubbing (abrasion) using wire brushes or sandpaper to mechanically scrape away (abrade) the epidermis *This procedure is commonly used to remove acne scars, tattoos, and scar tissue.*
fulguration fŭl-gū-RĀ-shŭn	Tissue destruction by means of high-frequency electric current; also called *electrodesiccation*
Surgical	
cryosurgery krī-ō-SĔR-jĕr-ē	Use of subfreezing temperature (commonly liquid nitrogen) to destroy or eliminate abnormal tissue, such as tumors, warts, and unwanted, cancerous, or infected tissue

(continued)

Diagnostic and Therapeutic Procedures—cont'd

Procedure	Description
incision and drainage (I&D)	Process of cutting through a lesion such as an abscess and draining its contents
skin graft	Surgical procedure to transplant healthy tissue by applying it to an injured site *Human, animal, or artificial skin can be used to provide a temporary covering or permanent layer of skin over a wound or burn.*
allograft ĂL-ō-grăft	Transplantation of healthy tissue from one person to another person; also called *homograft* *In an allograft, the skin donor is usually a cadaver. This type of skin graft is temporary and is used to protect the patient against infection and fluid loss. The allograft is frozen and stored in a skin bank until needed.*
autograft AW-tō-grăft	Transplantation of healthy tissue from one site to another site in the same individual
synthetic sĭn-THĔT-ĭk	Transplantation of artificial skin produced from collagen fibers arranged in a lattice pattern *The recipient's body does not reject synthetic skin (produced artificially) and healing skin grows into it as the graft gradually disintegrates.*
xenograft ZĔN-ō-grăft	Transplantation (dermis only) from a foreign donor (usually a pig) and transferred to a human; also called *heterograft* *A xenograft is used as a temporary graft to protect the patient against infection and fluid loss.*

Pharmacology

Various medications are available to treat skin disorders. (See Table 5–3.) Because of their superficial nature and location, many skin disorders respond well to topical drug therapy. Such mild, localized skin disorders as contact dermatitis, acne, poison ivy, and diaper rash can be effectively treated with topical agents available as over-the-counter products.

Widespread or particularly severe dermatological disorders may require systemic treatment. For example, poison ivy with large areas of open, weeping lesions may be difficult to treat with topical medication and may require a prescription-strength drug. In such a case, an oral steroid or antihistamine might be prescribed to relieve inflammation and severe itching.

Table 5-3   Drugs Used to Treat Skin Disorders

This table lists common drug classifications used to treat skin disorders, their therapeutic actions, and selected generic and trade names.

Classification	Therapeutic Action	Generic and Trade Names

antifungals	Alter the cell wall of fungi or disrupt enzyme activity, resulting in cell death
	
	Antifungals are used to treat ringworm (tinea corporis), athlete's foot (tinea pedis), and fungal infection of the nail (onychomycosis). When topical antifungals are not effective, oral or intravenous antifungal drugs may be necessary.
		nystatin
		NĬS-tă-tĭn
		  Mycostatin, Nyston
		
		itraconazole
		ĭt-ră-KŎN-ă-zōl
		  Sporanox

Table 5-3 **Drugs Used to Treat Skin Disorders—cont'd**

This table lists common drug classifications used to treat skin disorders, their therapeutic actions, and selected generic and trade names.

Classification	Therapeutic Action	Generic and Trade Names

antihistamines	Inhibit allergic reactions of inflammation, redness, and itching caused by the release of histamine
	
	In a case of severe itching, antihistamines may be given orally. As a group, these drugs are also known as antipruritics (pruritus means itching).
		diphenhydramine
		dī-fĕn-HĪ-dră-mēn
		  Benadryl
		
		loratadine
		lor-ĂH-tă-dēn
		  Claritin

antiseptics	Topically applied agents that inhibit growth of bacteria, thus preventing infections in cuts, scratches, and surgical incisions	**ethyl or isopropyl alcohol** ĔTH-ĭl ī-sō-PRŌ-pĭl **hydrogen peroxide** HĪ-drō-jĕn pĕ-RŎK-sīd

corticosteroids	Decrease inflammation and itching by suppressing the immune system's inflammatory response to tissue damage
	
	Topical corticosteroids are used to treat contact dermatitis, poison ivy, insect bites, psoriasis, seborrhea, and eczema. Oral corticosteroids may be prescribed for systemic treatment of severe or widespread inflammation or itching.
		hydrocortisone*
		hī-drō-KOR-tĭ-sōn
		  Certacort, Cortaid
		
		triamcinolone
		trī-ăm-SĬN-ō-lōn
		  Azmacort, Kenalog

keratolytics	Destroy and soften the outer layer of skin so that it is sloughed off or shed *Strong keratolytics remove warts and corns and aid in penetration of antifungal drugs. Milder keratolytics promote shedding of scales and crusts in eczema, psoriasis, seborrheic dermatitis, and other dry, scaly conditions. Weak keratolytics irritate inflamed skin, acting as a tonic to accelerate healing.*	**tretinoin** TRĔT-ĭ-noyn Retin-A, Vesanoid

parasiticides	Kill insect parasites, such as mites and lice
	
	Parasiticides are used to treat scabies (mites) and pediculosis (lice). The drug is applied as a cream or lotion to the body and as a shampoo to treat the scalp.
		lindane
		LĬN-dān
		  Kwell, Thion
		
		permethrin
		pĕr-MĔTH-rĭn
		  Nix

protectives	Cover, cool, dry, or soothe inflamed skin
	
	Protectives do not penetrate the skin or soften it. Rather, they allow the natural healing process to occur by forming a long-lasting film that protects the skin from air, water, and clothing.
		lotions
		  Cetaphil moisturizing lotion
		ointments
		  Vaseline

topical anesthetics	Block sensation of pain by numbing the skin layers and mucous membranes
	
	These topical drugs are administered directly by means of sprays, creams, gargles, suppositories, and other preparations. They provide temporary symptomatic relief of minor burns, sunburns, rashes, and insect bites.
		lidocaine
		LĪ-dō-kān
		  Xylocaine
		
		procaine
		PRŌ-kān
		  Novocain

*The suffixes -sone, -olone, and -onide are common to generic corticosteroids.

It is time to review diagnostic, symptomatic, procedure, and pharmacology terms by completing Learning Activity 5–5.

Abbreviations

This section introduces integumentary-related abbreviations and their meanings.

Abbreviation	Meaning	Abbreviation	Meaning
Bx, bx	biopsy	ID	intradermal
BCC	basal cell carcinoma	I&D	incision and drainage
CA	cancer; chronological age; cardiac arrest	IMP	impression (synonymous with diagnosis)
cm	centimeter	IV	intravenous
decub	decubitus (ulcer)	subcu, Sub-Q, subQ	subcutaneous (injection)
derm	dermatology	ung	ointment
FS	frozen section	XP, XDP	xeroderma pigmentosum

LEARNING ACTIVITIES

The following activities provide review of the integumentary system terms introduced in this chapter. Complete each activity and review your answers to evaluate your understanding of the chapter.

Learning Activity 5-1
Identifying Integumentary Structures

Label the following illustration using the terms listed below.

dermis	*papilla*	*stratum germinativum*
epidermis	*sebaceous (oil) gland*	*subcutaneous tissue*
hair follicle	*stratum corneum*	*sudoriferous (sweat) gland*
hair shaft		

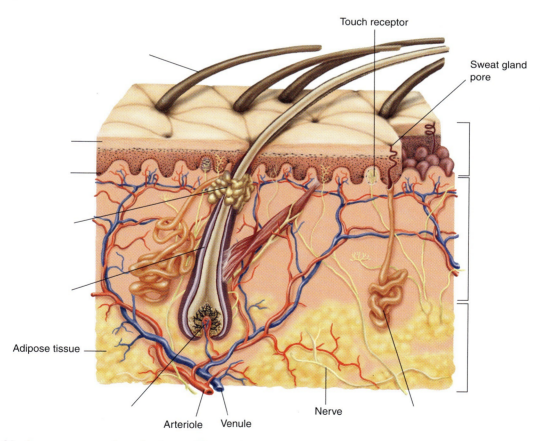

Check your answers by referring to Figure 5–1 on page 73. Review material that you did not answer correctly.

 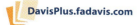 **DavisPlus.fadavis.com**

Enhance your study and reinforcement of word elements with the power of DavisPlus. Visit www.davisplus.fadavis.com/gylys/systems *for this chapter's flash-card activity. We recommend you complete the flash-card activity before completing Activity 5–2 below.*

Building Medical Words

Use *adip/o* or *lip/o* (fat) to build words that mean:

1. tumor consisting of fat _____
2. hernia containing fat _____
3. resembling fat _____
4. fat cell _____

Use *dermat/o* (skin) to build words that mean:

5. inflammation of the skin _____
6. instrument to incise the skin _____

Use *onych/o* (nail) to build words that mean:

7. tumor of the nails _____
8. softening of the nails _____
9. abnormal condition of the nails _____
10. abnormal condition of the nails caused by a fungus _____
11. abnormal condition of a hidden (ingrown) nail _____
12. disease of the nails _____

Use *trich/o* (hair) to build words that mean:

13. disease of the hair _____
14. abnormal condition of hair caused by a fungus _____

Use *–logy* or *–logist* to build words that mean:

15. study of the skin _____
16. specialist in skin (diseases) _____

Build surgical words that mean:

17. excision of fat (adipose tissue) _____
18. removal of a nail _____
19. incision of a nail _____
20. surgical repair (plastic surgery) of the skin _____

✔ *Check your answers in Appendix A. Review material that you did not answer correctly.*

Correct Answers _____ × 5 = _____ % Score

Identifying Skin Lesions

Label the following skin lesions on the lines provided, using the terms listed below.

bulla	*macule*	*pustule*	*vesicle*
excoriations	*nodule*	*tumor*	*wheal*
fissure	*papule*	*ulcer*	

PRIMARY LESIONS

FLAT LESIONS
Flat, discolored, circumscribed lesions of any size

Flat, pigmented, circumscribed area less than 1 cm in diameter.
Examples: freckle, flat mole, or rash that occurs in rubella.

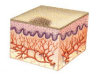

ELEVATED LESIONS

Solid   *Fluid-filled*

Solid, elevated lesion less than 1 cm in diameter that may be the same color as the skin or pigmented.
Examples: nevus, wart, pimple, ringworm, psoriasis, eczema.

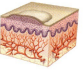

Elevated, circumscribed, fluid-filled lesion less than 0.5 cm in diameter.
Examples: poison ivy, shingles, chickenpox.

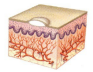

Palpable, circumscribed lesion; larger and deeper than a papule (0.6 to 2 cm in diameter); extends into the dermal area.
Examples: intradermal nevus, benign or malignant tumor.

Small, raised, circumscribed lesion that contains pus; usually less than 1 cm in diameter.
Examples: acne, furuncle, pustular psoriasis, scabies.

Solid, elevated lesion larger than 2 cm in diameter that extends into the dermal and subcutaneous layers.
Examples: lipoma, steatoma, dermatofibroma, hemangioma.

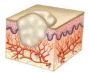

A vesicle or blister larger than 1 cm in diameter.
Examples: second-degree burns, severe poison oak, poison ivy.

Elevated, firm, rounded lesion with localized skin edema (swelling) that varies in size, shape, and color; paler in the center than its surrounding edges; accompanied by itching.
Examples: hives, insect bites, urticaria.

SECONDARY LESIONS

DEPRESSED LESIONS
Depressed lesions caused by loss of skin surface

Linear scratch marks or traumatized abrasions of the epidermis.
Examples: scratches, abrasions, chemical or thermal burns.

Small slit or crack-like sore that extends into the dermal layer; could be caused by continuous inflammation and drying.

An open sore or lesion that extends to the dermis and usually heals with scarring.
Examples: pressure sore, basal cell carcinoma.

 Check your answers by referring to Figure 5–3 on page 79. Review material that you did not answer correctly.

Learning Activity 5-4

Matching Burn and Oncology Terms

Match each term on the left with its meaning on the right.

1. _____ erythema		a. develops from keratinizing epidermal cells
2. _____ T0		b. noncancerous
3. _____ malignant		c. no evidence of metastasis
4. _____ first-degree burn		d. extensive damage to underlying connective tissue
5. _____ grading		f. determines degree of abnormal cancer cells compared with normal cells
6. _____ squamous cell carcinoma		e. no evidence of primary tumor
7. _____ benign		g. burn that heals without scar formation
8. _____ T1		h. cancerous; may be life-threatening
9. _____ M0		i. redness of skin
10. _____ third-degree burns		j. primary tumor size, small with minimal invasion

✓ *Check your answers in Appendix A. Review any material that you did not answer correctly.*

Correct Answers _____ × 10 = _____ % Score

Matching Diagnostic, Symptomatic, Procedure, and Pharmacology Terms

Match the following terms with the definitions in the numbered list.

alopecia	dermabrasion	keratolytics	scabies
antifungals	ecchymosis	parasiticides	tinea
autograft	fulguration	patch test	urticaria
chloasma	impetigo	pediculosis	vitiligo
corticosteroids	intradermal test	petechiae	xenograft

1. infestation with lice _____
2. skin depigmentation characterized by milk-white patches _____
3. fungal skin infection, also called ringworm _____
4. contagious skin disease transmitted by the itch mite _____
5. bacterial skin infection characterized by pustules that become crusted and rupture _____
6. allergic reaction of the skin characterized by elevated red patches called hives _____
7. hyperpigmentation of the skin, characterized by yellowish brown patches or spots _____
8. hemorrhagic spot or bruise on the skin _____
9. minute or small hemorrhagic spots on the skin _____
10. loss or absence of hair _____
11. topical agents to treat athlete's foot and onychomycosis _____
12. tissue destruction by means of high-frequency electric current _____
13. agents that decrease inflammation or itching _____
14. use of wire brushes or other abrasive materials to remove scars, tattoos, or fine wrinkles _____
15. agents that kill parasitic skin infestations _____
16. agents that soften the outer layer of skin so that it sloughs off _____
17. procedure in which extracts of suspected allergens are injected subcutaneously _____
18. procedure in which allergens are applied topically, usually on the forearm _____
19. skin graft taken from one site and applied to another site of the patient's body _____
20. skin graft taken from another species (usually a pig) to a human _____

✓ *Check your answers in Appendix A. Review material that you did not answer correctly.*

Correct Answers _____ × 5 = _____ **% Score**

MEDICAL RECORD ACTIVITIES

The two medical records included in the following activities use common clinical scenarios to show how medical terminology is used to document patient care. Complete the terminology and analysis sections for each activity to help you recognize and understand terms related to the integumentary system.

Medical Record Activity 5-1

Pathology report: Skin lesion

Terminology

Terms listed in the following table are taken from *Pathology report: Skin lesion* that follows. Use a medical dictionary such as *Taber's Cyclopedic Medical Dictionary*, the appendices of this book, or other resources to define each term. Then review the pronunciations for each term and practice by reading the medical record aloud.

Term	Definition
atypia ā-TĬP-ē-ă	
atypical ā-TĬP-ĭ-kăl	
basal cell layer BĀ-săl	
Bowen disease BŌ-ēn	
carcinoma kăr-sĭ-NŌ-mă	
dermatitis dĕr-mă-TĪ-tĭs	
dermis DĔR-mĭs	
dorsum DOR-sŭm	
epidermal hyperplasia ĕp-ĭ-DĔR-măl hī-pĕr-PLĀ-zē-ă	
fibroplasia fī-brō-PLĀ-sē-ă	
hyperkeratosis hī-pĕr-kĕr-ă-TŌ-sĭs	
infiltrate ĬN-fĭl-trāt	

Term	Definition
keratinocytes kĕ-RĂT-ĭ-nō-sīts	
lymphocytic lĭm-fō-SĬT-ĭk	
neoplastic nē-ō-PLĂS-tĭk	
papillary PĂP-ĭ-lăr-ē	
pathological păth-ō-LŎJ-ĭk-ăl	
solar elastosis SŌ-lăr ĕ-lăs-TŌ-sĭs	
squamous SKWĀ-mŭs	

Listen and Learn Online! *will help you master the pronunciation of selected medical words from this medical record activity. Visit* www.davisplus.com/gylys/systems *to find instructions on completing the* Listen and Learn Online! *exercise for this section and to practice pronunciations.*

PATHOLOGY REPORT: SKIN LESION

General Hospital

1511 Ninth Avenue ■■ **Sun City, USA 12345** ■■ **(555) 802-1887**

PATHOLOGY REPORT

Date: April 14, 20xx   Pathology: 43022
Patient: Franks, Robert   Room: 910
Physician: Dante Riox, MD

Specimen: Skin from (a) dorsum left wrist and (b) left forearm, ulnar, near elbow.

Clinical Diagnosis: Bowen disease versus basal cell carcinoma versus dermatitis.

Microscopic Description: (a) There is mild hyperkeratosis and moderate epidermal hyperplasia with full-thickness atypia of squamous keratinocytes. Squamatization of the basal cell layer exists. A lymphocytic inflammatory infiltrate is present in the papillary dermis. Solar elastosis is present. (b) Nests, strands, and columns of atypical neoplastic basaloid keratinocytes grow down from the epidermis into the underlying dermis. Fibroplasia is present. Solar elastosis is noted.

Pathological Diagnosis: (a) Bowen disease of left wrist; (b) nodular and infiltrating basal cell carcinoma of left forearm, near elbow.

Samantha Roberts, MD
Samantha Roberts, MD

sr:bg

D: 4-16-xx
T: 4-16-xx

Analysis

Review the medical record *Pathology report: Skin lesion* to answer the following questions.

1. In the specimen section, what does "skin on dorsum left wrist" mean?

_____

2. What was the inflammatory infiltrate?

_____

3. What was the pathologist's diagnosis for the left forearm?

_____

4. Provide a brief description of Bowen disease, the pathologist's diagnosis for the left wrist.

_____

Medical Record Activity 5-2

Patient referral letter: Onychomycosis

Terminology

Terms listed in the following table are taken from the *Patient referral letter: Onychomycosis* that follows. Use a medical dictionary such as *Taber's Cyclopedic Medical Dictionary*, the appendices of this book, or other resources to define each term. Then review the pronunciations for each term and practice by reading the medical record aloud.

Term	Definition
alkaline phosphatase ĂL-kă-lĭn FŎS-fă-tās	
bilaterally bī-LĂT-ĕr-ăl-ē	
CA	
debridement dā-brēd-MŎN	
hypertension hī-pĕr-TĚN-shŭn	
mastectomy măs-TĚK-tŏ-mē	
neurological noor-ō-LŎJ-ĭk-ăl	
onychomycosis ŏn-ĭ-kō-mī-KŌ-sĭs	

Term	Definition
Sporanox* SPŎR-ă-nŏks	
vascular VĂS-kū-lăr	

*Refer to Table 5–3 to determine the drug classification and the generic name for *Sporanox*.

 Listen and Learn Online! *will help you master the pronunciation of selected medical words from this medical record activity. Visit* www.davisplus.com/gylys/systems *to find instructions on completing the* Listen and Learn Online! *exercise for this section and to practice pronunciations.*

PATIENT REFERRAL LETTER: ONYCHOMYCOSIS

Physician Center

2422 Rodeo Drive ■■ **Sun City, USA 12345** ■■ **(555)788-2427**

May 3, 20xx

John Roberts, MD
1115 Forest Ave
Sun City, USA 12345

Dear Doctor Roberts:

Thank you for referring Alicia Gonzoles to my office. Mrs. Gonzoles presents to the office for evaluation and treatment of onychomycosis with no previous treatment. Past pertinent medical history does reveal hypertension and breast CA. Pertinent surgical history does reveal mastectomy.

Examination of patient's feet does reveal onychomycosis, 1–5 bilaterally. Vascular and neurological examinations are intact. Previous laboratory work was within normal limits except for an elevated alkaline phosphatase of 100.

Tentative diagnosis: Onychomycosis, 1–5 bilaterally

Treatment consisted of debridement of mycotic nails, bilateral feet, as well as dispensing a prescription for Sporanox Pulse Pack to be taken for 3 months to treat the onychomycotic infection.
I have also asked her to repeat her liver enzymes in approximately 4 weeks. Mrs. Gonzoles will make an appointment in 2 months for follow up, and I will keep you informed of any changes in her progress. If you have any questions, please feel free to contact me.

Sincerely yours,

Juan Perez, MD
Juan Perez, MD

jp:az

Analysis

Review the medical record *Patient referral letter: Onychomycosis* to answer the following questions.

1. What pertinent disorders were identified in the past medical history?

_____

2. What pertinent surgery was identified in the past surgical history?

_____

3. Did the doctor identify any problems in the vascular system or nervous system?

_____

4. What was the significant finding in the laboratory results?

_____

5. What treatment did the doctor employ for the onychomycosis?

_____

6. What did the doctor recommend regarding the abnormal laboratory finding?

_____

Digestive System

CHAPTER

6

Chapter Outline

Objectives

Upon completion of this chapter, you will be able to:

- Locate the major organs of the digestive system and describe their structure and function.
- Describe the functional relationship between the digestive system and other body systems.
- Recognize, pronounce, spell, and build words related to the digestive system.
- Describe pathological conditions, diagnostic and therapeutic procedures, and other terms related to the digestive system.
- Explain pharmacology related to the treatment of digestive disorders.
- Demonstrate your knowledge of this chapter by completing the learning and medical record activities.

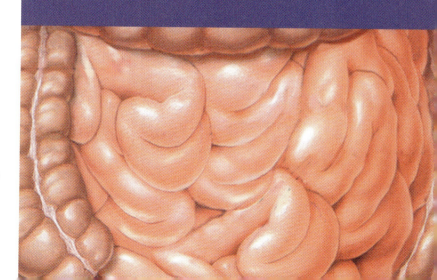

Anatomy and Physiology

The digestive system, also called the *gastrointestinal* **(GI)** system, consists of a digestive tube called the *GI tract* or *alimentary canal,* and several accessory organs whose primary function is to break down food, prepare it for absorption, and eliminate waste. The GI tract, extending from the mouth to the anus, varies in size and structure in several distinct regions:

- mouth
- pharynx (throat)
- esophagus
- stomach
- small intestine
- large intestine
- rectum
- anus.

Food passing along the GI tract is mixed with digestive enzymes and broken down into nutrient molecules, which are absorbed in the bloodstream. Undigested waste materials not absorbed by the blood are then eliminated from the body through defecation. Included in the digestive system are the accessory organs of digestion: the liver, gallbladder, and pancreas. (See Figure 6–1.)

Mouth

The process of digestion begins in the mouth. The mouth, also known as the (1) **oral cavity** or **buccal cavity,** is a receptacle for food. It is formed by the cheeks (**bucca**), lips, teeth, tongue, and hard and soft palates. Located around the oral cavity are three pairs of salivary glands, which secrete saliva. Saliva contains important digestive enzymes that help begin the chemical breakdown of food. In the mouth, food is broken down mechanically (by the teeth) and chemically (by saliva), and then formed into a **bolus.**

Teeth

The (2) **teeth** play an important role in initial stages of digestion by mechanically breaking down food (**mastication**) into smaller pieces as they mix it with saliva. Teeth are covered by a hard enamel, giving them a smooth, white appearance. Beneath the enamel is **dentin,** the main structure of the tooth. The innermost part of the tooth is the **pulp,** which contains nerves and blood vessels. The teeth are embedded in pink, fleshy tissue known as gums (**gingiva**).

Tongue

The (3) **tongue** assists in the chewing process by manipulating the bolus of food during chewing and moving it to the back of the mouth for swallowing (**deglutition**). The tongue also aids in speech production and taste. Rough projections on the surface of the tongue called *papillae* contain taste buds. The four basic taste sensations registered by chemical stimulation of the taste buds are sweet, sour, salty, and bitter. All other taste perceptions are combinations of these four

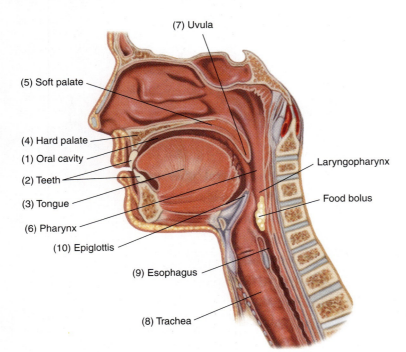

(7) Uvula

(5) Soft palate

(4) Hard palate

(1) Oral cavity

(2) Teeth

(3) Tongue

(6) Pharynx

(10) Epiglottis

(9) Esophagus

(8) Trachea

Laryngopharynx

Food bolus

Figure 6-1. Sagittal view of the head showing oral, nasal, and pharyngeal components of the digestive system.

Anatomy and Physiology Key Terms

This section introduces important terms, along with their definitions and pronunciations. Word analyses for selected terms are also provided.

Term	Definition
bilirubin bĭl-ĭ-ROO-bĭn	Orange-colored or yellowish pigment in bile *Bilirubin is formed principally by the breakdown of hemoglobin in red blood cells after termination of their normal lifespan.*
bolus BŌ-lŭs	Mass of masticated food ready to be swallowed
exocrine ĔKS-ō-krĭn *exo-:* outside, outward *-crine:* secrete	Denotes a gland that secretes its products through excretory ducts to the surface of an organ or tissue or into a vessel
sphincter SFĬNGK-tĕr	Circular band of muscle fibers that constricts a passage or closes a natural opening of the body *An example of a sphincter is the lower esophageal (cardiac) sphincter that constricts once food has passed into the stomach.*

Pronunciation Help	Long Sound	ā—rate	ē—rebirth	ī—isle	ō—over	ū—unite
	Short Sound	ă—alone	ĕ—ever	ĭ—it	ŏ—not	ŭ—cut

basic flavors. In addition, sense of taste is intricately linked with sense of smell, making taste perception very complex.

Hard and Soft Palates

The two structures forming the roof of the mouth are the (4) **hard palate** (anterior portion) and the (5) **soft palate** (posterior portion). The soft palate, which forms a partition between the mouth and the nasopharynx, is continuous with the hard palate. The entire oral cavity, like the rest of the GI tract, is lined with mucous membranes.

Pharynx, Esophagus, and Stomach

As the bolus is pushed by the tongue into the (6) **pharynx** (throat), it is guided by the soft, fleshy, V-shaped structure called the (7) *uvula.* The funnel-shaped pharynx serves as a passageway to the respiratory and GI tracts and provides a resonating chamber for speech sounds. The lowest portion of the pharynx divides into two tubes: one that leads to the lungs, called the (8) **trachea,** and one that leads to the stomach, called the (9) **esophagus.** A small flap of cartilage, called the (10) **epiglottis,** folds back to cover the trachea during swallowing,

forcing food to enter the esophagus. At all other times, the epiglottis remains upright, allowing air to freely pass through the respiratory structures.

The **stomach,** a saclike structure located in the left upper quadrant (LUQ) of the abdominal cavity, serves as a food reservoir that continues mechanical and chemical digestion. (See Figure 6–2.) The stomach extends from the (1) **esophagus** to the first part of the small intestine, the (2) **duodenum.** The terminal portion of the esophagus, the (3) **lower esophageal (cardiac) sphincter,** is composed of muscle fibers that constrict once food has passed into the stomach. It prevents the stomach contents from regurgitating back into the esophagus. The (4) **body** of the stomach, the large central portion, together with the (5) **fundus,** the upper portion, are mainly storage areas. Most digestion takes place in the funnel-shaped terminal portion, the (6) **pylorus.** The interior lining of the stomach is composed of mucous membranes and contains numerous macroscopic longitudinal folds called (7) **rugae** that gradually unfold as the stomach fills. Located within the rugae, digestive glands produce hydrochloric acid (HCl) and enzymes. Secretions from these glands coupled with the mechanical churning of the stomach turn the bolus into a semiliquid form called *chyme* that slowly leaves the stomach through the (8) **pyloric sphincter** to enter the duodenum. This sphincter regulates the speed and movement of chyme into the small intestine and prohibits back-flow. Food is propelled through the entire GI tract by coordinated, rhythmic muscle contractions called *peristalsis*.

Small Intestine

The small intestine is a coiled, 20-foot long tube that begins at the pyloric sphincter and extends at the large intestine. (See Figure 6–3.) It consists of three parts:

- (1) **duodenum,** the uppermost segment, which is about 10 inches long
- (2) **jejunum,** which is approximately 8 feet long
- (3) **ileum,** which is about 12 feet long

Digestion is completed in the small intestine with the help of additional enzymes and secretions from the (4) **pancreas** and (5) **liver.** Nutrients in chyme are absorbed through microscopic, finger-like projections called *villi*. Nutrients enter the bloodstream and lymphatic system for distribution to the rest of the body. At the terminal end of the small intestine, a sphincter muscle called the *ileocecal valve* allows undigested or unabsorbed material from the small intestine to pass into the large intestine and eventually be excreted from the body.

Large Intestine

The large intestine is about 5 feet long. It begins at the end of the ileum and extends to the anus. No digestion takes place in the large intestine. The only secretion is mucus in the colon, which lubricates fecal material so it can pass from the body. The large intestine has three main components: cecum, colon, and rectum. The first 2 or 3 inches of the large intestine is called the (6) **cecum,** a small pouch that hangs inferior to the ileocecal valve. Projecting downward from the cecum is a wormlike structures called the (7) **appendix.** The function of the appendix is unknown; however, problems arise if it becomes infected or inflamed. The cecum merges with the colon. The main functions of the colon are to absorb water and minerals and eliminate undigested material. The colon is divided into ascending, transverse, descending, and sigmoid portions:

- The (8) **ascending colon** extends from the cecum to the lower border of the liver and turns abruptly to form the (9) **hepatic flexure.**
- The colon continues across the abdomen to the left side as the (10) **transverse colon,** curving beneath the lower end of the (11) **spleen** to form the (12) **splenic flexure.**
- As the transverse colon turns downward, it becomes the (13) **descending colon.**
- The descending colon continues until it forms the (14) **sigmoid colon** and the (15) **rectum.** The rectum, the last part of the GI tract, terminates at the (16) **anus.**

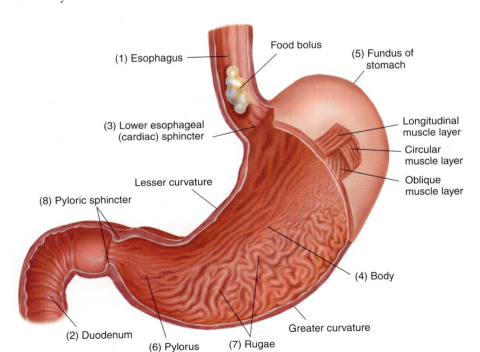

Figure 6-2. Anterior view of the stomach showing muscle layers and rugae of the mucosa.

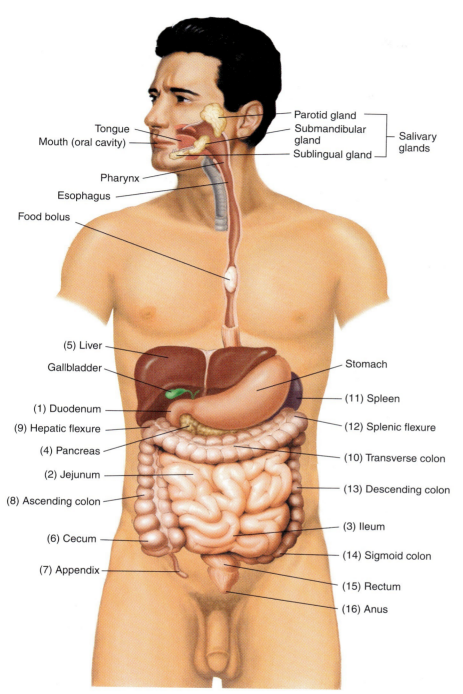

Tongue
Mouth (oral cavity)
Pharynx
Esophagus
Food bolus

Parotid gland
Submandibular gland
Sublingual gland
Salivary glands

Stomach

(5) Liver
Gallbladder
(1) Duodenum
(9) Hepatic flexure
(4) Pancreas
(2) Jejunum
(8) Ascending colon
(6) Cecum
(7) Appendix

(11) Spleen
(12) Splenic flexure
(10) Transverse colon
(13) Descending colon
(3) Ileum
(14) Sigmoid colon
(15) Rectum
(16) Anus

Figure 6-3. Anterior view of the trunk and digestive organs.

 It is time to review digestive structures by completing Learning Activity 6–1.

Accessory Organs of Digestion

Although the liver, gallbladder, and pancreas lie outside the GI tract, they play a vital role in the proper digestion and absorption of nutrients. (See Figure 6–4.)

Liver

The (1) **liver,** the largest glandular organ in the body, weighs approximately 3 to 4 lb. It is located beneath the diaphragm in the right upper quadrant (RUQ) of the abdominal cavity. The liver performs

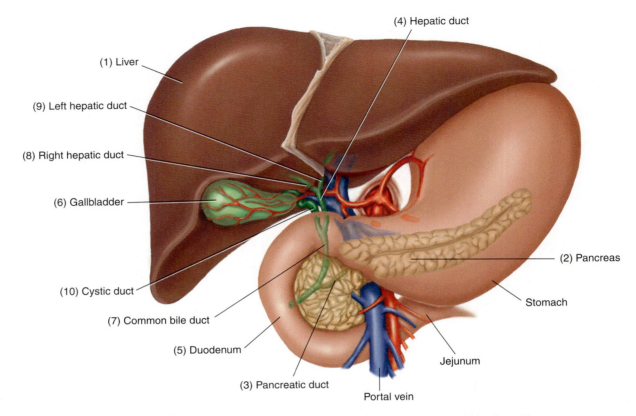

(4) Hepatic duct

(1) Liver

(9) Left hepatic duct

(8) Right hepatic duct

(6) Gallbladder

(10) Cystic duct

(7) Common bile duct

(5) Duodenum

(3) Pancreatic duct

Portal vein

(2) Pancreas

Stomach

Jejunum

Figure 6-4. Liver, gallbladder, pancreas, and duodenum with associated ducts and blood vessels.

many vital functions and death occurs if it ceases to function. Some of its important functions include:

- producing bile, used in the small intestine to emulsify and absorb fats
- removing **glucose** (sugar) from blood to synthesize **glycogen** (starch) and retain it for later use
- storing vitamins, such as B_{12}, A, D, E, and K
- destroying or transforming toxic products into less harmful compounds
- maintaining normal glucose levels in the blood
- destroying old **erythrocytes** and releasing **bilirubin**
- producing various blood proteins, such as prothrombin and fibrinogen, that aid in blood clotting.

Pancreas

The (2) **pancreas** is an elongated, somewhat flattened organ that lies posterior and slightly inferior to the stomach. It performs both endocrine and exocrine functions. As an **endocrine** gland, the pancreas secretes insulin directly into the bloodstream to maintain normal blood glucose levels. For a comprehensive discussion of the endocrine function of the pancreas, review Chapter 13. As an

exocrine gland, the pancreas produces digestive enzymes that pass into the duodenum through the (3) **pancreatic duct.** The pancreatic duct extends along the pancreas and, together with the (4) **hepatic duct** from the liver, enters the (5) **duodenum.** The digestive enzymes produced by the pancreas contain trypsin, which breaks down proteins; amylase, which breaks down carbohydrates; and lipase, which breaks down fat.

Gallbladder

The (6) **gallbladder,** a saclike structure on the inferior surface of the liver, serves as a storage area for bile, which is produced by the liver. When bile is needed for digestion, the gallbladder releases it into the duodenum through the (7) **common bile duct**. Bile is also drained from the liver through the (8) **right hepatic duct** and the (9) **left hepatic duct.** These two structures eventually form the hepatic duct. The (10) **cystic duct** of the gallbladder merges with the hepatic duct to form the common bile duct, which leads into the duodenum. Bile production is stimulated by hormone secretions, which are produced in the duodenum, as soon as food enters the small intestine. Without bile, fat digestion is not possible.

It is time to review anatomy of the accessory organs of digestion by completing Learning Activity 6–2.

Connecting Body Systems–Digestive System

The main function of the digestive system is to provide vital nutrients for growth, maintenance, and repair of all organs and body cells. Specific functional relationships between the digestive system and other body systems are discussed below.

Blood, lymph, and immune
- Liver regulates blood glucose levels.
- Digestive tract secretes acids and enzymes to provide a hostile environment for pathogens.
- Intestinal walls contain lymphoid nodules that help prevent invasion of pathogens.
- Digestive system absorbs vitamin K for blood clotting.

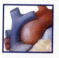

Cardiovascular
- Digestive system absorbs nutrients needed by the heart.

Endocrine
- Liver eliminates hormones from the blood to end their activity.
- Pancreas contains hormone-producing cells.

Female reproductive
- Digestive system provides adequate nutrition, including fats, to make conception and normal fetal development possible.
- Digestive system provides nutrients for repair of endometrium following menstruation.

Genitourinary
- Digestive system provides adequate nutrients in the development of viable sperm.
- Liver metabolizes hormones, toxins, and drugs to forms that can be excreted in urine.

Integumentary
- Digestive system supplies fats that provide insulation in the dermis and subcutaneous tissue.
- Digestive system absorbs nutrients for maintenance, growth, and repair of the skin.

Musculoskeletal
- Digestive system provides nutrients needed for energy fuel.
- Digestive system absorbs calcium needed for bone salts and muscle contraction.
- Liver removes lactic acid (resulting from muscle activity) from the blood.

Nervous
- Digestive system supplies nutrients for normal neural functioning.
- Digestive system provides nutrients for synthesis of neurotransmitters and electrolytes for transmission of a nervous impulse.
- Liver plays a role in maintaining glucose levels for neural function.

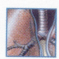

Respiratory
- Digestive system absorbs nutrients needed by cells in the lungs and other tissues in the respiratory tract.
- The pharynx is shared by the digestive and respiratory systems. The lowest portion of the pharynx divides into two tubes: one that leads to the lungs, called the trachea, and one that leads to the stomach, called the esophagus.

Medical Word Elements

This section introduces combining forms, suffixes, and prefixes related to the digestive system. Word analyses are also provided.

Element	Meaning	Word Analysis
Combining Forms		
Mouth		
or/o	mouth	**or**/al (OR-ăl): pertaining to the mouth *-al:* pertaining to
stomat/o		**stomat**/itis (stŏ-mă-TĪ-tĭs): inflammation of the mouth *-itis:* inflammation
gloss/o	tongue	**gloss**/ectomy (glŏs-ĔK-tō-mē): removal of all or part of the tongue *-ectomy:* excision, removal
lingu/o		**lingu**/al (LĬNG-gwăl): pertaining to the tongue *-al:* pertaining to
bucc/o	cheek	**bucc**/al (BŬK-ăl): pertaining to the cheek *-al:* pertaining to
cheil/o	lip	**cheil**/o/plasty (KĪ-lō-plăs-tē): surgical repair of a defective lip *-plasty:* surgical repair
labi/o		**labi**/al (LĀ-bē-ăl): pertaining to the lips, particularly the lips of the mouth *-al:* pertaining to
dent/o	teeth	**dent**/ist (DĔN-tĭst): specialist who diagnoses and treats diseases and disorders of teeth *-ist:* specialist
odont/o		orth/**odont**/ist (or-thō-DŎN-tĭst): dentist who specializes in correcting and preventing irregularities of abnormally positioned or aligned teeth *orth:* straight *-ist:* specialist
gingiv/o	gum(s)	**gingiv**/ectomy (jĭn-jĭ-VĔK-tō-mē): excision of diseased gingival tissue *-ectomy:* excision, removal ***Gingivectomy is performed as a surgical treatment for periodontal disease.***
sial/o	saliva, salivary gland	**sial**/o/lith (sī-ĂL-ō-lĭth): calculus formed in a salivary gland or duct *-lith:* stone, calculus
Esophagus, Pharynx, and Stomach		
esophag/o	esophagus	**esophag**/o/scope (ē-SŎF-ă-gō-skōp): instrument used to examine the esophagus *-scope:* instrument for examining
pharyng/o	pharynx (throat)	**pharyng**/o/tonsill/itis (fă-rĭng-gō-tŏn-sĭ-LĪ-tĭs): inflammation of the pharynx and tonsils *tonsill:* tonsils *-itis:* inflammation

Medical Word Elements—cont'd

Element	Meaning	Word Analysis
gastr/o	stomach	**gastr/algia** (găs-TRĂL-jē-ă): pain in the stomach; also called *stomachache* *-algia:* pain
pylor/o	pylorus	**pylor/o/spasm** (pī-LOR-ō-spăzm): involuntary contraction of the pyloric sphincter of the stomach, as in pyloric stenosis *-spasm:* involuntary contraction, twitching
Small Intestine		
duoden/o	duodenum (first part of small intestine)	**duoden/o/scopy** (dū-ŏd-ĕ-NŎS-kō-pē): visual examination of the duodenum *-scopy:* visual examination
enter/o	intestine (usually small intestine)	**enter/o/pathy** (ĕn-tĕr-ŎP-ă-thē): disease of the intestine *-pathy:* disease
jejun/o	jejunum (second part of small intestine)	**jejun/o/rrhaphy** (jĕ-joo-NOR-ă-fē): suture of the jejunum *-rrhaphy:* suture
ile/o	ileum (third part of small intestine)	**ile/o/stomy** (ĭl-ē-ŎS-tō-mē): creation of an opening between the ileum and the abdominal wall *-stomy*:* forming an opening (mouth) *An ileostomy creates an opening on the surface of the abdomen to allow feces to be discharged into a bag worn on the abdomen.*
Large Intestine		
append/o	appendix	**append/ectomy** (ăp-ĕn-DĔK-tō-mē): excision of the appendix *-ectomy:* excision, removal *Appendectomy is performed to remove a diseased appendix in danger of rupturing.*
appendic/o		**appendic/itis** (ă-pĕn-dĭ-SĪ-tĭs): inflammation of the appendix *-itis:* inflammation
col/o	colon	**col/o/stomy** (kō-LŎS-tō-mē): creation of an opening between the colon and the abdominal wall *-stomy*:* forming an opening (mouth) *A colostomy creates a place for fecal matter to exit the body other than through the anus.*
colon/o		**colon/o/scopy** (kō-lŏn-ŎS-kō-pē): visual examination of the colon *-scopy:* visual examination *Colonoscopy is performed with an elongated endoscope called a colonoscope.*
sigmoid/o	sigmoid colon	**sigmoid/o/tomy** (sĭg-moyd-ŎT-ō-mē): incision of the sigmoid colon *-tomy:* incision

(continued)

*When the suffix *-stomy* is used with a combining form that denotes an organ, it refers to a surgical opening to the outside of the body.

Medical Word Elements—cont'd

Element	Meaning	Word Analysis
Terminal End of Large Intestine		
rect/o	rectum	**rect/o**/cele (RĔK-tŏ-sēl): herniation or protrusion of the rectum; also called *proctocele* *-cele:* hernia, swelling
proct/o	anus, rectum	**proct/o**/logist (prŏk-TŎL-ō-jĭst): physician who specializes in treating disorders of the colon, rectum, and anus *-logist:* specialist in the study of
an/o	anus	peri/**an**/al (pĕr-ē-Ā-năl): pertaining to the area around the anus *peri-:* around *-al:* pertaining to
Accessory Organs of Digestion		
hepat/o	liver	**hepat/o**/megaly (hĕp-ă-tō-MĔG-ă-lē): enlargement of the liver *-megaly:* enlargement
pancreat/o	pancreas	**pancreat/o**/lysis (păn-krē-ă-TŎL-ĭ-sĭs): destruction of the pancreas by pancreatic enzymes *-lysis:* separation; destruction; loosening
cholangi/o	bile vessel	**cholangi**/ole (kō-LĂN-jē-ōl): small terminal portion of the bile duct *-ole:* small, minute
chol/e**	bile, gall	**chol/e**/lith (KŌ-lē-lĭth): gallstone *-lith:* calculus, stone *Gallstones are solid masses composed of bile and cholesterol that form in the gallbladder and common bile duct.*
cholecyst/o	gallbladder	**cholecyst**/ectomy (kō-lē-sĭs-TĔK-tō-mē): removal of the gallbladder *-ectomy:* excision, removal *Cholecystectomy is performed by laparoscopic or open surgery.*
choledoch/o	bile duct	**choledoch/o**/plasty (kō-LĔD-ō-kō-plăs-tē): surgical repair of the common bile duct *-plasty:* surgical repair
Suffixes		
-emesis	vomit	hyper/**emesis** (hī-pĕr-ĔM-ĕ-sĭs): excessive vomiting *hyper-:* excessive, above normal
-iasis	abnormal condition (produced by something specified)	chol/e/lith/**iasis** (kō-lē-lĭ-THĪ-ă-sĭs): presence or formation of gallstones in the gallbladder or common bile duct *chol/e:* bile, gall *lith:* stone, calculus *When gallstones form in the common bile duct, the condition is called* **choledocholithiasis.**

**The *e* in *chol/e* is an exception to the rule of using the connecting vowel *o.*

Medical Word Elements—cont'd

Element	Meaning	Word Analysis
-megaly	enlargement	hepat/o/**megaly** (hĕp-ă-tō-MĔG-ă-lē): enlargement of the liver *hepat/o:* liver *Hepatomegaly may be caused by hepatitis or infection, fatty infiltration (as in alcoholism), biliary obstruction, or malignancy.*
-orexia	appetite	an/**orexia** (ăn-ō-RĔK-sē-ă): loss of appetite *an–:* without, not *Anorexia can result from various conditions, such as adverse effects of drugs or various physical or psychological causes.*
-pepsia	digestion	dys/**pepsia** (dĭs-PĔP-sē-ă): epigastric discomfort felt after eating; also called *indigestion* *dys–:* bad; painful; difficult
-phagia	swallowing, eating	aer/o/**phagia** (ĕr-ō-FĀ-jē-ă): swallowing air *aer/o:* air
-prandial	meal	post/**prandial** (pōst-PRĂN-dē-ăl): following a meal *post–:* after, behind
-rrhea	discharge, flow	steat/o/**rrhea** (stē-ă-tō-RĒ-ă): excessive amount of fat discharged in fecal matter *-rrhea:* discharge, flow
Prefixes		
dia-	through, across	**dia**/rrhea (dī-ă-RĒ-ă): abnormally frequent discharge or flow of fluid fecal matter from the bowel *-rrhea:* discharge, flow
peri-	around	**peri**/sigmoid/itis (pĕr-ĭ-sĭg-moy-DĪ-tĭs): inflammation of peritoneal tissue around the sigmoid colon *peri–:* around *-itis:* inflammation
sub-	under, below	**sub**/lingu/al (sŭb-LĬNG-gwăl): pertaining to the area under the tongue *lingu:* tongue *-al:* pertaining to

 It is time to review medical word elements by completing Learning Activities 6–3 and 6–4. For audio pronunciations of the above-listed key terms, you can visit www.davisplus.fadavis.com/gylys/systems to download this chapter's Listen and Learn! *exercises or use the book's audio CD (if included).*

Pathology

Although some digestive disorders may be without symptoms (**asymptomatic**), many are associated with such symptoms as nausea, vomiting, bleeding, pain, and weight loss. Clinical signs, such as jaundice and edema, may indicate a hepatic disorder. Severe infection, drug toxicity, hepatic disease, and changes in fluid and electrolyte balance can cause behavioral abnormalities. Disorders of the GI tract or any of the accessory organs (liver, gallbladder, pancreas) may result in far-reaching metabolic or systemic problems that can eventually threaten life itself. Assessment of a suspected digestive disorder includes a thorough history and physical examination. A range of diagnostic tests assist in identifying abnormalities of the GI tract, liver, gallbladder, and pancreas.

For diagnosis, treatment, and management of digestive disorders, the medical services of a specialist may be warranted. **Gastroenterology** is the branch of medicine concerned with digestive diseases. The physician who specializes in the diagnoses and treatment of digestive disorders is known as a **gastroenterologist.** Gastroenterologists do not perform surgeries; however, under the broad classification of surgery, they do perform such procedures as liver biopsy and endoscopic examination.

Ulcer

An **ulcer** is a circumscribed open sore, on the skin or mucous membranes within the body. Peptic ulcers are the most common type of ulcer that occurs in the digestive system. There are two main types of peptic ulcers: gastric ulcers, which develop in the stomach, and duodenal ulcers, which develop in the duodenum, usually in the area nearest the stomach. A third type of ulceration that affects the digestive system is associated with a disorder called colitis. As the name implies, it occurs in the colon.

Peptic Ulcer Disease

Peptic ulcer disease (PUD) develops in the parts of the GI tract that are exposed to hydrochloric acid and pepsin, an enzyme secreted in the stomach that begins the digestion of proteins. Both of these products are found in gastric juice and normally act on food to begin the digestive process. The strong action of these digestive products can destroy the protective defenses of the mucous membranes of the stomach and duodenum, causing the lining to erode. However, current studies have identified the bacterium *Helicobacter pylori* as a leading cause of PUD. The spiral shape of this organism helps it to burrow into the mucosa, weakening it and making it more susceptible to the action of pepsin and stomach acid. Treatment includes antibiotics to destroy *H. pylori* and antacids to treat peptic ulcers. Patients are advised to avoid nonsteroidal anti-inflammatory drugs (NSAIDs), caffeine, smoking, and alcohol, which intensify (**exacerbate**) the symptoms of gastric ulcers. If left untreated, mucosal destruction produces a hole (**perforation**) in the wall lining with resultant bleeding from the damaged area.

Ulcerative Colitis

Ulcerative colitis, a chronic inflammatory disease of the large intestine and rectum, commonly begins in the rectum or sigmoid colon and extends upward into the entire colon. It is characterized by profuse, watery diarrhea containing varying amounts of blood, mucus, and pus. Ulcerative colitis is distinguished from other closely related bowel disorders by its characteristic inflammatory pattern. The inflammation involves only the mucosal lining of the colon, and the affected portion of the colon is uniformly involved, with no patches of healthy mucosal tissue evident. Ulcerative colitis is associated with a higher risk of colon cancer. Severe cases may require surgical creation of an opening (**stoma**) for bowel evacuation to a bag worn on the abdomen.

Hernia

A **hernia** is a protrusion of any organ, tissue, or structure through the wall of the cavity in which it is naturally contained. (See Figure 6–5.) In general, though, the term is applied to protrusions of abdominal organs (**viscera**) through the abdominal wall.

An (1) **inguinal hernia** develops in the groin where the abdominal folds of flesh meet the thighs. In initial stages, it may be hardly noticeable and appears as a soft lump under the skin, no larger than a marble. In early stages, an inguinal hernia is usually reducible; that is, it can be pushed gently back into its normal place. With this type of hernia, pain may be minimal. As time passes, pressure of the abdomen against the weak abdominal wall may increase the size of the opening as well as the size of the hernia lump. If the blood supply to the hernia is cut off because of pressure, a (2) **strangulated hernia** may develop leading to

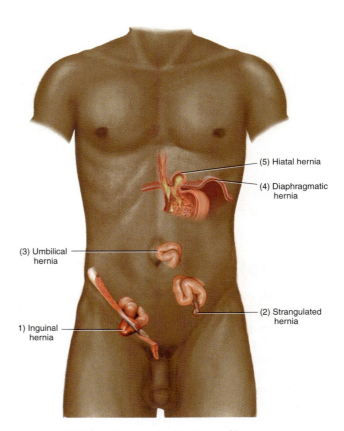

(5) Hiatal hernia

(4) Diaphragmatic hernia

(3) Umbilical hernia

(2) Strangulated hernia

1) Inguinal hernia

Figure 6-5. Common locations of hernias.

necrosis with gangrene. An (3) **umbilical hernia** is a protrusion of part of the intestine at the navel. It occurs more commonly in obese women and among those who have had several pregnancies. Hernias also occur in newborn infants (**congenital**) or during early childhood. If the defect has not corrected itself by age 2, the deformity can be surgically corrected. Treatment consists of surgical repair of the hernia (**hernioplasty**) with suture of the abdominal wall (**herniorrhaphy**).

Although hernias most commonly occur in the abdominal region, they may develop in the diaphragm. Two forms of this type include (4) **diaphragmatic hernia,** a congenital disorder, and (5) **hiatal hernia,** in which the lower part of the esophagus and the top of the stomach slides through an opening (**hiatus**) in the diaphragm into the thorax. With hiatal hernia, stomach acid backs up into the esophagus, causing heartburn, chest pain, and swallowing difficulty. Although many hiatal hernias are asymptomatic, if the disease continues for a prolonged period, it may cause **gastroesophageal reflux disease (GERD).**

Intestinal Obstruction

An intestinal obstruction is a partial or complete blockage in the small or large intestine that prevents forward flow of digestive products. Complete obstruction in any part of the intestine constitutes a medical emergency and requires rapid diagnosis and treatment within a 24-hour period to prevent death.

The two forms of intestinal obstructions include *mechanical blockage,* also called *ileus,* where contents of the intestine are prevented from moving forward due to an obstacle or barrier that blocks the lumen. The second form, *nonmechanical blockage,* also called *paralytic ileus,* where peristaltic movement is lacking or absent and contents are no longer propelled through the intestine.

Mechanical obstructions include tumors, scar tissues (**adhesions**), intestinal twisting (**volvolus**), intestinal "telescoping" where part of the intestine slips into another part just beneath it (**intussusceptions**), strangulated hernias, or the presence of foreign bodies, such as fruit pits and gallstones.

Nonmechanical blockages often result after abdominal surgeries or with spinal cord lesions where peristalsis or other neurogenic stimuli are affected. Other less common causes include thrombosis or embolism of mesenteric vessels and trauma or bacterial injury to the peritoneum.

The primary medical treatment for an intestinal obstruction is insertion of an intestinal tube. If the intestinal tube is ineffective in relieving the obstruction, surgery is indicated.

Hemorrhoids

Enlarged veins in the mucous membrane of the anal canal are called *hemorrhoids.* Often they may bleed, hurt, or itch. They may occur inside (**internal**) or outside (**external**) the rectal area. Hemorrhoids are usually caused by abdominal pressure, such as from straining during bowel movement, pregnancy, and standing or sitting for long periods. They may also be associated with some disorders of the liver or the heart.

A high-fiber diet as well as drinking plenty of water and juices plays a pivotal role in hemorrhoid prevention. Temporary relief from hemorrhoids can usually be obtained by cold compresses, sitz baths, stool softeners, or analgesic ointments. Treatment of an advanced hemorrhoidal condition involves surgical removal (**hemorrhoidectomy**).

Hepatitis

Hepatitis is an inflammatory condition of the liver. The usual causes include exposure to toxic substances, especially alcohol; obstructions in the bile ducts; metabolic diseases; autoimmune diseases; and bacterial or viral infections. A growing public health concern is the increasing incidence of viral hepatitis. Even though its mortality rate is low, the disease is easily transmitted and can cause significant morbidity and prolonged loss of time from school or employment.

Although forms of hepatitis range from hepatitis A through hepatitis E, the three most common forms are: hepatitis A, also called *infectious hepatitis;* hepatitis B, also called *serum hepatitis;* and hepatitis C. The most common causes of hepatitis A are ingestion of contaminated food, water, or milk. Hepatitis B and hepatitis C are usually transmitted by routes other than the mouth (**parenteral**), such as from blood transfusions and sexual contact. Because of patient exposure, health-care personnel are at increased risk for contracting hepatitis B, but a vaccine that provides immunity to hepatitis B is available. There is no vaccine available for hepatitis C. Patients with hepatitis C may remain asymptomatic for years or the disease may produce only mild flulike symptoms. Treatment for hepatitis includes antiviral drugs; however, there is no cure. As the disease progresses, scarring of the liver becomes so serious that liver transplantation is the only recourse.

One of the major symptoms of many liver disorders, including hepatitis and cirrhosis, is a yellowing of the skin, mucous membranes, and sclerae of the eyes (**jaundice, icterus**). This occurs because the liver is no longer able to remove bilirubin, a yellow compound formed when erythrocytes are destroyed. Jaundice may also result when the bile duct is blocked, causing bile to enter the bloodstream.

Diverticulosis

Diverticulosis is a condition in which small, blisterlike pockets (**diverticula**) develop in the inner lining of the large intestine and may balloon through the intestinal wall. These pockets occur most commonly in the sigmoid colon. They usually do not cause any problem unless they become inflamed (**diverticulitis**). (See Figure 6–6.) Signs and symptoms of diverticulitis include pain, often in the left lower quadrant (LLQ) of the abdomen; extreme constipation (**obstipation**) or diarrhea; fever; abdominal swelling; and occasional blood in bowel movements. The usual treatment for diverticulitis consists of bed rest, antibiotics, and a soft diet. In severe cases, however, excision of the diverticulum (**diverticulectomy**) may be advised.

Oncology

Although stomach cancer is rare in United States, it is common in many parts of the world where food preservation is problematic. It is an important medical problem because of its high mortality rate. Men are more susceptible to stomach cancer than women. The neoplasm nearly always develops from the epithelial or mucosal lining of the stomach in the form of a cancerous glandular tumor (**gastric adenocarcinoma**). Persistent indigestion is one of the important warning signs of stomach cancer. Other types of GI carcinomas include **esophageal** carcinomas, **hepatocellular** carcinomas, and **pancreatic** carcinomas.

Colorectal cancer arises from the epithelial lining of the large intestine. Signs and symptoms, which depend largely on the location of the malignancy, include changes in bowel habits, passage of blood and mucus in stools, rectal or abdominal pain, anemia, weight loss, obstruction, and perforation. An obstruction that develops suddenly may be the first symptom of cancer involving the colon between the cecum and the sigmoid. In this region, where bowel contents are liquid, a slowly developing obstruction will not become evident until the lumen is almost closed. Cancer of the sigmoid and rectum causes symptoms of partial obstruction with constipation alternating with diarrhea, lower abdominal cramping pain, and distention.

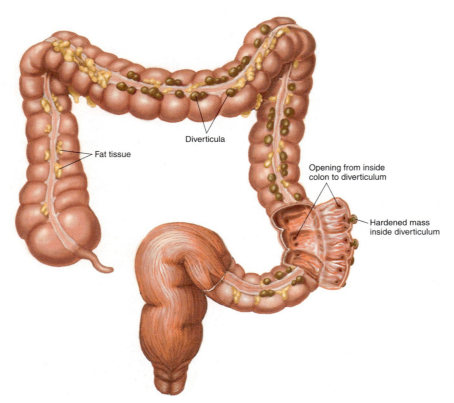

Diverticula

Fat tissue

Opening from inside colon to diverticulum

Hardened mass inside diverticulum

Figure 6-6. Diverticula of the colon.

Diagnostic, Symptomatic, and Related Terms

This section introduces diagnostic, symptomatic, and related terms and their meanings. Word analyses for selected terms are also provided.

Term	Definition
anorexia ăn-ō-RĔK-sē-ă *an-:* without, not *-orexia:* appetite	Lack or loss of appetite, resulting in the inability to eat *Anorexia should not be confused with anorexia nervosa, which is a complex psychogenic eating disorder characterized by an all-consuming desire to remain thin. Anorexia nervosa and a similar eating disorder called* **bulimia nervosa** *are discussed in Chapter 14.*
appendicitis ă-pĕn-dĭ-SĪ-tĭs *appendic:* appendix *-itis:* inflammation	Inflammation of the appendix, usually due to obstruction or infection *If left undiagnosed, appendicitis rapidly leads to perforation and peritonitis. Treatment is appendectomy within 24 to 48 hours of the first symptoms because delay usually results in rupture and peritonitis as fecal matter is released into the peritoneal cavity. (See Figure 6–7.)*

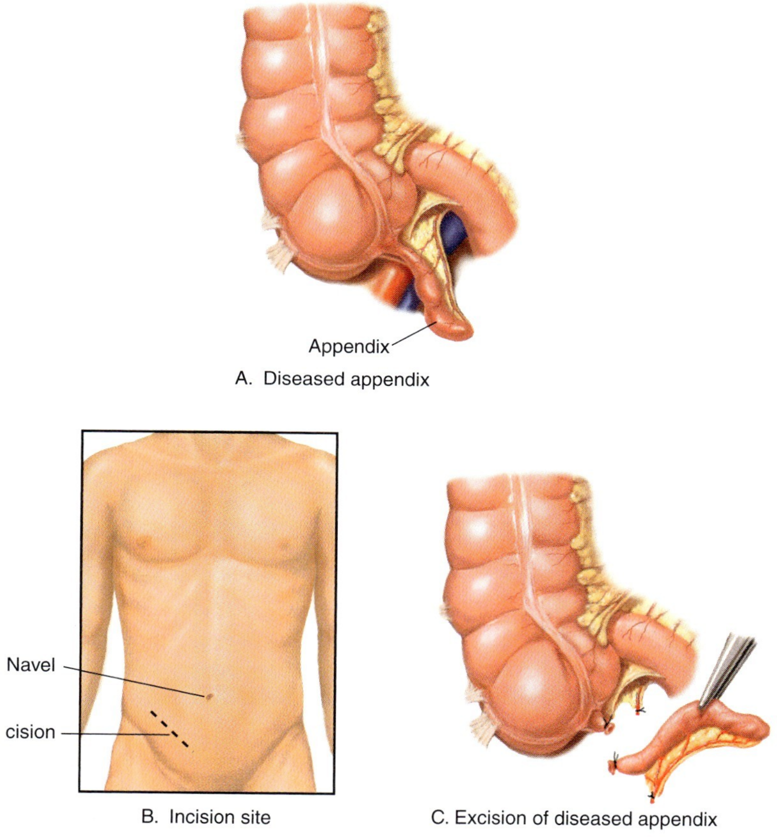

Appendix

A. Diseased appendix

Navel

cision

B. Incision site

C. Excision of diseased appendix

Figure 6-7. Appendectomy.

ascites ă-SĪ-tēz	Abnormal accumulation of fluid in the abdomen *Ascites is most commonly associated with cirrhosis of the liver, especially when caused by alcoholism. Failure of the liver to produce albumin (a protein that regulates the amount of fluid in the circulatory system), combined with portal hypertension forces fluid to pass from the circulatory system and accumulate in the peritoneum.*

(continued)

Diagnostic, Symptomatic, and Related Terms—cont'd

Term	Definition
borborygmus bŏr-bō-RĬG-mŭs	Rumbling or gurgling noises that are audible at a distance and caused by passage of gas through the liquid contents of the intestine
cachexia kă-KĔKS-ē-ă	Physical wasting that includes loss of weight and muscle mass; commonly associated with AIDS and cancer.
cholelithiasis kō-lē-lĭ-THĪ-ă-sĭs *chol/e:* bile, gall *lith:* stone, calculus *-iasis:* abnormal condition (produced by something specified)	Presence or formation of gallstones in the gallbladder or common bile duct *Cholelithiasis may or may not produce symptoms.* (See Figure 6–8.)

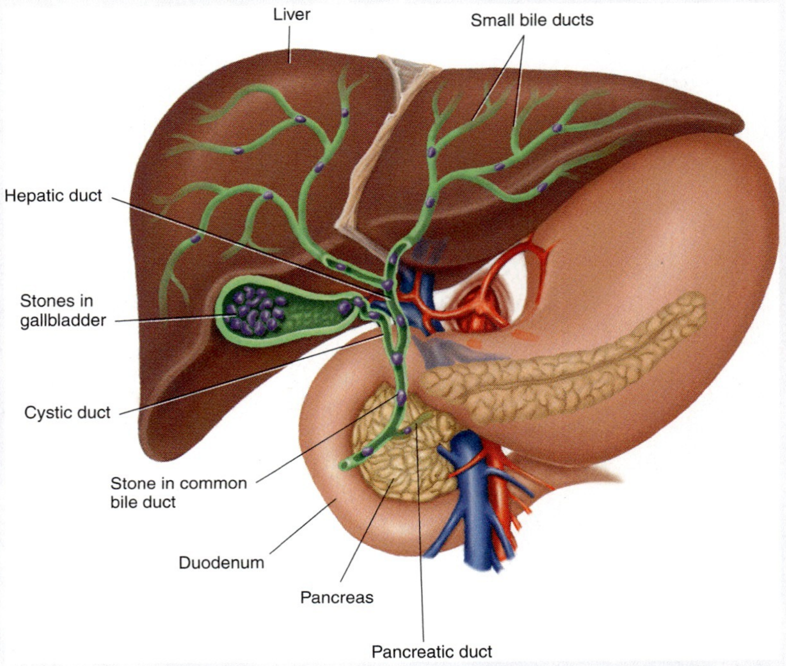

Figure 6-8. Sites of gallstones.

cirrhosis sĭr-RŌ-sĭs	Scarring and dysfunction of the liver cause by chronic liver disease *Cirrhosis is most commonly caused by chronic alcoholism. It may also be caused by toxins, infectious agents, metabolic diseases, and circulatory disorders. In this disorder, functional hepatic cells are replaced by nonfunctioning fibrous tissue that impairs the flow of blood and lymph within the liver, resulting in hepatic insufficiency.*
colic KŎL-ĭk	Spasm in any hollow or tubular soft organ especially in the colon, accompanied by pain
Crohn disease KRŌN	Chronic inflammation, usually of the ileum, but possibly affecting any portion of the intestinal tract; also called *regional enteritis* *Crohn disease is a chronic disease distinguished from closely related bowel disorders by its inflammatory pattern. It may cause fever, cramping, diarrhea, and weight loss.*
deglutition dē-gloo-TĬSH-ŭn	Act of swallowing

Diagnostic, Symptomatic, and Related Terms—cont'd

Term	Definition
dysentery DĬS-ĕn-tĕr-ē	Inflammation of the intestine, especially the colon, that may be caused by ingesting water or food containing chemical irritants, bacteria, protozoa, or parasites, which results in bloody diarrhea *Dysentery is common in underdeveloped countries and in times of disaster when sanitary living conditions, clean food, and safe water are not available.*
dyspepsia dĭs-PĔP-sē-ă *dys-:* bad; painful; difficult *-pepsia:* digestion	Epigastric discomfort felt after eating; also called *indigestion*
dysphagia dĭs-FĀ-jē-ă *dys-:* bad; painful; difficult *-phagia:* swallowing, eating	Inability or difficulty in swallowing; also called *aphagia*
eructation ĕ-rūk-TĀ-shŭn	Producing gas from the stomach, usually with a characteristic sound; also called *belching*
fecalith FĒ-kă-lĭth	Fecal concretion
flatus FLĀ-tŭs	Gas in the GI tract; expelling of air from a body orifice, especially the anus
gastroesophageal reflux disease (GERD) găs-trō-ĕ-s-ŏf-ă-JĒ-ăl RĒ-flŭks *gastr/o:* stomach *esophag:* esophagus *-eal:* pertaining to	Backflow of gastric contents into the esophagus due to a malfunction of the sphincter muscle at the inferior portion of the esophagus *GERD may occur whenever pressure in the stomach is greater than that in the esophagus and may be associated with heartburn, esophagitis, hiatal hernia, or chest pain.*
halitosis hăl-ĭ-TŌ-sĭs	Offensive, or "bad," breath
hematemesis hĕm-ăt-ĔM-ĕ-sĭs *hemat:* blood *-emesis:* vomiting	Vomiting of blood from bleeding in the stomach or esophagus *Hematemesis can be caused by an esophageal ulcer, esophageal varices (dilation of veins), or a gastric ulcer. Treatment requires correction of the underlying cause.*
irritable bowel syndrome (IBS)	Symptom complex marked by abdominal pain and altered bowel function (typically constipation, diarrhea, or alternating constipation and diarrhea) for which no organic cause can be determined; also called *spastic colon* *Contributing or aggravating factors of IBS include anxiety and stress.*
malabsorption syndrome măl-ăb-SORP-shŭn SĬN-drōm	Symptom complex of the small intestine characterized by the impaired passage of nutrients, minerals, or fluids through intestinal villi into the blood or lymph *Malabsorption syndrome may be associated with or due to a number of diseases, including those affecting the intestinal mucosa. It may also be due to surgery, such as gastric resection and ileal bypass, or antibiotic therapy.*

(continued)

Diagnostic, Symptomatic, and Related Terms—cont'd

Term	Definition
melena MĔL-ĕ-nă	Passage of dark-colored, tarry stools, due to the presence of blood altered by intestinal juices
obesity ō-BĒ-sĭ-tē	Excessive accumulation of fat that exceeds the body's skeletal and physical standards, usually an increase of 20 percent or more above ideal body weight. *Obesity may be due to excessive intake of food (exogenous) or metabolic or endocrine abnormalities (endogenous).*
morbid obesity ō-BĒ-sĭ-tē	Body mass index (BMI) of 40 or greater, which is generally 100 or more pounds over ideal body weight. *Morbid obesity is a disease with serious psychological, social, and medical ramifications and one that threatens necessary body functions such as respiration.*
obstipation ŏb-stĭ-PĀ-shŭn	Severe constipation; may be caused by an intestinal obstruction
oral leukoplakia OR-ăl loo-kō-PLĀ-kē-ă *leuk/o:* white *-plakia:* plaque	Formation of white spots or patches on the mucous membrane of the tongue, lips, or cheek caused primarily by irritation *Oral leukoplakia is a precancerous condition usually associated with pipe or cigarette smoking or ill-fitting dentures.*
peristalsis pĕr-ĭ-STĂL-sĭs	Progressive, wavelike movement that occurs involuntarily in hollow tubes of the body, especially the GI tract
pyloric stenosis pī-LOR-ĭk stĕ-NŌ-sĭs *pylor:* pylorus *-ic:* pertaining to *sten:* narrowing, stricture *-osis:* abnormal condition; increase (used primarily with blood cells)	Stricture or narrowing of the pyloric sphincter (circular muscle of the pylorus) at the outlet of the stomach, causing an obstruction that blocks the flow of food into the small intestine *The muscle fibers of the outlet are cut, without severing the mucosa, to widen the opening. After surgery in adults, a stomach tube remains in place and observation is maintained for signs of hemorrhage or blockage of the tube.*
regurgitation rē-gŭr-jĭ-TĀ-shŭn	Backward flowing, as in the return of solids or fluids to the mouth from the stomach
steatorrhea stē-ă-tō-RĒ-ă *steat/o:* fat *-rrhea:* discharge, flow	Passage of fat in large amounts in the feces due to failure to digest and absorb it *Steatorrhea may occur in pancreatic disease when pancreatic enzymes are not sufficient. It also occurs in malabsorption syndrome.*

 It is time to review pathological, diagnostic, symptomatic, and related terms by completing Learning Activity 6–5.

Diagnostic and Therapeutic Procedures

This section introduces procedures used to diagnose and treat digestive system disorders. Descriptions are provided as well as pronunciations and word analyses for selected terms.

Procedure	Description
Diagnostic Procedures	
Endoscopic	
endoscopy ĕn-DŎS-kō-pē *endo-:* in, within *-scopy:* visual examinination	Visual examination of a cavity or canal using a flexible fiberoptic instrument called an *endoscope* *The organ, cavity, or canal being examined dictates the name of the endoscopic procedure. (See Figure 4-6.) A camera and video recorder are commonly used during the procedure to provide a permanent record.*
upper GI	Endoscopy of the esophagus (esophagoscopy), stomach (gastroscopy), and duodenum (duodenoscopy) *Endoscopy of the upper GI tract is performed to identify tumors, esophagitis, gastroesophageal varices, peptic ulcers, and the source of upper GI bleeding. It is also used to confirm the presence and extent of varices in the lower esophagus and stomach in patients with liver disease.*
lower GI	Endoscopy of the colon (colonoscopy), sigmoid colon (sigmoidoscopy), and rectum and anal canal (proctoscopy) (See Figure 6-9.) *Endoscopy of the lower GI tract is used to identify pathological conditions in the colon. It may also be used to remove polyps. When polyps are discovered in the colon, they are retrieved and tested for cancer.*

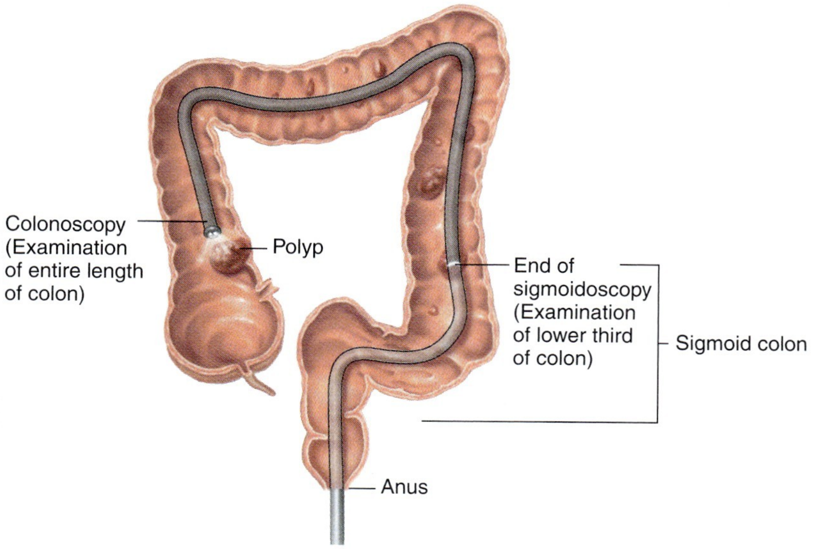

Figure 6-9. Colonoscopy and sigmoidoscopy.

Laboratory	
hepatitis panel hĕp-ă-TĪ-tĭs *hepat:* liver *-itis:* inflammation	Panel of blood tests that identify the specific virus—hepatitis A (HAV), hepatitis B (HBV), or hepatitis C (HCV)-causing hepatitis by testing serum using antibodies to each of these antigens

(continued)

Diagnostic and Therapeutic Procedures—cont'd

Procedure	Description
liver function tests (LFTs) LĬV-ĕr FŬNGK-shŭn	Group of blood tests that evaluate liver injury, liver function, and conditions often associated with the biliary tract *LFTs evaluate liver enzymes, bilirubin, and proteins produced by the liver.*
serum bilirubin SĒ-rŭm bĭl-ĭ-ROO-bĭn	Measurement of the level of bilirubin in the blood *Elevated serum bilirubin indicates excessive destruction of erythrocytes, liver disease, or biliary tract obstruction. Bilirubin is a breakdown product of hemoglobin and is normally excreted from the body as bile. Excessive bilirubin causes yellowing of the skin and mucous membranes, a condition called* jaundice.
stool culture	Test to identify microorganisms or parasites present in feces *Feces are examined microscopically after being placed in a growth medium.*
stool guaiac GWĪ-ăk	Applying a substance called guaiac to a stool sample to detect presence of occult (hidden) blood in the feces; also called *Hemoccult* (trade name of a modified guaiac test) *Stool test detects presence of blood in the feces that is not apparent on visual inspection. It also helps detect colon cancer and bleeding associated with digestive disorders.*
Radiographic	
barium enema (BE) BĂ-rē-ŭm ĔN-ĕ-mă	Radiographic examination of the rectum and colon following enema administration of barium sulfate (contrast medium) into the rectum; also called lower GI series *Barium is retained in the lower GI tract during fluoroscopic and radiographic studies. It is used for diagnosing obstructions, tumors, or other abnormalities of the colon. (See Figure 6-10.)*

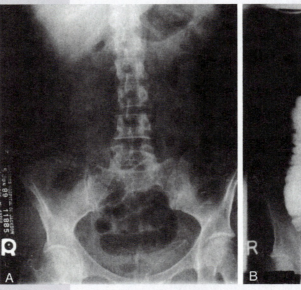 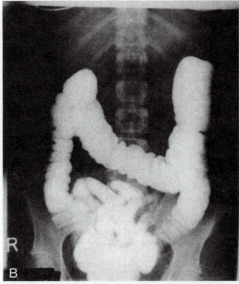

Figure 6-10. Barium enema done poorly (A) and correctly (B).

Diagnostic and Therapeutic Procedures—cont'd

Procedure	Description
barium swallow BĂ-rē-ŭm	Radiographic examination of the esophagus, stomach, and small intestine following oral administration of barium sulfate (contrast medium); also called *esophagram* and *upper GI series* *Barium swallow is used to diagnose structural defects of the esophagus and vessels, such as esophageal varices. It may also be used to locate swallowed objects.*
cholecystography kō-lē-sĭs-TŎG-ră-fē *chol/e:* bile, gall *cyst/o:* bladder *-graphy:* process of recording	Radiographic images taken of the gallbladder after administration of a contrast material containing iodine, usually in the form of a tablet *This test evaluates gallbladder function and identifies the presence of disease or gallstones.*
computed tomography (CT) kŏm-PŪ-tĕd tō-MŎG-ră-fē *tom/o:* to cut *-graphy:* process of recording	Imaging technique achieved by rotating an x-ray emitter around the area to be scanned and measuring the intensity of transmitted rays from different angles *In CT scanning, a computer is used to generate a detailed cross-sectional image that appears as a slice. (See Figure 4-5D.) In the digestive system, CT scans are used to view the gallbladder, bowel, liver, bile ducts, and pancreas. It is also used to diagnose tumors, cysts, inflammation, abscesses, perforation, bleeding, and obstructions.*
endoscopic retrograde cholangiopancreatography (ERCP) ĕn-dō-SKŎ-pĭk RĔT-rō-grād kō-lăn-jē-ō-păn-krē-ă-TŎG-ră-fē *cholangi/o:* bile vessel *pancreat/o:* pancreas *-graphy:* process of recording	Endoscopic procedure that provides radiographic visualization of the bile and pancreatic ducts to identify partial or total obstructions, as well as stones, cysts, and tumors. *In ERCP, a flexible fiberoptic duodenoscope is placed into the common bile duct. A radiopaque substance is instilled directly into the duct and serial x-ray films are taken.*
percutaneous transhepatic cholangiography (PTCP) pĕr-kū-TĀ-nē-ŭs trăns-hĕ-PĂT-ĭk kō-lăn-jē-ŎG-ră-fē *per-:* through *cutane:* skin *-ous:* pertaining to *trans-:* through, across *hepat:* liver *-ic:* pertaining to *cholangi/o:* bile vessel *-graphy:* process of recording	Radiographic examination of bile duct structures *Contrast medium is injected through a needle passed through the skin (percutaneous) and through the liver (transhepatic) directly into the hepatic duct. The bile duct can be viewed for obstructions, anatomical variations, and cysts.*
sialography sī-ă-LŎG-ră-fē *sial/o:* saliva, salivary glands *-graphy:* process of recording	Radiologic examination of the salivary glands and ducts *Sialography may be performed with or without a contrast medium.*

(continued)

Diagnostic and Therapeutic Procedures—cont'd

Procedure	Description
ultrasonography (US) ŭl-tră-sŏn-ŌG-ră-fē *ultra-:* excess, beyond *son/o:* sound *-graphy:* process of recording	Test that uses high-frequency sound waves (ultrasound) to analyze the reflected echos from anatomical structures and convert them into an image on a video monitor; also called *ultrasound, sonography, echo,* and *echogram* *US detects diseases and deformities in digestive organs, such as the gallbladder, liver, and pancreas. It is also used to locate abdominal masses outside the digestive organs.*
abdominal ăb-DŎM-ĭ-năl *abdomin:* abdomen *-al:* pertaining to	Ultrasound visualization of the abdominal aorta, liver, gallbladder, bile ducts, pancreas, kidneys, ureters, and bladder *An abdominal US is used to diagnose and locate cysts, tumors, and malformations as well as document the progression of various diseases and guide the insertion of instruments during surgical procedures.*

Surgical

biopsy (bx) BĪ-ŏp-sē liver	Representative tissue sample removed from a body site for microscopic examination, usually to establish a diagnosis Use of a large-bore needle to remove a core of liver tissue for histological examination

Therapeutic Procedures

Clinical

nasogastric intubation nā-zō-GĂS-trĭk ĭn-tū-BĀ-shŭn *nas/o:* nose *gastr:* stomach *-ic:* pertaining to	Procedure that involves insertion of a nasogastric tube through the nose into the stomach to relieve gastric distention by removing gas, food, or gastric secretions; to instill medication, food, or fluids; or to obtain a specimen for laboratory analysis

Surgical

anastomosis ă-năs-tō-MŌ-sĭs	Surgical joining of two ducts, vessels, or bowel segments to allow flow from one to another
ileorectal ĭl-ē-ō-RĔK-tăl *ile/o:* ileum *rect:* rectum *-al:* pertaining to	Surgical connection of the ileum and rectum after total colectomy, as is sometimes performed in the treatment of ulcerative colitis
intestinal ĭn-TĔS-tĭ-năl	Surgical connection of two portions of the intestines; also called *enteroenterostomy*

Diagnostic and Therapeutic Procedures—cont'd

Procedure	Description

bariatric surgery
băr-ē-Ă-trĭk

Group of procedures that treat morbid obesity, a condition which arises from severe accumulation of excess weight as fatty tissue, and the resultant health problems

Commonly employed bariatric surgeries include vertical banded gastroplasty and Roux-en-Y gastric bypass. (See Figure 6-11.)

vertical banded gastroplasty

Upper stomach near the esophagus is stapled vertically to reduce it to a small pouch. A band is then inserted that restricts food consumption and delays its passage from the pouch, causing a feeling of fullness.

Roux-en-Y gastric bypass (RGB)
rū-ĕn-Ē GĂS-trĭk

Stomach is first stapled to decrease it to a small pouch. Next, the jejunum is shortened and connected to the small stomach pouch, causing the base of the duodenum leading from the nonfunctioning portion of the stomach to form a Y configuration. This configuration decreases the pathway of food through the intestine, thus reducing absorption of calories and fats

RGB can be performed laparoscopically or as an open procedure (laparotomy), depending on the health of the pateint. RGB is the most commonly performed weight-loss surgery today.

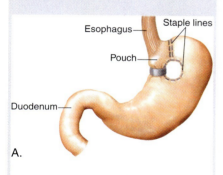

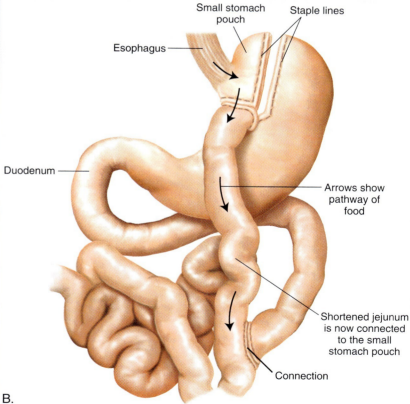

Figure 6-11. Bariatric surgery. (A) Vertical banded gastroplasty. (B) Roux-en-Y gastric bypass.

(continued)

Diagnostic and Therapeutic Procedures—cont'd

Procedure	Description
colostomy kō-LŎS-tō-mē *col/o:* colon	Creation of an opening of a portion of the colon through the abdominal wall to its outside surface in order to divert fecal flow to a colostomy bag (See Figure 6-12.)

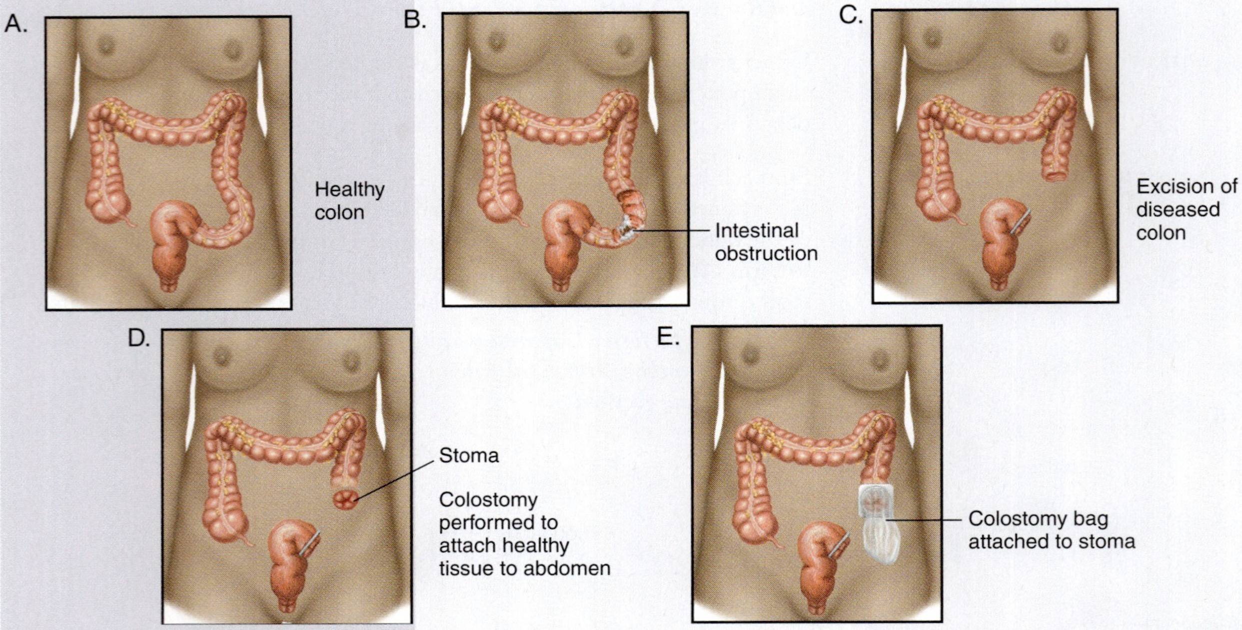

A.

Healthy colon

B.

Intestinal obstruction

C.

Excision of diseased colon

D.

Stoma

Colostomy performed to attach healthy tissue to abdomen

E.

Colostomy bag attached to stoma

Figure 6-12. Colostomy.

Procedure	Description
lithotripsy LĬTH-ō-trĭp-sē *lith/o:* stone, calculus *-tripsy:* crushing	Procedure for crushing a stone and eliminating its fragments either surgically or using ultrasonic shock waves
extracorporeal shockwave ĕks-tră-kor-POR-ē-ăl SHŎK-wāv	Use of shock waves as a noninvasive method to break up stones in the gallbladder or biliary ducts (See Figure 11-5.) *In extracorporeal shockwave lithotripsy (ESWL), ultrasound is used to locate the stone(s) and to monitor the destruction of the stones.*

Diagnostic and Therapeutic Procedures—cont'd

Procedure	Description
polypectomy pŏl-ĭ-PĔK-tō-mē *polyp:* small growth *-ectomy:* excision, removal	Excision of a polyp *When polyps are discovered during sigmoidoscopy or colonoscopy, they are excised for microscopic tissue examination for abnormal or cancerous cells. (See Figure 6-13.)* Polyps are removed from colon for examination **Figure 6-13.** Polypectomy.
pyloromyotomy pī-lō-rō-mī-ŎT-ō-mē *pylor/o:* pylorus *my/o:* muscle *-tomy:* incision	Incision of the longitudinal and circular muscles of the pylorus; used to treat hypertrophic pyloric stenosis

Pharmacology

Various pharmaceutical agents are available to counteract abnormal conditions that occur in the GI tract. Antacids counteract or decrease excessive stomach acid, the cause of heartburn, gastric discomfort, and gastric reflux. Antidiarrheals and antiemetics are prescribed to preserve water and electrolytes, which are essential for body hydration and homeostasis. Medications that increase or decrease peristalsis are used to regulate the speed at which food passes through the GI tract. These drugs include agents that relieve "cramping" (**antispasmodics**) and those that help in the movement of material through a sluggish bowel (**laxatives**). (See Table 6–1.)

Table 6-1 Drugs Used to Treat Digestive Disorders

This table lists common drug classifications used to treat digestive disorders, their therapeutic actions, and selected generic and trade names.

Classification	Therapeutic Action	Generic and Trade Names
antacids	Counteract or neutralize acidity, usually in the stomach *Antacids are used to treat and prevent heartburn and acid reflux.*	**calcium carbonate** KĂL-sē-ŭm KĂR-bŏn-āt Mylanta, Rolaids, Tums
antidiarrheals	Control loose stools and relieve diarrhea by absorbing excess water in the bowel or slowing peristalsis in the intestinal tract	**loperamide** lō-PĔR-ă-mīd Imodium **kaolin/pectin** KĀ-ō-lĭn PĔK-tĭn Donnagel-MB, Kapectolin

(continued)

Table 6-1	Drugs Used to Treat Digestive Disorders—cont'd		
Classification	**Therapeutic Action**	**Generic and Trade Names**	
antiemetics	Control nausea and vomiting by blocking nerve impulses to the vomiting center of the brain	**prochlorperazine** prō-klor-PĔR-ă-zēn Compazine, Compro	
	Some emetics act by hastening movement of food through the digestive tract.	**trimethobenzamide** trī-mĕth-ō-BĔN-ză-mīd T-Gen, Tigan	
antispasmodics	Decrease gastrointestinal (GI) spasms by slowing peristalsis and motility throughout the GI tract	**glycopyrrolate** glī-kō-PĬR-rō-lāt Robinul	
	Antispasmodics are prescribed for irritable bowel syndrome (IBS), spastic colon, and diverticulitis.	**propantheline** prō-PĂN-thĕ-lēn Pro-Banthine	
laxatives	Treat constipation by increasing peristaltic activity in the large intestine or increasing water and electrolyte secretion into the bowel to induce defecation	**senna, sennosides** SĔN-ă, SĔN-ō-sīdz Senokot, Senolax **psyllium** SĬL-ē-ŭm Metamucil, Natural Fiber Supplement	

Abbreviations

This section introduces digestive–related abbreviations and their meanings.

Abbreviation	Meaning	Abbreviation	Meaning
Common			
ABC	aspiration biopsy cytology	**EGD**	esophagogastroduodenoscopy
alk phos	alkaline phosphatase	**ERCP**	endoscopic retrograde cholangiopancreatography
ALT	alanine aminotransferase	**GB**	gallbladder
AST	angiotensin sensitivity	**GBS**	gallbladder series (x-ray studies)
Ba	barium	**GER**	gastroesophageal reflux
BaE, BE	barium enema	**GERD**	gastroesophageal reflux disease
BM	bowel movement	**GI**	gastrointestinal
BMI	body mass index	**HAV**	hepatitis A virus
CF	cystic fibrosis	**HBV**	hepatitis B virus
CT	computed tomography	**HCV**	hepatitis C virus

Abbreviations—cont'd

Abbreviation	Meaning	Abbreviation	Meaning
HDV	hepatitis D virus	PTHC	percutaneous transhepatic cholangeography
HEV	hepatitis E virus	stat, STAT	immediately
IBS	irritable bowel syndrome	PMH	past medical history
LFT	liver function test	PUD	peptic ulcer disease
NG	nasogastric	RGB	Roux-en-Y gastric bypass
PE	physical examination; pulmonary embolism	R/O	rule out

Medication time schedule

Abbreviation	Meaning	Abbreviation	Meaning
a.c.	before meals	qAM	every morning
b.i.d.	twice a day	q.d.	every day
hs	half strength	q.h.	every hour
h.s.	at bedtime	q.2h.	every 2 hours
NPO, n.p.o.	nothing by mouth	q.i.d.	four times a day
pc, p.c.	after meals	q.o.d.	every other day
p.o.	by mouth	qPM	every evening
p.r.n.	as required	t.i.d.	three times a day

It is time to review procedures, pharmacology, and abbreviations by completing Learning Activity 6–6.

LEARNING ACTIVITIES

The following activities provide review of the digestive system terms introduced in this chapter. Complete each activity and review your answers to evaluate your understanding of the chapter.

Learning Activity 6-1
Identifying Digestive Structures

Label the illustration on page 109 using the terms listed below.

anus	hepatic flexure	rectum
appendix	ileum	sigmoid colon
ascending colon	jejunum	spleen
cecum	liver	splenic flexure
descending colon	pancreas	transverse colon
duodenum		

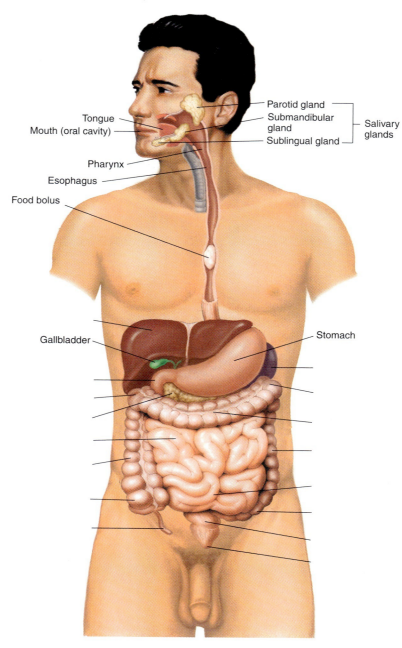

Tongue

Mouth (oral cavity)

Pharynx

Esophagus

Food bolus

Gallbladder

Parotid gland

Submandibular gland

Sublingual gland

Salivary glands

Stomach

Check your answers by referring to Figure 6–3 on page 109. Review material that you did not answer correctly.

Learning Activity 6-2
Identifying Accessory Organs of Digestion

Label the following illustration using the terms listed below.

common bile duct	*hepatic duct*	*pancreas*
cystic duct	*left hepatic duct*	*pancreatic duct*
duodenum	*liver*	*right hepatic duct*
gallbladder		

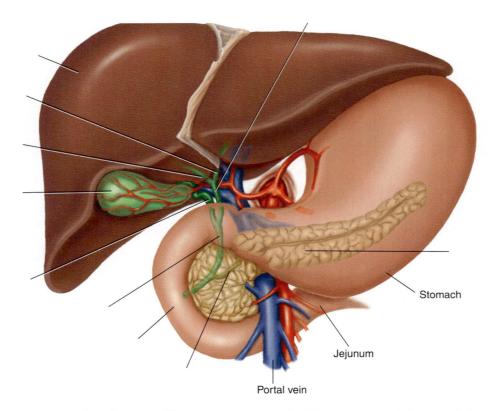

Stomach

Jejunum

Portal vein

 Check your answers by referring to Figure 6–4 on page 110. Review material that you did not answer correctly.

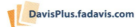 **DavisPlus.fadavis.com**

Enhance your study and reinforcement of word elements with the power of DavisPlus. Visit www.davisplus.fadavis.com/gylys/systems for this chapter's flash-card activity. We recommend you complete the flash-card activity before completing Activity 6–3 below.

Building Medical Words

Use *esophag/o* (esophagus) to build words that mean:

1. pain in the esophagus _____
2. spasm of the esophagus _____
3. stricture or narrowing of the esophagus _____

Use *gastr/o* (stomach) to build words that mean:

4. inflammation of the stomach _____
5. pain in the stomach _____
6. disease of the stomach _____

Use *duoden/o* (duodenum), *jejun/o* (jejunum), or *ile/o* (ileum) to build words that mean:

7. excision of all or part of the jejunum _____
8. relating to the duodenum _____
9. inflammation of the ileum _____
10. pertaining to the jejunum and ileum _____

Use *enter/o* (usually small intestine) to build words that mean:

11. inflammation of the small intestine _____
12. disease of the small intestine _____
13. inflammation of the small intestine and colon _____

Use *col/o* (colon) to build words that mean:

14. inflammation of the colon _____
15. pertaining to the colon and rectum _____
16. prolapse or downward displacement of the colon _____
17. disease of the colon _____

Use *proct/o* (anus, rectum) or *rect/o* (rectum) to build words that mean:

18. narrowing or constriction of the rectum _____
19. herniation of the rectum _____
20. paralysis of the anus (anal muscles) _____

Use *chol/e* (bile, gall) to build words that mean:

21. inflammation of the gallbladder _____
22. abnormal condition of a gallstone _____

Use *hepat/o* (liver) or *pancreat/o* (pancreas) to build words that mean:

23. tumor of the liver _____
24. enlargement of the liver _____
25. inflammation of the pancreas _____

✓ *Check your answers in Appendix A. Review material that you did not answer correctly.*

Correct Answers _____ ✕ 4 = _____ % Score

Learning Activity 6-4

Building Surgical Words

Build a surgical word that means:

1. excision of gums (tissue) _____
2. partial or complete excision of the tongue _____
3. repair of the esophagus _____
4. removal of part or all of the stomach _____
5. forming an opening between the stomach and jejunum _____
6. excision of (part of) the esophagus _____
7. forming an opening between the stomach, small intestine, and colon _____
8. surgical repair of the small intestine _____
9. fixation of the small intestine (to the abdominal wall) _____
10. suture of the bile duct _____
11. forming an opening into the colon _____
12. fixation of a movable liver (to the abdominal wall) _____
13. surgical repair of the anus or rectum _____
14. removal of the gallbladder _____
15. surgical repair of a bile duct _____

   ✔   *Check your answers in Appendix A. Review material that you did not answer correctly.*

Correct Answers _____ ✕ 6.67 = _____ % Score

Matching Pathological, Diagnostic, Symptomatic, and Related Terms

Match the following terms with the definitions in the numbered list.

anorexia	dysphagia	hematemesis
cachexia	dyspnea	lesion
cirrhosis	fecalith	melena
dyspepsia	halitosis	obstipation

1. vomiting blood _____
2. difficulty swallowing or inability to swallow _____
3. fecal concretion _____
4. "bad" breath _____
5. loss of appetite _____
6. poor digestion _____
7. degenerative liver disease _____
8. state of ill health, malnutrition, and wasting _____
9. intractable constipation _____
10. open sore _____

✔ *Check your answers in Appendix A. Review any material that you did not answer correctly.*

Correct Answers _____ × 10 = _____ % Score

Learning Activity 6-6
Matching Procedures, Pharmacology, and Abbreviations

Match the following terms with the definitions in the numbered list.

anastomosis	emetics	lower GI series	ultrasonography
antacids	endoscopy	proctosigmoidoscopy	upper GI series
antispasmodics	gastroscopy	PTHC	
bariatric	intubation	stat.	
bilirubin	laxatives	stool guaiac	
choledochoplasty	liver function tests	stomatoplasty	

1. percutaneous transhepatic radiographic examination of bile ducts _____
2. breakdown product of hemoglobin, excreted from the body as bile _____
3. agents that produce vomiting _____
4. agents that alleviate muscle spasms _____
5. surgical reconstruction of a bile duct _____
6. administration of barium enema while a series of radiographs are taken of the large intestine _____

7. visual examination of the stomach _____
8. surgical reconstruction of the mouth _____
9. insertion of a tube into any hollow organ _____
10. surgical formation of a passage or opening between two hollow viscera or vessels _____
11. detects presence of blood in the feces; also called Hemoccult _____
12. visual examination of a cavity or canal using a specialized lighted instrument _____
13. used to treat constipation _____
14. neutralize excess acid in the stomach and help to relieve gastritis and ulcer pain _____
15. procedure in which high-frequency sound waves produce images of internal body structures that are displayed on a monitor _____
16. measures the levels of certain enzymes, bilirubin, and various proteins _____
17. surgery that treats morbid obesity _____
18. immediately _____
19. endoscopic procedure for visualization of the rectosigmoid colon _____
20. barium solution swallowed for radiographic examination of the esophagus, stomach, and duodenum _____

✔ *Check your answers in Appendix A. Review material that you did not answer correctly.*

Correct Answers _____ × 5 = _____ % Score

MEDICAL RECORD ACTIVITIES

The two medical records included in the following activities use common clinical scenarios to show how medical terminology is used to document patient care. Complete the terminology and analysis sections for each activity to help you recognize and understand terms related to the digestive system.

Medical Record Activity 6-1
Chart Note: GI Evaluation

Terminology

Terms listed below come from the medical report *Chart Note: GI Evaluation* that follows. Use a medical dictionary such as *Taber's Cyclopedic Medical Dictionary*, the appendices of this book, or other resources to define each term. Then review the pronunciations for each term and practice by reading the medical record aloud.

Term	Definition
appendectomy* ăp-ĕn-DĔK-tō-mē	
cholecystectomy kō-lē-sĭs-TĔK-tō-mē	
cholecystitis kō-lē-sĭs-TĪ-tĭs	
cholelithiasis* kō-lē-lĭ-THĪ-ă-sĭs	
crescendo kră-SHĔN-dō	
decrescendo dā-kră-SHĔN-dō	
defecate DĔF-ĕ-kāt	
flatus FLĀ-tŭs	
heme-negative stool hēm-NĔG-ă-tĭv	
hepatomegaly hĕp-ă-tō-MĔG-ă-lē	
intermittent ĭn-tĕr-MĬT-ĕnt	
nausea NAW-sē-ă	

Term	Definition
PMH	
postoperative pōst-ŎP-ĕr-ă-tĭv	
R/O	
splenomegaly splē-nō-MĔG-ă-lē	
tonsillectomy tōn-sĭl-ĔK-tō-mē	

*Refer to Figure 6–5 and Figure 6–8 for a visual illustration of these terms.

 Listen and Learn Online! *will help you master pronunciations of selected medical words from this medical record activity. Visit* www.davisplus.com/gylys/systems *to find instructions on completing the* Listen and Learn Online! *exercise for this section and then to practice pronunciations.*

CHART NOTE: GI EVALUATION

Jones, Roberta
March 15, 20xx

Age: 50

HISTORY OF PRESENT ILLNESS: Patient's abdominal pain began 2 years ago when she first had intermittent, sharp epigastric pain. Each episode lasted 2 to 4 hours. Eventually, she was diagnosed as having cholecystitis with cholelithiasis and underwent cholecystectomy. Three to five large calcified stones were found.

POSTOPERATIVE COURSE: Her postoperative course was uneventful until 4 months ago when she began having continuous deep right-sided pain. This pain followed a crescendo pattern and peaked several weeks ago, at a time when family stress was also at its climax. Since then, the pain has been following a decrescendo pattern. It does not cause any nausea or vomiting, does not trigger any urge to defecate, and is not alleviated by passage of flatus. Her PMH is significant only for tonsillectomy, appendectomy, and the cholecystectomy. Her PE findings indicated that there was no hepatomegaly or splenomegaly. The rectal examination confirmed normal sphincter tone and heme-negative stool.

IMPRESSION: Abdominal pain. Rule out hepatomegaly and splenomegaly.

PLAN: Schedule a complete barium workup for possible obstruction.

Juan Perez, MD
Juan Perez, MD

bcg

Analysis

Review the medical record *Chart Note: GI Evaluation* to answer the following questions.

1. While referring to Figure 6–3, describe the location of the gallbladder in relation to the liver.

_____

2. Why did the patient undergo the cholecystectomy?

_____

3. List the patient's prior surgeries.

_____

4. How does the patient's most recent postoperative episode of discomfort (pain) differ from the initial pain she described?

_____

Operative Report: Esophagogastroduodenoscopy with Biopsy

Terminology

Terms listed below come from the medical report *Operative Report: Esophagogastroduodenoscopy with Biopsy* that follows. Use a medical dictionary such as *Taber's Cyclopedic Medical Dictionary*, the appendices of this book, or other resources to define each term. Then review the pronunciations for each term and practice by reading the medical record aloud.

Term	Definition
Demerol DĔM-ĕr-ŏl	
duodenal bulb dū-ō-DĒ-năl bŭlb	
duodenitis dū-ŏd-ĕ-NĪ-tĭs	
erythema ĕr-ĭ-THĒ-mă	
esophageal varices ĕ-sŏf-ă-JĒ-ăl VĂR-ĭ-sēz	
esophagogastro-duodenoscopy ĕ-SŎF-ă-gō-GĂS-trō-doo-ō-dĕn-ŎS-kō-pē	
etiology ē-tē-ŎL-ō-jē	
friability frī-ă-BĬL-ĭ-tē	
gastric antrum GĂS-trĭk ĂN-trŭm	
gastritis găs-TRĪ-tĭs	
hematemesis hĕm-ăt-ĔM-ĕ-sĭs	
lateral recumbent LĂT-ĕr-ăl rē-KŬM-bĕnt	
oximeter ŏk-SĬM-ĕ-tĕr	
punctate erythema PŬNK-tāt ĕr-ĭ-THĒ-mă	

Term	Definition
tomography tŏ-MŎG-ră-fē	
Versed VĔR-sĕd	
videoendoscope vĭd-ē-ō-ĔND-ō-skōp	

 Listen and Learn Online! *will help you master pronunciations of selected medical words from this medical record activity. Visit* www.davisplus.com/gylys/systems *to find instructions on completing the* Listen and Learn Online! *exercise for this section and then to practice pronunciations.*

OPERATIVE REPORT: ESOPHAGOGASTRODUODENOSCOPY WITH BIOPSY

General Hospital

1511 Ninth Avenue　■■　**Sun City, USA 12345**　■■　**(555) 802-1887**

OPERATIVE REPORT

Date:　May 14, 20xx　　　　　Physician:　Dante Riox, MD
Patient:　Franks, Roberta　　　　Room:　　703

PREOPERATIVE DIAGNOSIS: Hematemesis of unknown etiology.

POSTOPERATIVE DIAGNOSIS: Diffuse gastritis and duodenitis.

PROCEDURE: Esophagogastroduodenoscopy with biopsy.

SPECIMEN: Biopsies from gastric antrum and duodenal bulb.

ESTIMATED BLOOD LOSS: Nil.

COMPLICATIONS: None.

TIME UNDER SEDATION: 20 minutes.

PROCEDURE AND FINDINGS: After obtaining informed consent regarding the procedure, its risks, and its alternatives, the patient was taken to the GI lab, where she was placed on the examining table in the left lateral recumbent position. She was given nasal oxygen at 3 liters per minute and monitored with a pulse oximeter throughout the procedure. Through a previously inserted intravenous line, the patient was sedated with a total of 50 mg of Demerol intravenously plus 4 mg of Midazolam intravenously throughout the procedure. The Fujinon computed tomography scan videoendoscope was then readily introduced and the following organs evaluated.

　Esophagus: The esophageal mucosa appeared normal throughout. No other abnormalities were seen. Specifically, there was prior evidence of esophageal varices.
　Stomach: There was diffuse erythema with old blood seen within the stomach. No ulcerations, erosions, or fresh bleeding was seen. A representative biopsy was obtained from the gastric antrum and submitted to the pathology laboratory.
　Duodenum: Punctate erythema was noted in the duodenal bulb. There was some friability. No ulcerations, erosions, or active bleeding was seen. A bulbar biopsy was obtained. The second portion of the duodenum appeared normal.

The patient tolerated the procedure well. Patient was transferred to the recovery room in stable condition.

Dante Riox, MD
Dante Riox, MD

dr:bg

D: 5-14-20xx
T: 5-14-20xx

Analysis

Review the medical report *Operative Report: Esophagogastroduodenoscopy with Biopsy* to answer the following questions.

1. What caused the hematemesis?

_____

2. What procedures were carried out to determine the cause of bleeding?

_____

3. How much blood did the patient lose during the procedure?

_____

4. Were there any ulcerations or erosions found during the exploratory procedure that might account for the bleeding?

_____

5. What type of sedation was used during the procedure?

_____

6. What did the doctors find when they examined the stomach and duodenum?

_____

Respiratory System

Chapter Outline

Objectives

Upon completion of this chapter, you will be able to:

- Locate and describe the structures of the respiratory system.

- Describe the functional relationship between the respiratory system and other body systems.

- Pronounce, spell, and build words related to the respiratory system.

- Describe pathological conditions, diagnostic and therapeutic procedures, and other terms related to the respiratory system.

- Explain pharmacology related to the treatment of respiratory disorders.

- Demonstrate your knowledge of this chapter by completing the learning and medical record activities.

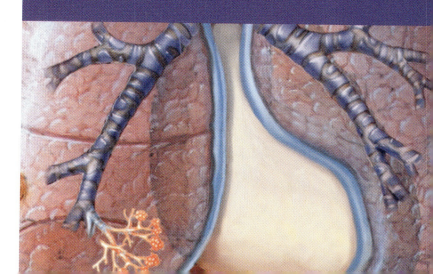

Anatomy and Physiology

The respiratory system is responsible for the exchange of **oxygen** (O_2) and **carbon dioxide** (CO_2). Oxygen is essential for life. It is carried to all cells of the body in exchange for CO_2, a waste product. The cardiovascular system helps in this vital function by providing blood vessels for carrying these gases.

Failure or deficiency in either system has the same effect on the body: disturbance of **homeostasis** and O_2 starvation in tissues that may cause death.

The lungs and airways bring in fresh, oxygen-enriched air and expel waste CO_2 by a process called *breathing,* or *ventilation.* Breathing helps regulate the **pH** (acidity-alkalinity) of the blood, thereby maintaining homeostasis.

Anatomy and Physiology Key Terms

This section introduces important respiratory system terms and their definitions. Word analyses for selected terms are also provided.

Term	Definition
carbon dioxide (CO_2) KĂR-bŏn dī-ŎK-sīd	Tasteless, colorless, odorless gas produced by body cells during the metabolic process *A product of cell respiration, CO_2 is carried by the blood to the lungs and exhaled.*
cartilage KĂR-tĭ-lĭj	Tough, elastic connective tissue that is more rigid than ligaments but less dense than bone *The tip of the nose and the outer ear are composed of cartilage.*
cilia SĬL-ē-ă	Any hairlike structure *Cilia in the trachea move particles upward to the pharynx, where they are removed by coughing, sneezing, or swallowing. This mechanism is called the cilia escalator. Habitual smoking destroys the cilia escalator.*
diffuse dĭ-FŪZ	Moving or spreading out of a substance at random, rather than by chemical reaction or application of external forces
homeostasis hŏ-mē-ō-STĀ-sĭs *homeo-:* same, alike *-stasis:* standing still	State in which the regulatory mechanisms of the body maintain a constant internal environment *The regulatory mechanisms of the body control temperature, acidity, and the concentration of salt, food, and waste products.*
mucous membrane MŪ-kŭs MĔM-brān *muc:* mucus *-ous:* pertaining to	Moist tissue layer lining hollow organs and cavities of the body that open to the environment; also called *mucosa*
oxygen (O_2) ŎK-sĭ-jĕn	Tasteless, odorless, colorless gas essential for human respiration *O_2 makes up about one fifth (by volume) of the atmosphere.*
pH	Symbol that indicates the degree of acidity or alkalinity of a substance *Increasing acidity is expressed as a number less than 7; increasing alkalinity as a number greater than 7, with 7 being neutral.*
septum SĔP-tŭm	Wall dividing two cavities, such as the nasal septum, which separates the two nostrils

Anatomy and Physiology Key Terms—cont'd

Term	Definition
serous membrane SĒR-ŭs MEM-brăn *ser:* serum *-ous:* pertaining to, relating to	Thin layer of tissue that covers internal body cavities, the cells of which secrete a fluid that keeps the membrane moist; also called *serosa*

Pronunciation Help	Long Sound	ā—rate	ē—rebirth	ī—isle	ō—over	ū—unite
	Short Sound	ă—lone	ĕ—ever	ĭ—it	ŏ—not	ŭ—cut

Upper Respiratory Tract

The breathing process begins with inhalation. (See Figure 7–1.) Air is drawn into the (1) **nasal cavity,** a chamber lined with mucous membranes and tiny hairs called *cilia* (singular, *cilium*). Here, air is filtered, heated, and moistened to prepare it for its journey to the lungs. The nasal cavity is divided into a right and left side by a vertical partition of cartilage called the *nasal* septum.

Olfactory neurons are receptors for the sense of smell. They are covered with a layer of mucus and located deep in the nasal cavity, embedded among the epithelial cells lining the nasal tract. Because they are located higher in the nasal passage than air normally travels during breathing, a person must sniff or inhale deeply to identify weak odors. Air passes from the nasal cavity to the throat (**pharynx**), a muscular tube that serves as a passageway for food and air. The pharynx consists of three sections: the (2) **nasopharynx,** posterior to the nose; the (3) **oropharynx,** posterior to the mouth; and the (4) **laryngopharynx,** superior to the larynx.

Within the nasopharynx is a collection of lymphoid tissue known as (5) **adenoids** (pharyngeal tonsils). The (6) **palatine tonsils,** more commonly known as *tonsils,* are located in the oropharynx. They protect the opening to the respiratory tract from microscopic organisms that may attempt entry by this route. The (7) **larynx** (voice box) contains the structures that make vocal sounds possible. A leaf-shaped structure on top of the larynx, the (8) **epiglottis,** seals off the air passage to the lungs during swallowing. This function ensures that food or liquids do not obstruct the flow of air to the lungs. The larynx is a short passage that joins the pharynx with the (9) **trachea** (windpipe). The trachea is composed of smooth muscle embedded with C-shaped rings of cartilage, which provide rigidity to keep the air passage open.

Lower Respiratory Tract

The trachea divides into two branches called (10) **bronchi** (singular, *bronchus*). One branch leads to the (11) **right lung** and the other to the (12) **left lung.** The inner walls of the trachea and bronchi are composed of mucous membrane (**mucosa**) embedded with cilia. This membrane traps incoming particles, and the cilia move the entrapped material upward into the pharynx, where it is coughed out, sneezed out, or swallowed. Like the trachea, bronchi contain C-shaped rings of cartilage.

Each bronchus divides into smaller and smaller branches, eventually forming (13) **bronchioles.** At the end of the bronchioles are tiny air sacs called (14) **alveoli** (singular, *alveolus*). An alveolus resembles a small balloon because it expands and contracts with inflow and outflow of air. The (15) **pulmonary capillaries** lie next to the thin tissue membranes of the alveoli. Carbon dioxide diffuses from the blood within the pulmonary capillaries and enters the alveolar spaces, while O_2 from the alveoli diffuses into the blood. After the exchange of gases, freshly oxygenated blood returns to the heart. It is now ready for delivery to all body tissues.

The lungs are divided into lobes: three lobes in the right lung and two lobes in the left lung. The space between the right and left lungs is called the (16) **mediastinum.** It contains the heart, aorta, esophagus, and bronchi. A serous membrane, the **pleura,** covers the lobes of the lungs and folds over to line the walls of the thoracic cavity. The membrane lying closest to the lung is the (17) **visceral pleura;** the membrane that lines the thoracic cavity is the (18) **parietal pleura.** The space between these two membranes is the (19) **pleural cavity.** It contains a small amount of lubricating fluid, which permits the visceral pleura to glide smoothly over the parietal pleura during breathing.

Ventilation depends on a pressure differential between the atmosphere and chest cavity. A large muscular partition, the (20) **diaphragm,** lies

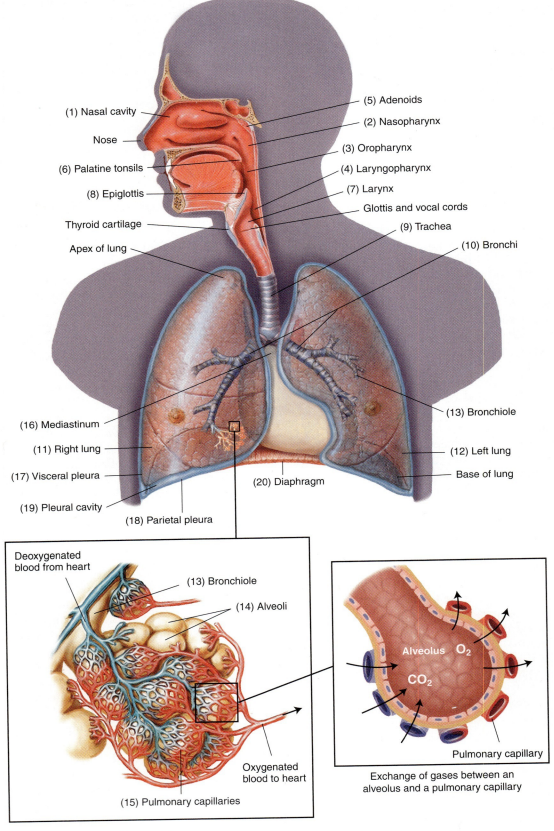

(1) Nasal cavity

(5) Adenoids

(2) Nasopharynx

Nose

(3) Oropharynx

(6) Palatine tonsils

(4) Laryngopharynx

(8) Epiglottis

(7) Larynx

Glottis and vocal cords

Thyroid cartilage

(9) Trachea

Apex of lung

(10) Bronchi

(16) Mediastinum

(13) Bronchiole

(11) Right lung

(12) Left lung

(17) Visceral pleura

Base of lung

(20) Diaphragm

(19) Pleural cavity

(18) Parietal pleura

Deoxygenated blood from heart

(13) Bronchiole

(14) Alveoli

Alveolus O_2

CO_2

Oxygenated blood to heart

Pulmonary capillary

(15) Pulmonary capillaries

Exchange of gases between an alveolus and a pulmonary capillary

Figure 7-1. Anterior view of the upper and lower respiratory tracts.

between the chest and abdominal cavities. The diaphragm assists in changing the volume of the thoracic cavity to produce the needed pressure differential for ventilation. When the diaphragm contracts, it partially descends into the abdominal cavity, thus decreasing the pressure within the chest and drawing air into the lungs (**inspiration**). When the diaphragm relaxes, it slowly reenters the thoracic cavity, thus increasing the pressure within the chest. As the pressure increases, air leaves the lungs (**expiration**). The intercostal muscles assist the diaphragm in changing the volume of the thoracic cavity by elevating and lowering the rib cage. (See Figure 7–2.)

Respiration

Respiration is the overall process by which O_2 is taken from air and carried to body cells for their use, while CO_2 and water, the waste products gen-

erated by these cells, are returned to the environment. Respiration includes four separate processes:

- **pulmonary ventilation,** more commonly called *breathing,* which is a largely involuntary action that moves air into (**inspiration**) and out of (**expiration**) the lungs in response to changes in blood O_2 and CO_2 levels and nervous stimulation of the diaphragm and intercostal muscles
- **external respiration,** which is the exchange of oxygen and carbon dioxide between the alveoli and the blood in the pulmonary capillaries
- **transport of respiratory gases,** which occurs when blood, aided by the cardiovascular system, transports CO_2 to the lungs and O_2 to body cells
- **internal respiration,** which is the exchange of O_2 and CO_2 between body cells and the blood in systemic capillaries.

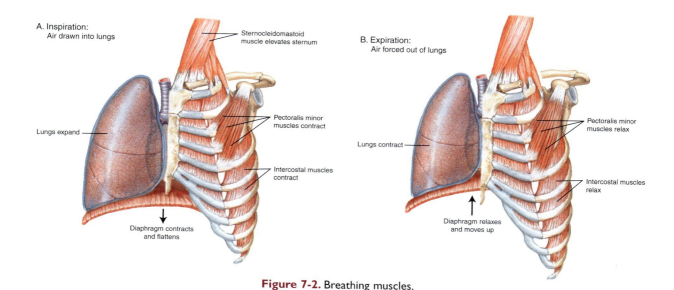

A. Inspiration:
Air drawn into lungs

Sternocleidomastoid muscle elevates sternum

Lungs expand

Pectoralis minor muscles contract

Intercostal muscles contract

Diaphragm contracts and flattens

B. Expiration:
Air forced out of lungs

Lungs contract

Pectoralis minor muscles relax

Intercostal muscles relax

Diaphragm relaxes and moves up

Figure 7-2. Breathing muscles.

Connecting Body Systems–Respiratory System

The main function of the respiratory system is to provide oxygen to the entire body and expel carbon dioxide from the body. Specific functional relationships between the respiratory system and other body systems are summarized below.

Blood, lymph, and immune
- Tonsils, adenoids, and other immune structures in the respiratory tract protect against pathogens that enter through respiratory passageways.

Cardiovascular
- Respiratory system provides O_2 and removes CO_2 from cardiac tissue.

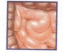

Digestive
- Respiratory system provides O_2 needed for digestive functions.
- Respiratory system removes CO_2 produced by the organs of digestion.
- Respiratory and digestive system share a common anatomic structure.

(continued)

Connecting Body Systems–Respiratory System—cont'd

Endocrine
- Respiratory system helps maintain a stable pH required for proper functioning of the endocrine glands.

Female reproductive
- Respiration rate increases in response to sexual activity.
- Fetal respiration occurs during pregnancy.

Genitourinary
- Respiratory system supplies O_2 and removes CO_2 to maintain proper functioning of urinary structures.
- Respiratory system helps maintain pH for gonadal hormone function.
- Respiratory system assists the urinary structures in regulating pH by removing CO_2.

Integumenary
- Respiratory system furnishes O_2 and disposes of CO_2 to maintain healthy skin.

Musculoskeletal
- Respiratory system provides O_2 for muscle contraction.
- Respiratory system eliminates CO_2 produced by muscles.
- Respiratory system provides O_2 for bone development.

Nervous
- Respiratory system provides O_2 for brain, spinal cord, and sensory organ functions.
- Respiratory system helps maintain a stable pH for neural function.

 It is time to review respiratory structures by completing Learning Activity 7–1.

Medical Word Elements

This section introduces combining forms, suffixes, and prefixes related to the respiratory system. Word analyses are also provided.

Element	Meaning	Word Analysis
Combining Forms		
Upper Respiratory Tract		
nas/o	nose	**nas**/al (NĀ-zl): pertaining to the nose *-al:* pertaining to
rhin/o		**rhin/o**/plasty (RĬ-nō-plăs-tē): surgical repair of the nose *-plasty:* surgical repair *Rhinoplasty is performed to correct birth defects or for cosmetic purposes.*
sept/o	septum	**sept/o**/plasty (SĔP-tō-plăs-tē): surgical repair of the septum *-plasty:* surgical repair *Septoplasty is commonly performed to correct a deviated septum.*
sinus/o	sinus, cavity	**sinus/o**/tomy (sī-nŭs-ŎT-ō-mē): incision of any of the sinuses *-tomy:* incision *Sinusotomy is performed to improve ventilation or drainage in unresponsive sinusitis.*
adenoid/o	adenoids	**adenoid**/ectomy (ăd-ĕ-noyd-ĔK-tō-mē): excision of adenoids *-ectomy:* excision, removal

Medical Word Elements—cont'd

Element	Meaning	Word Analysis
tonsill/o	tonsils	peri/**tonsill**/ar (pĕr-ĭ-TŎN-sĭ-lăr): pertaining to (the area) around the tonsils *peri-:* around *-ar:* pertaining to
pharyng/o	pharynx (throat)	**pharyng**/o/scope (făr-ĬN-gō-skōp): instrument for examining the pharynx *-scope:* instrument for examining
epiglott/o	epiglottis	**epiglott**/itis (ĕp-ĭ-glŏt-Ī-tĭs): inflammation of the epiglottis *-itis:* inflammation *Because the epiglottis seals the passageway traveled by air to and from the lungs, inflammation can lead to severe airway obstruction and death. Epiglottitis is treated as a medical emergency.*
laryng/o	larynx (voice box)	**laryng**/o/plegia (lă-rĭn-gō-PLĒ-jē-ă): paralysis of the (vocal cords and) larynx *-plegia:* paralysis
trache/o	trachea (windpipe)	**trache**/o/plasty (TRĀ-kē-ō-plăs-tē): surgical repair of the trachea *-plasty:* surgical repair *Tracheoplasty is performed to correct a narrow or stenotic trachea.*
Lower Respiratory Tract		
bronchi/o	bronchus (plural, bronchi)	**bronchi**/ectasis (brŏng-kē-ĔK-tă-sĭs): dilation of (one or more) bronchi *-ectasis:* dilation, expansion *Bronchiectasis is associated with various lung conditions and is commonly accompanied by chronic infection.*
bronch/o		**bronch**/o/scope (BRŎNG-kō-skōp): instrument for examining the bronchus or bronchi *-scope:* instrument for examining *A bronchoscope is a flexible tube that is passed through the nose or mouth and enables inspection of the lungs and collection of tissue biopsies and secretions for analysis.*
bronchiol/o	bronchiole	**bronchiol**/itis (brŏng-kē-ō-LĪ-tĭs): inflammation of the bronchioles *-itis:* inflammation
alveol/o	alveolus; air sac	**alveol**/ar (ăl-VĒ-ō-lăr): pertaining to the alveoli *-ar:* pertaining to
pleur/o	pleura	**pleur**/o/centesis (ploo-rō-sĕn-TĒ-sĭs): surgical puncture of the pleural cavity; also called *thoracocentesis* or *thoracentesis* *-centesis:* surgical puncture
pneum/o	air; lung	**pneum**/ectomy (nūm-ĔK-tō-mē): excision of (all or part of) a lung *-ectomy:* excision
pneumon/o		**pneumon**/ia (nū-MŌ-nē-ă): condition of inflammation of the lungs *-ia:* condition *The usual causes of pneumonia are infections due to bacteria, viruses, or other pathogenic organisms.*

(continued)

Medical Word Elements—cont'd

Element	Meaning	Word Analysis
pulmon/o	lung	**pulmon/o/logist** (pŭl-mŏ-NŎL-ŏ-jĭst): specialist in the study (and treatment) of lungs (and respiratory diseases) *-logist:* specialist in the study of
Other		
anthrac/o	coal, coal dust	**anthrac/osis** (ăn-thră-KŌ-sĭs): abnormal condition of coal dust (in the lungs) *-osis:* abnormal condition; increase (used primarily with blood cells) *Anthracosis is a chronic occupational disease found in coal miners and those associated with the coal industry.*
atel/o	incomplete; imperfect	**atel/ectasis** (ăt-ĕ-LĔK-tă-sĭs): incomplete expansion of the lung; also called *airless lung* or *collapsed lung* *-ectasis:* dilation, expansion
coni/o	dust	pneum/o/**coni**/osis (nū-mō-kō-nē-Ō-sĭs): condition of dust in the lungs *pneum/o:* air; lung *-osis:* abnormal condition; increase (used primarily with blood cells) *Pneumoconiosis is usually caused by mineral dusts of occupational or environmental origin. Forms of pneumoconiosis include silicosis, asbestosis, and anthracosis.*
cyan/o	blue	**cyan/osis** (sī-ă-NŌ-sĭs): abnormal condition of blueness *-osis:* abnormal condition; increase (used primarily with blood cells) *Cold temperatures, heart failure, lung diseases, and smothering cause unusual blueness of the skin and mucous membranes due to the build-up of carbon dioxide in the blood.*
lob/o	lobe	**lob/ectomy** (lō-BĔK-tō-mē): excision of a lobe *-ectomy:* excision *Lobectomies are performed when a malignancy is confined to a single lobe of any lobed organ, such as the lungs, liver, brain, and thyroid gland.*
orth/o	straight	**orth/o/pnea** (or-THŎP-nē-ă): breathing in a straight (or upright position) *-pnea:* breathing *Various lung disorders cause a patient to experience difficulty breathing in any position other than sitting or standing erect.*
ox/i	oxygen	**ox/i/meter** (ŏk-SĬM-ĕ-tĕr): instrument used for measuring oxygen *-meter:* instrument for measuring *An oximeter is usually attached to the tip of a finger but may also be placed on a toe or ear lobe. It provides a measurement of the oxygen saturation level of the blood.*
ox/o		hyp/**ox**/emia (hī-pŏks-Ē-mē-ă): deficiency of oxygen in blood *hyp-:* under, below, deficient *-emia:* blood condition
pector/o	chest	**pector/algia** (pĕk-tō-RĂL-jē-ă): pain in the chest; also called thoracalgia, *thoracodynia,* and *pectorodynia* *-algia:* pain
steth/o		**steth/o/scope** (STĔTH-ō-skōp): instrument used for examining the chest *-scope:* instrument for examining *A stethoscope enables evaluation of sounds in the chest as well as the abdomen.*

Medical Word Elements—cont'd

Element	Meaning	Word Analysis
thorac/o		**thorac/o**/pathy (thō-răk-ŎP-ă-thē): disease of the chest -*pathy:* disease
phren/o	diaphragm; mind	**phren/o**/spasm (FRĔN-ō-spăzm): involuntary contraction of the diaphragm -*spasm:* involuntary contraction, twitching
spir/o	breathe	**spir/o**/meter (spī-RŎM-ĕt-ĕr): instrument for measuring breathing -*meter:* instrument for measuring *A spirometer measures how much air the lungs can hold (vital capacity) as well as how much and how quickly air can be exhaled.*

Suffixes

Element	Meaning	Word Analysis
-capnia	carbon dioxide (CO_2)	hyper/**capnia** (hī-pĕr-KĂP-nē-ă): excessive CO_2 *hyper-:* excessive, above normal
-osmia	smell	an/**osmia** (ăn-ŎZ-mē-ă): without (the sense of) smell *an-:* without, not
-phonia	voice	dys/**phonia** (dĭs-FŌ-nē-ă): bad (impaired) voice quality *dys-:* bad; painful; difficult *Dysphonia includes hoarseness, voice fatigue, or decreased projection.*
-pnea	breathing	a/**pnea** (ăp-NĒ-ă): not breathing *a-:* without, not *Apnea is a temporary loss of breathing and includes sleep apnea, cardiac apnea, and apnea of the newborn.*
-ptysis	spitting	hem/o/**ptysis** (hē-MŎP-tĭ-sĭs): (coughing up or) spitting of blood *hem/o:* blood *Bloody sputum is usually a sign of a serious condition of the lungs.*
-thorax	chest	py/o/**thorax** (pī-ō-THŌ-răks): pus in the chest (cavity); also called *empyema* *py/o:* pus *Pyothorax is usually caused by a penetrating chest wound or spreading of infection from another part of the body.*

Prefixes

Element	Meaning	Word Analysis
brady-	slow	**brady**/pnea (brăd-ĭp-NĒ-ă): slow breathing -*pnea:* breathing
dys-	bad; painful; difficult	**dys**/pnea (dĭsp-NĒ-ă): difficult breathing -*pnea:* breathing *Dyspnea includes any discomfort or significant breathlessness.*
eu-	good, normal	**eu**/pnea (ūp-NĒ-ă): normal breathing -*pnea:* breathing *The normal range for a resting adult respiratory rate is 12 to 20 breaths/minute.*
tachy-	rapid	**tachy**/pnea (tăk-ĭp-NĒ-ă): rapid breathing -*pnea:* breathing

 It is time to review word elements by completing Learning Activity 7–2. For audio pronunciations of the above-listed key terms, you can visit www.davisplus.fadavis.com/gylys/systems *to download this chapter's* Listen and Learn! *exercises or use the book's audio CD (if included).*

Pathology

Common signs and symptoms of many respiratory disorders include cough (dry or productive), chest pain, altered breathing patterns, shortness of breath (SOB), cyanosis, and fever. Many disorders of the respiratory system, including bronchitis and emphysema, begin as an acute problem but become chronic over time. Chronic respiratory diseases are usually difficult to treat. Their damaging effects are commonly irreversible.

For diagnosis, treatment, and management of respiratory disorders, the medical services of a specialist may be warranted. **Pulmonology** is the medical specialty concerned with disorders of the respiratory system. The physician who treats these disorders is called a *pulmonologist*.

Chronic Obstructive Pulmonary Disease

Chronic obstructive pulmonary disease (COPD) includes respiratory disorders that produce a chronic partial obstruction of the air passages. The patient finds it difficult to breath (**dyspnea**) especially upon exertion and usually exhibits a chronic cough. The three major disorders included in COPD are asthma, chronic bronchitis, and emphysema. (See Figure 7–3.)

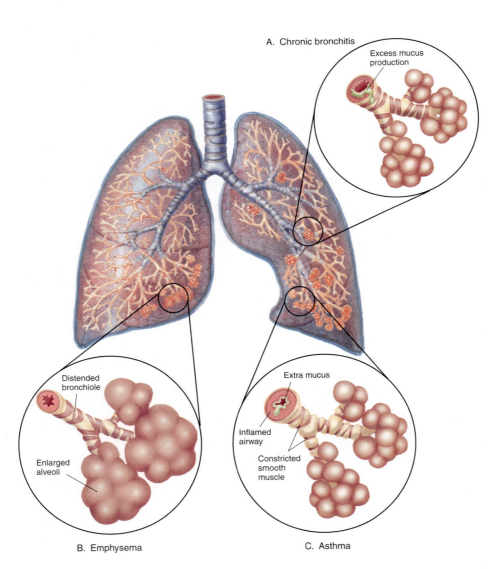

A. Chronic bronchitis

Excess mucus production

Distended bronchiole

Enlarged alveoli

B. Emphysema

Extra mucus

Inflamed airway

Constricted smooth muscle

C. Asthma

Figure 7-3. COPD. (A) Chronic bronchitis with inflamed airways and excessive mucus. (B) Emphysema with distended bronchioles and alveoli. (C) Asthma with narrowed bronchial tubes and swollen mucous membranes.

Asthma

Asthma produces spasms in the bronchial passages (**bronchospasms**) that may be sudden and violent (**paroxysmal**) and lead to dyspnea. Asthma is commonly caused by exposure to allergens or irritants. Other causes include stress, cold, and exercise. During recovery, coughing episodes produce large amounts of mucus (**productive cough**). Over time, the epithelium of the bronchial passages thickens, and breathing becomes more difficult. Treatment includes agents that loosen and break down mucus (**mucolytics**) and medications that expand the bronchi (**bronchodilators**) by relaxing their smooth muscles. If usual measures do not reverse the bronchospasms, the condition is referred to as *status asthmaticus.*

Chronic Bronchitis

Chronic bronchitis is an inflammation of the bronchi caused mainly by smoking and air pollution. However, other agents, such as viruses and bacteria may also cause the disorder. Bronchitis is characterized by swelling of the mucosa and a heavy, productive cough, commonly accompanied by chest pain. Patients usually seek medical help when they suffer exercise intolerance, wheezing, and shortness of breath (SOB). Bronchodilators and medications that aid in the removal of mucus (**expectorants**) help to widen air passages. Steroids may be prescribed if the disease progresses or becomes chronic.

Emphysema

Emphysema is characterized by decreased elasticity of the alveoli. The alveoli expand (**dilate**) but are unable to contract to their original size. The air that remains trapped in the chest results in a characteristic "barrel-chested" appearance. This disease commonly occurs with another respiratory disorder, such as asthma, tuberculosis, or chronic bronchitis. It is also found in long-term heavy smokers. Most emphysema sufferers find it easier to breathe when sitting upright or standing erect (**orthopnea**). As the disease progresses, relief even in the orthopneic position is not possible. Treatment for emphysema is similar to that of chronic bronchitis.

Influenza

Influenza (flu) is an acute infectious respiratory viral disease. Three major viral types are responsible: type A, type B, and type C. Type A is of primary concern because it is associated with worldwide epidemics (**pandemics**) and its causative organism is highly infectious (**virulent**). Influenza type A epidemics occur about every 2 to 3 years. Type B is usually limited geographically and tends to be less severe than type A. Both viruses undergo antigenic changes; consequently, new vaccines must be developed in anticipation of outbreaks. Type C is a mild flu and is not associated with epidemics.

The onset of the flu is usually rapid. Symptoms include fever, chills, headache, generalized muscle pain (**myalgia**), and loss of appetite, but recovery occurs in about 7 to 10 days. The flu virus rarely causes death. If death occurs, it is usually the result of a secondary pneumonia caused by bacteria or viruses that invade the lungs. Children should not use aspirin for relief of symptoms caused by viruses because there appears to be a relationship between Reye syndrome and the use of aspirin by children 2 to 15 years of age.

Pleural Effusions

Any abnormal fluid in the pleural cavity, the space between the visceral and parietal pleura, is called a *pleural effusion.* Normally, the pleural cavity contains only a small amount of lubricating fluid. However, some disorders may cause excessive fluid to collect in the pleural cavity. Two initial techniques used to diagnose pleural effusion are auscultation and percussion. **Auscultation** is the listening of sounds made by organs of the body using a stethoscope. **Percussion** is the gentle tapping the chest with the fingers and listening to the resultant sounds to determine the position, size, or consistency of the underlying structures. Chest x-ray (CXR) or magnetic resonance imaging (MRI) confirms the diagnosis.

Effusions are classified as transudates and exudates. A **transudate** is a noninflammatory fluid that resembles serum but with slightly less protein. It results from an imbalance in venous-arterial pressure or decrease of protein in blood. Both of these conditions allow serum to leak from the vascular system and collect in the pleural space. Common causes include left ventricular heart failure and liver disorders. An **exudate** is usually high in protein and often contains blood and immune cells. Common causes include tumors, infections, and inflammation. Various types of pleural effusions include serum (**hydrothorax**), pus (**empyema** or **pyothorax**), and blood (**hemothorax**). Although not considered a pleural effusion, air can enter the pleural space (**pneumothorax**), resulting in a partial or complete collapse of a lung. (See Figure 7–4.)

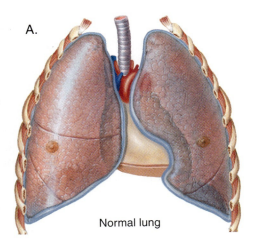

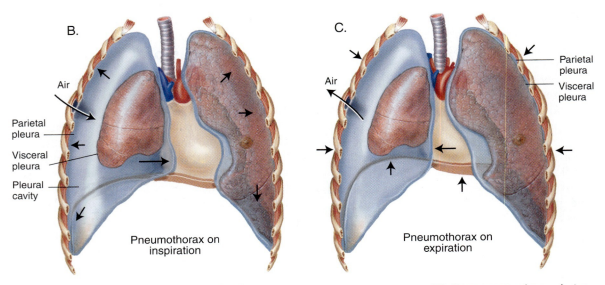

Figure 7-4. Pneumothorax. (A) Normal. (B) Open pneumothorax during inspiration. (C) Open pneumothorax during expiration.

Treatment consists of correcting the underlying cause of the effusion. Often a surgical puncture of the chest using a hollow-bore needle (**thoracocentesis, thoracentesis**) is undertaken to remove excess fluid for diagnostic or therapeutic purposes. (See Figure 7–5.) Sometimes chest tubes are inserted to drain fluid or remove air in pneumothorax.

Tuberculosis

Tuberculosis (TB) is a communicable disease caused by the bacterium *Mycobacterium tuberculosis*. TB spreads by droplets of respiratory secretions (**droplet nuclei**) from an infected individual when he/she coughs, laughs, or sneezes. The waxy coat of the TB organism keeps it alive (**viable**) and infec-

tious for 6 to 8 months outside the body. It also makes laboratory staining of this organism more challenging. Hence TB is also known as the *acid-fast bacillus* (AFB), a reference to its more complex method of laboratory staining.

The first time the TB organism enters the body (**primary tuberculosis**), the disease develops slowly. It eventually produces typical inflammatory nodules (**granulomas**) called *tubercles*. These granulomas usually remain dormant for years, during which time the patient is asymptomatic. When the immune system becomes impaired (**immunocompromised**) or when the patient is reexposed to the bacterium, a full-blown disease may develop.

Although primarily a lung disease, TB can infect the bones, genital tract, meninges, and peritoneum.

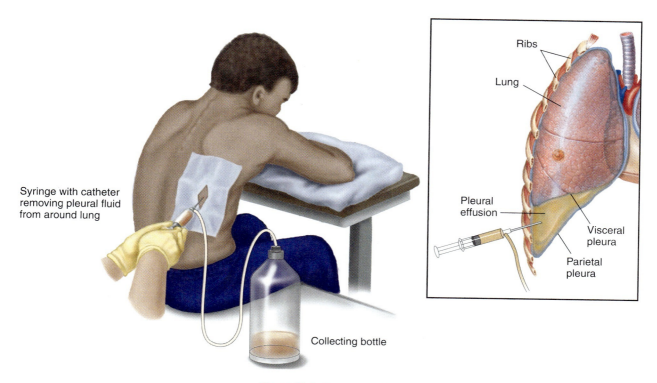

Syringe with catheter
removing pleural fluid
from around lung

Collecting bottle

Ribs

Lung

Pleural
effusion

Visceral
pleura

Parietal
pleura

Figure 7-5. Thoracentesis.

Some TB strains that infect AIDS patients have become resistant and do not respond to standard medications. Treatment may include using several antibiotics (**combination therapy**) at the same time.

Pneumonia

Pneumonia is any inflammatory disease of the lungs that may be caused by bacteria, viruses, or fungi. Chemicals or other agents can cause the lungs to become inflamed. A type of pneumonia associated with influenza is sometimes fatal. Other potentially fatal pneumonias may result from food or liquid inhalation (**aspiration pneumonias**). Some pneumonias affect only a lobe of the lung (**lobar pneumonia**), but some are more diffuse (**bronchopneumonia**). Chest pain, mucopurulent sputum, and spitting of blood (**hemoptysis**) are common signs and symptoms of the disease. If the air in the lungs is replaced by fluid and inflammatory debris, the lung tissue looses its spongy texture and become swollen and engorged (**consolidation**). Consolidation is associated primarily with bacterial pneumonias, not viral pneumonias.

Pneumocystis carinii pneumonia (PCP) is a type of pneumonia closely associated with AIDS. Recent evidence suggests that it is caused by a fungus that resides in or on most people (**normal flora**) but causes no harm as long as the individual remains healthy. When the immune system begins to fail, this organism becomes infectious (**opportunistic**). Diagnosis relies on examination of biopsied lung tissue or bronchial washings (**lavage**).

Cystic Fibrosis

Cystic fibrosis is a hereditary disorder of the exocrine glands that causes the body to secrete extremely thick (**viscous**) mucus. This thickened mucus clogs ducts of the pancreas and digestive tract. As a result, digestion is impaired and the patient may suffer from malnutrition. It also blocks ducts of the sweat glands, causing the skin to become highly "salty." In the lungs, mucus blocks airways and impedes natural disease-fighting mechanisms, causing repeated infections. Medication in the form of mists (**aerosols**) along with postural drainage provide relief.

An important diagnostic test called the *sweat test* measures the amount of salt excreted in sweat. When elevated, it indicates cystic fibrosis. Although the disease is fatal, improved methods of treatment have extended life expectancy, and patient survival is approximately 30 years.

Acute Respiratory Distress Syndrome

Acute respiratory distress syndrome (ARDS) is a condition in which the lungs no longer function effectively, threatening the life of the patient. It usually occurs as a result of very serious lung conditions, such as trauma, severe pneumonia, and other major infections that affect the entire body (**systemic infections**) or blood (**sepsis**). In ARDS, the alveoli fill with fluid (**edema**) caused by inflammation, and then collapse, making oxygen exchange impossible. Mechanical ventilation is commonly required to save the life of the patient.

Hyaline membrane disease (HMD), sometimes called *infant respiratory distress syndrome (IRDS)*, is a form of respiratory distress syndrome. It is most commonly seen in preterm infants or infants born to diabetic mothers. It is caused by insufficient **surfactant,** a phospholipid substance that helps keep alveoli open. With insufficient surfactant, the alveoli collapse and breathing becomes labored. Clinical signs may include blueness (**cyanosis**) of the extremities. Flaring of the nostrils (**nares**) and central cyanosis are typically present. Other signs include rapid breathing (**tachypnea**), intercostal retraction, and a characteristic grunt audible during exhalation. Radiography shows a membrane that has a ground-glass appearance (**hyaline membrane**), bilateral decrease in volume, and alveolar consolidation. Although severe cases of HMD result in death, some forms of therapy are effective.

Oncology

The most common form of lung cancer is bronchogenic carcinoma; also called *primary pulmonary cancer*. This cancer is usually associated with tobacco use. Cells of the bronchial epithelium divide repeatedly until the entire epithelium is involved. Within a short time, the epithelium begins to invade underlying tissues. As masses form, they block air passages and alveoli. Bronchogenic carcinoma spreads (**metastasizes**) rapidly to other areas of the body, including the lymph nodes, liver, bones, brain, and kidneys. Only about 10% of lung cancers are found in the early stages when the cure rate is high. Treatment of lung cancer includes surgery, radiation, and chemotherapy or a combination of these methods depending on specific cell type, how far the disease has spread, and the general health of the patient. Nevertheless, lung cancer is difficult to control and survival rates are very low.

Diagnostic, Symptomatic, and Related Terms

This section introduces diagnostic, symptomatic, and related terms and their meanings. Word analyses for selected terms are also provided.

Term	Definition
acidosis ăs-ĭ-DŌ-sĭs	Excessive acidity of body fluids *Respiratory acidosis is commonly associated with pulmonary insufficiency and the subsequent retention of carbon dioxide*
anosmia ăn-ŎZ-mē-ă *an-:* without, not *-osmia:* smell	Absence of the sense of smell *Anosmia usually occurs as a temporary condition resulting from an upper respiratory infection or a condition that causes intranasal swelling.*

Diagnostic, Symptomatic, and Related Terms—cont'd

Term	Definition

apnea
ăp-NĒ-ă
  a-: without, not
  -pnea: breathing

sleep

Temporary loss of breathing

There are three types of apnea: obstructive (enlarged tonsils and adenoids), central (failure of the brain to transmit impulses for breathing), and mixed (combination of obstructive and central apnea).
Sleeping disorder in which breathing stops repeatedly for more than 10 seconds, causing measurable blood deoxygenation. (See Figure 7-6.)

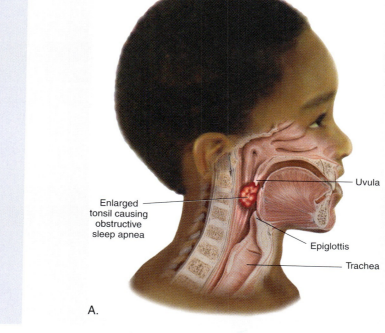

Uvula

Enlarged tonsil causing obstructive sleep apnea

Epiglottis

Trachea

A.

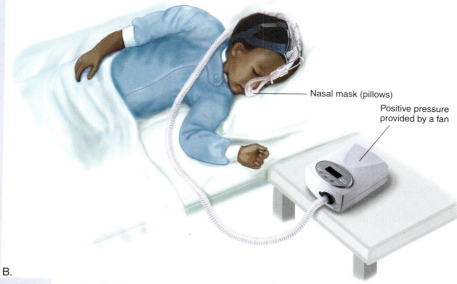

Nasal mask (pillows)

Positive pressure provided by a fan

B.

Figure 7-6. Sleep apnea. (A) Airway obstruction caused by enlarged tonsils, eventually leads to obstructive sleep apnea. (B) Continuous positive airway pressure (CPAP) machine used to treat sleep apnea.

(continued)

Diagnostic, Symptomatic, and Related Terms—cont'd

Term	Definition
asphyxia ăs-FĬK-sē-ă *a-:* without, not *-sphyxia:* pulse	Condition caused by insufficient intake of oxygen *Some common causes of asphyxia are drowning, electric shock, lodging of a foreign body in the respiratory tract, inhalation of toxic smoke, and poisoning.*
atelectasis ăt-ĕ-LĔK-tă-sĭs *atel:* incomplete; imperfect *-ectasis:* dilation, expansion	Collapsed or airless state of the lung, which may be acute or chronic and affect all or part of a lung *Atelectasis is a potential complication of some surgical procedures, especially those of the chest because breathing is commonly shallow after surgery to avoid pain from the surgical incision. In fetal atelectasis, the lungs fail to expand normally at birth.*
cheyne-Stokes respiration chān-stōks	Repeated breathing pattern characterized by fluctuation in the depth of respiration, first deeply, then shallow, then not at all *Cheyne-Stokes respirations are usually caused by diseases that affect the respiratory centers of the brain (such as heart failure and brain damage).*
compliance kŏm-PLĪ-ăns	Ease with which lung tissue can be stretched *Low compliance means lungs are less elastic; therefore, more effort is required to inflate the lungs.*
coryza kŏ-RĪ-ză	Head cold; upper respiratory infection (URI)
crackle KRĂK-ĕl	Abnormal respiratory sound heard on auscultation, caused by exudates, spasms, hyperplasia, or when air enters moisture-filled alveoli; also called *rale*
croup croop	Common childhood condition involving inflammation of the larynx, trachea, bronchial passages and, sometimes, lungs *Signs and symptoms include a resonant, barking cough with suffocative, difficult breathing; laryngeal spasms; and, sometimes, the narrowing of the top of the air passages.*
deviated nasal septum DĒ-vē-āt-ĕd NĀ-zl SĔP-tŭm	Displacement of cartilage dividing the nostrils
epiglottitis ĕp-ĭ-glŏt-Ī-tĭs *epiglott:* epiglottis *-itis:* inflammation	Severe, life-threatening infection of the epiglottis and supraglottic structures that occurs most commonly in children between 2 and 12 years of age *Signs and symptoms of epiglottitis include fever, dysphagia, inspiratory stridor, and severe respiratory distress. Intubation or tracheostomy may be required to open the obstructed airway.*
epistaxis ĕp-ĭ-STĂK-sĭs	Nosebleed; nasal hemorrhage
finger clubbing KLŬB-ĭng	Enlargement of the terminal phalanges of the fingers and toes, commonly associated with pulmonary disease
hypoxemia hī-pŏks-Ē-mē-ă *hyp-:* under, below, deficient *ox:* oxygen *-emia:* blood condition	Deficiency of oxygen in the blood *Hypoxemia is usually a sign of respiratory impairment.*

Diagnostic, Symptomatic, and Related Terms—cont'd

Term	Definition
hypoxia hī-PŎKS-ē-ă *hyp-:* under, below, deficient *-oxia:* oxygen	Deficiency of oxygen in tissues *Hypoxia is usually a sign of respiratory impairment.*
pertussis pĕr-TŬS-ĭs	Acute infectious disease characterized by a cough that has a "whoop" sound; also called *whooping* cough *Immunization of infants as part of the diphtheria-pertussis-tetanus (DPT) vaccination is effective in the prevention of pertussis.*
pleurisy PLOO-rĭs-ē *pleur:* pleura *-isy:* state of; condition	Inflammation of the pleural membrane characterized by a stabbing pain that is intensified by coughing or deep breathing; also called *pleuritis*
pneumoconiosis nū-mō-kō-nē-Ō-sĭs *pneum/o:* air; lung *coni:* dust *-osis:* abnormal condition; increase (used primarily with blood cells)	Disease caused by inhaling dust particles, including coal dust (anthracosis), stone dust (chalicosis), iron dust (siderosis), and asbestos particles (asbestosis)
pulmonary edema PŬL-mō-nĕ-rē ĕ-DĒ-mă *pulmon:* lung *-ary:* pertaining to	Accumulation of extravascular fluid in lung tissues and alveoli, caused most commonly by heart failure *Excessive fluid in the lungs induces coughing and dyspnea.*
pulmonary embolus PŬL-mō-nĕ-rē ĔM-bō-lŭs *pulmon:* lung *-ary:* pertaining to *embol:* plug *-us:* condition, structure	Blockage in an artery of the lungs caused by a mass of undissolved matter (such as a blood clot, tissue, air bubbles, and bacteria)
rhonchus RŎNG-kŭs	Abnormal breath sound heard on auscultation *A rhonchus is described as a course, rattling noise that resembles snoring, commonly suggesting secretions in the larger airways.*
stridor STRĪ-dor	High-pitched, harsh, adventitious breath sound caused by a spasm or swelling of the larynx or an obstruction in the upper airway *The presence of stridor requires immediate intervention.*
sudden infant death syndrome (SIDS)	Completely unexpected and unexplained death of an apparently normal, healthy infant, usually less than 12 months of age; also called *crib death* *The rate of SIDS has decreased more than 30% since parents have been instructed to place babies on their backs for sleeping rather than on their stomachs.*
wheeze HWĒZ	Whistling or sighing sound heard on auscultation that results from narrowing of the lumen of the respiratory passageway *Wheezing is a characteristic of asthma, croup, hay fever, obstructive emphysema, and other obstructive respiratory conditions.*

 It is time to review pathological, diagnostic, symptomatic, and related terms by completing Learning Activity 7–3.

Diagnostic and Therapeutic Procedures

This section introduces procedures used to diagnose and treat respiratory disorders. Descriptions are provided as well as pronunciations and word analyses for selected terms.

Procedure	Descripton
Diagnostic Procedures	
Clinical	
Mantoux test măn-TŪ	Intradermal test to determine tuberculin sensitivity based on a positive reaction where the area around the test site becomes red and swollen *A positive test suggests a past or present exposure to TB or past TB vaccination. However, the Mantoux test does not differentiate between active and inactive infection.*
oximetry ŏk-SĬM-ĕ-trē *ox/i:* oxygen *-metry:* act of measuring	Noninvasive method of monitoring the percentage of hemoglobin (Hb) saturated with oxygen; also called pulse oximetry *In oximetry, a probe is attached to the patient's finger or ear lobe and linked to a computer that displays the percentage of hemoglobin saturated with oxygen.*
polysomnography pŏl-ē-sŏm-NŎG-ră-fē *poly-:* many, much *somn/o:* sleep *-graphy:* process of recording	Test of sleep cycles and stages using continuous recordings of brain waves (EEGs), electrical activity of muscles, eye movement (electro-oculogram), respiratory rate, blood pressure, blood oxygen saturation, heart rhythm and, sometimes, direct observation of the person during sleep using a video camera
pulmonary function tests (PFTs) PŬL-mō-nĕ-rē *pulmon:* lung *-ary:* pertaining to	Multiple tests used to evaluate the ability of the lungs to take in and expel air as well as perform gas exchange across the alveolocapillary membrane
spirometry spī-RŎM-ĕ-trē *spir/o:* breathe *-metry:* act of measuring	Measurement of ventilatory ability by assessing lung capacity and flow, including the time necessary for exhaling the total volume of inhaled air *A spirometer produces a graphic record for placement in the patient's chart.*
Endoscopic	
bronchoscopy brŏng-KŎS-kō-pē *bronch/o:* bronchus *-scopy:* visual examination	Visual examination of the bronchi using an endoscope (flexible fiberoptic or rigid) inserted through the mouth and trachea for direct viewing of structures or for projection on a monitor (See Figure 7-7.) *Attachments on the bronchoscope can be used to suction mucus, remove foreign bodies, collect sputum, or perform biopsy.*
laryngoscopy lăr-ĭn-GŎS-kō-pē *laryng/o:* larynx (voice box) *-scopy:* visual examination	Visual examination of the larynx to detect tumors, foreign bodies, nerve or structural injury, or other abnormalities
mediastinoscopy mē-dē-ăs-tĭ-NŎS-kō-pē *mediastin/o:* mediastinum *-scopy:* visual examination	Visual examination of the mediastinal structures including the heart, trachea, esophagus, bronchus, thymus, and lymph nodes *The mediastinoscope is inserted through a small incision made above the sternum. The attached camera projects images on a monitor. Additional incisions may be made if nodes are removed or other diagnostic or therapeutic procedures are performed.*

Diagnostic and Therapeutic Procedures—cont'd

Procedure	Descripton

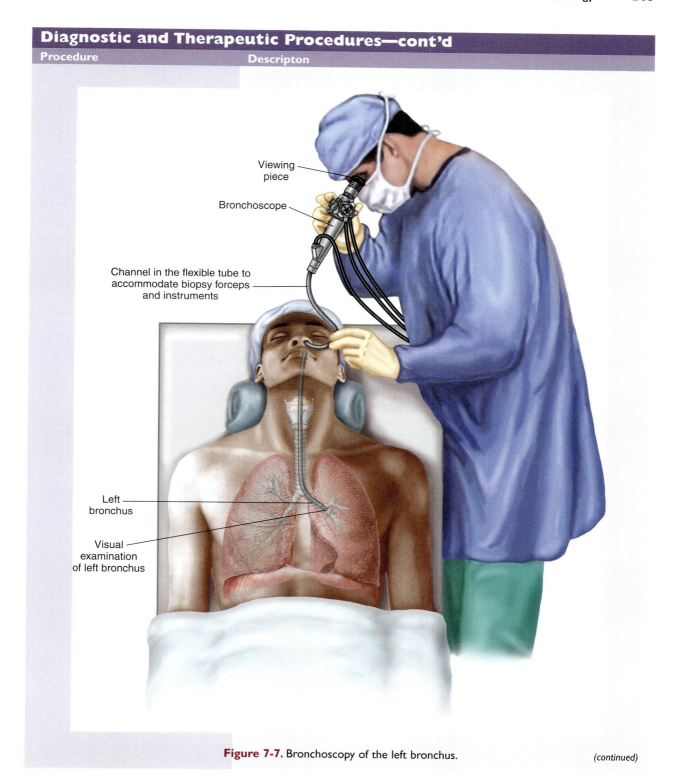

Viewing piece

Bronchoscope

Channel in the flexible tube to accommodate biopsy forceps and instruments

Left bronchus

Visual examination of left bronchus

Figure 7-7. Bronchoscopy of the left bronchus.

(continued)

Diagnostic and Therapeutic Procedures—cont'd

Procedure	Descripton
Laboratory	
arterial blood gas (ABG) ăr-TĒ-rē-ăl	Test that measures partial pressure of oxygen (Po_2), carbon dioxide (Pco_2), pH (acidity or alkalinity), and bicarbonate level of an arterial blood sample *ABG analysis evaluates pulmonary gas exchange and helps guide treatment of acid–base imbalances.*
sputum culture SPŪ-tŭm	Microbial test used to identify disease-causing organisms of the lower respiratory tract, especially those that cause pneumonias
sweat test	Measurement of the amount of salt (sodium chloride) in sweat *A sweat test is used almost exclusively in children to confirm cystic fibrosis.*
throat culture	Test used to identify pathogens, especially group A streptococci *Untreated streptococcal infections may lead to serious secondary complications, including kidney and heart disease.*
Radiographic	
radiography rā-dē-ŎG-ră-fē *radi/o:* radiation, x-ray; radius (lower arm bone on thumb side) *-graphy:* process of recording	Process of producing images using an x-ray passed through the body or area and captured on a film
thoracic (chest) thō-RĂS-ĭk *thorac:* chest *-ic:* pertaining to, relating to	Images of the chest taken from anteroposterior (AP) projection, posteroanterior (PA) projection, lateral projection, or a combination of these projections *Chest radiography is used to diagnose rib fractures and lung diseases, including atelectasis, masses, pneumonia, and emphysema.*
scan	Imaging procedure that gathers information about a specific organ or structure of the body. In some cases, small amounts of injected radionuclide (tracer) are used to enhance images
lung	Nuclear scanning test primarily used to detect pulmonary emboli *Lung scan is commonly performed to detect the presence of a blood clot that may be interfering with blood flow in or to the lung.*

Diagnostic and Therapeutic Procedures—cont'd

Procedure	Descripton

Therapeutic Procedures

Clinical

aerosol therapy
ĂR-ō-sŏl THĔR-ă-pē

Lung treatment using various techniques to deliver medication in mist form directly to the lungs or air passageways. Techniques include nebulizers, metered-dose inhalers (MDIs), and dry powder inhalers (DPIs)

Nebulizers change liquid medications into droplets to be inhaled through a mouthpiece. (See Figure 7-8.) MDIs deliver a specific amount when activated. Children and the elderly can use a spacer to synchronize inhalation with medication release. (See Figure 7-9.) A DPI is activated by a quick inhalation by the user.

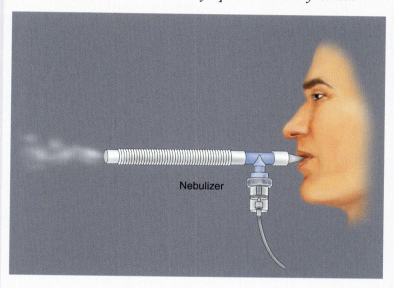

Nebulizer

Figure 7-8. Nebulizer.

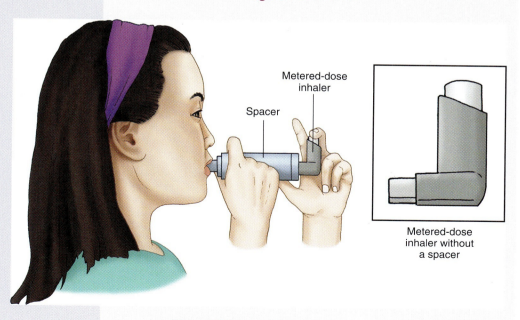

Spacer

Metered-dose inhaler

Metered-dose inhaler without a spacer

Figure 7-9. Metered-dose inhaler.

(continued)

Diagnostic and Therapeutic Procedures—cont'd

Procedure	Descripton
lavage lă-VĂZH	Irrigating or washing out of an organ, stomach, bladder, bowel, or body cavity with a stream of water or other fluid *Lavage of the paranasal sinuses is usually performed to remove mucopurulent material in an immunosuppressed patient or one with known sinusitis that has failed medical management.*
antral ĂN-trăl	Irrigation of the antrum (maxillary sinus) in chronic or nonresponsive sinusitis
postural drainage PŎS-tū-răl	Positioning a patient so that gravity aids in the drainage of secretions from the bronchi and lobes of the lungs
Surgical	
pleurectomy ploor-ĔK-tō-mē *pleur:* pleura *-ectomy:* excision, removal	Excision of part of the pleura, usually parietal *Pleurectomy is performed to reduce pain caused by a tumor mass or to prevent the recurrence of pleural effusion but is generally ineffective in the treatment of malignancy of the pleura.*
pneumectomy nūm-ĔK-tō-mē *pneum:* air; lung *-ectomy:* excision, removal	Excision of a lung *The removal of a lobe of the lung is called a **lobectomy***
rhinoplasty RĪ-nō-plăs-tē *rhin/o:* nose *-plasty:* surgical repair	Reconstructive surgery of the nose to correct deformities or for cosmetic purposes
septoplasty sĕp-tō-PLĂS-tē *sept/o:* septum *-plasty:* surgical repair	Surgical repair of a deviated nasal septum usually performed when the septum is encroaching on the breathing passages or nasal structures *Common complications of a deviated septum include interference with breathing and a predisposition to sinus infections.*
thoracentesis thō-ră-sĕn-TĒ-sĭs	Surgical puncture and drainage of the pleural cavity; also called *pleurocentesis* or *thoracocentesis* *Thoracentesis is performed as a diagnostic procedure to determine the nature and cause of an effusion or as a therapeutic procedure to relieve the discomfort caused by the effusion.* (See Figure 7–5.)
tracheostomy trā-kē-ŎS-tō-mē	Surgical procedure in which an opening is made in the neck and into the trachea into which a breathing tube may be inserted (See Figure 7–10.)

Diagnostic and Therapeutic Procedures—cont'd

Procedure	Descripton

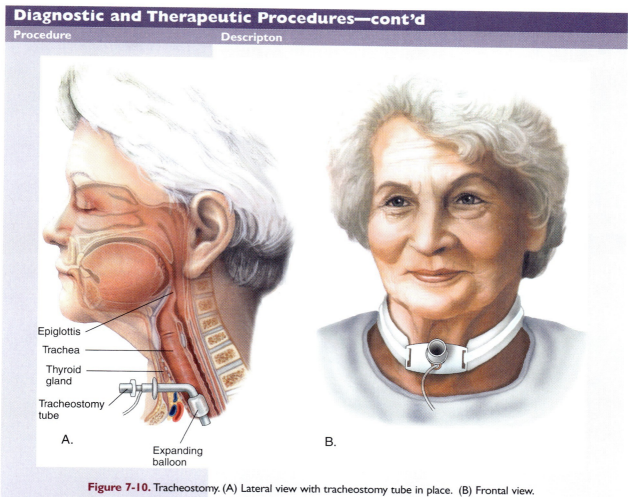

Epiglottis

Trachea

Thyroid gland

Tracheostomy tube

A.

Expanding balloon

B.

Figure 7-10. Tracheostomy. (A) Lateral view with tracheostomy tube in place. (B) Frontal view.

Pharmacology

In addition to antibiotics used to treat respiratory infections, there are several classes of drugs that treat pulmonary disorders. (See Table 7–1.) Bronchodilators are especially significant in the treatment of COPD and exercise-induced asthma. They relax smooth muscles of the bronchi, thus increasing airflow. Some bronchodilators are delivered as a fine mist directly to the airways via aerosol delivery devices, including nebulizers and metered-dose inhalers (MDIs). Another method of delivering medications directly to the lungs is dry-powder inhalers (DPIs) that dispense medications in the form of a powder. Steroidal and nonsteroidal anti-inflammatory drugs are important in the control and management of many pulmonary disorders.

Table 7-1	Drugs Used to Treat Respiratory Disorders

This table lists common drug classifications used to treat respiratory disorders, their therapeutic actions, and selected generic and trade names.

Classification	Therapeutic Action	Generic and Trade Names
antihistamines	Block histamines from binding with histamine receptor sites in tissues *Histamines cause sneezing, runny nose, itchiness, and rashes.*	**fexofenadine** fĕks-ō-FĔN-ă-dēn Allegra **loratadine** lor-ĂH-tă-dēn Claritin
antitussives	Relieve or suppress coughing by blocking the cough reflex in the medulla of the brain *Antitussives alleviate nonproductive dry coughs and should not be used with productive coughs.*	**hydrocodone** hī-drō-KŌ-dŏn Hycodan **dextromethorphan** dĕk-strō-MĔTH-or-făn Vicks Formula 44
bronchodilators	Stimulate bronchial muscles to relax, thereby expanding air passages, resulting in increased air flow *Bronchodilators are used to treat chronic symptoms and prevent acute attacks in respiratory diseases, such as asthma and COPD. Pharmacological agents may be delivered by an inhaler either orally or intravenously.*	**albuterol** ăl-BŪ-tĕr-ăl Proventil, Ventolin **salmeterol** săl-mē-TĔR-ŏl Serevent
corticosteroids	Act on the immune system by blocking production of substances that trigger allergic and inflammatory actions *Corticosteroids are available as nasal sprays, in metered-dose-inhalers (inhaled steroids) and in oral forms (pills or syrups) to treat chronic lung conditions such as asthma and COPD.*	**beclomethasone dipropionate** bĕ-klō-MĔTH-ă-sōn dī-PRŌ-pĕ-ō-năt Vanceril, Beclovent **triamcinolone** trī-ăm-SĬN-ō-lōn Azmacort
decongestants	Constrict blood vessels of nasal passages and limit blood flow, which causes swollen tissues to shrink so that air can pass more freely through the passageways *Decongestants are commonly prescribed for allergies and colds and are usually combined with antihistamines in cold remedies. They can be administered orally or topically as nasal sprays and nasal drops.*	**oxymetazoline** ŏks-ē-mĕt-ĂZ-ō-lēn Dristan **pseudoephedrine** soo-dō-ĕ-FĔD-rĭn Drixoral, Sudafed
expectorants	Liquify respiratory secretions so that they are more easily dislodged during coughing episodes *Expectorants are prescribed for productive coughs.*	**guaifenesin** gwī-FĔN-ĕ-sĭn Robitussin, Organidin

Abbreviations

This section introduces respiratory-related abbreviations and their meanings.

Abbreviation	Meaning	Abbreviation	Meaning
ABG	arterial blood gas(es)	MRI	magnetic resonance imaging
AFB	acid-fast bacillus (TB organism)	NMT	nebulized mist treatment
AP	anteroposterior	O_2	oxygen
ARDS	acute respiratory distress syndrome	PA	posteroanterior; pernicious anemia
CO_2	carbon dioxide	P_{CO_2}	partial pressure of carbon dioxide
COPD	chronic obstructive pulmonary disease	PCP	*Pneumocystis carinii* pneumonia; primary care physician; phencyclidine (hallucinogen)
CPAP	continuous positive airway pressure	PFT	pulmonary function test
CPR	cardiopulmonary resuscitation	pH	symbol for degree of acidity or alkalinity
CT	computed tomography	PND	paroxysmal nocturnal dyspnea
CXR	chest x-ray, chest radiograph	PO_2	partial pressure of oxygen
DPI	dry power inhaler	RD	respiratory distress
DPT	diphtheria, pertussis, tetanus	RDS	respiratory distress syndrome
EEG	encephalogram, encephalography	SaO_2	arterial oxygen saturation
FVC	forced vital capacity	SIDS	sudden infant death syndrome
Hb, Hgb	hemoglobin	SOB	shortness of breath
HMD	hyaline membrane disease	T&A	tonsillectomy and adenoidectomy
Hx	history	TB	tuberculosis
IPPB	intermittent positive-pressure breathing	TPR	temperature, pulse, and respiration
IRDS	infant respiratory distress syndrome	URI	upper respiratory infection
MDI	metered dose inhaler	VC	vital capacity

 It is time to review procedures, pharmacology, and abbreviations by completing Learning Activity 7–4.

LEARNING ACTIVITIES

The following activities provide review of the respiratory system terms introduced in this chapter. Complete each activity and review your answers to evaluate your understanding of the chapter.

Learning Activity 7-1
Identifying Respiratory Structures

Label the following illustration using the terms listed below.

adenoids	larynx	parietal pleura
alveoli	left lung	pleural cavity
bronchi	mediastinum	pulmonary capillaries
bronchiole	nasal cavity	right lung
diaphragm	nasopharynx	trachea
epiglottis	oropharynx	visceral pleura
laryngopharynx	palatine tonsils	

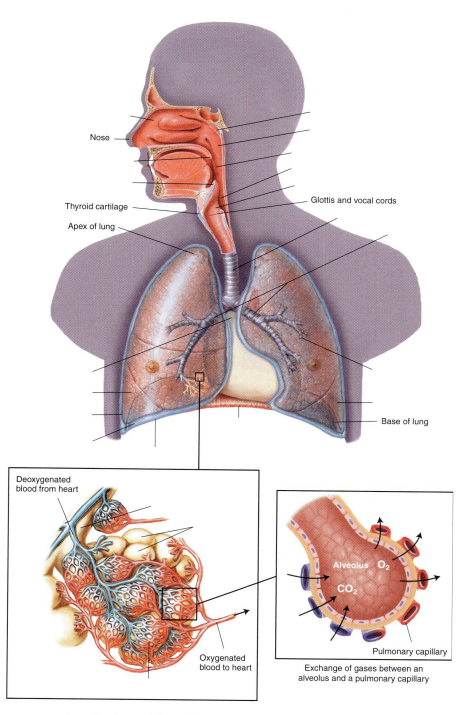

Nose

Thyroid cartilage

Apex of lung

Glottis and vocal cords

Base of lung

Deoxygenated
blood from heart

Oxygenated
blood to heart

Alveolus O$_2$

CO$_2$

Pulmonary capillary

Exchange of gases between an
alveolus and a pulmonary capillary

*Check your answers by referring to Figure 7–1 on page 150. Review material that you did
not answer correctly.*

 DavisPlus.fadavis.com

Enhance your study and reinforcement of word elements with the power of DavisPlus. Visit www.
davisplus.fadavis.com/gylys/systems *for this chapter's flash-card activity. We recommend you
complete the flash-card activity before completing activity 7–2 below.*

Learning Activity 7-2
Building Medical Words

Use *rhin/o* (nose) to build words that mean:

1. discharge from the nose _____
2. inflammation of (mucous membranes of the) nose _____

Use *laryng/o* (larynx [voice box]) to build words that mean:

3. visual examination of larynx _____
4. inflammation of larynx _____
5. stricture or narrowing of the larynx _____

Use *bronch/o* or *bronchi/o* (bronchus) to build words that mean:

6. dilation or expansion of the bronchus _____
7. disease of the bronchus _____
8. spasm of the bronchus _____

Use *pneumon/o* or *pneum/o* (air; lung) to build words that mean:

9. air in the chest (pleural space) _____
10. inflammation of lungs _____

Use *pulmon/o* (lung) to build words that mean:

11. specialist in lung (diseases) _____
12. pertaining to the lung _____

Use *-pnea* (breathing) to build words that mean:

13. difficult breathing _____
14. slow breathing _____
15. rapid breathing _____
16. absence of breathing _____

Build surgical words that mean:

17. surgical repair of the nose _____
18. surgical puncture of the chest _____
19. removal of a lung _____
20. forming an opening (mouth) in the trachea _____

✓ *Check your answers in Appendix A. Review material that you did not answer correctly.*

Correct Answers _____ × 5 = _____ % Score

Learning Activity 7-3
Matching Pathological, Diagnostic, Symptomatic, and Related Terms

Match the following terms with the definitions in the numbered list.

anosmia	consolidation	empyema	pneumoconiosis
apnea	coryza	epistaxis	pulmonary edema
atelectasis	crackle	hypoxemia	stridor
auscultation	deviated septum	pertussis	surfactant
compliance	emphysema	pleurisy	tubercles

1. _____ collapsed or airless lung
2. _____ pus in the pleural cavity
3. _____ phospholipid that allows the lungs to expand with ease
4. _____ loss of sponginess of lungs due to engorgement
5. _____ listening to the chest sounds using a stethoscope
6. _____ absence or decrease in the sense of smell
7. _____ deficiency of oxygen in the blood
8. _____ granulomas associated with tuberculosis
9. _____ temporary loss of breathing
10. _____ disease characterized by a decrease in alveolar elasticity
11. _____ ease with which lung tissue can be stretched
12. _____ nosebleed; nasal hemorrhage
13. _____ excessive fluid in the lungs that induces cough and dyspnea
14. _____ abnormal respiratory sound associated with exudates, spasms, or hyperplasia
15. _____ displacement of the cartilage dividing the nostrils
16. _____ head cold; upper respiratory infection
17. _____ condition in which dust particles are found in the lungs
18. _____ inflammation of the pleural membrane
19. _____ abnormal sound caused by spasms or swelling of larynx
20. _____ whooping cough

✓ *Check your answers in Appendix A. Review material that you did not answer correctly.*

Correct Answers _____ × 5 = _____ % Score

Learning Activity 7-4
Matching Procedures, Pharmacology, and Abbreviations

Match the following terms with the definitions in the numbered list.

ABGs	antral lavage	Mantoux test	radiography
aerosol therapy	decongestant	oximetry	rhinoplasty
AFB	expectorant	pneumectomy	septoplasty
antihistamine	laryngoscopy	polysomnography	sweat test
antitussive	lung scan	pulmonary function tests	throat culture

1. _____ imaging procedure that uses radionuclide to evaluate blood flow in the lungs

2. _____ test of sleep cycles and stages

3. _____ producing images using an x-ray machine

4. _____ washing or irrigating sinuses

5. _____ sneezing, runny nose, itchiness, and rashes

6. _____ relieves or suppresses coughing

7. _____ used primarily in children to confirm cystic fibrosis

8. _____ noninvasive test used to monitor percentage of hemoglobin saturated with oxygen

9. _____ TB organism

10. _____ inhalation of medication directly into the respiratory system via a nebulizer

11. _____ decreases mucous membrane swelling by constricting blood vessels

12. _____ intradermal test to determine tuberculin sensitivity

13. _____ laboratory tests to assess gases and pH of arterial blood

14. _____ reduces the viscosity of sputum to facilitate productive coughing

15. _____ used to identify pathogens, especially group A streptococci

16. _____ multiple tests used to determine the ability of lungs and capillary membranes to exchange oxygen

17. _____ visual examination of the voice box to detect tumors and other abnormalities

18. _____ surgery to correct a deviated nasal septum

19. _____ excision of the entire lung

20. _____ reconstructive surgery of the nose, commonly for cosmetic purposes

✓ *Check your answers in Appendix A. Review any material that you did not answer correctly.*

Correct Answers _____ × 5 = _____ % Score

MEDICAL RECORD ACTIVITIES

The two medical records included in the following activities use common clinical scenarios to show how medical terminology is used to document patient care. Complete the terminology and analysis sections for each activity to help you recognize and understand terms related to body structure.

Medical Record Activity 7-1
SOAP Note: Respiratory Evaluation

Terminology

Terms listed below come from the *SOAP Note: Respiratory Evaluation* that follows. Use a medical dictionary such as *Taber's Cyclopedic Medical Dictionary*, the appendices of this book, or other resources to define each term. Then review the pronunciations for each term and practice by reading the medical record aloud.

Term	Definition
anteriorly ăn-TĔR-ē-or-lē	
bilateral bī-LĂT-ĕr-ăl	
COPD	
exacerbation ĕks-ăs-ĕr-BĀ-shŭn	
heart failure	
Hx	
hypertension hī-pĕr-TĔN-shŭn	
interstitial ĭn-tĕr-STĬSH-ăl	
PE	

peripheral vascular
  disease
pĕr-ĬF-ĕr-ăl VĂS-
  kū-lăr	

pleural PLOO-răl	
posteriorly pŏs-TĔR-ē-or-lē	
rhonchi RŎNG-kī	

Term	Definition
SOB	
wheezes HWĒZ-ĕz	

 Listen and Learn Online! *will help you master the pronunciation of selected medical words from this medical record activity. Visit* www.davisplus.com/gylys/systems *to find instructions on completing the* Listen and Learn Online! *exercise for this section and to practice pronunciations.*

SOAP NOTE: RESPIRATORY EVALUATION

Emergency Department Record

Date: February 1, 20xx
Patient: Flowers, Richard

Time Registered: 1345 hours
Physician: Samara Batichara, MD

Chief Complaint: SOB

Medications: Vytorin 10/20 mg daily; Toprol-XL 50 mg daily; Azmacort 2 puffs t.i.d; Proventil 2 puffs q.6 h.

S: This 49-year-old man with Hx of COPD is admitted because of exacerbation of SOB over the past few days. Patient was a heavy smoker and states that he quit smoking for a short while but now smokes 3-4 cigarettes a day. He has a Hx of difficult breathing, hypertension, COPD, and peripheral vascular disease. He underwent triple bypass surgery in 19xx.

O: T: 98.9 F. BP: 180/90. Pulse: 80 and regular. R: 20 and shallow. PE indicates scattered bilateral wheezes and rhonchi heard anteriorly and posteriorly. When compared with a portable chest film taken 22 months earlier, the current study most likely indicates interstitial vascular congestion. Some superimposed inflammatory change cannot be excluded. There may also be some pleural reactive change.

A: 1. Acute exacerbation of chronic obstructive pulmonary disease.
    2. Heart failure.
    3. Hypertension.
    4. Peripheral vascular disease.

P: Admit to hospital.

Samara Batichara, MD
Samara Batichara, MD

SB:icc

D: 2/1/20xx
T: 2/1/20xx

Analysis

Review the medical record *SOAP Note: Respiratory Evaluation* to answer the following questions.

1. What symptom caused the patient to seek medical help?

   _____

2. What was the patient's previous history?

   _____

3. What were the abnormal findings of the physical examination?

   _____

4. What changes were noted from the previous film?

   _____

5. What are the present assessments?

   _____

6. What new diagnosis was made that did not appear in the previous medical history?

   _____

Medical Record Activity 7-2
SOAP Note: Chronic Interstitial Lung Disease

Terminology

Terms listed below come from the *SOAP Note: Chronic Interstitial Lung Disease* that follows. Use a medical dictionary such as *Taber's Cyclopedic Medical Dictionary*, the appendices of this book, or other resources to define each term. Then review the pronunciations for each term and practice by reading the medical record aloud.

Term	Definition	
ABG		
adenopathy ăd-ĕ-NŎP-ă-thē		
basilar crackles BĂS-ĭ-lăr KRĂK-ĕlz		
cardiomyopathy kăr-dē-ō-mī-ŎP-ă-thē		
chronic KRŎN-ĭk		

Term	Definition
diuresis dī-ū-RĒ-sĭs	
dyspnea dĭsp-NĒ-ă	
fibrosis fī-BRŌ-sĭs	
interstitial ĭn-tĕr-STĬSH-ăl	
kyphosis kī-FŌ-sĭs	
Lasix LĀ-sĭks	
neuropathy nū-RŎP-ă-thē	
PCO_2	
pedal edema PĔD-ĕl ē-DĒ-mă	
pH	
PO_2	
pulmonary fibrosis PŬL-mō-nĕ-rē fī-BRŌ-sĭs	
renal insufficiency RĒ-năl ĭn-sŭ-FĬSH-ĕn-sē	
rhonchi RŎNG-kī	
silicosis sĭl-ĭ-KŌ-sĭs	
thyromegaly thī-rō-MĔG-ă-lē	

Listen and Learn Online! *will help you master the pronunciation of selected medical words from this medical record activity. Visit* www.davisplus.com/gylys/systems *to find instructions on completing the* Listen and Learn Online! *exercise for this section and to practice pronunciations.*

SOAP NOTE: CHRONIC INTERSTITIAL LUNG DISEASE

09/01/20xx

O'Malley, Robert

SUBJECTIVE: Patient is an 84-year-old male with chief complaint of dyspnea with activity and pedal edema. He carries the dx cardiomyopathy, renal insufficiency, COPD, and pulmonary fibrosis. He also has peripheral neuropathy, which has improved with Elavil therapy.

OBJECTIVE: BP: 140/70. Pulse: 76. Neck is supple without thyromegaly or adenopathy. Mild kyphosis without scoliosis is present. Chest reveals basilar crackles without wheezing or rhonchi. Cardiac examination shows trace edema without clubbing or murmur. Abdomen is soft and non-tender. ABGs on room air demonstrate a Po_2 of 55, Pco_2 of 45, and pH of 7.42.

ASSESSMENT: Chronic interstitial lung disease, likely a combination of pulmonary fibrosis and heart failure. We do believe he would benefit from further diuresis, which was implemented by Dr. Lu. Should there continue to be concerns about his volume status or lack of response to Lasix therapy, then he might benefit from right heart catheterization.

PLAN: Supplemental oxygen will be continued. We plan no change in his pulmonary medication at this time and will see him in return visit in 4 months. He has been told to contact us should he worsen in the interim.

Samara Batichara, MD
Samara Batichara, MD

SB:icc

Analysis

Review the medical record *SOAP Note: Chronic Interstitial Lung Disease* to answer the following questions.

1. When did the patient notice dyspnea?

   _____

2. Other than the respiratory system, what other body systems are identified in the history of present illness?

   _____

3. What were the findings regarding the neck?

   _____

4. What was the finding regarding the chest?

   _____

5. What appears to be the likely cause of the chronic interstitial lung disease?

   _____

6. What did the cardiac examination reveal?

   _____

Cardiovascular System

CHAPTER

8

Chapter Outline

Objectives

Upon completion of this chapter, you will be able to:

- Locate and describe the structures of the cardiovascular system.
- Describe the functional relationship between the cardiovascular system and other body systems.
- Identify, pronounce, spell, and build words related to the cardiovascular system.
- Describe pathological conditions, diagnostic and therapeutic procedures, and other terms related to the cardiovascular system.
- Explain pharmacology related to the treatment of cardiovascular disorders.
- Demonstrate your knowledge of this chapter by completing the learning and medical record activities.

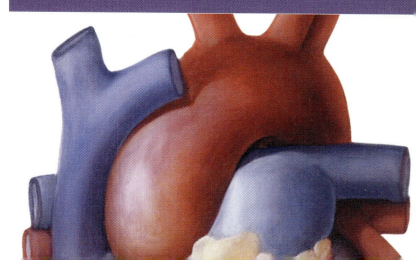

Anatomy and Physiology

The cardiovascular (CV) system is composed of the heart and blood vessels. The heart is a hollow, muscular organ lying in the mediastinum, the center of the thoracic cavity between the lungs. The pumping action of the heart propels blood containing oxygen, nutrients, and other vital products from the heart to body cells through a vast network of blood vessels called *arteries*. Arteries branch into smaller vessels until they become microscopic vessels called *capillaries*. It is at the capillary level that exchange of products occurs between body cells and blood. Capillaries merge to form larger blood vessels called *venules*, which then combine to form *veins*, the vessels that return blood to the heart to begin the cycle again. Millions of body cells rely on the cardiovascular system for their survival. When this transportation system fails, life at the cellular level is not possible and, ultimately, the organism will die.

Vascular System

Three major types of vessels—(1) **artery**, (2) **capillary**, and (3) **vein**—carry blood throughout the body. (See Figure 8–1.) Each type of vessel differs in structure depending on its function.

Arteries

Arteries carry blood from the heart to all cells of the body. Because blood is propelled thorough the arteries by the pumping action of the heart, the walls of the arteries must be strong and flexible enough to withstand the surge of blood that results from each contraction of the heart.

The walls of large arteries have three layers to provide toughness and elasticity. The (4) **tunica externa** is the outer coat composed of connective tissue that provides strength and flexibility. The (5) **tunica media** is the middle layer composed of smooth muscle. Depending on the needs of the body, this muscle can alter the size of the (7) **lumen**

Anatomy and Physiology Key Terms

This section introduces important terms and their definitions and pronunciation.

Term	Definition
autonomic nervous system (ANS) aw-tō-NŎM-ĭk NĔR-vĕs	Portion of the nervous system that regulates involuntary actions, such as heart rate, digestion, and peristalsis
leaflet	Thin, flattened structure; term used to describe the leaf-shaped structures that compose a heart valve
lumen LŪ-mĕn	Tubular space or channel within any organ or structure of the body; space within an artery, vein, intestine, or tube
regurgitation rē-gŭr-jĭ-TĀ-shŭn	Backflow or ejecting of contents through an opening
sphincter SFĬNGK-tĕr	Circular muscle found in a tubular structure or hollow organ that constricts or dilates to regulate passage of substances through its opening
vasoconstriction văs-ō-kŏn-STRĬK-shŭn	Narrowing of the lumen of a blood vessel that limits blood flow, usually as a result of diseases, medications, or physiological processes
vasodilation văs-ō-dī-LĀ-shŭn	Widening of the lumen of a blood vessel caused by the relaxing of the muscles of the vascular walls
viscosity vĭs-KŎS-ĭ-tē	State of being sticky or gummy *A solution that has high viscosity is relatively thick and flows slowly.*

Pronunciation Help	Long Sound	ā—rate	ē—rebirth	ī—isle	ō—over	ū—unite
	Short Sound	ă—alone	ĕ—ever	ĭ—it	ŏ—not	ŭ—cut

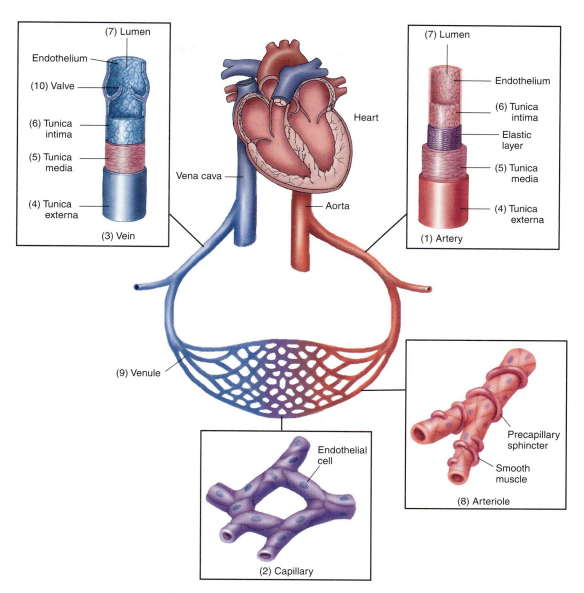

Figure 8-1. Vascular structures.

of the vessel. When it contracts, it causes **vasoconstriction,** resulting in decreased blood flow. When it relaxes, it causes **vasodilation,** resulting in increase blood flow. The (6) **tunica intima** is the thin, inner lining of the lumen of the vessel, composed of endothelial cells that provide a smooth surface on the inside of the vessel.

The surge of blood felt in the arteries when blood is pumped from the heart is referred to as a *pulse.* Because of the pressure against arterial walls associated with the pumping action of the heart, a cut or severed artery may lead to profuse bleeding.

Arterial blood (except for that found in the pulmonary artery) contains a high concentration of oxygen (**oxygenated**) and appears bright red in color. Oxygenated blood travels to smaller arteries

called (8) **arterioles** and, finally, to the smallest vessels, the capillaries.

Capillaries

Capillaries are microscopic vessels that join the arterial system with the venous system. Although they seem like the most insignificant of the three vessel types owing to their microscopic size, they are actually the most important because of their function. Because capillary walls are composed of only a single layer of endothelial cells, they are very thin. This thinness enables the exchange of water, respiratory gases, macromolecules, metabolites, and wastes between the blood and adjacent cells. The vast number of capillaries branching from arterioles causes blood to flow very slowly, providing sufficient time for exchange of necessary substances.

Blood flow through the highly branched capillary system is partially regulated by the contraction of smooth muscle precapillary **sphincters** that lead into the capillary bed. When tissues require more blood, these sphincters open; when less blood is required, they close. Once the exchange of products is complete, blood enters the venous system for its return cycle to the heart.

Veins

Veins return blood to the heart. They are formed from smaller vessels called (9) **venules** that develop from the union of capillaries. Because the extensive network of capillaries absorbs the propelling pressure exerted by the heart, veins use other methods to return blood to the heart, including:

- skeletal muscle contraction
- gravity
- respiratory activity
- valves.

The (10) **valves** are small structures within veins that prevent the backflow of blood. Valves are found mainly in the extremities and are especially important for returning blood from the legs to the heart because blood must travel a long distance against the force of gravity to reach the heart from the legs. Large veins, especially in the abdomen, contain smooth muscle that propels blood toward the heart by peristalsis.

Blood carried in veins (except for the blood in the pulmonary veins) contains a low concentration of oxygen (**deoxygenated**) with a corresponding high concentration of carbon dioxide. Deoxygenated blood takes on a characteristic purple color. Blood continuously circulates from the heart to the lungs so that carbon dioxide can be exchanged for oxygen.

Heart

The **heart** is a muscular pump that propels blood to entire body through a closed vascular system. It is found in a sac called the *pericardium*. The heart is composed of three distinct tissue layers:

- **endocardium,** a serous membrane that lines the four chambers of the heart and its valves and is continuous with the endothelium of the arteries and veins
- **myocardium,** the muscular layer of the heart
- **epicardium,** the outermost layer of the heart.

The heart is divided into four chambers. (See Figure 8–2.) The two upper chambers, the (1) **right**

atrium and (2) **left atrium,** collect blood. The two lower chambers, the (3) **right ventricle** and (4) **left ventricle,** pump blood from the heart. The right ventricle pumps blood to the lungs (**pulmonary circulation**) for oxygenation, and the left ventricle pumps oxygenated blood to the entire body (**systemic circulation**).

Deoxygenated blood from the body returns to the right atrium by way of two large veins: the (5) **superior vena cava,** which collects and carries blood from the upper body; and the (6) **inferior vena cava,** which collects and carries blood from the lower body. From the right atrium, blood passes through the (7) **tricuspid valve,** consisting of three **leaflets,** to the right ventricle. When the heart contracts, blood leaves the right ventricle by way of the (8) **left pulmonary artery** and (9) **right pulmonary artery** and travels to the lungs. During contraction of the ventricle, the tricuspid valve closes to prevent a backflow of blood to the right atrium. The (10) **pulmonic valve** (or *pulmonary semilunar valve*) prevents **regurgitation** of blood into the right ventricle from the pulmonary artery. In the lungs, the pulmonary artery branches into millions of capillaries, each lying close to an alveolus. Here, carbon dioxide in the blood is exchanged for oxygen that has been drawn into the lungs during inhalation.

Pulmonary capillaries unite to form four pulmonary veins—two (11) **right pulmonary veins** and two (12) **left pulmonary veins.** These vessels carry oxygenated blood back to the heart. They deposit blood in the left atrium. From there, blood passes through the (13) **mitral (bicuspid) valve,** consisting of two leaflets to the left ventricle. Upon contraction of the ventricles, the oxygenated blood leaves the left ventricle through the largest artery of the body, the (14) **aorta.** The aorta contains the (15) **aortic semilunar valve (aortic valve)** that permits blood to flow in only one direction—from the left ventricle to the aorta. The aorta branches into many smaller arteries that carry blood to all parts of the body. Some arteries derive their names from the organs or areas of the body they vascularize. For example, the splenic artery vascularizes the spleen and the renal arteries vascularize the kidneys.

It is important to understand that oxygen in the blood passing through the chambers of the heart cannot be used by the myocardium as a source of oxygen and nutrients. Instead, an arterial system composed of the coronary arteries branches from the aorta and provides the heart with its own blood supply. The artery vascularizing the right side of the heart is the (16) **right coronary artery.** The artery vascularizing the left side of the heart is the (17) **left coronary artery.** The left coronary artery

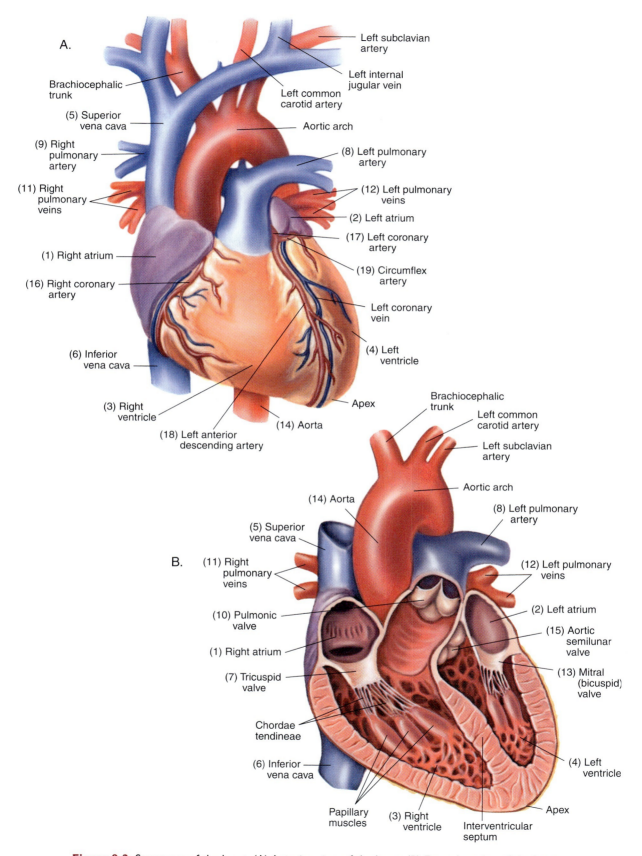

A.

Left subclavian artery

Left internal jugular vein

Left common carotid artery

Brachiocephalic trunk

(5) Superior vena cava

Aortic arch

(9) Right pulmonary artery

(8) Left pulmonary artery

(11) Right pulmonary veins

(12) Left pulmonary veins

(2) Left atrium

(1) Right atrium

(17) Left coronary artery

(16) Right coronary artery

(19) Circumflex artery

Left coronary vein

(6) Inferior vena cava

(4) Left ventricle

(3) Right ventricle

Apex

(14) Aorta

(18) Left anterior descending artery

Brachiocephalic trunk

Left common carotid artery

Left subclavian artery

Aortic arch

(14) Aorta

(8) Left pulmonary artery

(5) Superior vena cava

B.

(11) Right pulmonary veins

(12) Left pulmonary veins

(10) Pulmonic valve

(2) Left atrium

(1) Right atrium

(15) Aortic semilunar valve

(7) Tricuspid valve

(13) Mitral (bicuspid) valve

Chordae tendineae

(6) Inferior vena cava

(4) Left ventricle

Apex

Papillary muscles

(3) Right ventricle

Interventricular septum

Figure 8-2. Structures of the heart. (A) Anterior view of the heart. (B) Frontal section of the heart.

divides into the (18) **left anterior descending artery** and the (19) **circumflex artery.** If blood flow in the coronary arteries is diminished, damage to the heart muscle may result. When severe damage occurs, part of the heart muscle may die.

Conduction System of the Heart

Within the heart, a specialized cardiac tissue known as *conduction tissue* has the sole function of initiating and spreading contraction impulses. (See Figure 8–3.) This tissue consists of four masses of highly specialized cells that possess characteristics of nervous and cardiac tissue:

- sinoatrial (SA) node
- atrioventricular (AV) node
- bundle of His (AV bundle)
- Purkinje fibers.

The (1) **sinoatrial (SA) node** is located in the upper portion of the right atrium and possesses its own intrinsic rhythm. Without being stimulated by external nerves, it has the ability to initiate and propagate each heartbeat, thereby setting the basic pace for the cardiac rate. For this reason, the SA node is commonly known as the *pacemaker* of the heart. Cardiac rate may be altered by impulses from the **autonomic nervous system.** Such an arrangement allows outside influences to accelerate or decelerate heart rate. For example, the heart beats more quickly during physical exertion and more slowly during rest. Each electrical impulse discharged by the SA node is transmitted to the (2) **atrioventricular (AV) node,** causing the atria to contract. The AV node is located at the base of the right atrium. From this point, a tract of con-

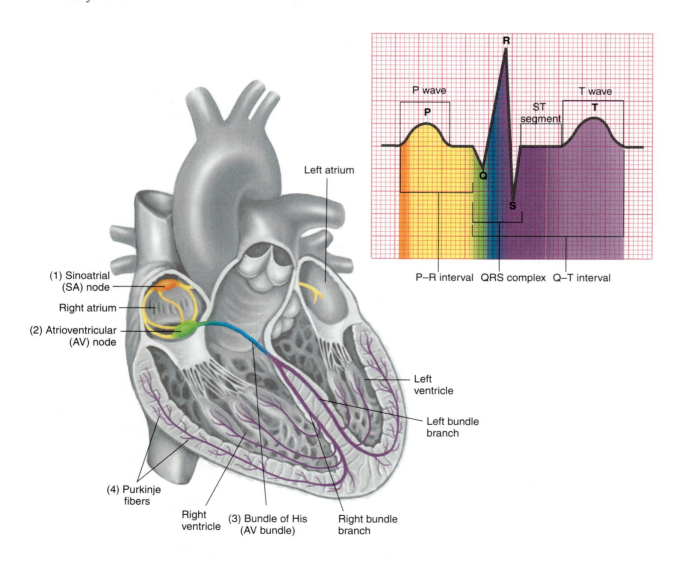

Figure 8-3. Conduction system.

duction fibers called the (3) **bundle of His** (AV bundle), composed of a right and left branch, relays the impulse to the (4) **Purkinje fibers.** These fibers extend up the ventricle walls. The Purkinje fibers transmit the impulse to the right and left ventricles, causing them to contract. Blood is now forced from the heart through the pulmonary artery and aorta. Thus, the sequence of the four structures responsible for conduction of a contraction impulse is:

SA node → AV node → bundle of His → Purkinje fibers

Impulse transmission through the conduction system generates weak electrical currents that can be detected on the surface of the body. An instrument called an *electrocardiograph* records these electrical impulses, using a needle, or stylus, that records the activity on graph paper. The needle deflection of the electrocardiograph produces waves or peaks designated by the letters P, Q, R, S, and T, each of which is associated with a specific electrical event:

- The **P wave** is the depolarization (contraction) of the atria.
- The **QRS complex** is the depolarization (contraction) of the ventricles.
- The **T wave**, which appears a short time later, is the repolarization (recovery) of the ventricles.

Blood Pressure

Blood pressure (BP) measures the force of blood against the arterial walls during two phases of a heartbeat: the contraction phase (**systole**) when the blood is forced out of the heart, and the relaxation phase (**diastole**) when the ventricles are filling with blood. Systole produces the maximum force; diastole, the weakest. These measurements are recorded as two figures separated by a diagonal line. Systolic pressure is given first, followed by diastolic pressure. For instance, a blood pressure of 120/80 mm Hg means a systolic pressure of 120 with a diastolic pressure of 80. A consistently elevated blood pressure is

called *hypertension;* decreased blood pressure is called *hypotension.*

Several factors influence blood pressure:

- resistance of blood flow in blood vessels
- pumping action of the heart
- **viscosity,** or thickness, of blood
- elasticity of arteries
- quantity of blood in the vascular system.

Fetal Circulation

Blood circulation through a fetus is, by necessity, different from that of a newborn infant. The process of gas exchange, the procurement of nutrients, and the elimination of metabolic wastes occur in the placenta. This remarkable structure delivers nutrients and oxygen from the mother to the fetus and removes waste products from the fetus and delivers them to the mother for disposal. The placenta develops during pregnancy and is expelled after the delivery of the infant.

There are several important structures involved in fetal circulation. (See Figure 8–4.) The (1) **umbilical cord**, containing (2) two **arteries**, carries deoxygenated blood from the fetus to the (3) **placenta.** After oxygenation in the placenta, blood returns to the fetus via the (4) **umbilical vein.** Most of the blood in the umbilical vein enters the (5) **inferior vena cava** through the (6) **ductus venosus**, where it is delivered to the (7) **right atrium.** Some of this blood passes to the (8) **right ventricle;** however, most of it passes to the (9) **left atrium** through a small opening in the atrial septum called the (10) **foramen ovale,** which closes shortly after birth. From the left atrium, blood enters the (11) **left ventricle** and finally exits the heart through the aorta, where it travels to the head and upper extremities. Because fetal lungs are nonfunctional, most of the blood in the pulmonary arteries is shunted through a connecting vessel called the (12) **ductus arteriosus** to the aorta. Immediately after birth, the ductus arteriosus withers and closes off. As circulation increases in the neonate, the increase of blood flow to the right atrium forces the foramen ovale to close. Normal circulation is now fully established.

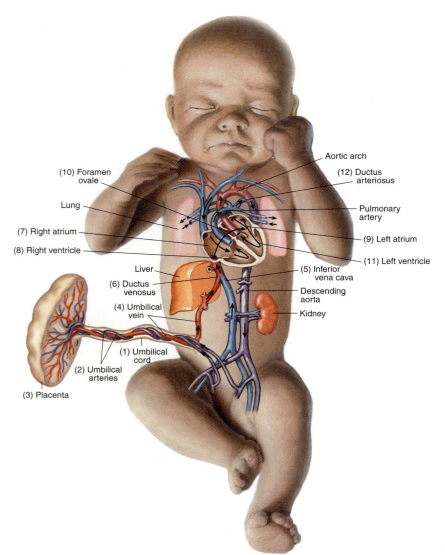

(10) Foramen
ovale

Lung

(7) Right atrium

(8) Right ventricle

Liver

(6) Ductus
venosus

(4) Umbilical
vein

(1) Umbilical
cord

(2) Umbilical
arteries

(3) Placenta

Aortic arch

(12) Ductus
arteriosus

Pulmonary
artery

(9) Left atrium

(11) Left ventricle

(5) Inferior
vena cava

Descending
aorta

Kidney

Figure 8-4. Fetal circulation.

Connecting Body Systems–Cardiovascular System

The main function of the cardiovascular system is to provide a network of vessels though which blood is pumped by the heart to all body cells. Specific functional relationships between the cardiovascular system and other body systems are discussed below.

Blood, lymph, and immune
- Cardiovascular system transports the products of the immune system.

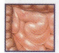

Digestive
- Cardiovascular system delivers hormones that affect glandular activity of the digestive tract.
- Cardiovascular system provides vasculature to the walls of the small intestine for absorption of nutrients.

Endocrine
- Cardiovascular system delivers oxygen and nutrients to endocrine glands.
- Cardiovascular system transports hormones from glands to target organs.

Female reproductive
- Cardiovascular system transports hormones that regulate the menstrual cycle.
- Cardiovascular system influences the normal function of sex organs, especially erectile tissue.

Connecting Body Systems-Cardiovascular System—cont'd

- Cardiovascular system provides the vessels of the placenta during pregnancy for the exchange of nutrients and waste products.

Genitourinary

- Cardiovascular system transports reproductive hormones.
- Cardiovascular system influences the normal function of sex organs, especially erectile tissue.
- Cardiovascular system delivers dissolved wastes to the kidneys for excretion in urine.

Integumentary

- Cardiovascular system provides blood vessels in the skin to regulate body temperature
- Cardiovascular system transports clotting factors to the skin to control bleeding.
- Cardiovascular system carries immune agents to sites of skin wounds and infections.

Musculoskeletal

- Cardiovascular system removes heat and waste products generated by muscle contraction.
- Cardiovascular system delivers oxygen for energy to sustain muscle contraction.
- Cardiovascular system delivers calcium and nutrients and removes metabolic wastes from skeletal structures.
- Cardiovascular system delivers hormones that regulate skeletal growth.

Nervous

- Cardiovascular system carries electrolytes for transmission of electrical impulses.

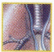

Respiratory

- Cardiovascular system transports oxygen and carbon dioxide between lungs and tissues

 It is time to review cardiovascular structures by completing Learning Activity 8–1.

Medical Word Elements

This section introduces combining forms, suffixes, and prefixes related to the cardiovascular system. Word analyses are also provided.

Element	Meaning	Word Analysis
Combining Forms		
aneurysm/o	widened blood vessel	**aneurysm/o/rrhaphy** (ăn-ū-rĭz-MOR-ă-fē): suture of an aneurysm *-rrhaphy:* suture
angi/o	vessel (usually blood or lymph)	**angi/o/plasty** (ĂN-jē-ō-plăs-tē): surgical repair of a vessel *-plasty:* surgical repair *Angioplasty includes any endovascular procedure that reopens narrowed blood vessels and restores blood flow.*
vascul/o		**vascul/itis** (văs-kū-LĪ-tĭs): inflammation of (blood) vessels *-itis:* inflammation
aort/o	aorta	**aort/o/stenosis** (ā-or-tō-stě-NŌ-sĭs): narrowing of the aorta *-stenosis:* narrowing, stricture
arteri/o	artery	**arteri/o/rrhexis** (ăr-tē-rē-ō-RĚK-sĭs): rupture of an artery *-rrhexis:* rupture

(continued)

Medical Word Elements—cont'd

Element	Meaning	Word Analysis
arteriol/o	arteriole	**arteriol**/itis (ăr-tēr-ē-ō-LĪ-tĭs): inflammation of an arteriole *-itis:* inflammation
atri/o	atrium	**atri/o**/megaly (ā-trē-ō-MĔG-ă-lē): enlargement of the atrium *-megaly:* enlargement
ather/o	fatty plaque	**ather**/oma (ăth-ĕr-Ō-mă): tumor of fatty plaque *-oma:* tumor *Atheromas are formed when fatty plaque builds up on the inner lining of arterial walls. As calcium and other minerals are absorbed by plaque, the vessel hardens.*
cardi/o	heart	**cardi/o**/megaly (kăr-dē-ō-MĔG-ă-lē): enlargement of the heart *-megaly:* enlargement
electr/o	electricity	**electr/o**/cardi/o/gram (ē-lĕk-trō-KĂR-dē-ō-grăm): record of the electrical (impulses) of the heart *cardi/o:* heart *-gram:* record, recording *An electrocardiogram is commonly used to diagnose abnormalities of the heart.*
embol/o	embolus (plug)	**embol**/ectomy (ĕm-bō-LĔK-tō-mē): removal of an embolus *-ectomy:* excision, removal *An embolectomy is the removal of a clot or other foreign material from a blood vessel. Most emboli are blood clots (thrombi) that have been transported from a distant vessel by the blood.*
hemangi/o	blood vessel	**hemangi**/oma (hē-măn-jē-Ō-mă): tumor of blood vessels *-oma:* tumor *Infantile hemangiomas are also called* **birthmarks.** *They are not considered malignant and usually disappear over time.*
my/o	muscle	**my/o**/cardi/al (mī-ō-KĂR-dē-ăl): pertaining to heart muscle *cardi:* heart *-al:* pertaining to, relating to
phleb/o	vein	**phleb**/ectasis (flĕ-BĔK-tă-sĭs): expansion of a vein *-ectasis:* dilation, expansion
ven/o		**ven/o**/stasis (vē-nō-STĀ-sĭs): standing still of (blood in a) vein; also called *phlebostasis* *-stasis:* standing still
scler/o	hardening; sclera (white of eye)	arteri/o/**scler**/osis (ăr-tē-rē-ō-sklĕ-RŌ-sĭs): abnormal condition of hardening of the artery *arteri/o:* artery *-osis:* abnormal condition; increase (used primarily with blood cells) *The most common cause of arteriosclerosis is the presence of an atheroma in the vessel. Other common causes include smoking, diabetes, high blood pressure, obesity, and familial tendency.*

Medical Word Elements—cont'd

Element	Meaning	Word Analysis
sept/o	septum	**sept/o**/stomy (sĕp-TŎS-tō-mē): forming an opening in a septum *-stomy:* forming an opening (mouth) *Septostomy is a temporary procedure performed to increase systemic oxygenation in infants with congenital heart defects until corrective surgery can be performed.*
sphygm/o	pulse	**sphygm/**oid (SFĬG-moyd): resembling a pulse *-oid:* resembling
sten/o	narrowing, stricture	**sten/o**/tic (stĕ-NŎT-ĭk): pertaining to a narrowing or stricture *-tic:* pertaining to
thromb/o	blood clot	**thromb/o**/lysis (thrŏm-BŎL-ĭ-sĭs): destruction of a blood clot *-lysis:* separation; destruction; loosening *In thrombolysis, enzymes that destroy blood clots are infused into the occluded vessel.*
ventricul/o	ventricle (of the heart or brain)	**ventricul/**ar (vĕn-TRĬK-ū-lăr): pertaining to a ventricle (chamber of the heart or brain) *-ar:* pertaining to
Suffixes		
-gram	record, writing	arteri/o/**gram** (ăr-TĒ-rē-ō-grăm): record of an artery *arteri/o:* artery *An arteriogram is used to visualize almost any artery, including those of the heart, head, kidneys, lungs, and other organs.*

-graph	instrument for recording	electr/o/cardi/o/**graph** (ē-lĕk-trō-KĂR-dē-ō-grăf): instrument for recording electrical (activity) of the heart
		  electr/o: electricity
		  cardi/o: heart

-graphy	process of recording	angi/o/**graphy** (ăn-jē-ŎG-ră-fē): process of recording (an image of) a vessel *angi/o:* vessel (usually blood or lymph) *Angiography is commonly used to identify atherosclerosis and diagnose heart and peripheral vascular disease.*
-sphyxia	pulse	a/**sphyxia** (ăs-FĬK-sē-ă): without a pulse; also called *suffocation* *a-:* without, not *The term **asphyxia** usually refers to a death caused by anoxia.*
-stenosis	narrowing, stricture	aort/o/**stenosis** (ā-or-tō-stĕ-NŌ-sĭs): narrowing of the aorta *aort/o:* aorta
Prefixes		
brady-	slow	**brady/**cardia (brăd-ē-KĂR-dē-ă): slow heart (beat) *-cardia:* heart condition *Bradycardia is usually defined as a heart rate less than 55 beats per minute when resting.*

endo-	in, within	**endo/**vascul/ar (ĕn-dō-VĂS-kū-lăr): relating to (the area) within a vessel
		  vascul: vessel
		  -ar: pertaining to

(continued)

Medical Word Elements—cont'd

Element	Meaning	Word Analysis
extra-	outside	**extra**/vascul/ar (ĕks-tră-VĂS-kū-lăr): relating to the (area) outside a vessel *vascul:* vessel *-ar:* pertaining to
peri-	around	**peri**/cardi/al (pĕr-ĭ-KĂR-dē-ăl): pertaining to (the area) around the heart *cardi:* heart *-al:* pertaining to, relating to
tachy	rapid	**tachy**/cardia (tăk-ē-KĂR-dē-ă): rapid heart (beat) *-cardia:* heart condition *Tachycardia is defined as a heart rate greater than 100 beats per minute.*
trans-	across	**trans**/sept/al (trăns-SĔP-tăl): across the septum *sept:* septum *-al:* pertaining to

It is time to review medical word elements by completing Learning Activity 8–2. For audio pronunciations of the above-listed key terms, you can visit www.davisplus.fadavis.com/gylys/systems to download this chapter's Listen and Learn! *exercises or use the book's audio CD (if included).*

Pathology

Many cardiac disorders, especially coronary artery disease, and valvular disorders are associated with a genetic predisposition. Thus, a complete history as well as a physical examination is essential in the diagnosis of cardiovascular disease. Although some of the most serious cardiovascular diseases have few signs and symptoms, when they occur they may include chest pain (**angina**), palpitations, breathing difficulties (**dyspnea**), cardiac irregularities (**arrhythmias**) and loss of consciousness (**syncope**). The location, duration, pattern of radiation, and severity of pain are important qualities indifferentiating the various forms of cardiovascular disease and are sometimes characteristic of specific disorders. Because of the general nature of the signs and symptoms of cardiovascular disorders, invasive and noninvasive tests are usually required to confirm or rule out a suspected disease.

For diagnosis, treatment, and management of cardiovascular disorders, the medical services of a specialist may be warranted. **Cardiology** is the medical specialty concerned with disorders of the cardiovascular system. The physician who treats these disorders is called a *cardiologist*.

Arteriosclerosis

Arteriosclerosis is a hardening of arterial walls that causes them to become thickened and brittle. This hardening results from a build-up of a plaquelike substance composed of cholesterol, lipids, and cellular debris (**atheroma**). Over time, it builds up on the inside lining (**tunica intima**) of the arterial walls. Eventually, the plaque hardens (**atherosclerosis**), causing the vessel to lose elasticity. (See Figure 8–5.) The lumen narrows as the plaque becomes larger. After a while, it becomes difficult for blood to pass through the blocked areas. Tissues distal to the occlusion become ischemic. In many instances, blood hemorrhages into the plaque and forms a clot (**thrombus**) that may dislodge. When a thrombus travels though the vascular system it is called an *embolus* (plural, *emboli*). Emboli in venous circulation may cause death. Emboli in arterial circulation commonly lodge in a capillary bed and cause localized tissue death (**infarct**). Sometimes plaque weakens the vessel wall to such an extent that it forms a bulge (**aneurysm**) that may rupture. (See Figure 8–6.)

Arteriosclerosis usually affects large- or medium-sized arteries, including the abdominal aorta; the

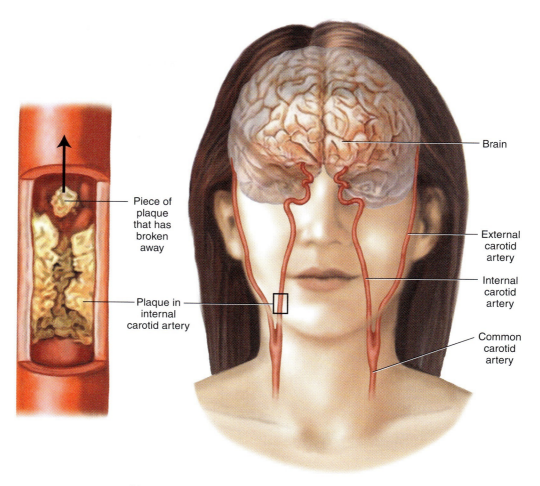

Figure 8-5. Atherosclerosis of the internal carotid artery.

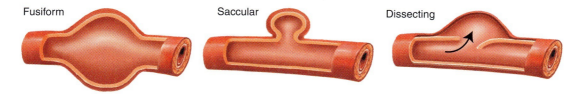

Figure 8-6. Aneurysms.

coronary, cerebral, and renal arteries; and major arteries of the legs (**femoral arteries**). One of the major risk factors for developing arteriosclerosis is an elevated cholesterol level (**hypercholesterolemia**). Other major risk factors include age, family history, smoking, hypertension, and diabetes.

Treatment for arthrosclerosis varies depending on the location and symptoms. In one method, occluding material and plaque are removed from the innermost layer of the artery (**endarterectomy**). (See Figure 8–7.) In this procedure, the surgeon opens the site and removes the plaque, there-

by resuming normal blood flow. Physicians commonly use endarterectomy to treat carotid artery disease, peripheral arterial disease, and diseases of the renal artery and aortic arch.

Coronary Artery Disease

In order for the heart to function effectively, it must receive an uninterrupted supply of blood. This blood is delivered to the heart muscle by way of the coronary arteries. Failure of the coronary arteries to deliver an adequate supply of blood to

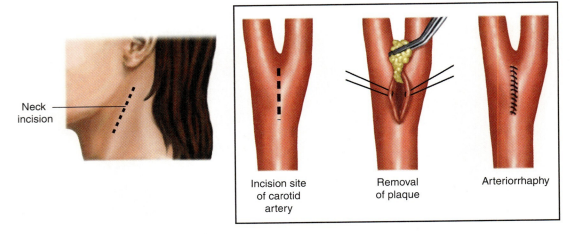

Neck incision

Incision site of carotid artery

Removal of plaque

Arteriorrhaphy

Figure 8-7. Endarterectomy of the common carotid artery.

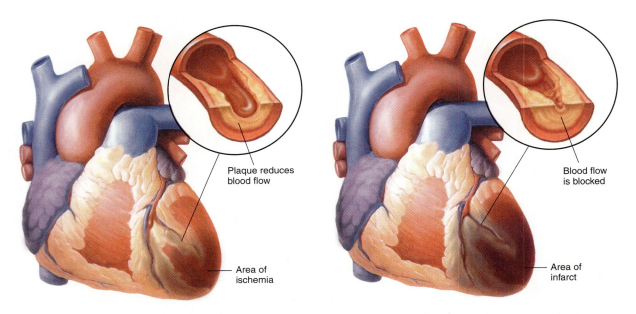

Plaque reduces blood flow

Area of ischemia

Blood flow is blocked

Area of infarct

Figure 8-8. Occlusions. (A) Partial occlusion. (B) Total occlusion.

the myocardium is called *coronary artery disease* **(CAD)**. Its major cause is the accumulation of plaque which causes the walls of the artery to harden (**arteriosclerosis**). With partial occlusion, localized areas of the heart experience oxygen deficiency (**ischemia**). When the occlusion is total or almost total, the affected area of the heart muscle dies (**infarction**). (See Figure 8–8.) The clinical signs and symptoms of myocardial infarction (MI) typically include intense chest pain (**angina**), profuse sweating (**diaphoresis**), paleness (**pallor**), and labored breathing (**dyspnea**). Arrhythmia with an abnormally rapid heart rate (**tachycardia**) or an abnormally slow heart rate (**bradycardia**) may also accompany an MI.

As the heart muscle undergoes necrotic changes, it releases several highly specific cardiac enzymes, including troponin T, troponin I, and creatinine kinase (CK). The rapid elevation of these enzymes at predictable times following MI helps differentiate MI from pericarditis, abdominal aortic aneurysm (AAA), and acute pulmonary embolism.

When angina cannot be controlled with medication, surgical intervention may be necessary. In **percutaneous transluminal coronary angioplasty (PTCA),** a deflated balloon is passed through a small incision in the skin and into the diseased blood vessel. When the balloon inflates, it presses the occluding material against the lumen walls to force open the channel. (See Figure 8–9.) After the

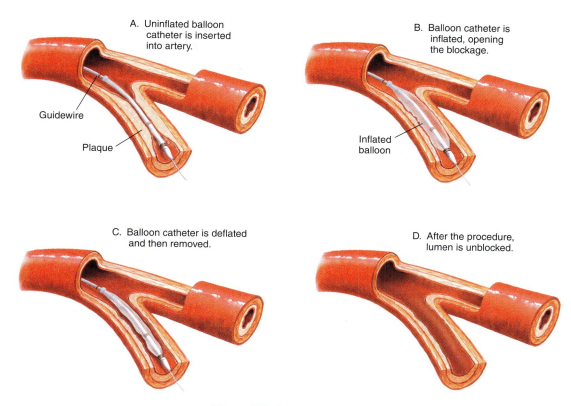

A. Uninflated balloon catheter is inserted into artery.

Guidewire

Plaque

B. Balloon catheter is inflated, opening the blockage.

Inflated balloon

C. Balloon catheter is deflated and then removed.

D. After the procedure, lumen is unblocked.

Figure 8-9. Balloon angioplasty.

procedure, the physician deflates and removes the balloon. Sometimes, the physician will place a hollow, thin mesh tube (**stent**) on the balloon and position it against the artery wall. It remains in place after the balloon catheter is removed and keeps the artery opened.

A more invasive procedure involves rerouting blood around the occluded area using a vein graft that bypasses the obstruction (**coronary artery bypass graft [CABG]**). One end of the graft vessel is sutured to the aorta and the other end is sutured to the coronary artery below the blocked area. This graft reestablishes blood flow to the heart muscle. (See Figure 8–10.)

Endocarditis

Endocarditis is an inflammation of the inner lining of the heart and its valves. It may be noninfective in nature, caused by thrombi formation, or infective, caused by various microorganisms. Although the infecting organism can be viral or fungal, the usual culprit is a bacterium. Congenital valvular defects, scarlet fever, rheumatic fever, calcified bicuspid or aortic valves, mitral valve prolapse, and prosthetic

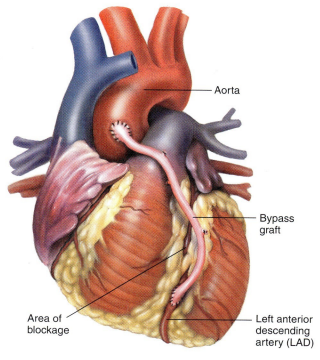

Aorta

Bypass graft

Area of blockage

Left anterior descending artery (LAD)

Figure 8-10. Coronary artery bypass graft.

valves are predisposing factors. Bacteria traveling in the bloodstream (**bacteremia**) may lodge in the weakened heart tissue and form small masses called *vegetations* composed of fibrin and platelets. Vegetations usually collect on the leaflets of the valves and their cords, causing a backflow of blood (**regurgitation**) or scarring. Vegetations may dislodge (**embolize**) and travel to the brain, lungs, kidneys, or spleen.   Scaring of the valves may cause them to narrow (**stenosis**) or not close properly (**insufficiency**). Although medications may prove helpful, if heart failure develops as a result of damaged heart valves, surgery may be the only option. Whenever possible, the original valve is repaired. When the damage is extensive, a mechanical or bioprosthetic valve may be used.

Patients who are susceptible to endocarditis are given antibiotic treatment to protect against infection prior to invasive procedures (**prophylactic treatment**). Because many bacteria normally found in the mouth are also responsible for endocarditis, prophylactic treatment is essential for tooth removal, root canal procedures, and even routine cleaning.

Varicose Veins

Varicose veins are enlarged, twisted, superficial veins. They develop when the valves of the veins do not function properly (**incompetent**) and fail to prevent the backflow of blood. (See Figure 8–11.) Blood accumulates and the vein becomes engorged and distended. Excess fluid eventually seeps from the vein, causing swelling in surrounding tissues (**edema**). Varicose veins may develop in almost any part of the body, including the esophagus (**varices**) and rectum (**hemorrhoids**), but occur most commonly in the greater and lesser saphenous veins of the lower legs. Types of varicose veins include reticular veins, which appear as small blue veins seen through the skin, and "spider" veins (**teleangiectases**), which look like short, fine lines, starburst clusters, or weblike mazes.

Varicose veins of the legs are not typically painful but may be unsightly in appearance. However, if open lesions or pain is present, treatment includes laser ablation, microphlebectomies, sclerotherapy, and occasionally, ligation and stripping for heavily damaged or diseased veins. The same methods are used as an elective procedure to improve the appearance of the legs. Treatment of mild cases of varicose veins includes use of elastic stockings and rest periods during which the legs are elevated.

Oncology

Although rare, the most common primary tumor of the heart is composed of mucous connective tissue (**myxoma**); however, these tumors tend to be benign. Although some myxomas originate in the endocardium of the heart chambers, most arise in the left atrium. Occasionally, they impede mitral valve function and cause a decrease in exercise tolerance, dyspnea, fluid in the lungs (**pulmonary edema**), and systemic problems, including joint

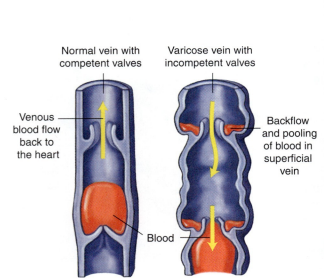

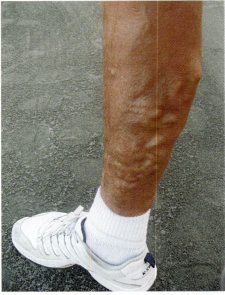

Figure 8-11. Healthy and unhealthy veins and valves. (A) Valve function in competent and incompetent valves. (B) Varicose veins.

pain (**arthralgia**), malaise, and anemia. These tumors are usually identified and located by two-dimensional echocardiography. When present, they should be excised surgically.

Most malignant tumors of the heart are the result of a malignancy originating in another area of the body (**primary tumor**) that has spread (**metastasized**) to the heart. The most common type originates in a darkly pigmented mole or tumor (**malignant melanoma**) of the skin. Other primary sites of malignancy that metastasize to the heart are bone marrow and lymphatic tissue. Treatment of the metastatic tumor of the heart involves treating the primary tumor.

Diagnostic, Symptomatic, and Related Terms

This section introduces diagnostic, symptomatic, and related terms and their meanings. Word analyses for selected terms are also provided

Term	Definition
aneurysm ĂN-ū-rĭzm	Localized abnormal dilation of a vessel, usually an artery
arrest	Condition of being stopped or bringing to a stop

cardiac
KĂR-dē-ăk
  cardi: heart
  -ac: pertaining to, relating to
circulatory
SĔR-kū-lă-tor-ē
	Loss of effective cardiac function, which results in cessation of circulation
	Cardiac arrest (CA) may be due to ventricular fibrillation or asystole in which there is no observable myocardial activity.
	Cessation of the circulation of blood due to ventricular standstill or fibrillation

arrhythmia ă-RĬTH-mē-ă	Inability of the heart to maintain a normal sinus rhythm, possibly including a rapid or slow beat or "skipping" a beat; also called *dysrhythmia*
bruit brwē	Soft blowing sound heard on auscultation, possibly due to vibrations associated with the movement of blood, valvular action, or both; also called *murmur*

cardiomyopathy
kăr-dē-ō-mī-ŎP-ă-thē
  cardi/o: heart
  my/o: muscle
  -pathy: disease
	Any disease or weakening of heart muscle that diminishes cardiac function
	Causes of cardiomyopathy include viral or bacterial infections, metabolic disorders, or general systemic disease.

catheter KĂTH-ĕ-tĕr	Thin, flexible, hollow plastic tube that is small enough to be threaded through a vein, artery, or tubular structure
coarctation kō-ărk-TĀ-shŭn	Narrowing of a vessel, especially the aorta

deep vein thrombosis (DVT)
thrŏm-BŌ-sĭs
  thromb: blood clot
  -osis: abnormal condition;
    increased (used primarily
    with blood cells)
	Blood clot that forms in the deep veins of the body, especially those in the legs or thighs
	In DVT, blood clots may break away from the vein wall and travel in the body. If they lodge in the lung, the condition is called pulmonary embolism. Pulmonary embolism may be life threatening if a large portion of the lung is damaged.

ejection fraction (EF)	Calculation of how much blood a ventricle can eject with one contraction *The left ventricular EF averages 50% to 70% in healthy hearts but can be markedly reduced if part of the heart muscle dies, as evident after an MI or in cardiomyopathy or valvular heart disease.*

(continued)

Diagnostic, Symptomatic, and Related Terms—cont'd

Term	Definition
heart failure (HF)	Failure of the heart to supply an adequate amount of blood to tissues and organs *HF is commonly caused by impaired coronary blood flow, cardiomyopathies, and heart valve disease.*
embolus ĔM-bō-lŭs *embol:* embolus (plug) *-us:* condition, structure	Mass of undissolved matter (foreign object, air, gas, tissue, thrombus) circulating in blood or lymphatic channels until it becomes lodged in a vessel
fibrillation fĭ-brĭl-Ā-shŭn	Quivering or spontaneous muscle contractions, especially of the heart, causing ineffectual contractions *Fibrillation is commonly corrected with a defibrillator.*
hemostasis hē-mō-STĀ-sĭs *hem/o:* blood *-stasis:* standing still	Arrest of bleeding or circulation
hyperlipidemia hī-pĕr-lĭp-ĭ-DĔ-mē-ă *hyper-:* excessive, above normal *lipid:* fat *-emia:* blood condition	Excessive amounts of lipids (cholesterol, phospholipids, and triglycerides) in the blood *The term* **hypercholesterolemia** *refers to elevation of cholesterol in the blood. It has been associated with an increased risk of atherosclerosis.*
hypertension (HTN) hī-pĕr-TĔN-shŭn *hyper-:* excessive, above normal *-tension:* to stretch	Common disorder characterized by elevated blood pressure persistently exceeding 140 mm Hg systolic or 90 mm Hg diastolic
primary	HTN in which there is no identifiable cause; also called *essential hypertension* *Primary hypertension is the most common form of hypertension and is associated with obesity, a high serum sodium level, hypercholesterolemia, or family history.*
secondary	HTN that results from an underlying, identifiable, commonly correctable cause
hypertensive heart disease hī-pĕr-TĔN-sĭv	Any heart disorder caused by prolonged hypertension, including left ventricular hypertrophy, coronary artery disease, cardiac arrhythmias, and heart failure
implantable cardioverter-defibrillator (ICD) KĂR-dē-ō-vĕr-tĕr-dē-FĬB-rĭ-lā-tor	Implantable battery-powered device that monitors and automatically corrects ventricular tachycardia or fibrillation by sending electrical impulses to the heart (See Figure 8-12.) *In ventricular fibrillation, the heart quivers rather than beats, and blood is not pumped to the brain. Unless treatment is received within 5 to 10 minutes, ventricular fibrillation causes death.*
infarct ĬN-fărkt	Area of tissue that undergoes necrosis following cessation of blood supply

Diagnostic, Symptomatic, and Related Terms—cont'd

Term	Definition

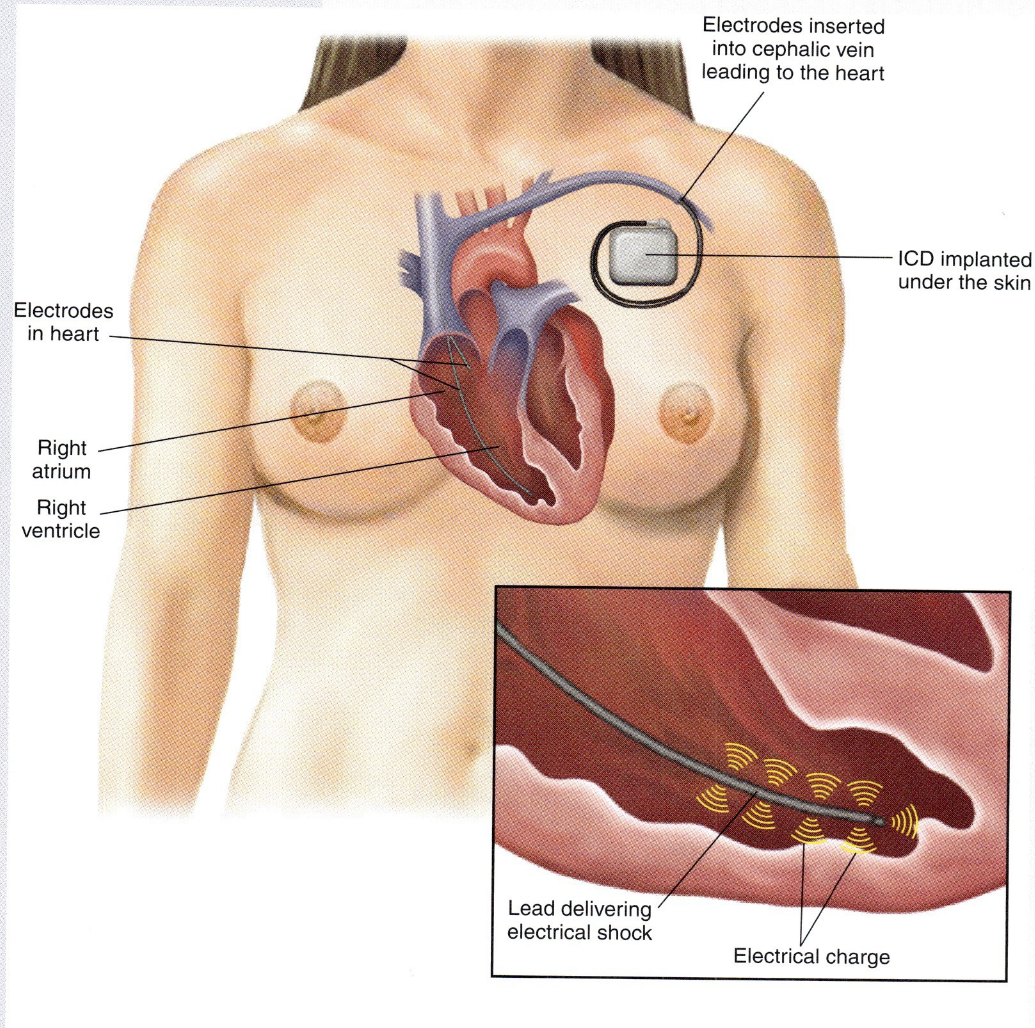

Electrodes inserted into cephalic vein leading to the heart

ICD implanted under the skin

Electrodes in heart

Right atrium

Right ventricle

Lead delivering electrical shock

Electrical charge

Figure 8-12. Implantable cardioverter-defibrillator (ICD).

Term	Definition
ischemia ĭs-KĒ-mē-ă	Local and temporary deficiency of blood supply due to circulatory obstruction
mitral valve prolapse (MVP) MĪ-trăl, PRŌ-lăps	Common and occasionally serious condition in which the leaflets of the mitral valve prolapse into the left atrium during systole causing a characteristic murmur heard on auscultation *Common signs and symptoms of MVP include palpitations of the heart and, occasionally, panic attacks with pounding heartbeat. Because of the possibility of valve infection, prophylactic treatment with antibiotics is suggested before undergoing invasive procedures such as dental work.*
radioisotope rā-dē-ō-Ī-sō-tōp	Chemical radioactive material used as a tracer to follow a substance through the body or a structure

(continued)

Diagnostic, Symptomatic, and Related Terms—cont'd

Term	Definition
palpitation păl-pĭ-TĀ-shŭn	Sensation that the heart is not beating normally, possibly including "thumping," "fluttering," "skipped beats," or a pounding feeling in the chest *Although most palpitations are harmless, those caused by arrhythmias may be serious. Medical attention should be sought if palpitations are accompanied by pain, dizziness, overall weakness, or shortness of breath.*
patent ductus arteriosus PĂT-ĕnt DŬK-tŭs ăr-tē-rē-Ō-sŭs	Failure of the ductus arteriosus to close after birth, allowing blood to flow from the aorta into the pulmonary (lung) artery
perfusion pĕr-FŪ-zhŭn	Circulation of blood through tissues or the passage of fluids through vessels of an organ
tetralogy of Fallot tĕ-TRĂL-ō-jē, făl-Ō	Congenital anomaly consisting of four elements: (1) pulmonary artery stenosis; (2) interventricular septal defect; (3) transposition of the aorta, so that both ventricles empty into the aorta; (4) right ventricular hypertrophy caused by increased workload of the right ventricle
stent stĕnt	Slender or threadlike device used to hold open vessels, tubes, or obstructed arteries *Stents are used to support tubular structures that are being anastomosed or to induce or maintain patency within these tubular structures.*
thrombus THRŎM-bŭs *thromb:* blood clot *-us:* condition; structure	Blood clot that obstructs a vessel

 It is time to review pathological, diagnostic, symptomatic, and related terms by completing Learning Activity 8–3.

Diagnostic and Therapeutic Procedures

This section introduces procedures used to diagnose and treat cardiovascular disorders. Descriptions are provided as well as pronunciations and word analyses for selected terms

Procedure	Description
Diagnostic Procedures	
Clinical	
cardiac catheterization (CC) KĂR-dē-ăk kăth-ĕ-tĕr-ĭ-ZĀ-shŭn *cardi:* heart *-ac:* pertaining to, relating to	Passage of a catheter into the heart through a vein or artery to provide a comprehensive evaluation of the heart (See Figure 8-13.) *CC gathers information about the heart, such as blood supply through the coronary arteries and blood flow and pressure in the chambers of the heart as well as enabling blood sample collection and x-rays of the heart.*
electrocardiogram (ECG, EKG) ē-lĕk-trō-KĂR-dē-ō-grăm *electr/o:* electricity *cardi/o:* heart *-gram:* record, writing	Graphic line recording that shows the spread of electrical excitation to different parts of the heart using small metal electrodes applied to the chest, arms, and legs *ECGs help diagnose abnormal heart rhythms and myocardial damage.*

Diagnostic and Therapeutic Procedures—cont'd

Procedure	Description

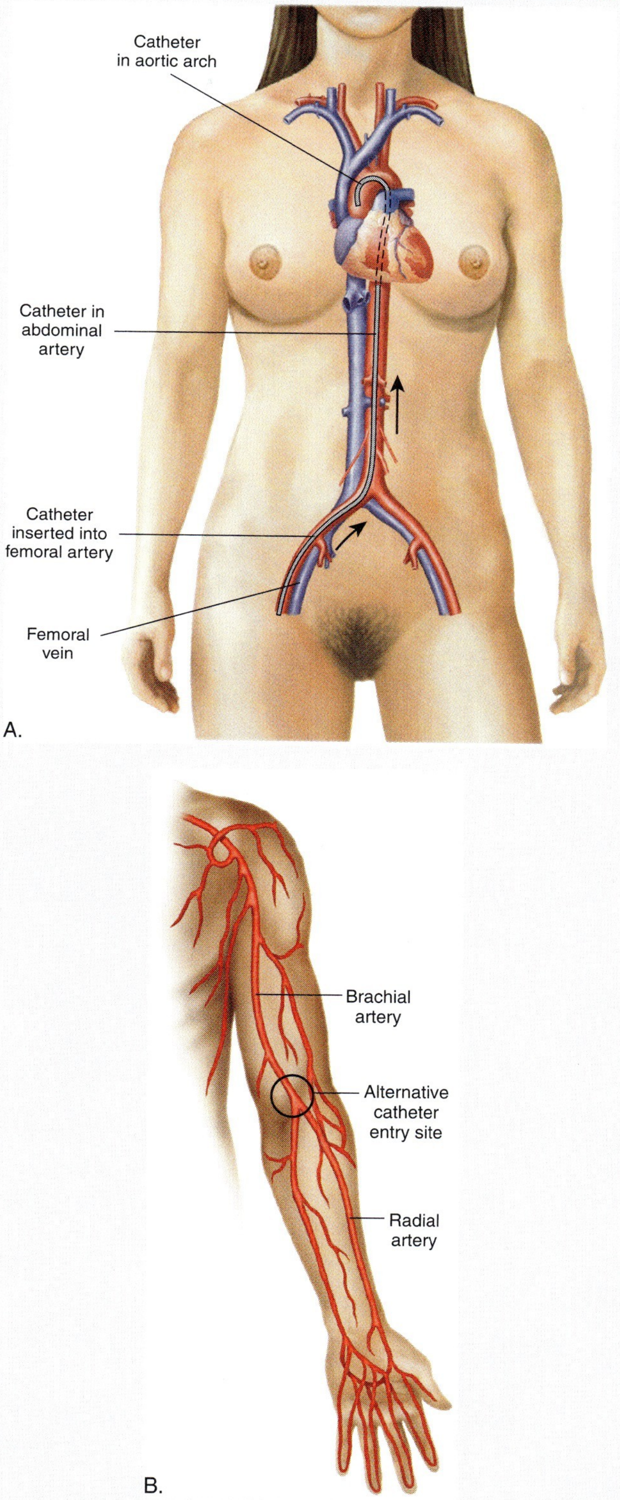

Catheter
in aortic arch

Catheter in
abdominal
artery

Catheter
inserted into
femoral artery

Femoral
vein

A.

Brachial
artery

Alternative
catheter
entry site

Radial
artery

B.

Figure 8-13. Cardiac catheterization. (A) Catheter insertion in femoral vein or artery. (B) Catheter insertion in brachial or radial artery.

(continued)

Diagnostic and Therapeutic Procedures—cont'd

Procedure	Description
Holter monitor test HŌL-tĕr MŎN-ĭ-tor	ECG taken with a small portable recording system capable of storing up to 24 hours of ECG tracings (See Figure 8-14.) *Holter monitoring is particularly useful in obtaining a cardiac arrhythmia record that would be missed during an ECG of only a few minutes' duration.*

Figure 8-14. Holter monitor.

Procedure	Description
stress test	ECG taken under controlled exercise stress conditions *A stress test may show abnormal ECG tracings that do not appear during an ECG taken when the patient is resting.*
nuclear	ECG that utilizes a radioisotope to evaluate coronary blood flow *In a nuclear stress test, the radioisotope is injected at the height of exercise. The area not receiving sufficient oxygen is visualized by decreased uptake of the isotope.*

Laboratory

Procedure	Description
cardiac enzyme studies KĂR-dē-ăk ĔN-zīm	Blood test that measures troponin T, troponin I, and creatinine kinase (CK-MB) *Cardiac enzymes are released into the bloodstream from damaged heart muscle tissue. Their presence in a blood specimen is consistent with myocardial damage.*
lipid panel LĬP-ĭd	Series of tests (total cholesterol, high density lipoprotein, low density lipoprotein, and triglycerides) used to assess risk factors of ischemic heart disease

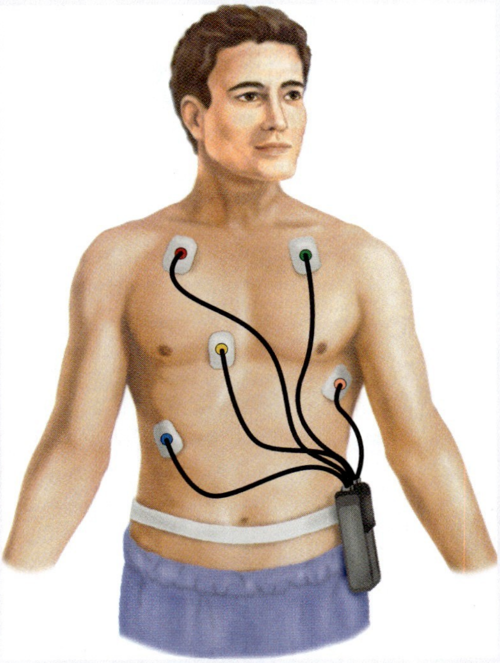

Diagnostic and Therapeutic Procedures—cont'd

Procedure	Description
Radiographic	
angiography ăn-jē-ŎG-ră-fē *angi/o:* vessel (usually blood or lymph) *-graphy:* process of recording	Radiographic imaging of the heart and blood vessels after injection of a contrast dye
coronary KOR-ō-nă-rē ăn-jē-ŎG-ră-fē	Angiography to determine the degree of obstruction of the arteries that supply blood to the heart *In coronary angiography, a catheter is inserted into the femoral artery and threaded to the aorta. The contrast dye outlines the coronary arteries and shows narrowing, stenosis, or blockage.*
digital subtraction ăn-jē-ŎG-ră-fē	Angiography in which two radiographic images are obtained, the first one without contrast material and the second one after a contrast material has been injected, and then compared by a computer that digitally subtracts (removes) the images of soft tissues, bones, and muscles, leaving only the image of vessels with contrast
aortography ā-or-TŎG-ră-fē *aort/o:* aorta *-graphy:* process of recording	Radiological examination of the aorta and its branches following injection of a contrast medium via a catheter
echocardiography (ECHO) ĕk-ō-kăr-dē-ŎG-ră-fē *echo-:* repeated sound *cardi/o:* heart *-graphy:* process of recording	Noninvasive diagnostic method that uses ultrasound to visualize internal cardiac structures and produce images of the heart *A transducer is placed on the chest to direct ultra–high-frequency sound waves toward cardiac structures. Reflected echoes are then converted to electrical impulses and displayed on a screen.*
Doppler ultrasound DŎP-lĕr	Noninvasive adaptation of ultrasound technology in which blood flow velocity is assessed in different areas of the heart *Sound waves strike moving red blood cells and are reflected back to a recording device that graphically records blood flow through cardiac structures.*
magnetic resonance imaging (MRI) măg-NĔT-ĭk RĔZ-ĕn-ăns ĬM-ĭj-ĭng	Noninvasive technique that uses radiowaves and a strong magnetic field, rather than an x-ray beam, to produce multiplanar cross-sectional images of blood vessels *MRI provide information about aneurysms, cardiac structures, and cardiac output. Magnetic resonance angiography (MRA) is a type of MRI that provides highly detailed images of the blood vessels. MRA is used to view arteries and blockages within the arteries. A radiopaque contrast dye can be injected to provide greater detail of body structures.*
multiple-gated acquisition (MUGA)	Nuclear procedure that uses radioactive tracers to produce movie-like images of the structures of the heart, including the myocardium and the mitral and tricuspid valves *The MUGA scan shows the motion of the heart wall muscle and the ventricle's ability to eject blood (ejection fraction).*

(continued)

Diagnostic and Therapeutic Procedures—cont'd

Procedure	Description
phonocardiography fō-nō-kăr-dē-ŎG-ră-fē *phon/o:* voice, sound *cardi/o:* heart *-graphy:* process of recording	Imaging technique that provides a graphic display of heart sounds and murmurs during the cardiac cycle *In phonocardiography, a transducer sends ultrasonic pulses through the chest wall and the echoes are converted into images on a monitor to assess overall cardiac performance.*
scintigraphy sĭn-TĬG-ră-fē	Diagnostic test that uses radiation emitted by the body after an injection of radioactive substances to create images of various organs or identify body functions and diseases *Scintigraphy identifies infarcted or scarred areas of the heart that show up as "cold spots" (areas of reduced radioactivity), taken when the patient is at rest.*
thallium study (resting) THĂL-ē-ŭm	Scintigraphy procedure that uses injected radioactive thallium and records the uptake of the isotope with a gamma camera to produce an image *A stress thallium study is commonly performed at the same time as a resting study, and the two images are compared to further identify abnormalities.*
sclerotherapy sklĕr-ō-THĔR-ă-pē *scler/o:* hardening; sclera (white of the eye) *-therapy:* treatment	Injection of a chemical irritant (sclerosing agent) into a vein to produce inflammation and fibrosis that destroys the lumen of the vein *Sclerotherapy is commonly performed to treat varicose veins and sometimes telangiectasias.*
venography vē-NŎG-ră-fē *ven/o:* vein *-graphy:* process of recording	Radiography of a vein after injection of a contrast medium to detect incomplete filling of a vein, which indicates obstruction *Venography is used primarily to locate blood clots in veins of the leg.*

Therapeutic Procedures

Clinical

cardioversion KĂR-dē-ō-vĕr-zhŭn *cardi/o:* heart *-version:* turning	Procedure to restore normal rhythm of the heart by applying a controlled electrical shock to the exterior of the chest
embolization ĕm-bō-lĭ-ZĀ-shŭn *embol:* plug *-izaton:* process (of)	Technique used to block blood flow to a site by passing a catheter to the area and injecting a synthetic material or medication specially designed to occlude the blood vessel *Embolization may serve to eliminate an abnormal communication between an artery and a vein, stop bleeding, or close vessels that are supporting tumor growth.*

Surgical

angioplasty ĂN-jē-ō-plăs-tē *angi/o:* vessel (usually blood or lymph) *-plasty:* surgical repair	Procedure that alters a vessel through surgery or dilation of the vessel using a balloon catheter
coronary artery bypass graft (CABG) KOR-ō-nă-rē ĂR-tĕr-ē	Surgical procedure that uses a vessel graft from another part of the body to bypass the blocked part of a coronary artery and restore blood supply to the heart muscle

Diagnostic and Therapeutic Procedures—cont'd

Procedure	Description
percutaneous transluminal coronary angioplasty (PTCA) pĕr-kū-TĀ-nē-ŭs trăns-LŪ-mĭ-năl KOR-ō-nă-rē ĂN-jē-ō-plăs-tē *per-:* through *cutane:* skin *-ous:* pertaining to, relating to	Dilation of an occluded vessel using a balloon catheter under fluoroscopic guidance *In PTCA, the physician inserts a catheter transcutaneously, inflates the balloon thereby dilating the narrowed vessel, and commonly positions a stent to hold the vessel open.*
atherectomy ăth-ĕr-ĔK-tō-mē *ather:* fatty plaque *-ectomy:* excision, removal	Removal of material from an occluded vessel using a specially designed catheter fitted with a cutting or grinding device
biopsy BĪ-ŏp-sē	Removal and examination of a small piece of tissue for diagnostic purposes
arterial ăr-TĒ-rē-ăl *arteri:* artery *-al:* pertaining to, relating to	Removal and examination of a segment of an arterial vessel wall to confirm inflammation of the wall or arteritis, a type of vasculitis
catheter ablation KĂTH-ĕ-tĕr ăb-LĀ-shŭn	Destruction of conduction tissue of the heart to interrupt the abnormal conduction pathway causing the arrhythmia, thus allowing normal heart rhythm to resume *Catheter ablation is usually performed under fluoroscopic guidance.*
commissurotomy kŏm-ĭ-shūr-ŎT-ō-mē	Surgical separation of the leaflets of the mitral valve, which have fused together at their "commissures" (points of touching) *Many candidates for commissurotomy are now treated with balloon mitral valvuloplasty.*
laser ablation LĀ-zĕr ăb-LĀ-shŭn	Procedure used to remove or treat varicose veins *In laser ablation, the laser's heat coagulates blood inside the vessel, causing it to collapse and seal. Later, the vessels dissolve within the body, becoming less visible, or disappear altogether.*
ligation and stripping lī-GĀ-shŭn, STRĬP-ĭng	Tying a varicose vein (ligation) followed by removal (stripping) of the affected segment *Ligation and stripping are procedures performed for heavily damaged or diseased veins. Usual treatment for varicose veins is laser ablation in combination with microphlebectomies and sclerotherapy.*
open heart surgery	Surgical procedure performed on or within the exposed heart, usually with the assistance of a heart-lung machine *During the operation, the heart-lung machine takes over circulation to allow surgery on the resting (nonbeating) heart. After the heart has been restarted and is beating, the patient is disconnected from the heart-lung machine. Types of open heart surgery include coronary artery bypass graft, valve replacement, and heart transplant.*

(continued)

Diagnostic and Therapeutic Procedures—cont'd

Procedure	Description
pericardiocentesis pĕr-ĭ-kăr-dē-ō-sĕn-TĒ-sĭs *peri-:* around *cardi/o:* heart *-centesis:* surgical puncture	Puncturing of the pericardium to remove excess fluid from the pericardial sac or to test for protein, sugar, and enzymes or determine the causative organism of pericarditis
thrombolysis thrŏm-BŎL-ĭ-sĭs *thromb/o:* blood clot *-lysis:* separation; destruction; loosening intravascular ĭn-tră-VĂS-kū-lăr *intra-:* in, within *vascul/o:* vessel *-ar:* pertaining to, relating to	Destruction of a blood clot using anticlotting agents called *clot-busters,* such as tissue plasminogen activator *Prompt thrombolysis can restore blood flow to tissue before serious irreversible damage occurs. However, many thrombolytic agents also pose the risk of hemorrhage.* Infusion of a thrombolytic agent into a vessel to dissolve a blood clot
valvotomy văl-VŎT-ō-mē *valv/o:* valve *-tomy:* incision	Incision of a valve to increase the size of the opening; used in treating mitral stenosis
venipuncture VĔN-ĭ-pŭnk-chŭr	Puncture of a vein by a needle attached to a syringe or catheter to withdraw a specimen of blood; also called *phlebotomy*

Pharmacology

A healthy, functional cardiovascular system is needed to ensure adequate blood circulation and efficient delivery of oxygen and nutrients to all parts of the body. When any part of the cardiovascular system malfunctions or becomes diseased, drug therapy plays an integral role in establishing and maintaining perfusion and homeostasis.

Medications are used to treat a variety of cardiovascular conditions, including angina pectoris, myocardial infarction, heart failure (HF), arrhythmias, hypertension, hyperlipidemia, and vascular disorders. (See Table 8–1.) Many of the cardiovascular drugs treat multiple problems simultaneously.

Table 8-1   Drugs Used to Treat Cardiovascular Disorders

This table lists common drug classifications used to treat cardiovascular disorders, their therapeutic actions, and selected generic and trade names.

Classification	Therapeutic Action	Generic and Trade Names
angiotensin-converting enzyme inhibitors	Lower blood pressure by inhibiting the conversion of angiotensin I (an inactive enzyme) to angiotensin II (a potent vasoconstrictor). *Angiotensin-converting enzyme (ACE) inhibitors are used to treat hypertension alone or with other agents and aid in the management of heart failure.*	**benazepril** bĕn-Ā-ză-prĭl Lotensin **captopril** KĂP-tō-prĭl Capoten

Table 8-1	**Drugs Used To Treat Cardiovascular Disorders—cont'd**	
Classification	**Therapeutic Action**	**Generic and Trade Names**
antiarrhythmics	Prevent, alleviate, or correct cardiac arrhythmias (dysrhythmias) by stabilizing the electrical conduction of the heart. *Anitarrhythmics are used to treat atrial and ventricular dysrhythmias.*	**flecainide** flĕ-KĀ-nĭd Tambocor
beta-blockers	Block the effect of adrenaline on beta receptors, which slow nerve pulses that pass through the heart, thereby causing a decrease heart rate and contractility. *Beta-blockers are prescribed for hypertension, angina, and arrhythmias (dysrhythmias).*	**atenolol** ă-TĔN-ō-lŏl Tenormin **metoprolol** mĕ-TŌ-prō-lŏl Lopressor, Toprol-XL
calcium channel blockers	Block movement of calcium (required for blood vessel contraction) into myocardial cells and arterial walls, causing heart rate and blood pressure to decrease *Calcium channel blockers are used to treat angina pectoris, hypertension, arrhythmias, and heart failure.*	**amlodipine** ăm-LŌ-dĭ-pēn Norvasc **diltiazem** dĭl-TĪ-ă-zĕm Cardizem CD **nifedipine** nī-FĔD-ĭ-pēn Adalat CC, Procardia
diuretics	Act on kidneys to increase excretion of water and sodium. *Diuretics reduce fluid build-up in the body, including fluid in the lungs, a common symptom of heart failure. Diuretics are also used to treat hypertension.*	**furosemide** fū-RŌ-sĕ-mīd Lasix
nitrates	Dilate blood vessels of the heart, causing an increase in the amount of oxygen delivered to the myocardium, and decrease venous return and arterial resistance, which decreases myocardial oxygen demand and relieves angina. *Nitrates can be administered in several ways: sublingually as a spray or tablet, orally as a tablet, transdermally as a patch, topically as an ointment, or intravenously in an emergency setting.*	**nitroglycerin** nī-trō-GLĬS-ĕr-ĭn Nitrolingual, Nitrogard, Nitrostat
statins	Lower cholesterol in the blood and reduce its production in the liver by blocking the enzyme that produces it. *Vitorin, a statin drug, combined with a cholesterol absorption inhibitor not only lowers cholesterol in the blood and reduces its production in the liver, but also decreases absorption of dietary cholesterol from the intestine. Hypercholesterolemia is a major factor in development of heart disease.* Dilate arteries in skeletal muscles, thus improving peripheral blood flow.	**atorvastatin** ăh-tŏr-vă-STĂ-tĭn Lipitor **simvastatin** SĬM-vă-stă-tĭn Zocor **simvastatin and ezetimibe** SĬM-vă-stă-tĭn, ĕ-ZĔ-tĭ-mīb Vytorin

(continued)

Table 8-1	**Drugs Used to Treat Cardiovascular Disorders—cont'd**		
Classification	**Therapeutic Action**		**Generic and Trade Names**
peripheral vasodilators	Peripheral vasodilators treat peripheral vascular diseases, diabetic peripheral vascular insufficiency, and Raynaud disease.		**cyclandelate** sĭ-KLĂN-dĕ-lāt Cyclan **isoxsuprine** ī-SŎK-sū-prēn Vasodilan

Abbreviations

This section introduces cardiovascular-related abbreviations and their meanings.

Abbreviation	Meaning	Abbreviation	Meaning
AAA	abdominal aortic aneurysm	CHD	coronary heart disease
ACE	angiotensin-converting enzyme (inhibitor)	Chol	cholesterol
AF	atrial fibrillation	CK	creatine kinase (cardiac enzyme); conductive keratoplasty
AS	aortic stenosis	CPR	cardiopulmonary resuscitation
ASD	atrial septal defect	CV	cardiovascular
ASHD	arteriosclerotic heart disease	DES	drug-eluting stent
AST	angiotensin sensitivity test	DOE	dyspnea on exertion
AV	atrioventricular; arteriovenous	DSA	digital subtraction angiography
BBB	bundle-branch block	DVT	deep vein thrombosis, deep venous thrombosis
BP, B/P	blood pressure	ECG, EKG	electrocardiogram; electrocardiography
CA	cancer; chronological age; cardiac arrest	ECHO	echocardiogram echocardiography; echo-encephalogram, echoencephalography
CABG	coronary artery bypass graft	EF	ejection fraction
CAD	coronary artery disease	ETT	exercise tolerance test
CC	cardiac catheterization	HDL	high-density lipoprotein
CCU	coronary care unit	HF	heart failure

Abbreviations—cont'd

Abbreviation	Meaning	Abbreviation	Meaning
HTN	hypertension	MUGA	Multiple-gated acquisition (scan)
ICD	implantable cardioverter defibrillator	MVP	mitral valve prolapse
IV	intravenous	NSR	normal sinus rhythm
LA	left atrium	PAC	premature atrial contraction
LD	lactate dehydrogenase; lactic acid dehydrogenase (cardiac enzyme)	PTCA	percutaneous transluminal coronary angioplasty
LDL	low-density lipoprotein	PVC	premature ventricular contraction
LV	left ventricle	RA	right atrium
MI	myocardial infarction	RV	residual volume; right ventricle
MR	mitral regurgitation	SA, S-A	sinoatrial
MRA	magnetic resonance angiogram; magnetic resonance angiography	SOB	shortness of breath
MRI	magnetic resonance imaging	VSD	ventricular septal defect
MS	musculoskeletal; multiple sclerosis; mitral stenosis; mental status	VT	ventricular tachycardia

It is time to review procedures, pharmacology, and abbreviations by completing Learning Activity 8–4.

LEARNING ACTIVITIES

The following activities provide review of the cardiovascular system terms introduced in this chapter. Complete each activity and review your answers to evaluate your understanding of the chapter.

Learning Activity 8-1
Identifying Cardiovascular Structures

Label the following illustration using the terms listed below.

aorta	left coronary artery	right coronary artery
circumflex artery	left pulmonary artery	right pulmonary artery
inferior vena cava	left pulmonary veins	right pulmonary veins
left anterior descending artery	left ventricle	right ventricle
left atrium	right atrium	superior vena cava

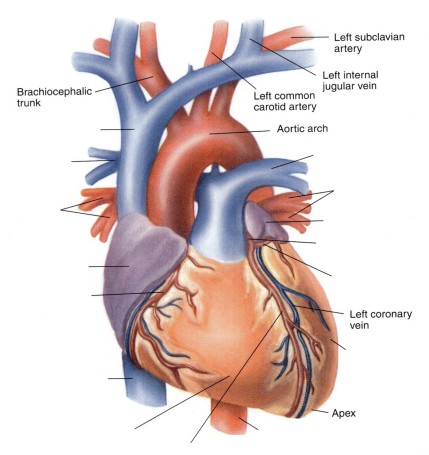

 Check your answers by referring to Figure 8–2A on page 189. Review material that you did not answer correctly.

Label the following illustration using the terms listed below.

aorta	*left pulmonary veins*	*right pulmonary veins*
aortic semilunalr valve	*left ventricle*	*right ventricle*
inferior vena cava	*mitral (bicuspid) valve*	*superior vena cava*
left atrium	*pulmonic valve*	*tricuspid valve*
left pulmonary artery	*right atrium*	

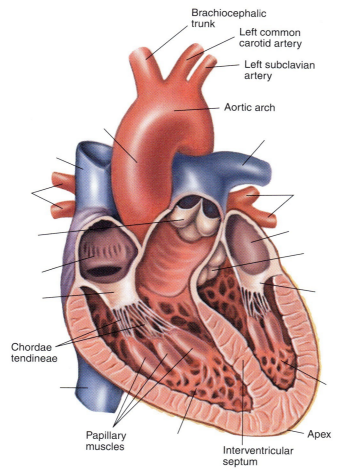

Brachiocephalic trunk

Left common carotid artery

Left subclavian artery

Aortic arch

Chordae tendineae

Papillary muscles

Interventricular septum

Apex

☑ *Check your answers by referring to Figure 8–2B on page 189. Review material that you did not answer correctly.*

 DavisPlus.fadavis.com

Enhance your study and reinforcement of word elements with the power of DavisPlus. Visit www. davisplus.fadavis.com/gylys/systems *for this chapter's flash-card activity. We recommend you complete the flash-card activity before completing Activity 8–2 below.*

Learning Activity 8-2
Building Medical Words

Use *ather/o* (fatty plaque) to build words that mean:

1. tumor of fatty plaque _____
2. hardening of fatty plaque _____

Use *phleb/o* (vein) to build words that mean:

3. inflammation of a vein (wall) _____
4. abnormal condition of a blood clot in a vein _____

Use *ven/o* (vein) to build words that mean:

5. pertaining to a vein _____
6. spasm of a vein _____

Use *cardi/o* (heart) to build words that mean:

7. specialist in the study of the heart _____
8. rupture of the heart _____
9. poisonous to the heart _____
10. enlargement of the heart _____

Use *angi/o* (vessel) to build words that mean:

11. softening of a vessel (wall) _____
12. tumor of a vessel _____

Use *thromb/o* (blood clot) to build words that mean:

13. beginning or formation of a blood clot _____
14. abnormal condition of a blood clot _____

Use *aort/o* (heart) to build words that mean:

15. abnormal condition of narrowing or stricture of the aorta _____
16. process of recording the aorta _____

Build surgical words that mean:

17. puncture of the heart _____
18. suture of an artery _____
19. removal of an embolus _____
20. separation, destruction, or loosening of a blood clot _____

✓ *Check your answers in Appendix A. Review material that you did not answer correctly.*

Correct Answers _____ ✕ 5 = _____ % Score

Matching Pathological, Diagnostic, Symptomatic, and Related Terms

Match the following terms with the definitions in the numbered list.

aneurysm	bruit	diaphoresis	incompetent	perfusion
angina	catheter	embolus	infarct	stent
arrest	coarctation	hyperlipidemia	ischemia	varices
arrhythmia	deep vein thrombosis	hypertension	palpitation	vegetations

1. area of tissue that undergoes necrosis _____

2. chest pain _____

3. inability of a valve to close completely _____

4. small masses of inflammatory material found on the leaflets of valves _____

5. varicose veins of the esophagus _____

6. soft, blowing sound heard on auscultation; murmur _____

7. thin, flexible, hollow tube that can be inserted into a vessel or cavity (vein or artery) of the body _____

8. sensation of the heart not beating normally _____

9. blood clot that often forms in the legs and thighs and may lead to pulmonary thrombosis _____

10. localized abnormal dilation of a vessel _____

11. mass of undissolved matter circulating in blood or lymph channels _____

12. inability of the heart to maintain a steady beat _____

13. condition of being stopped or bringing to a stop _____

14. profuse sweating _____

15. slender or threadlike device used to support tubular structures or hold arteries open during and after angioplasty _____

16. common disorder characterized by persistent elevated blood pressure _____

17. excessive amounts of lipids in the blood _____

18. narrowing of a vessel, especially the aorta _____

19. local and temporary deficiency of blood supply due to circulatory obstruction _____

20. circulation of blood through tissues _____

✓ *Check your answers in Appendix A. Review any material that you did not answer correctly.*

Correct Answers _____ × 5 = _____ % Score

Learning Activity 8-4
Matching Procedures, Pharmacology, and Abbreviations

Match the following terms with the definitions in the numbered list.

angioplasty	catheter ablation	embolization	scintigraphy
arterial biopsy	commissurotomy	Holter monitor test	statins
atherectomy	coronary angiography	ligation and stripping	stress test
CABG	diuretics	nitrates	thrombolysis
cardiac enzyme studies	echocardiography	PTCA	venipuncture

1. 24-hour ECG tracing taken with a small, portable recording system _____
2. noninvasive ultrasound diagnostic test used to visualize internal cardiac structures _____
3. radiological examination of the blood vessels of and around the heart _____
4. agents used to treat angina _____
5. drugs that have powerful lipid-lowering properties _____
6. management of edema associated with heart failure and hypertension _____
7. include troponin T, troponin I, and creatinine kinase _____
8. injection and detection of radioactive isotopes to create images and identify function and disease
   _____
9. ECG taken under controlled exercise stress conditions _____
10. tying of a varicose vein and subsequent removal _____
11. surgical separation of the leaflets of the mitral valve _____
12. removal of a small segment of an artery for diagnostic purposes _____
13. destruction of conductive tissue of the heart to interrupt abnormal contractions _____
14. technique used to block flow to a site by injecting an occluding agent _____
15. procedure that alters a vessel through surgery or dilation _____
16. dilation of an occluded vessel using a balloon catheter _____
17. surgery that creates a bypass around a blocked segment of a coronary artery _____
18. removal of occluding material using a cutting or grinding device _____
19. incision or puncture of a vein to remove blood or introduce fluids _____
20. destruction of a blood clot _____

✔ *Check your answers in Appendix A. Review any material that you did not answer correctly.*

Correct Answers _____ × 5 = _____ % Score

MEDICAL RECORD ACTIVITIES

The two medical records included in the following activities use common clinical scenarios to show how medical terminology is used to document patient care. Complete the terminology and analysis sections for each activity to help you recognize and understand terms related to the cardiovascular system.

Medical Record Activity 8-1
Chart Note: Acute Myocardial Infarction

Terminology

Terms listed in the following table are taken from *Chart Note: Acute Myocardial Infarction* that follows. Use a medical dictionary such as *Taber's Cyclopedic Medical Dictionary,* the appendices of this book, or other resources to define each term. Then review the pronunciations for each term and practice by reading the medical record aloud.

Term	Definition
acute	
cardiac enzymes KĂR-dē-ăk ĔN-zīmz	
CCU	
ECG	
heparin HĔP-ă-rĭn	
infarction ĭn-FĂRK-shŭn	
inferior	
ischemia ĭs-KĒ-mē-ă	
lateral LĂT-ĕr-ăl	
MI	
myocardial mī-ō-KĂR-dē-ăl	
partial thromboplastin time thrŏm-bō-PLĂS-tĭn	

Term	Definition	
streptokinase strĕp-tō-KĪ-nās		
substernal sŭb-STĔR-năl		

 Listen and Learn Online! *will help you master the pronunciation of selected medical words from this medical record activity. Visit* www.davisplus.com/gylys/systems *to find instructions on completing the* Listen and Learn Online! *exercise for this section and to practice pronunciations.*

CHART NOTE: ACUTE MYOCARDIAL INFARCTION

March 15, 20xx

Gately, Mary

PRESENT ILLNESS: Patient is a 68–year-old woman hospitalized for acute anterior myocardial infarction. She has a history of sudden onset of chest pain. Approximately 2 hours before hospitalization, she had severe substernal pain with radiation to the back. ECG showed evidence of abnormalities. She was given streptokinase and treated with heparin at 800 units per hour. She will be evaluated with a partial thromboplastin time and cardiac enzymes in the morning.

PAST HISTORY: Patient was seen in 20xx, with history of an inferior MI in 19xx, but she was stable and underwent a treadmill test. Test results showed no ischemia and she had no chest pain. Her records confirmed an MI with enzyme elevation and evidence of a previous inferior MI.

IMPRESSION: Acute lateral anterior myocardial infarction and a previous healed inferior myocardial infarction. At this time patient is stable, is in coronary care unit, and will be given appropriate followup and supportive care.

PLAN: At this time the patient is stable, is in CCU and will be given appropriate followup and supportive care.

Juan Perez, MD
Juan Perez, MD

D: 03-15-20xx
T: 03-15-20xx

Ibg

Analysis

Review the medical record *Chart Note: Acute Myocardial Infarction* to answer the following questions.

1. How long had the patient experienced chest pain before she was seen in the hospital?

_____

2. Did the patient have a previous history of chest pain?

_____

3. Initially, what medications were administered to stabilize the patient?

_____

4. What two laboratory tests will be used to evaluate the patient?

_____

5. During the current admission, what part of the heart was damaged?

_____

6. Was the location of damage to the heart for this admission the same as for the initial MI?

_____

Medical Record Activity 8-2

Operative Report: Right Temporal Artery Biopsy

Terms listed in the following table are taken from *Operative Report: Right Temporal Artery Biopsy* that follows. Use a medical dictionary such as *Taber's Cyclopedic Medical Dictionary,* the appendices of this book, or other resources to define each term. Then review the pronunciations for each term and practice by reading the medical record aloud.

Term	Definition
arteritis ăr-tĕ-RĪ-tĭs	
Betadine BĀ-tă-dīn	
biopsy BĪ-ŏp-sē	
dissected dĭ-SĔKT-ĕd	
distally DĬS-tă-lē	
incised ĭn-SĪZD	
IV	
ligated LĪ-gā-tĕd	
palpable PĂL-pă-b'l	

Term	Definition
preauricular prē-aw-RĬK-ū-lăr	
proximally PRŎK-sĭ-mă-lē	
superficial fascia soo-pĕr-FĬSH-ăl FĂSH-ē-ă	
supine sū-PĪN	
temporal TĔM-por-ăl	
Xylocaine ZĪ-lō-kān	

 Listen and Learn Online! *will help you master the pronunciation of selected medical words from this medical record activity. Visit* www.davisplus.com/gylys/systems *to find instructions on completing the* Listen and Learn Online! *exercise for this section and to practice pronunciations.*

OPERATIVE REPORT: RIGHT TEMPORAL ARTERY BIOPSY

General Hospital

1511 Ninth Avenue ■■ **Sun City, USA 12345** ■■ **(555) 8022-1887**

OPERATIVE REPORT

Date: May 14, 20xx   Physician: Dante Riox, MD

Patient: Gonzolez, Roberto   Room: 703

PREOPERATIVE DIAGNOSIS: Rule out right temporal arteritis.

POSTOPERATIVE DIAGNOSIS: Rule out right temporal arteritis.

PROCEDURE: Right temporal artery biopsy.

SPECIMEN: 1.5-cm segment of right temporal artery.

ESTIMATED BLOOD LOSS: Nil.

COMPLICATIONS: None.

TIME UNDER SEDATION: 25 minutes.

PROCEDURE AND FINDINGS: Informed consent was obtained. Patient was taken to the surgical suite and placed in the supine position. IV sedation was administered. Patient was turned to his left side and the preauricular area was prepped for surgery using Betadine. Having been draped in sterile fashion, 1% Xylocaine was infiltrated along the palpable temporal artery and a vertical incision was made. Dissection was carried down through the subcutaneous tissue and superficial fascia, which was incised. The temporal artery was located and dissected proximally and distally. Then the artery was ligated with 6–0 Vicryl proximally and distally and a large segment of approximately 1.5 cm was removed. The specimen was sent to the pathology laboratory and then superficial fascia was closed with interrupted stitches of 6–0 Vicryl and skin was closed with interrupted stitches of 6–0 Prolene. A sterile dressing was applied. Patient tolerated the procedure well and was transferred to the postanesthesia care unit in stable condition.

Dante Riox, MD
Dante Riox, MD

dr:bg

D: 5-14-20xx
T: 5-14-20xx

Analysis

Review the medical record *Operative Report: Right Temporal Artery Biopsy* to answer the following questions.

1. Why was the right temporal artery biopsied?

2. In what position was the patient placed?

3. What was the incision area?

4. How was the temporal artery located for administration of Xylocaine?

5. How was the dissection carried out?

6. What was the size of the specimen?

Blood, Lymph, and Immune Systems

Chapter Outline

Objectives

Upon completion of this chapter, you will be able to:

- Identify and describe the components of blood.
- Locate and identify the structures associated with the lymphatic system.
- List the cells associated with the acquired immune response and describe their function.
- Describe the functional relationship between the blood, lymph, and immune systems and other body systems.
- Recognize, pronounce, spell, and build words related to the blood, lymph, and immune systems.
- Describe pathological conditions, diagnostic and therapeutic procedures, and other terms related to the blood, lymph, and immune systems.
- Explain pharmacology related to the treatment of blood, lymph, and immune disorders.
- Demonstrate your knowledge of this chapter by completing the learning and medical record activities.

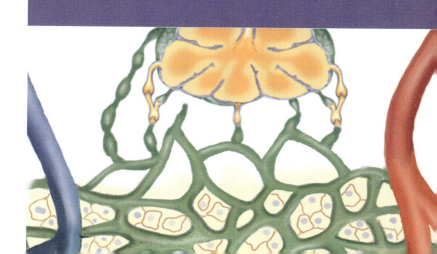

Anatomy and Physiology

The blood, lymph, and immune systems share common cells, structures, and functions. Blood provides immune cells that locate, identify, and destroy disease-causing agents. These immune cells actively engage in the destruction of the invading agent or produce substances that seek out and tag the agent for destruction. Immune cells rely on lymph vessels and blood vessels to deliver their protective devices to the entire body. Furthermore, immune cells use lymph structures (the spleen and lymph nodes) for permanent or temporary lodging sites. They also use these structures to monitor the **extracellular fluid** of the body as it filters through the nodes. When immune cells identify disease-causing agents passing through the nodes, they destroy them before they cause disease in the **host.** The lymph system returns extracellular fluid, lymph, and immune substances back to the circulatory system as plasma to be ready once again for redelivery to the entire body. Although blood, lymph, and immune systems are discussed separately, their functions and structures overlap.

Blood

Blood is connective tissue composed of a liquid medium called *plasma* in which solid components are suspended. It accounts for approximately 8% of the total weight of the body. The solid components of blood include:

- red blood cells (**erythrocytes**)
- white blood cells (**leukocytes**)
- platelets (**thrombocytes**). (See Figure 9–1.)

Anatomy and Physiology Key Terms

This section introduces important blood, lymph, and immune system terms and their definitions. Word analyses for selected terms are also provided.

Term	Definition
antibody ĂN-tĭ-bŏd-ē	Protective protein produced by B lymphocytes in response to presence of a foreign substance called an *antigen*
antigen ĂN-tĭ-jĕn	Substance recognized as harmful to the host and stimulates formation of antibodies in an immunocompetent individual
bile pigments BĪL	Substances derived from the breakdown of hemoglobin, produced by the liver, and excreted in the form of bile *Interference with the excretion of bile may lead to jaundice.*
cytokines SĪ-tō-kīnz	Chemical substances produced by certain cells that initiate, inhibit, increase, or decrease activity in other cells *Cytokines are important chemical communicators in the immune response, regulating many activities associated with immunity and inflammation.*
extracellular fluid ĕks-tră-SĔL-ū-lăr	All body fluids found outside cells, including interstitial fluid, plasma, lymph, and cerebrospinal fluid *Extracellular fluid provides a stable external environment for body cells.*
host	Organism that maintains or harbors another organism
immunocompetent ĭm-ū-nō-KŎM-pĕ-tĕnt	Ability to develop an immune response, or the ability to recognize antigens and respond to them
natural killer cells	Specialized lymphocytes that kill abnormal cells by releasing chemicals that destroy the cell membrane causing its intercellular fluids to leak out *Natural killer (NK) cells destroy virally infected cells and tumor cells.*

Pronunciation Help	Long Sound	ā—rate	ē—rebirth	ī—isle	ō—over	ū—unite
	Short Sound	ă—alone	ĕ—ever	ĭ—it	ŏ—not	ŭ—cut

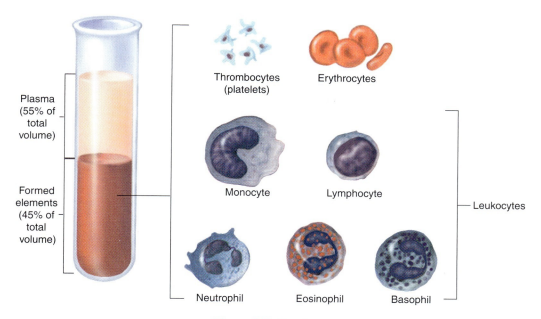

Figure 9-1. Blood composition.

In adults, blood cells are formed in the bone marrow of the skull, ribs, sternum, vertebrae, pelvis and the ends of the long bones of the arms and legs. Blood cells develop from an undifferentiated cell called a *stem cell.* The development and maturation of blood cells is called *hematopoiesis,* or *hemopoiesis.* (See Figure 9–2.) Red blood cell development is called *erythropoiesis;* white blood cell development, *leukopoiesis;* and platelet development, *thrombopoiesis.* After blood cells mature, they leave the bone marrow and enter the circulatory system.

Red blood cells transport oxygen and carbon dioxide. White blood cells provide defenses against diseases and other harmful substances and aid in tissue repair. Platelets provide mechanisms for blood coagulation. Although blood makes up only about 8% of all body tissues, it is essential to life.

Red Blood Cells

Red blood cells (RBCs), or **erythrocytes,** are the most numerous of the circulating blood cells. During erythropoiesis, RBCs decrease in size and, just before reaching maturity, the nucleus is extruded. Small fragments of nuclear material may remain in the immature RBC and appear as a fine, lacy net. This immature RBC is called a *reticulocyte.* Although some reticulocytes are found in circulation, most lose their nuclear material prior to entering the circulatory system as mature erythrocytes. During erythropoiesis, RBCs develop a specialized iron-containing compound called *hemo-*

globin that gives them their red color. Hemoglobin carries oxygen to body tissues and exchanges it for carbon dioxide. When mature, RBCs are shaped like biconcave disks.

RBCs live about 120 days and then rupture, releasing hemoglobin and cell fragments. Hemoglobin breaks down into an iron compound called *hemosiderin* and several bile pigments. Most hemosiderin returns to the bone marrow and is reused in a different form to manufacture new blood cells. The liver eventually excretes bile pigments.

White Blood Cells

White blood cells (WBCs), or **leukocytes,** protect the body against invasion by pathogens and foreign substances, remove debris from injured tissue, and aid in the healing process. While RBCs remain in the bloodstream, WBCs migrate through endothelial walls of capillaries and venules and enter tissue spaces by a process called *diapedesis.* (See Figure 9–3.) There they initiate inflammation and the immune response if they encounter sites of injury or infection. WBCs are divided into two groups: granulocytes and agranulocytes depending on the presence or absence of granules in the cytoplasm.

Granulocytes

There are three types of **granulocytes:** neutrophils, eosinophils, and basophils. Their names are derived from the type of dye that stains their

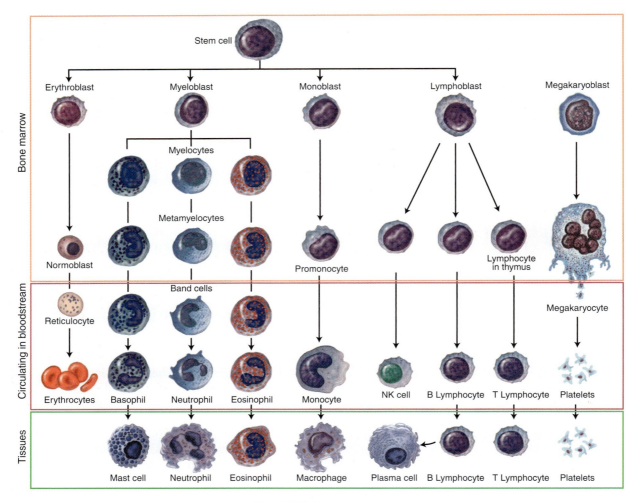

Figure 9-2. Hematopoiesis.

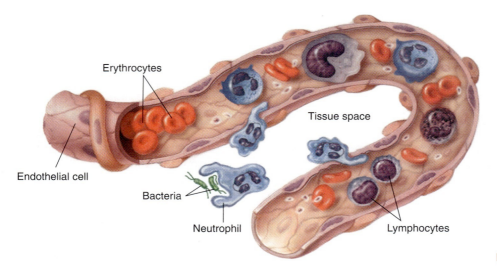

Figure 9-3. Diapedesis.

cytoplasmic granules when a blood smear is prepared in the laboratory for examination:

- **Neutrophils** are the most numerous circulating leukocyte. Their granules stain with a neutral dye, giving them their lilac color. Neutrophils are motile and highly phagocytic, permitting them to ingest and devour bacteria and other particulate matter. They are the first cell to appear at a site of injury or infection to begin the work of phagocytizing foreign material. (See Figure 9–4.) Their importance in body protection cannot be underestimated. A person with a serious deficiency of this blood cell type will die despite protective attempts by other body defences.
- **Eosinophils** contain granules that stain with a red acidic dye called *eosin*. Eosinophils protect the body by releasing many substances that neutralize toxic compounds, especially of a chemical nature. Eosinophils increase in number during allergic reactions and animal parasite infestations.
- **Basophils** contain granules that readily stain with a purple alkaline (basic) dye. Basophils release histamines and heparin when tissue is

damaged. **Histamines** initiate the inflammatory process by increasing blood flow. As more blood flows to the damaged area, it carries with it additional nutrients, immune substances, and immune cells that help in damage containment and tissue repair. **Heparin** is an anticoagulant and acts to prevent blood from clotting at the injury site.

In their mature forms, all three types of granulocytes commonly exhibit a nucleus with at least two lobes, and in neutrophils, sometimes as many as six lobes (**polymorphonuclear**).

Agranulocytes

Agranulocytes arise in the bone marrow from stem cells. Their nuclei do not form lobes. Thus, they are commonly called *mononuclear leukocytes.* There are two types of agranulocytes: monocytes and lymphocytes.

- **Monocytes** are mildly phagocytic when found within blood vessels. However, they remain in the vascular channels only a short time. When they exit, they transform into **macrophages,** avid phagocytes

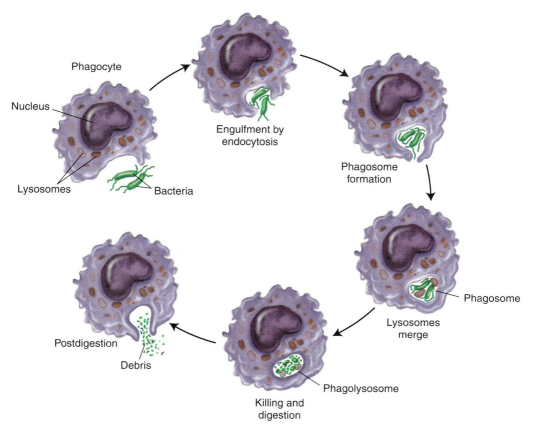

Figure 9-4. Phagocytosis.

capable of ingesting pathogens, dead cells, and other debris found at sites of inflammation. Macrophages play a chief role in many activities associated with specific immunity.

- **Lymphocytes** include B cells, T cells, and natural killer cells. B cells and T cells provide a specialized type of defence called the *specific immune response.* This mode of protection is custom-made and aimed at a specific antigen. Its dual action includes humoral immunity and cellular immunity. Natural killer (NK) cells provide a generalized defence and respond whenever a potentially dangerous or abnormal cell is encountered. They "kill" by releasing potent chemicals that rupture the cell membrane of abnormal cells. NK cells are highly effective against cancer cells and cells harboring pathogens. These cells have the ability to kill over and over again before they die. (See Table 9-1.)

Platelets

Platelets are the smallest formed elements found in blood. Although they are sometimes called *thrombocytes,* they are not true cells, as this term erroneously suggests, but merely fragments of cells. Platelets initiate blood clotting (**hemostasis**) when injury occurs. Hemostasis is not a single reaction, but a series of interlinked reactions, each requiring a specific factor. If any one of the factors is absent, a clot will not form. Initially, the damaged blood vessel constricts and platelets become "sticky." They aggregate at the injury site and provide a barrier to contain blood loss. Clotting factors in platelets and injured tissue release **thromboplastin**, a substance that initiates clot formation. In the final step of coagulation, **fibrinogen** (a soluble blood protein) becomes insoluble and forms fibrin strands that act as a net, entrapping blood cells. This jellylike mass of blood cells and fibrin is called a *thrombus* or *blood clot.*

Plasma

Plasma is the liquid portion of blood in which blood cells are suspended. When blood cells are removed, plasma appears as a thin, almost colorless fluid. It is composed of about 92% water and contains such products as **plasma proteins** (albumins, globulins, and fibrinogen), gases, nutrients, salts, hormones, and waste materials. Plasma makes possible the chemical communication between body cells by transporting body products throughout the body.

Blood serum is a product of blood plasma. If fibrinogen and clotting elements are removed from plasma, the resulting fluid is called *serum.* If a blood sample clots in a test tube, the resulting fluid that remains after the clot is removed is serum, because fibrinogen and other clotting elements have been expended to form the clot.

Blood Groups

Human blood is divided into four groups, A, B, AB, and O, based on the presence or absence of specific antigens on the surface of RBCs. (See Table 9–2.) In each of these four blood groups, the plasma does not contain the antibody against the antigen that is present on the RBCs. Rather, the plasma contains the opposite antibodies. These

Table 9-1	**Protective Actions of White Blood**

This chart lists the two main categories of white blood cells along with their cellular components and their protective actions.

Cell Type	Protective Action
Granulocytes	
Neutrophils	Phagocytosis
Eosinophils	Allergy, animal parasites
Basophils	Inflammation mediators, anticoagulant properties
Agranulocytes	
Monocytes	Phagocytosis
Lymphocytes	
• B cells	Humoral immunity
• T cells	Cellular immunity
• Natural killer cells	Destruction without specificity

Table 9-2 **ABO System**			
The table below lists the four blood types along with their respective antigens and antibodies and the percentage of the population that have each type.			
Blood Type	**Antigen (RBC)**	**Antibody (plasma)**	**% Population**
A	A	anti-B	41
B	B	anti-A	10
AB	A and B	none	4
O	neither A nor B	anti-A and anti-B	45

antibodies occur naturally; that is, they are present or develop shortly after birth even though there has been no previous exposure to the antigen.

In addition to antigens of the four blood groups, there are numerous other antigens that may be present on RBCs. One such antigen group includes the Rh blood factor. This particular factor is implicated in **hemolytic disease of the newborn (HDN)**, caused by an incompatibility between maternal and fetal blood.

Blood groups are medically important in transfusions, transplants, and maternal-fetal incompatibilities. Although hematologists have identified more than 300 different blood antigens, most of these are not of medical concern.

Lymph System

The lymph system consists of a fluid called *lymph* (in which lymphocytes and monocytes are suspended), a network of transporting vessels called *lymph vessels,* and a multiplicity of other structures, including nodes, spleen, thymus, and tonsils. Functions of the lymph system include:

• maintaining fluid balance of the body by draining extracellular fluid from tissue spaces and returning it to the blood
• transporting lipids away from the digestive organs for use by body tissues
• filtering and removing unwanted or infectious products in lymph nodes.
(See Figure 9–5.)

Lymph vessels begin as closed-ended capillaries in tissue spaces and terminate at the right lymphatic duct and the thoracic duct in the chest cavity. As whole blood circulates, a small amount of plasma seeps from (1) **blood capillaries**. This fluid, now called *extracellular (interstitial* or *tissue) fluid,* resembles plasma but contains slightly less protein. Extracellular fluid carries needed products

to tissue cells while removing their wastes. As extracellular fluid moves through tissues, it also collects cellular debris, bacteria, and particulate matter. Extracellular fluid returns to blood capillaries to become plasma or enters (2) **lymph capillaries** to become lymph. Lymph passes into larger and larger vessels on its return trip to the bloodstream. Before it reaches its final destination, it first enters (3) **lymph nodes**. These nodes serve as depositories for cellular debris. In the node, macrophages phagocytize bacteria and other harmful material while T cells and B cells exert their protective influence. When a local infection exists, the number of bacteria entering a node is so great and the destruction by T cells and B cells so powerful that the node commonly enlarges and becomes tender.

Lymph vessels from the right chest and arm join the (4) **right lymphatic duct.** This duct drains into the (5) **right subclavian vein,** a major vessel in the cardiovascular system. Lymph from all other areas of the body enters the (6) **thoracic duct** and drains into the (7) **left subclavian vein.** Lymph is redeposited into the circulating blood and becomes plasma. This cycle continually repeats itself.

The (8) **spleen** resembles lymph nodes because it acts like a filter removing cellular debris, bacteria, parasites, and other infectious agents. However, the spleen also destroys old RBCs and serves as a repository for healthy blood cells. The (9) **thymus** is located in the upper part of the chest (**mediastinum**). It partially controls the immune system by transforming certain lymphocytes into T cells, the lymphocytes responsible for cellular immunity. The (10) **tonsils** are masses of lymphatic tissue located in the pharynx. They act as filters to protect the upper respiratory structures from invasion by pathogens.

Immune System

Although exposed to a vast number of harmful substances, most people suffer relatively few diseases throughout their lifetime. Numerous body

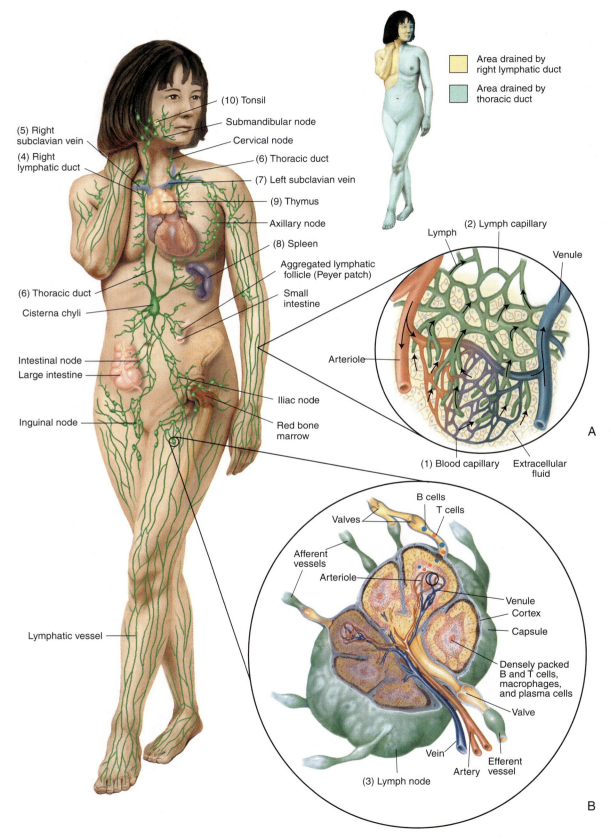

Area drained by right lymphatic duct

Area drained by thoracic duct

(10) Tonsil
Submandibular node
(5) Right subclavian vein
Cervical node
(4) Right lymphatic duct
(6) Thoracic duct
(7) Left subclavian vein
(9) Thymus
Axillary node
(8) Spleen
Aggregated lymphatic follicle (Peyer patch)
(6) Thoracic duct
Small intestine
Cisterna chyli
Intestinal node
Large intestine
Iliac node
Inguinal node
Red bone marrow
Lymphatic vessel

Lymph
(2) Lymph capillary
Venule
Arteriole
(1) Blood capillary
Extracellular fluid
A

B cells
T cells
Valves
Afferent vessels
Arteriole
Venule
Cortex
Capsule
Densely packed B and T cells, macrophages, and plasma cells
Valve
Vein
Efferent vessel
Artery
(3) Lymph node
B

Figure 9-5. Lymph system. (A) Capillary. (B) Lymph node.

defenses called *resistance* work together to protect against disease. Resistance includes physical barriers (skin and mucous membranes) and chemical and cellular barriers (tears, saliva, gastric juices, and neutrophils). Because these barriers are present at birth, they are said to be *innate* barriers. Another form of resistance called the *acquired immune response* develops after birth. This form of resistance is by far the most complex in structure and function. It continuously develops throughout life as a result of exposure to one disease after another. With each exposure, the immune system of an immunocompetent individual identifies the invading antigen, musters a unique response to destroy it, and then retreats with a memory of both the invader and the method of destruction. In the event of a second encounter by the same invader, the immune system is armed and ready to destroy it before it can cause disease. The WBCs responsible for the specific immune response include monocytes and lymphocytes.

Monocytes

After a brief stay in the vascular system, monocytes enter tissue spaces and become highly phagocytic **macrophages.** In this form, they consume large numbers of pathogens, including bacteria and viruses. After macrophages engulf a pathogen, they process it in such a way that the highly specific antigenic properties of the pathogen are placed on the cell surface of the macrophage. Thus, the macrophage becomes an **antigen-presenting cell (APC).** The APC awaits an encounter with a lymphocyte capable of responding to that specific antigen. When this occurs, the specific immune system begins the operations required for the systematic destruction of the antigen.

Lymphocytes

Two types of **lymphocytes,** T cells and B cells, are the active cells of the acquired immune response. Each cell type mediates a specific type of immunity, either humoral or cellular.

Humoral Immunity

Humoral immunity is the component of the specific immune system that protects primarily against extracellular antigens, such as bacteria and viruses that have not yet entered a cell. Humoral immunity is mediated by B cells, which originate and mature in the bone marrow. During maturation, each B cell develops receptors for a specific antigen and then enters the circulatory system. Upon an

encounter with its specific antigen, the B cell produces a clone of cells called *plasma cells.* Plasma cells produce highly specific proteins called *antibodies.* Antibodies travel throughout the body in plasma, tissue fluid, and lymph. When an antibody encounters its specific antigen, it attaches to it and forms an **antigen-antibody complex.** Once the antigen-antibody complex is formed, the antigen is inactivated, neutralized, or tagged for destruction. After all antigens have been destroyed, memory B cells migrate to lymph tissue and remain available for immediate recall if that same antigen is encountered again.

Cellular Immunity

Cellular immunity is the component of the specific immune system that protects primarily against intracellular antigens such as viruses and cancer cells. Cellular immunity is mediated by T cells. These cells originate in the bone marrow but migrate and mature in the thymus. The four types of T cells include the cytotoxic T cell (T_C), helper T cell (T_H), suppressor T cell (T_S), and memory T cell (T_M). The **cytotoxic T cell** is the cell that actually destroys the invading antigen. It determines the antigen's specific weakness and uses this weakness as a point of attack to destroy it. The **helper T cell** is essential to the proper functioning of both humoral and cellular immunity. It uses chemical messengers called cytokines to activate, direct, and regulate the activity of most of the other components of the immune system, especially B cells. If the number of helper T cells is deficient, the immune system essentially shuts down and the patient becomes a victim of even the most harmless organisms. The **suppressor T cell** monitors the progression of infection. When infection resolves, the suppressor T cell "shuts down" the immune response. Finally, like the humoral response, the cellular response also produces memory cells. These **memory T cells** find their way to the lymph system and remain there long after the encounter with the antigen, ready for combat if the antigen reappears. (See Table 9–3.)

The memory component is unique to the acquired immune response. Memory B and T cells are able to "recall" how they previously disposed of a particular antigen and are able to repeat the process. The repeat performance is immediate, powerful, and sustained. Disposing of the antigen during the second and all subsequent exposures is extremely rapid and much more effective than it was during the first exposure. This "repeat performance" is called the *anamnestic response.*

| Table 9-3 | **Lymphocytes and Immune Response** |

The chart below lists the lymphocytes involved in humoral and cellular immunity along with their functions and sites of origin and maturation.

Lymphocyte	Function	Origin	Maturation
Humoral immunity			
B lymphocytes		Bone marrow	Bone marrow
• Plasma cells	• Antibody formation for destruction of extracellular antigens		
• Memory cells	• Provides active immunity		
Cellular immunity			
T lymphocytes		Bone marrow	Thymus, immune system
• Cytotoxic T cell (T_C)	• Destruction of infected cells and cancer cells		
• Helper T cell (T_H)	• Assistance for B cells, cytotoxic T cells and other components of the immune system		
• Suppressor T cell (T_S)	• Suppression (shutting down) of humoral and cellular response when infection resolves		
• Memory T cell (T_M)	• Active immunity		

Connecting Body Systems-Blood, Lymph, and Immune Systems

The main functions of the blood, lymph, and immune systems are to provide a medium for the transport and exchange of products throughout the body and to protect and repair cells that are damaged by disease or trauma. Specific functional relationships between the blood, lymph, and immune systems and other body systems are summarized below.

Cardiovascular
• Blood delivers oxygen to the heart needed for contraction.
• Lymphatic system returns interstitial fluid to the vascular system to maintain blood volume.
• Immune system protects against infections.

Digestive
• Blood transports products of digestion to nourish body cells.
• Immune system provides surveillance mechanisms to detect and destroy cancer cells in the digestive tract.
• An innate component of the immune system, the acidic environment of the stomach helps control pathogens of the digestive tract.

Endocrine
• Blood and lymph systems transport hormones to target organs.
• Immune system protects against infection in endocrine glands.

Female reproductive
• Blood, lymph, and immune systems transport nourishing and defensive products across the placental barrier for the developing fetus.
• Immune system provides specific defense against pathogens that enter the body through the reproductive tract.
• Immune system supplies antibodies for breast milk that protect the baby until its immune system is established.

(continued)

Connecting Body Systems-Blood, Lymph, and Immune Systems—cont'd

Musculoskeletal

- Blood removes lactic acid that accumulates in muscles during strenuous exercise.
- Blood transports calcium to bones for strength and healing.
- Lymph system maintains interstitial fluid balance in muscle tissue.
- Immune system aids in repair of muscle tissue following trauma.

Nervous

- Immune system responds to nervous stimuli in order to identify injury or infection sites and initiate tissue defense and repair.
- Plasma and lymph provide the medium in which nervous stimuli cross from one neuron to another.
- Lymph system removes excess interstitial fluid from tissues surrounding nerves.

Respiratory

- Red blood cells transport respiratory gases to and from the lungs.

- Tonsils harbor immune cells that combat pathogens that enter through the nose and mouth.

Genitourinary

- Immune system provides surveillance against cancer cells.
- Blood transports waste products, especially urea, to the kidneys for removal via the production of urine.
- Blood in peritubular capillaries recaptures essential products that have been filtered by the nephron.

Integumentary

- Blood provides leukocytes, especially neutrophils, to the integumentary system when breaches or injury occur in the skin.
- Lymph system supplies antibodies to the dermis for defense against pathogens.
- Blood found in the skin, the largest organ of the body, helps maintain temperature homeostasis.

 It is time to review lymph structures by completing Learning Activity 9–1.

Medical Word Elements

This section introduces combining forms, suffixes, and prefixes related to the blood, lymph, and immune systems. Word analyses are also provided.

Element	Meaning	Word Analysis
Combining Forms		
aden/o	gland	**aden**/oid (ĂD-ĕ-noyd): resembling a gland *-oid:* resembling
agglutin/o	clumping, gluing	**agglutin**/ation (ă-gloo-tĭ-NĀ-shŭn): process of clumping *-ation:* process (of)
bas/o	base (alkaline, opposite of acid)	**bas/o**/phil (BĀ-sō-fĭl): attraction to base (alkaline dyes) *-phil:* attraction for *The granules of the basophil appear dark blue when stained with a dye used in hematology.*

blast/o	embryonic cell	erythr/o/**blast**/osis (ĕ-rĭth-rō-blăs-TŌ-sĭs): abnormal increase of embryonic red (cells)
		  erythr/o: red
		  -osis: abnormal condition; increase (used primarily with blood cells)
		
		Erythroblastosis fetalis is a potentially fatal disease of newborns occurring when a blood incompatibility exists between mother and fetus.

(continued)

Medical Word Elements—cont'd

Element	Meaning	Word Analysis
chrom/o	color	**hypo/chrom/ic** (hī-pō-KRŌM-ĭk): under coloration *hypo-:* under, below *-ic:* pertaining to *Hypochromic cells are erythrocytes that contain inadequate hemoglobin. These cells are commonly associated with iron-deficiency anemia.*
eosin/o	dawn (rose-colored)	**eosin/o/phil** (ē-ō-SĬN-ō-fĭl): attraction for rose colored (dye) *-phil:* attraction for *The granules of an eosinophil appear rose-colored when stained with eosin, a dye used in hematology.*
erythr/o	red	**erythr/o/cyte** (ĕ-RĬTH-rō-sīt): red cell *-cyte:* cell *An erythrocyte is a red blood cell.*
granul/o	granule	**granul/o/cyte** (GRĂN-ū-lō-sīt): cell (containing) granulocytes (in the cytoplasm) *-cyte:* cell
hem/o	blood	**hem/o/phobia** (hē-mō-FŌ-bē-ă): fear of blood *-phobia:* fear *People who suffer from hemophobia commonly faint at the sight of blood.*
hemat/o		**hemat/oma** (hē-mă-TŌ-mă): blood tumor *-oma:* tumor *A hematoma is a mass of extravasated, usually clotted blood caused by a break or leak in a blood vessel. It may be found in any organ, tissue, or space within the body.*
immun/o	immune, immunity, safe	**immun/o/logy** (ĭm-ū-NŎL-ō-jē): study of immunity *-logy:* study of *Immunology includes the study of autoimmune diseases, hypersensitivities, and immune deficiencies.*
kary/o	nucleus	**kary/o/lysis** (kăr-ē-ŎL-ĭ-sĭs): destruction of the nucleus *-lysis:* separation; destruction; loosening *Karyolysis results in cell death.*
nucle/o		**mono/nucle/ar** (mŏn-ō-NŪ-klē-ăr): pertaining to a single nucleus *mono-:* one *-ar:* pertaining to
leuk/o	white	**leuk/emia** (loo-KĒ-mē-ă): white blood condition *-emia:* blood condition *Leukemia causes a profoundly elevated white blood cell count and a very low red blood cell count.*
lymphaden/o	lymph gland (node)	**lymphaden/o/pathy** (lĭm-făd-ĕ-NŎP-ă-thē): disease of lymph nodes *-pathy:* disease *Lymphadenopathy is characterized by changes in the size, consistency, or number of lymph nodes.*

Medical Word Elements—cont'd

Element	Meaning	Word Analysis
lymph/o	lymph	**lymph/**oid (LĬM-foyd): resembling lymph *-oid:* resembling
lymphangi/o	lymph vessel	**lymphangi/**oma (lĭm-făn-jē-Ō-mă): tumor (composed of) lymph vessels *-oma:* tumor
morph/o	form, shape, structure	**morph/o/**logy (mor-FŎL-ō-jē): study of form, shape, and structure *-logy:* study of
myel/o	bone marrow; spinal cord	**myel/o/**gen/ic (mī-ĕ-lō-JĔN-ĭk): relating to the origin in bone marrow *gen:* forming, producing, origin *-ic:* pertaining to *Granulocytes are formed in the bone marrow and are thus considered* **myelogenic.**
neutr/o	neutral, neither	**neutr/o/**phil/ic (nū-trō-FĬL-ĭk): pertaining to an attraction for neutral dyes *-phil:* attraction for *-ic:* pertaining to, relating to *A neutrophil is a leukocyte whose granules stain easily with neutral dyes.*
phag/o	swallowing, eating	**phag/o/**cyte (FĂG-ō-sīt): cell that eats (foreign material) *-cyte:* cell *The neutrophil is phagocytic and protects the body by consuming foreign substances that may cause disease or injury.*
plas/o	formation, growth	a/**plas/**tic (ā-PLĂS-tĭk): pertaining to a failure to form *a-:* without, not *-tic:* pertaining to *Aplastic anemia is a failure of the bone marrow to produce adequate blood cells.*
poikil/o	varied, irregular	**poikil/o/**cyte (POY-kĭl-ō-sīt): cell that is irregular or varied (in shape) *cyte:* cell
reticul/o	net, mesh	**reticul/o/**cyte (rĕ-TĬK-ū-lō-sīt): cell (that contains a) net or meshwork *-cyte:* cell *A reticulocyte is an immature erythrocyte that contains strands of nuclear material. This material appears as a tiny net when observed microscopically.*
ser/o	serum	**ser/o/**logy (sē-RŎL-ō-jē): study of serum *-logy:* study of *Serology includes the study of antigens and antibodies in serum as well as sources other than serum, including plasma, saliva, and urine.*
sider/o	iron	**sider/o/**penia (sĭd-ĕr-ō-PĒ-nē-ă): deficiency of iron *-penia:* decrease, deficiency *Sideropenia usually results from inadequate iron uptake or from hemorrhage.*
splen/o	spleen	**splen/o/**rrhagia (splē-nō-RĀ-jē-ă): bursting forth of the spleen *-rrhagia:* bursting forth *Splenorrhagia is a hemorrhage from a ruptured spleen.*

(continued)

Medical Word Elements—cont'd

Element	Meaning	Word Analysis
Combining Forms		
thromb/o	blood clot	**thromb/**osis (thrŏm-BŌ-sĭs): abnormal condition of a blood clot *-osis:* abnormal condition; increase (used primarily with blood cells) *Thrombosis is the formation of blood clots in the blood vessels.*
thym/o	thymus gland	**thym/o/**pathy (thī-MŎP-ă-thē): disease of the thymus gland *-pathy:* disease
xen/o	foreign, strange	**xen/o/**graft (ZĔN-ō-grăft): foreign transplantation, also called *heterograft* *-graft:* transplantation *A xenograft is a cross-species transplant, such as a pig heart valve to a human recipient. A xenograft is used as a temporary measure when there is insufficient tissue available from the patient or other human donors.*
Suffixes		
-blast	embryonic cell	erythr/o/**blast** (ĕ-RĬTH-rō-blăst): embryonic red cell *erythr/o:* red
-emia	blood condition	an/**emia** (ă-NĒ-mē-ă): without blood *an-:* without, not *Anemia is any condition characterized by a reduction in the number of red blood cells or a deficiency in their hemoglobin.*
-globin	protein	hem/o/**globin** (HĒ-mō-glō-bĭn): blood protein *hem/o:* blood *Hemoglobin is an iron-containing protein found in RBCs that transports oxygen and gives blood its red color.*
-graft	transplantation	auto/**graft** (AW-tō-grăft): self transplantation *auto-:* self, own *An autograft is a surgical transplantation of tissue from one location of the body to another in the same individual.*
-osis	abnormal condition; increase (used primarily with blood cells)	leuk/o/cyt/**osis** (loo-kō-sī-TŌ-sĭs): abnormal increase in white (blood) cells *leuk/o:* white *cyt:* cell
-penia	decrease, deficiency	erythr/o/**penia** (ĕ-rĭth-rō-PĒ-nē-ă): abnormal decrease in red (blood cells) *erythr/o:* red
-phil	attraction for	neutr/o/**phil** (NŪ-trō-fĭl): attraction for a neutral (dye) *neutr/o:* neutral, neither *Neutrophils are the most numerous type of leukocyte. They provide phagocytic protection for the body.*
-phoresis	carrying, transmission	electr/o/**phoresis** (ē-lĕk-trō-fō-RĒ-sĭs): carrying an electric (charge) *electr/o:* electricity *Electrophoresis is a laboratory technique used to separate proteins based on their electrical charge, size, and shape. It is a commonly employed technique used in deoxyribonucleic acid (DNA) testing.*

Medical Word Elements—cont'd

Element	Meaning	Word Analysis
-phylaxis	protection	ana/**phylaxis** (ăn-ă-fĭ-LĂK-sĭs): against protection *ana-:* against, up, back *Anaphylaxis is an exaggerated, life-threatening hypersensitivity reaction to a previously encountered antigen. It is treated as a medical emergency.*
-poiesis	formation, production	hem/o/**poiesis** (hē-mō-poy-Ē-sĭs): formation of blood *hem/o:* blood
-stasis	standing still	hem/o/**stasis** (hē-mō-STĀ-sĭs): standing still of blood *hem/o:* blood *Hemostasis is the control or arrest of bleeding, commonly using chemical agents.*

Prefixes

Element	Meaning	Word Analysis
a-	without, not	**a**/morph/ic (ā-MOR-fĭk): without a (definite) form *morph:* form, shape, structure *ic:* pertaining to
allo-	other, differing from the normal	**allo**/graft (ĂL-ō-grăft): transplantation differing from the normal; also called *homograft* *-graft:* transplantation *An allograft is a transplant between two individuals who are not identical twins but are genetically compatible.*
aniso-	unequal, dissimilar	**aniso**/cyt/osis (ăn-ī-sō-sĭ-TŌ-sĭs): abnormal increase in cells that are unequal *cyt:* cell *-osis:* abnormal condition; increase (used primarily with blood cells) *Anisocytosis generally refers to red blood cells that vary is size from normal (normocytic) to abnormally large (macrocytic) or abnormally small (microcytic).*
iso-	same, equal	**iso**/chrom/ic (ī-sō-KRŌM-ĭk): pertaining to the same color *chrom:* color *ic:* pertaining to
macro-	large	**macro**/cyte (MĂK-rō-sīt): large (red) cell *-cyte:* cell
micro-	small	**micro**/cyte (MĪ-krō-sīt): small (red) cell *-cyte:* cell
mono-	one	**mono**/nucle/osis (mŏn-ō-nū-klē-Ō-sĭs): abnormal increase of mononuclear (cells) *nucle:* nucleus *-osis:* abnormal condition; increase (used primarily with blood cells) *In infectious mononucleosis, there is an increase in monocytes and lymphocytes.*
poly-	many, much	**poly**/morph/ic (pŏl-ē-MOR-fĭk): pertaining to many forms or shapes *morph:* form, shape, structure *-ic:* pertaining to

 It is time to review medical word elements by completing Learning Activity 9–2. For audio pronunciations of the above-listed key terms, you can visit www.davisplus.fadavis.com/gylys/systems *to download this chapter's* Listen and Learn! *exercises or use the book's audio CD (if included).*

Pathology

Pathology associated with blood includes anemias, leukemias, and coagulation disorders. These groups of disorders typically share common signs and symptoms that generally include paleness, weakness, shortness of breath, and heart palpitations. Lymphatic disorders are commonly associated with edema and lymphadenopathy. In these disorders, tissues are swollen with enlarged, tender nodes. Immunopathies include abnormally heightened immune responses to antigens (allergies, hypersensitivities, and autoimmune disorders) or abnormally depressed responses (immunodeficiencies and cancers). Many immunological disorders are manifested in other body systems. For example, asthma and hay fever are immunological disorders that affect the respiratory system; atopic dermatitis and eczema are immunological disorders that affect the integumentary system. Some of the most devastating diseases, such as rheumatoid arthritis, and AIDS, are caused by disordered immunity.

For diagnosis, treatment, and management of diseases that affect blood and blood-forming organs, the medical services of a specialist may be warranted. **Hematology** is the branch of medicine that studies blood cells, blood-clotting mechanisms, bone marrow, and lymph nodes. The physician who specializes in this branch of medicine is called a *hematologist*. **Allergy and immunology** is the branch of medicine involving disorders of the immune system, including asthma and anaphylaxis, adverse reactions to drugs, autoimmune diseases, organ transplantations, and malignancies of the immune system. The physician who specializes in this combined branch of medicine is called an *allergist* and *immunologist*.

Anemias

Anemia is any condition in which the oxygen-carrying capacity of blood is deficient. It is not a disease but rather a symptom of various diseases. It results when there is a decrease in the number of circulating RBCs (**erythropenia**), the amount of hemoglobin (**hypochromasia**) within them, or in the volume of packed erythrocytes (**hematocrit**). Some of the causes of anemias include excessive blood loss, excessive blood-cell destruction, decreased blood formation, and faulty hemoglobin production.

Anemia commonly causes changes in the appearance of RBCs when observed microscopically. In healthy individuals, RBCs fall within a normal range for size (**normocytic**) and amount

of hemoglobin (**normochromic**). Variations in these normal values include RBCs that are excessively large (**macrocytic**), are excessively small (**microcytic**), or have decreased amounts of hemoglobin (**hypochromic**). Signs and symptoms associated with most anemias include difficulty breathing (**dyspnea**), weakness, rapid heartbeat (**tachycardia**), paleness (**pallor**), low blood pressure (**hypotension**) and, commonly, a slight fever. (See Table 9–4.)

Acquired Immune Deficiency Syndrome (AIDS)

Acquired immune deficiency syndrome (AIDS) is an infectious disease caused by the human immunodeficiency virus (HIV), which slowly destroys the immune system. The immune system becomes so weak (**immunocompromised**) that, in the final stage of the disease, the patient falls victim to infections that usually do not affect healthy individuals (**opportunistic infections**). Symptoms of AIDS begin to appear gradually, and include swollen lymph glands (**lymphadenopathy**), malaise, fever, night sweats, and weight loss. **Kaposi sarcoma,** a neoplastic disorder, and *Pneumocystis* **pneumonia** (PCP) are two diseases closely associated with AIDS.

Transmission of HIV occurs primarily through body fluids—mostly blood, semen, and vaginal secretions. The virus attacks the most important cell in the immune system, the helper T cell. Once infected by HIV, the helper T cell becomes a "mini-factory" for the replication of the virus. More importantly, the virus destroys the helper T cell, which impacts the effective functioning of the humoral and cellular arms of the immune system, ultimately causing the patient's death.

Although there is no cure for HIV, treatments are available that can slow the development of the virus and the progression of the disease. These medications have serious adverse effects; however, once the decision for medical management is made, the patient should continue treatment. Failure to do so causes the virus to become highly resistant to current treatment options.

Allergy

An **allergy** is an acquired abnormal immune response. It requires initial exposure (**sensitization**) to an allergen (**antigen**). Subsequent exposures to the allergen produce increasing allergic reactions that cause a broad range of inflammatory changes.

Table 9-4 — Common Anemias

This table lists various types of anemia along with descriptions and causes for each.

Type of Anemia	Description	Causes
Aplastic (hypoplastic)	• Associated with bone marrow failure • Diminished numbers of red blood cells (RBCs), white blood cells (WBCs), and platelets due to bone marrow suppression • Serious form of anemia that may be fatal	Commonly caused by exposure to cytotoxic agents, radiation, hepatitis virus, and certain medications
Folic-acid deficiency anemia	• RBCs are large and deformed with a diminished production rate and life span	Caused by insufficient folic acid intake due to poor diet, impaired absorption, prolonged drug therapy, or increased requirements (pregnancy or rapid growth as seen in children)
Hemolytic	• Associated with premature destruction of RBCs • Usually accompanied by jaundice	Caused by the excessive destruction of red blood cells or such disorders as erythroblastosis and sickle cell anemia
Hemorrhagic	• Associated with loss of blood volume • Normal levels achieved with correction of the underlying disorder	Commonly caused by acute blood loss (as in trauma), childbirth, or chronic blood loss (as in bleeding ulcers)
Iron-deficiency anemia	• Most common type of anemia worldwide	Caused by a greater demand on stored iron than can be supplied, commonly as a result of inadequate dietary iron intake or malabsorption of iron
Pernicious anemia	• Chronic, progressive disorder found mostly in people older than age 50 • Treated with B_{12} injections	Caused by low levels of vitamin B_{12} in peripheral red blood cells that may be the result of a lack of intrinsic factor in the stomach, which then inhibits absorption of vitamin B_{12}
Sickle cell anemia	• Most common genetic disorder in people of African descent • Characterized by RBCs that become crescent and irregularly shaped when oxygen levels are low, thus preventing cells from entering capillaries and resulting in severe pain and internal bleeding	Caused by a defect in the gene responsible for hemoglobin synthesis (A person must have both genes for the disease to manifest. Those with only one gene for the trait are carriers of the disease.)

Common signs and symptoms include hives (**urticaria**), eczema, allergic rhinitis, asthma and, in the extreme, **anaphylactic shock,** a life-threatening condition.

The offending allergens are identified by allergy sensitivity tests. In one such test, small scratches are made on the patient's back and a liquid suspension of the allergen is introduced into the scratch. If antibodies to the allergen are present in the patient, the scratch becomes red, swollen, and hardened (**indurated**).

A treatment called **desensitization** reduces the sensitivity of the patient to the offending allergen. This treatment involves repeated injections of highly diluted solutions containing the allergen. The initial concentration of the solution is too weak to cause symptoms. Additional exposure to higher concentrations promotes tolerance of the allergen.

Autoimmune Disease

Autoimmunity is the failure of the body to distinguish accurately between "self" and "nonself." In this abnormal response, the immune system attacks the antigens found on its own cells to such an extent that tissue injury results. Types of autoimmune disorders range from those that affect only a single organ to those that affect many organs and tissues (**multisystemic**).

Myasthenia gravis is an autoimmune disorder that affects the neuromuscular junction. Muscles of the limbs and eyes and those affecting speech and swallowing are usually involved. Other autoimmune diseases include rheumatoid arthritis (RA), idiopathic thrombocytopenic purpura (ITP), vasculitis, and systemic lupus erythematosus (SLE).

Treatment consists of attempting to reach a balance between suppressing the immune response to avoid tissue damage, while still maintaining the immune mechanism sufficiently to protect against disease. Most autoimmune diseases have periods of flare-up (**exacerbations**) and latency (**remissions**). Autoimmune diseases are usually chronic, requiring lifelong care and monitoring, even when the person may look or feel well. Currently, few autoimmune diseases can be cured; however, with treatment, those afflicted can live relatively normal lives.

Edema

Edema is an abnormal accumulation of fluids in the intercellular spaces of the body. A major cause of edema is a decrease in the blood protein level (**hypoproteinemia**), especially albumin, which controls the amount of plasma leaving the vascular channels. Other causes of edema include poor lymph drainage, high sodium intake, increased capillary permeability, and heart failure.

Edema limited to a specific area (**localized**) may be relieved by elevation of that body part and application of cold packs. Systemic edema may be treated with medications that promote urination (**diuretics**).

Closely associated with edema is a condition called **ascites,** in which fluid collects within the peritoneal or pleural cavity. The chief causes of ascites are interference in venous return in cardiac disease, obstruction of lymphatic flow, disturbances in electrolyte balance, and liver disease.

Hemophilia

Hemophilia is a hereditary disorder in which the blood-clotting mechanism is impaired. There are two main types of hemophilia: **hemophilia A,** a deficiency in clotting factor VIII, and **hemophilia B**, a deficiency in clotting factor IX. The degree of deficiency varies from mild to severe. The disease is sex-linked and found most commonly in men. Women are carriers of the trait but generally do not have symptoms of the disease.

Mild symptoms include nosebleeds, easy bruising, and bleeding from the gums. Severe symptoms produce areas of blood seepage (**hematomas**) deep within muscles. If blood enters joints (**hemarthrosis**), it is associated with pain and, possibly, permanent deformity. Uncontrolled bleeding in the body may lead to shock and death. Treatment consists of intravenous administration of the deficient factor. The amount of factor replaced depends on the seriousness of the hemorrhage and the amount of blood lost.

Infectious Mononucleosis

Infectious mononucleosis is one of the acute infections caused by the Epstein-Barr virus (EBV). It is usually found in young adults and tends to appear in early spring and fall. Saliva and respiratory secretions have been implicated as significant infectious agents, hence the name "kissing disease." Sore throat, fever, and enlarged cervical lymph nodes characterize this disease. Other signs and symptoms include gum infection (**gingivitis**), headache, tiredness, loss of appetite (**anorexia**), and general malaise. In most cases, the disease resolves spontaneously and without complications. In some cases, however, the liver and spleen enlarge (**hepatomegaly/splenomegaly**). Less common clinical findings include hemolytic anemia with jaundice and thrombocytopenia. Recovery usually ensures a lasting immunity.

Oncology

Oncological disorders associated with the blood, lymph, and immune systems include leukemia, Hodgkin disease, and Kaposi sarcoma.

Leukemia

Leukemia is an oncological disorder of the blood-forming organs, characterized by an overgrowth (**proliferation**) of blood cells. With this condition, malignant cells replace healthy bone marrow cells. The disease is generally categorized by the type of leukocyte population affected: granulocytic (**myelogenous**) or lymphocytic.

The various types of leukemia may be further classified as **chronic** or **acute**. In the acute form, the cells are highly embryonic (**blastic**) with few mature forms, resulting in severe anemia, infections, and bleeding disorders. This form of leukemia is life threatening. Although there is a proliferation of blastic cells in chronic forms of leukemia, there are usually enough mature cells to carry on the functions of the various cell types.

Although the causes of leukemia are unknown, viruses, environmental conditions, high-dose radiation, and genetic factors have been implicated. Bone marrow aspiration and bone marrow biopsy are used to diagnose leukemia. Treatment includes chemotherapy, radiation, biological therapy, bone marrow transplant, or a combination of these modalities. Left untreated, leukemias are fatal.

Hodgkin Disease

Hodgkin disease, also called *Hodgkin lymphoma,* is a malignant disease of the lymph system, primarily the lymph nodes. Although malignancy usually remains only in neighboring nodes, it may spread to the spleen, GI tract, liver, or bone marrow.

Hodgkin disease usually begins with a painless enlargement of lymph nodes, typically on one side of the neck, chest, or underarm. Other symptoms include severe itching (**pruritus**), weight loss, progressive anemia, and fever. If nodes in the neck become excessively large, they may press on the trachea, causing difficulty in breathing (**dyspnea**), or on the esophagus, causing difficulty in swallowing (**dysphagia**).

Radiation and chemotherapy are important methods of controlling the disease. Newer methods of treatment include bone marrow transplants. Treatment is highly effective.

Kaposi Sarcoma

Kaposi sarcoma is a malignancy of connective tissue, including bone, fat, muscle, and fibrous tissue. It is closely associated with AIDS and is commonly fatal because the tumors readily metastasize to other organs. Its close association with HIV has resulted in this disorder being classified as one of several "AIDS-defining conditions." The lesions emerge as purplish brown macules and develop into plaques and nodules. The lesions initially appear over the lower extremities and tend to spread symmetrically over the upper body, particularly the face and oral mucosa. Treatment for AIDS-related Kaposi sarcoma is usually palliative, relieving the pain and discomfort that accompany the lesions, but there is little evidence that it prolongs life.

Diagnostic, Symptomatic, and Related Terms

This section introduces diagnostic, symptomatic, and related terms and their meanings. Word analyses for selected terms are also provided.

Term	Definition
anisocytosis ăn-ī-sō-sī-TŌ-sĭs *an-:* without, not *iso-:* same, equal *cyt:* cell *-osis:* abnormal condition; increase (used primarily with blood cells)	Condition of marked variation in the size of erythrocytes when observed on a blood smear *With anisocytosis, the blood smear shows macrocytes (large RBCs) and microcytes (small RBCs) as well as normocytes (normal-size RBCs).*
ascites ă-SĪ-tēz	Accumulation of serous fluid in the peritoneal or pleural cavity
bacteremia băk-tĕr-Ē-mē-ă *bacter:* bacteria *-emia:* blood condition	Presence of viable bacteria circulating in the bloodstream usually transient in nature
graft rejection grăft	Destruction of a transplanted organ or tissue by the recipient's immune system

Diagnostic, Symptomatic, and Related Terms—cont'd

Term	Definition
graft-versus-host disease (GVHD) GRĂFT	Condition that occurs following bone marrow transplant in which the immune cells in the transplanted marrow produce antibodies against the host's tissues *GVHD can be acute or chronic. The acute form appears within 2 months of the transplant; the chronic form usually appears within 3 months. GVHD may also occur as a reaction to blood transfusion.*
hematoma hēm-ă-TŌ-mă *hemat:* blood *-oma:* tumor	Localized accumulation of blood, usually clotted, in an organ, space, or tissue due to a break in or severing of a blood vessel
hemoglobinopathy hē-mō-glō-bĭ-NŎP-ă-thē *hem/o:* blood *globin/o:* protein *-pathy:* disease	Any disorder caused by abnormalities in the hemoglobin molecule *One of the most common hemoglobinopathies is sickle cell anemia.*
hemolysis hē-MŎL-ĭ-sĭs *hem/o:* blood *-lysis:* separation; destruction; loosening	Destruction of RBCs with a release of hemoglobin that diffuses into the surrounding fluid
hemostasis hē-mō-STĀ-sĭs *hem/o:* blood *-stasis:* standing still	Arrest of bleeding or circulation
immunity ĭ-MŪ-nĭ-tē	State of being protected against infectious diseases
active	Immunity produced by the person's own immune system *Active immunity is generally long lived because memory cells are formed. Its two types include natural active immunity, resulting from recovery from a disease, and artificial active immunity, resulting from an immunizing vaccination.*
passive	Immunity in which antibodies or other immune substances formed in one individual are transferred to another individual to provide immediate, temporary immunity *Passive immunity is short lived because memory cells are not transferred to the recipient. Two types of passive immunity include natural passive immunity, where medical intervention is not required (infant receiving antibodies through breast milk) and artificial passive immunity, where antibodies, antitoxins, or toxoids (generally produced in sheep or horses) are transfused or injected into the patient to provide immediate protection.*
lymphadenopathy lĭm-făd-ĕ-NŎP-ă-thē *lymph:* lymph *aden/o:* gland *-pathy:* disease	Any disease of the lymph nodes *In localized lymphadenopathy, only one area of the body is affected. In systemic lymphadenopathy, two or more noncontiguous areas of the body are affected.*

Diagnostic, Symptomatic, and Related Terms—cont'd

Term	Definition
lymphosarcoma lĭm-fō-săr-KŌ-mă *lymph/o:* lymph *sarc:* flesh (connective tissue) *–oma:* tumor	Malignant neoplastic disorder of lymphatic tissue (not related to Hodgkin disease)
septicemia sĕp-tĭ-SĒ-mē-ă	Serious, life-threatening bloodstream infection that may arise from other infections throughout the body, such as pneumonia, urinary tract infection, meningitis, or infections of the bone or GI tract; also called *blood infection* or *blood poisoning* *Septicemia is characterized by chills, fever, tachycardia, tachypnea, confusion, hypotension, and ecchymoses. If left untreated, it may lead to shock and death.*
serology sē-RŎL-ō-jē *ser/o:* serum *–logy:* study of	Laboratory test to detect the presence of antibodies, antigens, or immune substances
titer TĪ-tĕr	Blood test that measures the amount of antibodies in blood; commonly used as an indicator of immune status

 It is time to review pathological, diagnostic, symptomatic, and related terms by completing Learning Activity 9–3.

Diagnostic and Therapeutic Procedures

This section introduces procedures used to diagnose and treat blood, lymph, and immune disorders. Descriptions are provided as well as pronunciations and word analyses for selected terms.

Procedure	Description
Diagnostic Procedures	
Laboratory	
blood culture	Test to determine the presence of pathogens in the bloodstream
complete blood count (CBC)	Series of tests that includes hemoglobin; hematocrit; RBC, WBC, and platelet counts; differential WBC count; RBC indices; and RBC and WBC morphology
differential count (diff) dĭf-ĕr-ĔN-shăl	Test that enumerates the distribution of WBCs in a stained blood smear by counting the different kinds of WBCs and reporting each as a percentage of the total examined *Because differential values change considerably in pathology, this test is commonly used as a first step in diagnosing a disease.*
erythrocyte sedimentation rate (ESR) ĕ-RĬTH-rō-sīt sĕd-ĭ-mĕn-TĀ-shŭn *erythr/o:* red *–cyte:* cell	Measurement of the distance RBCs settle to the bottom of a test tube under standardized condition; also called *sed rate* *Elevated ESR is associated with inflammatory diseases, cancer, and pregnancy, but decreases in liver disease. The more elevated the sed rate, the more severe is the inflammation.*

(continued)

Diagnostic and Therapeutic Procedures—cont'd

Procedure	Description
hemoglobin (Hgb) value HĒ-mō-glō-bĭn *hem/o:* blood *-globin:* protein	Measurement of the amount of hemoglobin found in a whole blood sample *Hgb values decrease in anemia and increase in dehydration, polycythemia vera, and thrombocytopenia purpura.*
hematocrit (Hct) hē-MĂT-ō-krĭt	Measurement of the percentage of RBCs in a whole blood sample
Monospot	Non specific rapid serological test for infectious mononucleosis; also called *the heterophile antibody test*
partial thromboplastin time (PTT) thrŏm-bō-PLĂS-tĭn	Test that measures the length of time it takes blood to clot. It screens for deficiencies of some clotting factors and monitors the effectiveness of anticoagulant (heparin) therapy; also called *activated partial thromboplastin time (APTT)* *PTT is valuable for preoperative screening of bleeding tendencies.*
prothrombin time (PT) prō-THRŎM-bĭn	Test that measures the time it takes for the plasma portion of blood to clot. It is used to evaluate portions of the coagulation system; also called *pro time* *PT is commonly used to manage patients receiving the anticoagulant warfarin (Coumadin).*
red blood cell (RBC) indices	Mathematical calculation of the size, volume, and concentration of hemoglobin for an RBC
Schilling test	Test used to assess the absorption of radioactive vitamin B_{12} by the digestive system *Schilling test is the definitive test for diagnosing pernicious anemia because vitamin B_{12} is not absorbed in this disorder and passes from the body by way of stool.*
Radiographic	
lymphadenography lĭm-făd-ĕ-NŎG-ră-fē *lymph:* lymph *aden/o:* gland *-graphy:* process of recording	Radiographic examination of lymph nodes after injection of a contrast medium
lymphangiography lĭm-făn-jē-ŎG-ră-fē *lymph:* lymph *angi/o:* vessel *-graphy:* process of recording	Radiographic examination of lymph vessels or tissues after injection of contrast medium
Surgical	
aspiration ăs-pĭ-RĀ-shŭn bone marrow bōn MĂR-ō	Drawing in or out by suction Procedure using a syringe with a thin aspirating needle inserted (usually in the pelvic bone and rarely the sternum) to withdraw a small sample of bone marrow fluid for microscopic evaluation (See Figure 9–6.)

Diagnostic and Therapeutic Procedures—cont'd

Procedure	Description

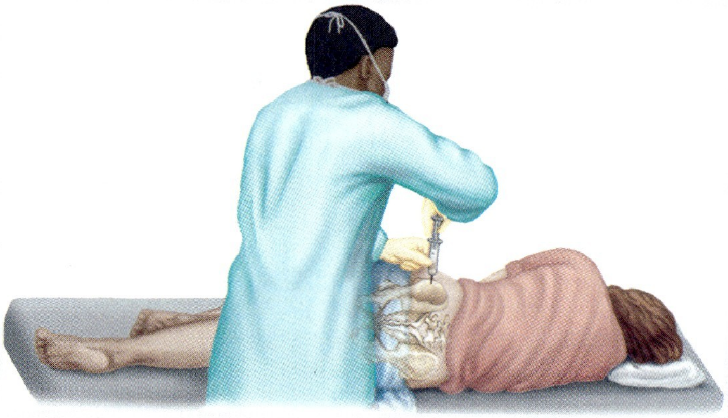

Figure 9-6. Bone marrow aspiration.

biopsy (bx)
BĪ-ŏp-sē

Representative tissue sample removed from a body site for microscopic examination, usually to establish a diagnosis

bone marrow
bōn MĂR-ō

Removal of a small core sample of tissue from bone marrow for examination under a microscope and, possibly, for analysis using other tests

sentinel node
SĔNT-ĭ-nĕl NŌD

Removal of the first lymph node (the *sentinel node*) that receives drainage from cancer-containing areas and the one most likely to contain malignant cells

If the sentinel node does not contain malignant cells, there may be no need to remove additional lymph nodes.

Therapeutic Procedures

Surgical

lymphangiectomy
lĭm-făn-jē-ĔK-tō-mē
lymph: lymph
angi: vessel
-ectomy: excision

Removal of a lymph vessel

transfusion
trăns-FŪ-zhŭn

Infusion of blood or blood components into the bloodstream

autologous
aw-TŎL-ō-gŭs

Transfusion prepared from the recipient's own blood

homologous
hō-MŎL-ō-gŭs

Transfusion prepared from another individual whose blood is compatible with that of the recipient

transplantation

Grafting of living tissue from its normal position to another site or from one person to another

autologous bone marrow
aw-TŎL-ō-gŭs bōn MĂR-ō

Harvesting, freezing (cryopreserving), and reinfusing the patient's own bone marrow to treat bone marrow hypoplasia following cancer therapy

homologous bone marrow
hō-MŎL-ō-gŭs bōn MĂR-ō

Transplantation of bone marrow from one individual to another to treat aplastic anemia, leukemia, and immunodeficiency disorders

Pharmacology

Various drugs are prescribed to treat blood, lymph, and immune systems disorders. (See Table 9–5.) These drugs act directly on individual components of each system. For example, anticoagulants are used to prevent clot formation but are ineffective in destroying formed clots. Instead, thrombolytics are used to dissolve clots that obstruct coronary, cerebral, or pulmonary arteries and, conversely, hemostatics are used to prevent or control hemorrhage. In addition, chemotherapy and radiation are commonly used to treat diseases of the blood and immune system. For example, antineoplastics prevent cellular replication to halt the spread of cancer in the body; antivirals prevent viral replication within cells and have been effective in slowing the progression of HIV and AIDS.

Table 9-5	Drugs used to Treat Blood, Lymph, and Immune Disorders

This table lists common drug classifications used to treat blood, lymph, and immune disorders, their therapeutic actions, and selected generic and trade names.

Classification	Therapeutic Action	Generic and Trade Names

anticoagulants	Prevent blood clot formation by inhibiting the synthesis or inactivating one or more clotting factors
	
	These drugs prevent deep vein thrombosis (DVT) and postoperative clot formation and decrease the risk of stroke.
		heparin
		HĔP-ă-rĭn
		  heparin sodium
		warfarin
		WĂR-făr-ĭn
		  Coumadin

antifibrinolytics	Neutralize fibrinolytic chemicals in the mucous membranes of the mouth, nose, and urinary tract to prevent the breakdown of blood clots *Antifibrinolytics are commonly used to treat serious bleeding following certain surgeries and dental procedures especially in patients with medical problems such as hemophilia*	**aminocaproic acid** ă-mē-nō-kă-PRŌ-ĭk ĂS-ĭd Amicar

antimicrobials	Destroy bacteria, fungi, and protozoa, depending on the particular drug, generally by interfering with the functions of their cell membrane or their reproductive cycle
	
	HIV patients are commonly treated prophylactically with antimicrobials to prevent development of Pneumocystis carinii pneumonia (PCP).
		trimethoprim, sulfamethoxazole
		trĭ-MĔTH-ō-prĭm,
		sŭl-fă-mĕth-ŎK-să-zōl
		  Bactrim, Septra
		pentamidine
		pĕn-TĂM-ĭ-dēn
		  NebuPent, Pentam-300

antivirals	Prevent replication of viruses within host cells
	
	Antivirals are used in treatment of HIV infection and AIDS.
		nelfinavir
		nĕl-FĬN-ă-vēr
		  Viracept
		lamivudine/zidovudine
		lă-MĬV-ū-dēn-
		zī-DŌ-vū-dēn
		  Combivir

Table 9-5	Drugs used to Treat Blood, Lymph, and Immune Disorders—cont'd		
Classification	**Therapeutic Action**	**Generic and Trade Names**
fat-soluble vitamins	Prevent and treat bleeding disorders resulting from a lack of prothrombin, which is commonly caused by vitamin K deficiency	**phytonadione** fī-tō-nă-DĪ-ōn Vitamin K1 Mephyton
thrombolytics	Dissolve blood clots by destroying their fibrin strands *Thrombolytics are used to break apart, or lyse, thrombi, especially those that obstruct coronary, pulmonary, and cerebral arteries.*	**alteplase** ĂL-tĕ-plās Activase, t-PA **streptokinase** strĕp-tō-KĪ-nās Streptase

Abbreviations

This section introduces blood, lymph, and immune system abbreviations and their meanings.

Abbreviation	Meaning	Abbreviation	Meaning
AB, Ab, ab	antibody, abortion	**EBV**	Epstein-Barr virus
A, B, AB, O	blood types in ABO blood group	**eos**	eosinophil (type of white blood cell)
AIDS	acquired immune deficiency syndrome	**ESR**	erythrocyte sedimentation rate
ALL	acute lymphocytic leukemia	**Hb, Hgb**	hemoglobin
AML	acute myelogenous leukemia	**HCT, Hct**	hematocrit
APC	Antigen-presenting cell	**HDN**	hemolytic disease of the newborn
APTT	activated partial thromboplastin time	**HIV**	human immunodeficiency virus
baso	basophil (type of white blood cell)	**Igs**	immunoglobulins
CBC	complete blood count	**ITP**	idiopathic thrombocytopenic purpura
CLL	chronic lymphocytic leukemia	**IV**	intravenous
CML	chronic myelogenous leukemia	**lymphos**	lymphocytes
diff	differential count (white blood cells)	**MCH**	mean cell hemoglobin (average amount of hemoglobin per cell)

Abbreviations—cont'd

Abbreviation	Meaning	Abbreviation	Meaning
MCHC	mean cell hemoglobin concentration (average concentration of hemoglobin in a single red cell)	PT	prothrombin time, physical therapy
MCV	mean cell volume (average volume or size of a single red blood cell)	PTT	partial thromboplastin time
ml, mL	milliliter (1/1000 of a liter)	RA	right atrium; rheumatoid arthritis
NK cell	natural killer cell	RBC, rbc	red blood cell
PA	posteroanterior; pernicious anemia; pulmonary artery	sed	sedimentation
PCP	*Pneumocystis* pneumonia; primary care physician; phencyclidine (hallucinogen)	segs	segmented neutrophils
PCV	packed cell volume	SLE	systemic lupus erythematosus
poly, PMN, PMNL	polymorphonuclear leukocyte	WBC, wbc	white blood cell

It is time to review procedures, pharmacology, and abbreviations by completing Learning Activity 9–4.

LEARNING ACTIVITIES

The following activities provide review of the blood, lymph, and immune system terms introduced in this chapter. Complete each activity and review your answers to evaluate your understanding of the chapter.

Learning Activity 9-1
Identifying Lymph Structures

Label the following illustration using the terms listed below.

blood capillary	lymph node	spleen	tonsil
left subclavian vein	right lymphatic duct	thoracic duct	
lymph capillary	right subclavian vein	thymus	

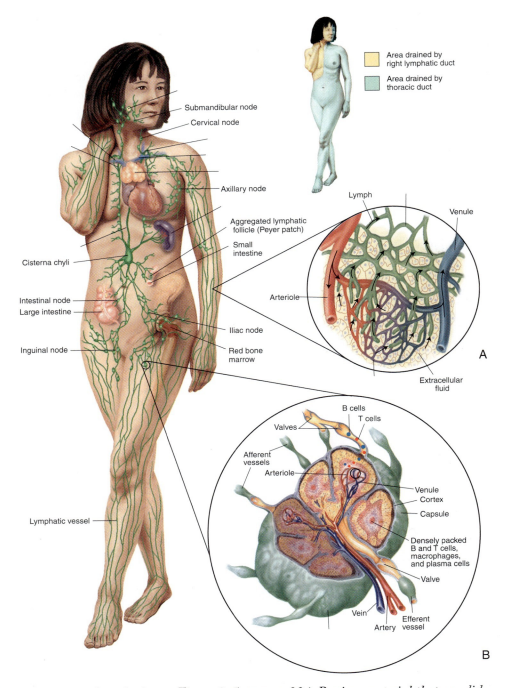

Submandibular node
Cervical node
Axillary node
Aggregated lymphatic follicle (Peyer patch)
Small intestine
Cisterna chyli
Intestinal node
Large intestine
Inguinal node
Iliac node
Red bone marrow
Lymphatic vessel

Area drained by right lymphatic duct
Area drained by thoracic duct

Lymph
Venule
Arteriole
Extracellular fluid

A

B cells
T cells
Valves
Afferent vessels
Arteriole
Venule
Cortex
Capsule
Densely packed B and T cells, macrophages, and plasma cells
Valve
Vein
Artery
Efferent vessel

B

✓ *Check your answers by referring to Figure 9–5 on page 234. Review material that you did not answer correctly.*

DavisPlus.fadavis.com

Enhance your study and reinforcement of word elements with the power of DavisPlus. Visit www.davisplus.fadavis.com/gylys/systems *for this chapter's flash-card activity. We recommend you complete the flash-card activity before completing activity 9–2 below.*

Building Medical Words

Use *–osis* (abnormal condition; increase [used primarily with blood cells]) to build words that mean:

1. abnormal increase in erythrocytes _____
2. abnormal increase in leukocytes _____
3. abnormal increase in lymphocytes _____
4. abnormal increase in reticulocytes _____

Use *–penia* (deficiency, decrease) to build words that mean:

5. decrease in leukocytes _____
6. decrease in erythrocytes _____
7. decrease in thrombocytes _____
8. decrease in lymphocytes _____

Use *–poiesis* (formation, production) to build words that mean:

9. production of blood _____
10. production of white cells _____
11. production of thormbocytes _____

Use *immun/o* (immune, immunity, safe) to build words that mean:

12. specialist in study of immunity _____
13. study of immunity _____

Use *splen/o* (spleen) to build words that mean:

14. herniation of the spleen _____
15. destruction of the spleen _____

Build surgical words that mean:

16. excision of the spleen _____
17. removal of the thymus _____
18. destruction of the thymus _____
19. incision of the spleen _____
20. fixation of (a displaced) spleen _____

Check your answers in Appendix A. Review any material that you did not answer correctly.

Correct Answers _____ × 5 = _____ % Score

Learning Activity 9-3
Matching Pathological, Diagnostic, Symptomatic, and Related Terms

Match the following terms with the definitions in the numbered list.

active	exacerbations	hemophilia	myelogenous
anisocytosis	graft rejection	immunocompromised	normocytic
aplastic anemia	hematoma	infectious mononucleosis	opportunistic infection
artificial	hemoglobinopathy	Kaposi sarcoma	passive
bacteremia	hemolysis	lymphadenopathy	septicemia

1. _____ periods of flare-up
2. _____ any disorder due to abnormalities in the hemoglobin molecule
3. _____ presence of bacteria in blood
4. _____ associated with bone marrow failure
5. _____ type of immunity where memory cells are formed
6. _____ malignancy of connective tissue commonly associated with HIV
7. _____ used to denote an erythrocyte that is normal in size
8. _____ swollen or diseased lymph glands
9. _____ term that denotes a weakened immune system
10. _____ blood-clotting disorder
11. _____ common viral disorder caused by the Epstein-Barr virus
12. _____ leukemia that affects granulocytes
13. _____ type of immunity where memory cells are not transferred to the recipient
14. _____ type of passive immunity where medical intervention is required
15. _____ destruction of erythrocytes with the release of hemoglobin
16. _____ localized accumulation of blood in tissue; blood clot
17. _____ destruction of a transplanted organ or tissue by the recipient's immune system
18. _____ condition of marked variation in the size of erythrocytes
19. _____ disease that normally does not infect a healthy individual
20. _____ blood infection

✔ *Check your answers in Appendix A. Review any material that you did not answer correctly.*

Correct Answers _____ × 5 = _____ % Score

Learning Activity 9-4
Matching Procedures, Pharmacology, and Abbreviations

Match the following terms with the definitions in the numbered list.

anticoagulants	homologous	RBC indices
aspiration	lymphadenography	sentinel
autologous	lymphangiectomy	Shilling
differential	Monospot	thrombolytics
hematocrit	RBC	WBC

1. _____ drawing in or out by suction

2. _____ measurement of erythrocytes expressed as a percentage in a whole blood sample

3. _____ serologic test for infectious mononucleosis

4. _____ used to prevent blood clot formation

5. _____ leukocyte

6. _____ term used to describe a transplantation from another individual

7. _____ removal of a lymph vessel

8. _____ mathematical calculation of the size, volume, and concentration of hemoglobin for an average RBC

9. _____ definitive test for pernicious anemia

10. _____ radiographic examination of lymph nodes

11. _____ term used to describe a transfusion from the recipient's own blood

12. _____ first lymph node that receives drainage from cancer containing areas

13. _____ erythrocyte

14. _____ used to dissolve blood clots

15. _____ test to enumerate the distribution of WBCs in a stained blood smear

✔ *Check your answers in Appendix A. Review any material that you did not answer correctly.*

Correct Answers _____ × 6.67 = _____ % Score

MEDICAL RECORD ACTIVITIES

The two medical records included in the following activities use common clinical scenarios to show how medical terminology is used to document patient care. Complete the terminology and analysis sections for each activity to help you recognize and understand terms related to the blood, lymph, and immune systems.

Medical Record Activity 9-1
Discharge Summary: Sickle Cell Crisis

Terms listed in the following table are taken from *Discharge Summary: Sickle Cell Crisis* that follows. Use a medical dictionary such as *Taber's Cyclopedic Medical Dictionary*, the appendices of this book, or other resources to define each term. Then review the pronunciations for each term and practice by reading the medical record aloud.

Term	Definition
ambulating ĂM-bū-lāt-ĭng	
analgesia ăn-ăl-JĒ-zē-ă	
anemia ă-NĒ-mē-ă	
crisis KRĪ-sĭs	
CT	
hemoglobin HĒ-mō-glō-bĭn	
ileus ĬL-ē-ŭs	
infarction ĭn-FĂRK-shŭn	
morphine MOR-fēn	
sickle cell SĬK-ăl SĔL	
splenectomy splē-NĔK-tō-mē	
Vicodin VĪ-kō-dĭn	

Listen and Learn Online! *will help you master the pronunciation of selected medical words from this medical record activity. Visit* www.davisplus.com/gylys/systems *to find instructions on completing the* Listen and Learn Online! *exercise for this section and to practice pronunciations.*

DISCHARGE SUMMARY: SICKLE CELL CRISIS

General Hospital

1511 Ninth Avenue ■■ **Sun City, USA 12345** ■■ **(555) 802-1887**

DISCHARGE SUMMARY

July 6, 20xx

ADMISSION DATE: June 21, 20xx   DISCHARGE DATE: June 23, 20xx

ADMITTING AND DISCHARGE DIAGNOSES:
1. Sickle cell crisis.
2. Abdominal pain.

PROCEDURES: Two units of packed red blood cells and CT scan of the abdomen.

REASON FOR ADMISSION: This is a 46-year-old African American man who reports a history of sickle cell anemia, which results in abdominal cramping when he is in crisis. His hemoglobin was 6 upon admission. He says his baseline runs 7 to 8. The patient states that he has not had a splenectomy. He describes the pain as mid abdominal and cramplike. He denied any chills, fevers, or sweats.

HOSPITAL COURSE BY PROBLEM:
Problem 1. Sickle cell crisis. Patient was admitted to a medical/surgical bed, and placed on oxygen and IV fluids. He received morphine for analgesia, as well as Vicodin. At discharge, his abdominal pain had resolved; however, he reported weakness. He was kept for an additional day for observation.

Problem 2. CT scan was performed on the belly and showed evidence of ileus in the small bowel with somewhat dilated small-bowel loops and also an abnormal enhancement pattern in the kidney. The patient has had no nausea or vomiting. He is moving his bowels without any difficulty. He is ambulating. He even goes outside to smoke cigarettes, which he has been advised not to do. Certainly, we should obtain some information on his renal function and have his regular doctor assess this problem.

DISCHARGE INSTRUCTIONS: Patient advised to stop smoking and to see his regular doctor for follow-up on renal function.

Michael R. Saadi, MD
Michael R. Saadi, MD

MRS:dp

D: 6-21-20xx
T: 6-21-20xx

Patient: Evans, Joshua   Physician: Michael R. Saadi, MD
Room #: 609 P   Patient ID#: 532657

Analysis

Review the medical record *Discharge Summary: Sickle Cell Crisis* to answer the following questions.

1. What blood product was administered to the patient?

_____

2. Why was this blood product given to the patient?

_____

3. Why was a CT scan performed on the patient?

_____

4. What were the three findings of the CT scan?

_____

5. Why should the patient see his regular doctor?

_____

Medical Record Activity 9-2

Discharge Summary: PCP and HIV

Terminology

Terms listed in the following table are taken from *Discharge Summary: PCP and HIV* that follows. Use a medical dictionary such as *Taber's Cyclopedic Medical Dictionary*, the appendices of this book, or other resources to define each term. Then review the pronunciations for each term and practice by reading the medical record aloud.

Term	Definition
alveolar lavage ăl-VĒ-ō-lăr lă-VĂZH	
Bactrim BĂK-trĭm	
bronchoscopy brŏng-KŎS-kō-pē	
diffuse dĭ-FŪS	
HIV	
human immuno- deficiency virus ĭm-ū-nō-dē-FĬSH- ĕn-sē	
infiltrate ĬN-fĭl-trāt	

Term	Definition
Kaposi sarcoma KĂP-ō-sē săr-KŌ-mă	
leukoencephalopathy loo-kō-ĕn-sĕf-ă-LŎP- ă-thē	
multifocal mŭl-tĭ-FŌ-kăl	
PCP	
PMN	
Pneumocystis pneumonia nū-mō-SĬS-tĭs nū-MŌ-nē-ă	
thrush THRŬSH	
vaginal candidiasis VĂJ-ĭn-ăl kăn-dĭ-DĪ- ă-sĭs	

Listen and Learn Online! *will help you master the pronunciation of selected medical words from this medical record activity. Visit* www.davisplus.com/gylys/systems *to find instructions on completing the* Listen and Learn Online! *exercise for this section and to practice pronunciations.*

DISCHARGE SUMMARY: PCP AND HIV

General Hospital

1511 Ninth Avenue ■■ Sun City, USA 12345 ■■ (544) 802-1887

DISCHARGE SUMMARY

March 5, 20xx

Age: 31

ADMISSION DATE: March 5, 20xx

DISCHARGE DATE: March 6, 20xx

ADMITTING AND DISCHARGE DIAGNOSES:
1. *Pneumocystis* pneumonia.
2. Human immunodeficiency virus infection.
3. Wasting.

SOCIAL HISTORY: Patient's husband is deceased from AIDS 1 year ago with progressive multifocal leukoencephalopathy and Kaposi sarcoma. She denies any history of intravenous drug use, transfusion, and identifies three lifetime sexual partners.

PAST MEDICAL HISTORY: Patient's past medical history is significant for HIV and several episodes of diarrhea, sinusitis, thrush, and vaginal candidiasis. She gave a history of a 10-pound weight loss. The chest x-ray showed diffuse lower lobe infiltrates, and she was diagnosed with presumptive *Pneumocystis* pneumonia and placed on Bactrim. She was admitted for a bronchoscopy with alveolar lavage to confirm the diagnosis.

PROCEDURE: The antiretroviral treatment was reinitiated, and she was counseled as to the need to strictly adhere to her therapeutic regimen.

DISCHARGE INSTRUCTIONS: Complete medication regimen. Patient discharged to the care of Dr. Amid Shaheen.

Michael R. Saadi, MD
Michael R. Saadi, MD

MRS:dp

D: 3-05-20xx
T: 3-06-20xx

Patient: Smart, Joann
Room #: 540

Physician: Michael R. Saadi, MD
Patient ID#: 532850

Analysis

Review the medical record *Discharge Summary: PCP and HIV* to answer the following questions.

1. How do you think the patient acquired the HIV infection?

2. What were the two diagnoses of the husband?

3. What four disorders in the medical history are significant for HIV?

4. What was the x-ray finding?

5. What two procedures are going to be performed to confirm the diagnosis of PCP pneumonia?

Musculoskeletal System

CHAPTER

10

Chapter Outline

Objectives

Upon completion of this chapter, you will be able to:

- Locate and describe the structures of the musculoskeletal system.
- Recognize, pronounce, spell, and build words related to the musculoskeletal system.
- Describe pathological conditions, diagnostic and therapeutic procedures, and other terms related to the musculoskeletal system.
- Explain pharmacology related to the treatment of musculoskeletal disorders.
- Demonstrate your knowledge of this chapter by completing the learning and medical record activities.

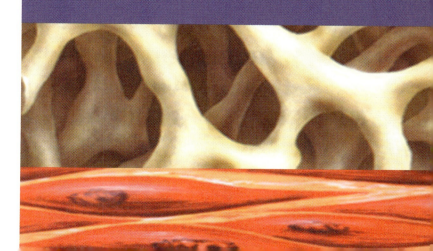

Anatomy and Physiology

The musculoskeletal system includes muscles, bones, joints, and related structures, such as the tendons and connective tissue that function in support and movement of body parts and organs.

Muscles

Muscle tissue is composed of contractile cells or fibers that provide movement of an organ or body part. Muscles contribute to posture, produce body heat, and act as a protective covering for internal organs. Muscles make up the bulk of the body. They have the ability to be excited by a stimulus, contract, relax, and return to their original size and shape. Whether muscles are attached to bones or to internal organs and blood vessels, their primary responsibility is movement. (See Table 10–1.) Apparent motion provided by muscles include walking and talking. Less apparent motions include the passage and elimination of food through the digestive system, propulsion of blood through the arteries, and contraction of the bladder to eliminate urine. (See Figure 10–1.)

There are three types of muscle tissue in the body:

- **Skeletal muscles,** also called **voluntary** or **striated muscles**, are muscles whose action is under voluntary control. Some examples of voluntary muscles are muscles that move the eyeballs, tongue, and bones.
- **Cardiac muscle** is found only in the heart. It is unique for its branched interconnections, and makes up most of the wall of the heart. Cardiac muscle shares similarities with both skeletal and smooth muscles. Like skeletal muscle, it is striated, but it produces rhythmic involuntary contractions like smooth muscle.
- **Smooth muscles,** also called **involuntary** or **visceral muscles**, are muscles whose actions are involuntary. They are found principally in the visceral organs, walls of arteries and respiratory passages, and urinary and reproductive ducts. The contraction of smooth muscle is controlled by the autonomic (involuntary) nervous system. (See Figure 10–2.)

Anatomy and Physiology Key Terms

This section introduces important terms along with their definitions and pronunciations. Word analyses are also provided.

Term	Definition
appendage ă-PĔN-dĭj	Any body part attached to a main structure *Examples of appendages include the arms and legs.*
articulation ăr-tĭk-ū-LĀ-shŭn	Place of union between two or more bones; also called *joint*
cancellous	Spongy or porous structure, as found at the ends of long bones
cruciate ligaments KROO-shē-āt *cruci:* cross *-ate:* having the form of; possessing	Ligaments that cross each other forming an X within the notch between the femoral condyles *Along with other structures, the cruciate ligaments help secure and stabilize the knee.*
hematopoiesis hĕm-ă-tō-poy-Ē-sĭs *hemat/o:* blood *-poiesis:* formation, production	Production and development of blood cells, normally in the bone marrow

Pronunciation Help	Long Sound	ā—rate	ē—rebirth	ī—isle	ō—over	ū—unite
	Short Sound	ă—alone	ĕ—ever	ĭ—it	ŏ—not	ŭ—cut

Table 10-1	**Body Movements Produced by Muscle Action**

This chart lists body movements and the resulting muscle action. With the exception of rotation, these movements are in pairs of opposing functions.

Motion	Action
Adduction	Moves closer to the midline
Abduction	Moves away from the midline
Flexion	Decreases the angle of a joint
Extension	Increases the angle of a joint
Rotation	Moves a bone around its own axis
Pronation	Turns the palm down
Supination	Turns the palm up
Inversion	Moves the sole of the foot inward
Eversion	Moves the sole of the foot outward
Dorsiflexion	Elevates the foot
Plantar flexion	Lowers the foot (points the toes)

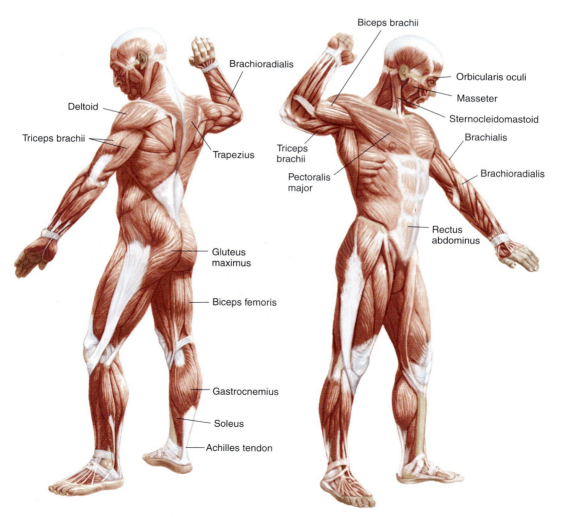

Figure 10-1. Selected muscles of the body.

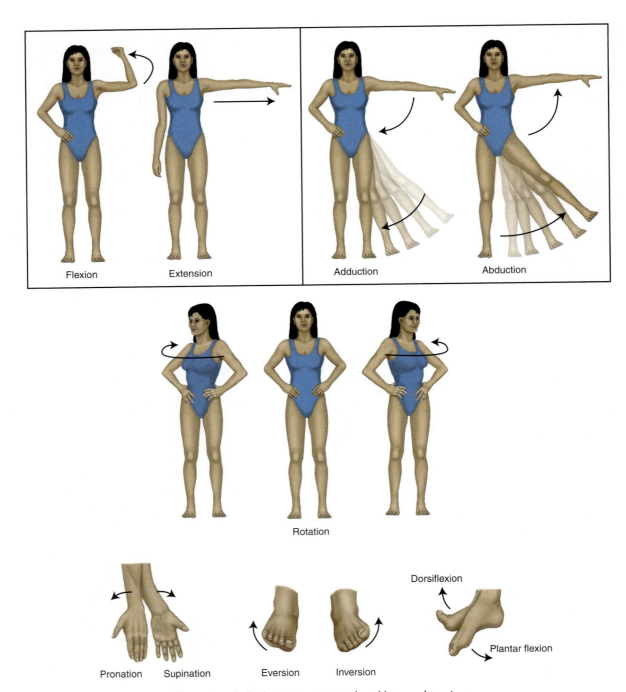

Figure 10-2. Body movements produced by muscle action.

Attachments

Muscles attach to bones by fleshy or fibrous attachments. In **fleshy attachments,** muscle fibers arise directly from bone. Although these fibers distribute force over wide areas, they are weaker than a fibrous attachment. In **fibrous attachments,** the connective tissue converges at the end of the muscle to become continuous and indistinguishable from the periosteum. When the fibrous attachment spans a large area of a particular bone, the attachment is called an *aponeurosis*. Such attachments are found in the lumbar region of the back. In some instances, this connective tissue penetrates the bone itself. When connective tissue fibers form a cord or strap, it is referred to as a *tendon*. This arrangement localizes a great deal of force in a small area of bone. **Ligaments** are flexible bands of fibrous tissue that are highly adapted for resisting strains and are one of the principal mechanical factors that hold bones close together in a synovial joint. An example are the **cruciate ligaments** of the knee that help to prevent anterior-posterior displacement of the articular surfaces and to secure articulating bones when we stand.

 It is time to review muscle structures by completing Learning Activity 10–1.

Bones

Bones provide the framework of the body, protect internal organs, store calcium and other minerals, and produce blood cells within bone marrow **(hematopoiesis).** Together with soft tissue, most vital organs are enclosed and protected by bones. For example, bones of the skull protect the brain; the rib cage protects the heart and lungs. In addition to support and protection, the skeletal system carries out a number of other important functions. Movement is possible because bones provide points of attachment for muscles, tendons, and ligaments. As muscles contract, tendons and ligaments pull on bones and cause skeletal movement. Bone marrow, found within the larger bones, is responsible for hematopoiesis, continuously producing millions of blood cells to replace those that have been destroyed. Bones serve as a storehouse for minerals, particularly phosphorus and calcium. When the body experiences a need for a certain mineral, such as calcium during pregnancy, and a sufficient dietary supply is not available, calcium is withdrawn from the bones.

Bone types

There are four principal types of bone:

- **Short bones** are somewhat cube shaped. They consist of a core of spongy bone, also known as *cancellous bone,* enclosed in a thin surface layer of compact bone. Examples of short bones include the bones of the ankles, wrists, and toes.
- **Irregular bones** include the bones that cannot be classified as short or long because of their complex shapes. Examples of irregular bones include vertebrae and the bones of the middle ear.
- **Flat bones** are exactly what their name suggests. They provide broad surfaces for muscular attachment or protection for internal organs. Examples of flat bones include bones of the skull, shoulder blades, and sternum.
- **Long bones** are found in the **appendages** (extremities) of the body, such as the legs, arms, and fingers. (See Figure 10–3.) The parts of a long bone include:

– The (1) **diaphysis** is the shaft or long, main portion of a bone. It consists of (2) **compact bone** that forms a cylinder and surrounds a central canal called the (3) **medullary cavity.** The medullary cavity, also called *marrow cavity*, contains fatty yellow marrow in adults and consists primarily of fat cells and a few scattered blood cells.

– The (4) **distal epiphysis** and (5) **proximal epiphysis** (plural, *epiphyses*) are the two ends of the bones. Both ends have a somewhat bulbous shape to provide space for muscle and ligament attachments near the joints. The epiphyses are covered with (6) **articular cartilage,** a type of elastic connective tissue that provides a smooth surface for movement of joints. It also reduces friction and absorbs shock at the freely movable joints. In addition, the epiphyses are made up largely of a porous chamber of (7) **spongy bone** surrounded by a layer of compact bone. Within spongy bone is red bone marrow, which is richly supplied with blood and consists of immature and mature blood cells in various stages of development. In an adult, production of red blood cells (**erythropoiesis**) occurs in red bone marrow. Red bone marrow is also responsible for the formation of white blood cells (**leukopoiesis**) and platelets.

– The (8) **periosteum,** a dense, white, fibrous membrane, covers the remaining surface of the bone. It contains numerous blood and lymph vessels and nerves. In growing bones, the inner layer contains the bone-forming cells known as **osteoblasts.** Because blood vessels and osteoblasts are located here, the periosteum provides a means for bone repair and general bone nutrition. Bones that lose periosteum through injury or disease usually scale or die. The periosteum also serves as a point of attachment for muscles, ligaments, and tendons.

 It is time to review bone structures by completing Learning Activity 10–2.

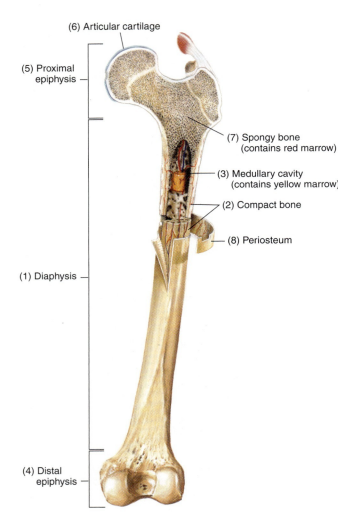

(6) Articular cartilage

(5) Proximal epiphysis

(7) Spongy bone (contains red marrow)

(3) Medullary cavity (contains yellow marrow)

(2) Compact bone

(8) Periosteum

(1) Diaphysis

(4) Distal epiphysis

Figure 10-3. Longitudinal structure of a long bone.

Surface Features of Bones

Surfaces of bones are rarely smooth but rather consist of projections, depressions, and openings that provide sites for muscle and ligament attachment. They also provide pathways and openings for blood vessels, nerves, and ducts. Various types of projections are evident in bones, some of which serve as points of **articulation.** Surfaces of bones may be rounded, sharp, or narrow or have a large ridge. Depressions and openings are cavities and holes in a bone. They provide pathways and openings for blood vessels, nerves, and ducts. (See Table 10–2.)

Divisions of the Skeletal System

The skeletal system of a human adult consists of 206 individual bones. However, only the major bones are discussed. For anatomical purposes, the human skeleton is divided into the axial skeleton and appendicular skeleton. (See Figure 10–4.)

Axial Skeleton

The axial skeleton is divided into three major regions: skull, rib cage, and vertebral column. It contributes to the formation of body cavities and provides protection for internal organs, such as the brain, spinal cord, and organs enclosed in the thorax. The axial skeleton is distinguished with bone color in Figure 10–4.

Skull

The bony structure of the skull consists of cranial bones and facial bones. (See Figure 10–5.) With the exception of one facial bone, all other bones of the skull are joined together by sutures. Sutures are

Table 10-2	**Surface Features of Bones**			

This chart lists the most common types of projections, depressions, and openings along with the bones involved, descriptions, and examples for each. Becoming familiar with these terms will help you identify parts of individual bones described in medical reports related to orthopedics.

Surface Type	Bone Marking	Description	Example
Projections			
• Nonarticulating surfaces	• Trochanter	• Very large, irregularly shaped process found only on the femur	• Greater trochanter of the femur
• Sites of muscle and ligament attachment	• Tubercle	• Small, rounded process	• Tubercle of the femur
	• Tuberosity	• Large, rounded process	• Tuberosity of the humerus

Table 10-2	**Surface Features of Bones—cont'd**			
	Surface Type	**Bone Marking**	**Description**	**Example**
	Articulating surfaces			
	• Projections that form joints	• Condyle	• Rounded, articulating knob	• Condyle of the humerus
		• Head	• Prominent, rounded, articulating end of a bone	• Head of the femur
	Depressions and openings			
	• Sites for blood vessel, nerve, and duct passage	• Foramen	• Rounded opening through and nerves a bone to accommodate blood vessels	• Foramen of the skull through which cranial nerves pass
		• Fissure	• Narrow, slitlike opening	• Fissure of the sphenoid bone
		• Meatus	• Opening or passage into a bone	• External auditory meatus of the temporal bone
		• Sinus	• Cavity or hollow space in a bone	• Cavity of the frontal sinus con taining a duct that carries secre- tions to the upper part of the nasal cavity

the lines of junction between two bones, especially of the skull, and are usually immovable.

Cranial Bones
Eight bones, collectively known as the ***cranium (skull)***, enclose and protect the brain and the organs of hearing and equilibrium. Cranial bones are connected to muscles to provide head movements, chewing motions, and facial expressions.

An infant's skull contains an unossified membrane, or soft spot (incomplete bone formation), lying between the cranial bones called a ***fontanel***. The pulse of blood vessels can be felt under the skin in those areas. The chief function of the fontanels is to allow the bones to move as the fetus passes through the birth canal during the delivery process. With age, the fontanels begin to fuse together and become immobile in early childhood.

The (1) **frontal bone** forms the anterior portion of the skull (**forehead**) and the roof of the bony cavities that contain the eyeballs. One (2) **parietal bone** is situated on each side of the skull just behind the frontal bone. Together they form the upper sides and roof of the cranium. Each parietal bone meets the frontal bone along the (3) **coronal suture**. A single (4) **occipital bone** forms the back and base of the skull. It contains an opening in its base through which the spinal cord passes. Two (5) **temporal bone(s),** one on each side of the skull, form part of the lower cranium. Each temporal bone has a complicated shape that contains

various cavities and recesses associated with the internal ear, the essential part of the organ of hearing. The temporal bone projects downward to form the **mastoid process,** which provides a point of attachment for several neck muscles. The (6) **sphenoid bone,** located at the middle part of the base of the skull, forms a central wedge that joins with all other cranial bones, holding them together. A very light and spongy bone, the (7) **ethmoid bone,** forms most of the bony area between the nasal cavity and parts of the orbits of the eyes.

Facial Bones
All facial bones, with the exception of the (8) **mandible** (lower jaw bone), are joined together by sutures and are immovable. Movement of the mandible is needed for speaking and chewing (**mastication**). The (9) **maxillae,** paired upper jawbones, are fused in the midline by a suture. They form the upper jaw and **hard palate** (roof of the mouth). If the maxillary bones do not fuse properly before birth, a congenital defect called ***cleft palate*** results. The maxillae (singular, *maxilla*) and the mandible contain sockets for the roots of the teeth. Two thin, nearly rectangular bones, the (10) **nasal bones,** lie side-by-side and are fused medially, forming the shape and the bridge of the nose. Two paired (11) **lacrimal bones** are located at the corner of each eye. These thin, small bones unite to form the groove for the lacrimal sac and canals through which the tear ducts pass into the nasal cavity. The

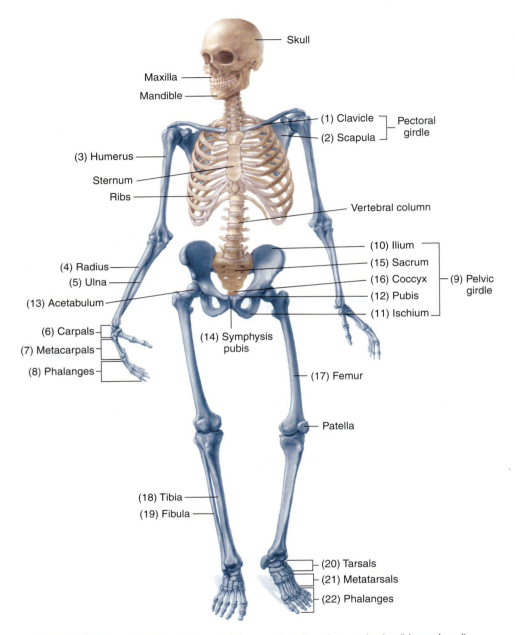

Figure 10-4. Anterior view of the axial (bone colored) and appendicular (blue colored) skeleton.

paired (12) **zygomatic bones** are located on the side of the face below the eyes and form the higher portion of the cheeks below and to the sides of the eyes. The zygomatic bone is commonly referred to as the *cheekbone*. The (13) **vomer** is a single, thin bone that forms the lower part of the nasal septum.

Other important structures, the **paranasal sinuses,** are cavities located within the cranial and facial bones. As their name implies, the frontal, ethmoidal, sphenoidal, and maxillary sinuses are named after the bones in which they are located.

(See Figure 10–6.) The paranasal sinuses open into the nasal cavities and are lined with **ciliary epithelium** that is continuous with the mucosa of the nasal cavities. When sinuses are unable to drain properly, a feeling of being "stuffed up" ensues. This commonly occurs during upper respiratory infections (URI) or with allergies.

Thorax

The internal organs of the chest (**thorax**), including the heart and lungs, are enclosed and protected by a bony rib cage. The thorax consists

A.

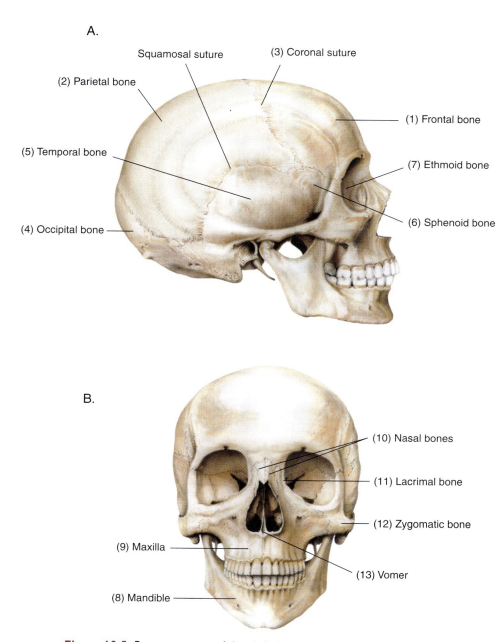

Squamosal suture

(3) Coronal suture

(2) Parietal bone

(1) Frontal bone

(5) Temporal bone

(7) Ethmoid bone

(4) Occipital bone

(6) Sphenoid bone

B.

(10) Nasal bones

(11) Lacrimal bone

(12) Zygomatic bone

(9) Maxilla

(13) Vomer

(8) Mandible

Figure 10-5. Bony structures of the skull. (A) Cranial bones. (B) Facial bones.

of 12 pairs of ribs, all attached to the spine. (See Figure 10–7.) The first seven pairs, the (1) **true ribs,** are attached directly to the (2) **sternum** by a strip of (3) **costal cartilage.** The costal cartilage of the next five pairs of ribs is not fastened directly to the sternum, so these ribs are known as (4) **false ribs.** The last two pairs of false ribs are not joined, even indirectly, to the sternum but attach posteriorly to the thoracic vertebrae. These last two pairs of false ribs are known as (5) **floating ribs.**

Vertebral Column

The vertebral column of the adult is composed of 26 bones called ***vertebrae*** (singular, *vertebra*). The vertebral column supports the body and provides a protective bony canal for the spinal cord. A healthy, normal spine has four curves that help make it resilient and maintain balance. The cervical and lumbar regions curve forward, whereas the thoracic and sacral regions curve backward. Abnormal curves may be due to a congenital defect, poor posture, or bone disease. (See Figure 10–8.)

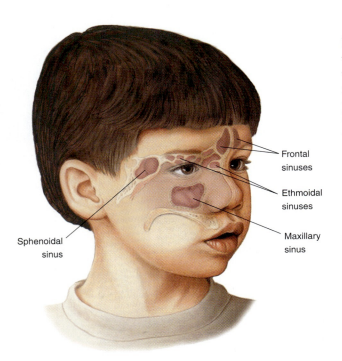

Figure 10-6. Paranasal sinuses.

The vertebral column consists of five regions of bones, each deriving its name from its location within the spinal column. The seven (1) **cervical vertebrae** form the skeletal framework of the neck. The first cervical vertebra, the (2) **atlas,** supports the skull. The second cervical vertebra, the (3) **axis,** makes possible the rotation of the skull on the neck. Under the seventh cervical vertebra are 12 (4) **thoracic vertebrae,** which support the chest and serve as a point of articulation for the ribs. The next five vertebrae, the (5) **lumbar vertebrae,** are situated in the lower back area and carry most of the weight of the torso. Below this area are five sacral vertebrae, which are fused into a single bone in the adult and are referred to as the (6) **sacrum.** The tail of the vertebral column consists of four or five fragmented fused vertebrae referred to as the (7) **coccyx.**

Vertebrae are separated by flat, round structures, the (8) **intervertebral disks,** which are composed of a fibrocartilaginous substance with a gelatinous mass in the center (*nucleus pulposus*). When disk material protrudes into the neural canal, pressure on the adjacent spinal root nerve causes pain. This condition occurs most commonly in the lower

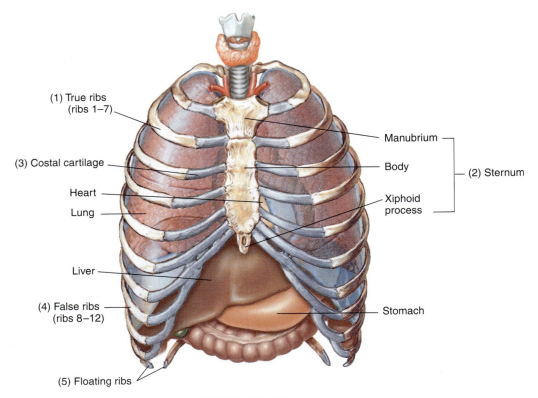

Figure 10-7. Thorax.

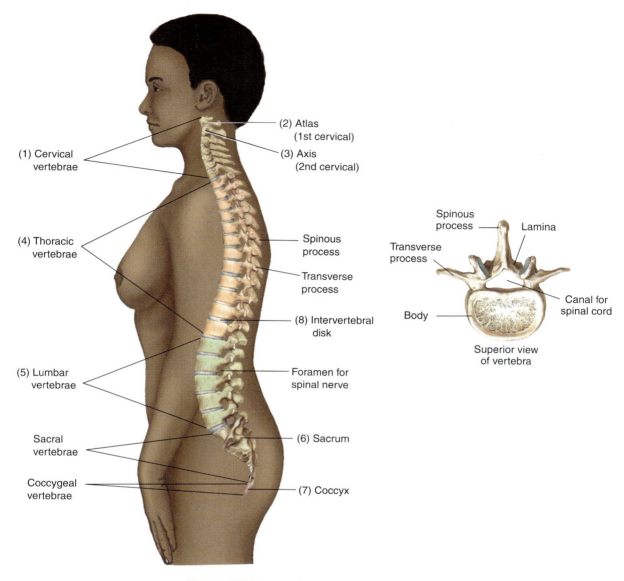

(1) Cervical vertebrae

(2) Atlas (1st cervical)

(3) Axis (2nd cervical)

(4) Thoracic vertebrae

Spinous process

Transverse process

(8) Intervertebral disk

(5) Lumbar vertebrae

Foramen for spinal nerve

Sacral vertebrae

(6) Sacrum

Coccygeal vertebrae

(7) Coccyx

Spinous process

Lamina

Transverse process

Canal for spinal cord

Body

Superior view of vertebra

Figure 10-8. Lateral view of the vertebral column.

spine and is referred to as ***herniation of an intervertebral disk, herniated nucleus pulposus (HNP), ruptured disk, prolapsed disk,*** or ***slipped disk.*** (See Figure 10–9.)

Appendicular Skeleton

The appendicular skeleton consists of bones of the upper and lower limbs and their girdles that attach the limbs to the axial skeleton. The appendicular skeleton is distinguished with a blue color in Figure 10–4. The difference between the axial and appendicular skeletons is that the axial skeleton protects internal organs and provides central support for the body; the appendicular skeleton enables the body

to move. The ability to walk, run, or catch a ball is possible because of the movable joints of the limbs that make up the appendicular skeleton.

Pectoral (Shoulder) Girdle

The pectoral girdle consists of two bones, the anterior (1) **clavicle** (collar bone) and the posterior (2) **scapula** (triangular shoulder blade). The primary function of the pectoral girdle is to attach the bones of the upper limbs to the axial skeleton and provide attachments for muscles that aid upper limb movements. The paired pectoral structures and their associated muscles form the shoulders of the body.

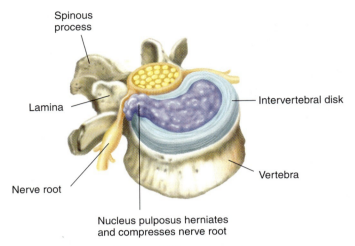

Spinous
process

Lamina

Intervertebral disk

Nerve root

Vertebra

Nucleus pulposus herniates
and compresses nerve root

Figure 10-9. Herniated disk.

Upper Limbs

The skeletal framework of each upper limb includes the arm, forearm, and hand. Anatomically speaking, the arm is only that part of the upper limb between the shoulder and elbow. Each appendage consists of a (3) **humerus** (upper arm bone), which articulates with the (4) **radius** and (5) **ulna** at the elbow. The radius and ulna form the skeleton of the forearm. The bones of the hand include eight (6) **carpals** (wrist); five radiating (7) **metacarpals** (palm); and ten radiating (8) **phalanges** (fingers).

Pelvic (Hip) Girdle

The (9) **pelvic girdle** is a basin-shaped structure that attaches the lower limbs to the axial skeleton. Along with its associated ligaments, it supports the trunk of the body and provides protection for the visceral organs of the pelvis (lower organs of digestion and urinary and reproductive structures).

Male and female **pelves** (singular, *pelvis*) differ considerably in size and shape but share the same basic structures. Some of the differences are attributable to the function of the female pelvis during childbearing. The female pelvis is shallower than the male pelvis but wider in all directions. The female pelvis not only supports the enlarged uterus as the fetus matures but also provides a large opening to allow the infant to pass through during birth. Even so, female and male pelves are divided into the (10) **ilium,** (11) **ischium,** and (12) **pubis.** These three bones are fused together in the adult to form a single bone called the **innominate (hip) bone.** The ilium travels inferiorly to form part of the (13) **acetabulum** (the deep socket of the hip joint) and medially to join the pubis. The bladder is located behind the (14) **symphysis pubis;** the rectum is in the curve of the (15) **sacrum** and (16) **coccyx.** In the female, the uterus, fallopian tubes, ovaries, and vagina are located between the bladder and the rectum.

Lower Limbs

The lower limbs support the complete weight of the erect body and are subjected to exceptional stresses, especially in running or jumping. To accommodate for these types of forces, the lower limb bones are stronger and thicker than comparable bones of the upper limbs. The difference between the upper and lower limb bones is that the lighter bones of the upper limbs are adapted for mobility and flexibility; the massive bones of the lower limbs are specialized for stability and weight bearing.

There are three parts of each lower limb: the thigh, the leg, and the foot. The thigh consists of a single bone called the (17) **femur.** It is the largest, longest, and strongest bone in the body. The leg is formed by two parallel bones: the (18) **tibia** and the (19) **fibula.** The seven (20) **tarsals** (ankle bones) resemble metacarpals (wrist bones) in structure. Lastly, the bones of the foot include the (21) **metatarsals,** which consists of five small long bones numbered 1 to 5 beginning with the great toe on the medial side of the foot, and the much smaller (22) **phalanges** (toes).

Joints or Articulations

To allow for body movements, bones must have points where they meet (**articulate**). These articulating points form joints that have various degrees of mobility. Some are freely movable (**diarthroses**), others are only slightly movable (**amphiarthroses**), and the remaining are immovable (**synarthroses**). All three types are necessary for smooth, coordinated body movements.

Joints that allow movement are called *synovial joints.* The ends of the bones that comprise these joints are encased in a sleevelike extension of the periosteum called the *joint capsule.* This capsule binds the articulating bones to each other. In most synovial joints, the capsule is strengthened by ligaments that lash the bones together, providing additional strength to the joint capsule. A membrane called the *synovial membrane* surrounds the inside of the capsule. It secretes a lubricating fluid (**synovial fluid**) within the entire joint capsule. The ends of each of the bones are covered with a smooth layer of cartilage that serves as a cushion.

 It is time to review skeletal structures by completing Learning Activity 10–3.

Connecting Body Systems–Musculoskeletal System

The main function of the musculoskeletal system is to provide support, protection, and movement of body parts. Specific functional relationships between the musculoskeletal system and other body systems are summarized below.

 Blood, lymph, and immune
- Muscle action pumps lymph through lymphatic vessels.
- Bone marrow provides a place for cells of the immune system to develop.

 Cardiovascular
- Bone helps regulate blood calcium levels, important to heart function.

 Digestive
- Muscles play an important role in swallowing and propelling food through the digestive tract.
- Muscles of the stomach mechanically break down food to prepare it for chemical digestion.

 Endocrine
- Exercising skeletal muscles stimulate release of hormones to increase blood flow.

 Female reproductive
- Skeletal muscles are important in sexual activity and during delivery of the fetus.

- Bones provide a source of calcium during pregnancy and lactation if dietary intake is lacking or insufficient.
- Pelvis helps support the enlarged uterus during pregnancy.

 Genitourinary
- Skeletal muscles are important in sexual activity.
- Bones work in conjunction with the kidneys to help regulate blood calcium levels.
- Skeletal muscles help control urine elimination.

 Integumentary
- Involuntary muscle contractions (shivering) help regulate body temperature.

 Nervous
- Bones protect the brain and spinal cord.

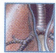 **Respiratory**
- Muscles and ribs work together in the breathing process.

Medical Word Elements

This section introduces combining forms, suffixes, and prefixes related to the musculoskeletal system. Word analyses are also provided.

Element	Meaning	Word Analysis
Combining Forms		
Skeletal System		
General		
ankyl/o	stiffness; bent, crooked	**ankyl**/osis (ăng-kĭ-LŌ-sĭs): abnormal condition of stiffness -*osis:* abnormal condition; increase (used primarily with blood cells) *Ankylosis results in immobility and stiffness of a joint. It may be the result of trauma, surgery, or disease and most commonly occurs in rheumatoid arthritis.*
arthr/o	joint	**arthr**/itis (ăr-THRĪ-tĭs): inflammation of a joint -*itis:* inflammation
kyph/o	humpback	**kyph**/osis (kī-FŌ-sĭs): abnormal condition of a humpback posture -*osis:* abnormal condition; increase (used primarily with blood cells)
lamin/o	lamina (part of vertebral arch)	**lamin**/ectomy (lăm-ĭ-NĔK-tō-mē): excision of the lamina -*ectomy:* excision, removal *Laminectomy is usually performed to relieve compression of the spinal cord or to remove a lesion or herniated disk.*
lord/o	curve, swayback	**lord**/osis (lor-DŌ-sĭs): abnormal condition of a swayback posture -*osis:* abnormal condition; increase (used primarily with blood cells)
myel/o	bone marrow; spinal cord	**myel**/**o**/cyte (MĪ-ĕl-ō-sīt): bone marrow cell -*cyte:* cell
orth/o	straight	**orth**/**o**/ped/ist (or-thō-PĒ-dĭst): specialist in treatment of musculoskeletal disorders *ped:* foot; child -*ist:* specialist *Initially, an orthopedist corrected deformities and straightened children's bones. In today's medical practice, however, the orthopedist treats musculoskeletal disorders and associated structures in persons of all ages.*
oste/o	bone	**oste**/oma (ŏs-tē-Ō-mă): tumor composed of bone -*oma:* tumor *Osteomas are benign bony tumors.*
ped/o	foot; child	**ped**/**o**/graph (PĔD-ō-grăf): instrument for recording the foot -*graph:* instrument for recording *A pedograph is an instrument for recording an imprint of the foot on paper, and the gait (manner of walking).*
ped/i		**ped**/**i**/cure (PĔD-ĭ-kūr): care of feet
scoli/o	crooked, bent	**scoli**/osis (skō-lē-Ō-sĭs): abnormal bending of the spine -*osis:* abnormal condition; increase (used primarily with blood cells)
thorac/o	chest	**thorac**/**o**/dynia (thō-răk-ō-DĬN-ē-ă): pain in the chest -*dynia:* pain

Medical Word Elements—cont'd

Element	Meaning	Word Analysis
Specific Bones		
acromi/o	acromion (projection of scapula)	**acromi**/al (ăk-RŌ-mē-ăl): pertaining to the acromion *-al:* pertaining to
brachi/o	arm	**brachi**/algia (brā-kē-ĂL-jē-ă): pain in the arm *-algia:* pain
calcane/o	calcaneum (heel bone)	**calcane/o**/dynia (kăl-kăn-ō-DĬN-ē-ă): pain in the heel *-dynia:* pain
carp/o	carpus (wrist bone)	**carp/o**/ptosis (kăr-pŏp-TŌ-sĭs): wrist drop *-ptosis:* prolapse, downward displacement
cephal/o	head	**cephal**/ad (SĚF-ă-lăd): toward the head *-ad:* toward
cervic/o	neck; cervix uteri (neck of uterus)	**cervic/o**/dynia (sĕr-vĭ-kō-DĬN-ē-ă): pain in the neck; also called *cervical neuralgia* *-dynia:* pain
clavicul/o	clavicle (collar bone)	**clavicul**/ar (klă-VĬK-ū-lăr): pertaining to the clavicle *-ar:* pertaining to
cost/o	Ribs	**cost**/ectomy (kŏs-TĚK-tō-mē): excision of a rib *-ectomy:* excision, removal
crani/o	cranium (skull)	**crani/o**/tomy (krā-nē-ŎT-ō-mē): incision of the cranium *-tomy:* incision
dactyl/o	fingers; toes	**dactyl**/itis (dăk-tĭl-Ī-tĭs): inflammation of fingers or toes *-itis:* inflammation
femor/o	femur (thigh bone)	**femor**/al (FĚM-or-ăl): pertaining to the femur *-al:* pertaining to
fibul/o	fibula (smaller bone of lower leg)	**fibul/o**/calcane/al (fĭb-ū-lō-kăl-KĀ-nē-ăl): pertaining to the fibula and calcaneus *calcane:* calcaneum (heel bone) *-al:* pertaining to
humer/o	humerus (upper arm bone)	**humer/o**/scapul/ar (hū-měr-ō-SKĂP-ū-lăr): relating to the humerus and scapula *scapul:* scapula (shoulder blade) *-ar:* pertaining to
ili/o	ilium (lateral, flaring portion of hip bone)	**ili/o**/pelv/ic (ĭl-ē-ō-PĚL-vĭk): pertaining to the iliac area of the pelvis *pelv:* pelvis *-ic:* pertaining to
ischi/o	ischium (lower portion of hip bone)	**ischi/o**/dynia (ĭs-kē-ō-DĬN-ē-ă): pain in the ischium *-dynia:* pain

(continued)

Medical Word Elements—cont'd

Element	Meaning	Word Analysis
lumb/o	loins (lower back)	**lumb/o**/dynia (lŭm-bō-DĬN-ē-ă): pain in lumbar region of the back; also called *lumbago* *-dynia:* pain
metacarp/o	metacarpus (hand bones)	**metacarp**/ectomy (mĕt-ă-kăr-PĔK-tō-mē): excision of metacarpal bone(s) *-ectomy:* excision, removal
metatars/o	metatarsus (foot bones)	**metatars**/algia (mĕt-ă-tăr-SĂL-jē-ă): pain in the metatarsus *-algia:* pain *Metatarsalgia emanates from the heads of the metatarsus and worsens with weight bearing or palpation.*
patell/o	patella (kneecap)	**patell**/ectomy (păt-ĕ-LĔK-tō-mē): removal of the patella *-ectomy:* excision, removal
pelv/i	pelvis	**pelv/i**/metry* (pĕl-VĬM-ĕt-rē): act of measuring the pelvis *-metry:* act of measuring *Pelvimetry is routinely performed in obstetrical management.*
pelv/o		**pelv**/ic (PĔL-vĭk): pertaining to the pelvis *-ic:* petaining to
phalang/o	phalanges (bones of the fingers and toes)	**phalang**/ectomy (făl-ăn-JĔK-tō-mē): excision of phalanges *-ectomy:* excision, removal
pod/o	foot	**pod**/iatry (pō-DĪ-ă-trē): treatment of the feet *-iatry:* medicine, treatment
pub/o	pelvis bone (anterior part of pelvic bone)	**pub/o**/coccyg/eal (pū-bō-kŏk-SĬJ-ē-ăl): pertaining to the pubis and the coccyx *coccyg:* coccyx (tailbone) *-eal:* pertaining to
radi/o	radiation, x-ray; radius (lower arm bone on thumb side)	**radi**/al (RĀ-dē-ăl): pertaining to the radius *-al:* pertaining to
spondyl/o	vertebrae (backbone)	**spondyl**/itis (spŏn-dĭl-Ī-tĭs): inflammation of the vertebrae *-itis:* inflammation *The combining form* **spondyl/o** *is used to describe diseases and conditions.*
vertebr/o		inter/**vertebr**/al (ĭn-tĕr-VĔRT-ĕ-brĕl): relating to the area between two vertebrae *inter-:* between *-al:* pertaining to *The combining form* **vertebr/o** *is used to indicate anatomical terms.*
stern/o	sternum (breastbone)	**stern**/ad (STĔR-năd): toward the sternum *-ad:* toward

*The *i* in *pelv/i/metry* is an exception to the rule of using the connecting vowel *o*.

Medical Word Elements—cont'd

Element	Meaning	Word Analysis
tibi/o	tibia (larger bone of lower leg)	**tibi/o**/femor/al (tĭb-ē-ō-FĔM-or-ăl) pertaining to the tibia and femur *femor:* femur *-al:* pertaining to
Muscular System		
leiomy/o	smooth muscle (visceral)	**leiomy/**oma (lī-ō-mī-Ō-mă): tumor of smooth muscle *-oma:* tumor
muscul/o	muscle	**muscul/**ar (MŬS-kū-lăr): pertaining to muscles *-ar:* pertaining to
my/o		**my/**oma (mī-Ō-mă): tumor of muscle (tissue) *-oma:* tumor
rhabd/o	rod-shaped (striated)	**rhabd/**oid (RĂB-doyd): resembling a rod *-oid:* resembling
rhabdomy/o	rod-shaped (striated) muscle	**rhabdomy/**oma (răb-dō-mī-Ō-mă): tumor composed of striated muscular tissue *-oma:* tumor
Related Structures		
chondr/o	cartilage	**chondr/**itis (kŏn-DRĪ-tĭs): inflammation of cartilage *-itis:* inflammation
fasci/o	band, fascia (fibrous membrane supporting and separating muscles)	**fasci/o**/plasty (FĂSH-ē-ō-plăs-tē): surgical repair of fascia *-plasty:* surgical repair
fibr/o	fiber, fibrous tissue	**fibr/**oma (fī-BRŌ-mă): tumor of fibrous tissue *-oma:* tumor
synov/o	synovial membrane, synovial fluid	**synov/**ectomy (sĭn-ō-VĔK-tō-mē): removal of a synovial membrane *-ectomy:* excision, removal
ten/o	tendon	**ten/o**/desis (tĕn-ŌD-ĕ-sĭs): surgical binding or fixation of a tendon *-desis:* binding, fixation (of a bone or joint)
tend/o		**tend/o**/plasty (TĔN-dō-plăs-tē): surgical repair of a tendon *-plasty:* surgical repair
tendin/o		**tendin/**itis (tĕn-dĭn-Ī-tĭs): inflammation of a tendon *-itis:* inflammation
Suffixes		
-asthenia	weakness, debility	my/**asthenia** (mī-ăs-THĒ-nē-ă): weakness of muscle (and abnormal fatigue) *my:* muscle

(continued)

Medical Word Elements—cont'd

Element	Meaning	Word Analysis
-blast	embryonic cell	my/o/**blast** (MĪ-ō-blăst): embryonic cell that develops into muscle *my/o:* muscle
-clasia	to break; surgical fracture	oste/o/**clasia** (ŏs-tē-ō-KLĀ-zē-ă): surgical fracture of a bone *oste/o:* bone *Osteoclasia is the intentional fracture of a bone to correct a deformity and is also called* **osteoclasis.**
-clast	to break	oste/o/**clast** (ŎS-tē-ō-klăst): cell that breaks down bone *oste/o:* bone *An osteoclast destroys the matrix of bone. Osteoblasts and osteoclasts work together to maintain a constant bone size in adults.*
-desis	binding, fixation (of a bone or joint)	arthr/o/**desis** (ăr-thrō-DĒ-sĭs): binding together of a joint *arthr/o:* joint
-malacia	softening	chondr/o/**malacia** (kŏn-drō-măl-Ā-shē-ă): softening of cartilage *chondr/o:* cartilage *Chondromalacia is a softening of the articular cartilage, usually involving the patella.*
-physis	growth	epi/**physis** (ĕ-PĬF-ĭ-sĭs): growth upon (the end of a long bone) *epi–:* above, upon *The epiphyses are the enlarged proximal and distal ends of a long bone.*
-porosis	porous	oste/o/**porosis** (ŏs-tē-ō-pŏ-RŌ-sĭs): porous bone *oste/o:* bone *Osteoporosis is a disorder characterized by loss of bone density. It may cause pain, especially in the lower back; pathological fractures; loss of stature; and hairline fractures.*
-scopy	visual examination	arthr/o/**scopy** (ăr-THRŎS-kō-pē): visual examination of a joint *arthr/o:* joint *Arthroscopy is an endoscopic examination of the interior of a joint. It is performed by inserting small surgical instruments to remove and repair damaged tissue, such as cartilage fragments or torn ligaments.*
Prefixes		
a-	without, not	**a**/trophy (ĂT-rō-fē): without nourishment *-trophy:* development, nourishment *Atrophy is a wasting or decrease in size or physiological activity of a part of the body because of disease or other influences.*
dys-	bad; painful; difficult	**dys**/trophy (DĬS-trō-fē): disorder caused by defective nutrition or metabolism *-trophy:* development, nourishment
sub-	under, below	**sub**/patell/ar (sŭb-pă-TĔL-ăr): pertaining to below the patella *patell:* patella (kneecap) *-ar:* pertaining to

Medical Word Elements—cont'd

Element	Meaning	Word Analysis
supra-	above; excessive; superior	**supra**/cost/al (soo-pră-KŎS-tăl): pertaining to above the ribs *cost:* ribs *-al:* pertaining to
syn-	union, together, joined	**syn**/dactyl/ism (sĭn-DĂK-tĭl-ĭzm): condition of joined fingers or toes *dactyl:* fingers, toes *-ism:* condition *Syndactylism is a fusion of two or more fingers or toes.*

It is time to review medical word elements by completing Learning Activity 10–4. For audio pronunciations of the above-listed key terms, you can visit www.davisplus.fadavis.com/gylys/systems to download this chapter's Listen and Learn! *exercises or use the book's audio CD (if included).*

Pathology

Joints are especially vulnerable to constant wear and tear. Repeated motion, disease, trauma, and aging affect joints as well as muscles and tendons. Overall, disorders of the musculoskeletal system are more likely to be caused by injury than disease. Other disorders of structure and bone strength—such as osteoporosis, which occurs primarily in elderly women—affect the health of the musculoskeletal system.

For diagnosis, treatment, and management of musculoskeletal disorders, the medical services of a specialist may be warranted. **Orthopedics** is the branch of medicine concerned with prevention, diagnosis, care, and treatment of musculoskeletal disorders. The physician who specializes in the diagnoses and treatment of musculoskeletal disorders is known as an *orthopedist.* These physicians employ medical, physical, and surgical methods to restore function that has been lost as a result of musculoskeletal injury or disease. Another physician who specializes in treating joint disease is the **rheumatologist.** Still another physician, a **Doctor of Osteopathy (DO),** maintains that good health requires proper alignment of bones, muscles, ligaments, and nerves. Like the medical doctor, osteopathic physicians combine manipulative procedures with state-of-the-art methods of medical treatment, including prescribing drugs and performing surgeries.

Bone Disorders

Disorders involving the bones include fractures, infections, osteoporosis, and spinal curvatures.

Fractures

A broken bone is called a *fracture.* The different types of fractures are classified by extent of damage. (See Figure 10–10.) A (1) **closed (simple) fracture** is one in which the bone is broken but no external wound exists. An (2) **open (compound) fracture** involves a broken bone and an external wound that leads to the site of fracture. Fragments of bone commonly protrude through the skin. A (3) **complicated fracture** is one in which a broken bone has injured an internal organ, such as when a broken rib pierces a lung. In a (4) **comminuted fracture,** the bone has broken or splintered into pieces. An (5) **impacted fracture** occurs when the bone is broken and one end is wedged into the interior of another bone. An (6) **incomplete fracture** occurs when the line of fracture does not completely transverse the entire bone. A (7) **greenstick fracture** is when the broken bone does not extend through the entire thickness of the bone; that is, one side of the bone is broken and one side of the bone is bent. It occurs most often in children as part of the bone is still composed of flexible cartilage. The term *greenstick* refers to new branches on a tree that bend rather than break. A greenstick fracture is also known as an incomplete fracture. A (8) **Colles fracture**, a break at the lower end of the radius, occurs just above the wrist. It causes displacement of the hand and usually occurs as a result of flexing a hand to cushion a fall. A **hairline fracture** is a minor fracture in which all portions of the bone are in perfect alignment. The fracture is seen on radiographic examination as a very thin hairline between the two segments but not extending entirely through the bone. **Pathological (spontaneous)**

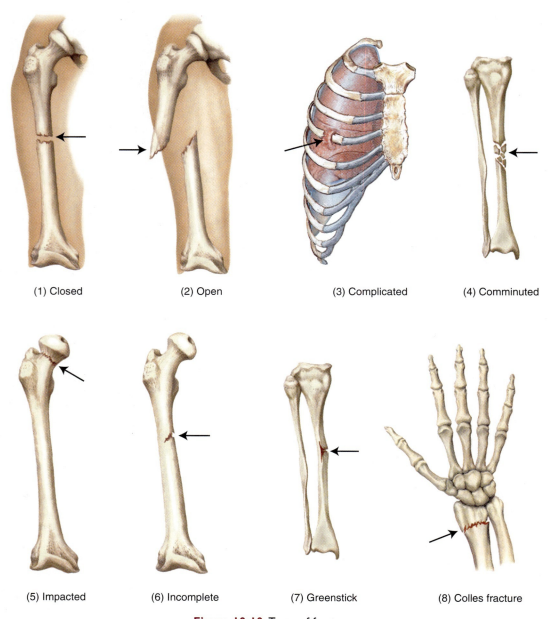

(1) Closed   (2) Open   (3) Complicated   (4) Comminuted

(5) Impacted   (6) Incomplete   (7) Greenstick   (8) Colles fracture

Figure 10-10. Types of fractures.

fractures are usually caused by a disease process such as a neoplasm or osteoporosis.

Unlike other repairs of the body, bones sometimes require months to heal. Several factors influence the rate at which fractures heal. Some fractures need to be immobilized to ensure that bones unite soundly in their proper position. In most cases, this is achieved with bandages, casts, traction, or a fixation device. Certain fractures, particularly those with bone fragments, require surgery to reposition and fix bones securely, so that surrounding tissues heal. In addition to promoting healing, immobilization prevents further injury and reduces pain.

Some bones have a natural tendency to heal more rapidly than others. For instance, the long bones of the arms usually mend twice as fast as those of the legs. Age also plays an important role in bone fracture healing rate; older patients require more time for healing. In addition, an adequate blood supply to the injured area and the nutritive state of the individual are crucial to the healing process.

Infections

Infection of the bone and bone marrow is called **osteomyelitis.** It may be acute or chronic. Bone infections are primarily caused by pus-forming (**pyogenic**) bacteria. The disease usually begins with local trauma to the bone causing a blood clot (**hematoma**). Bacteria from an acute infection in another area of the body find their way to the injured bone and establish the infection.

Most bone infections are more difficult to treat effectively than soft tissue infections. Eventually, some bone infections result in destruction (**necrosis**) of the bone and stiffening or freezing of the joints (**ankylosis**). Osteomyelitis may be acute or chronic. With early treatment, prognosis for acute osteomyelitis is good; prognosis for the chronic form of the disease is poor.

Paget disease, also known as *osteitis deformans,* is a chronic inflammation of bones resulting in thickening and softening of bones. It can occur in any bone but most commonly affects the long bones of the legs, the lower spine, the pelvis, and the skull. This disease is found in persons over age 40. Although a variety of causes have been proposed, a slow virus (not yet isolated) is currently thought to be the most likely cause.

Osteoporosis

Osteoporosis is a common metabolic bone disorder in the elderly, particularly in postmenopausal women and especially women older than age 60. It is characterized by decreased bone density that occurs when the rate of bone resorption (loss of substance) exceeds the rate of bone formation. Among the many causes of osteoporosis are disturbances of protein metabolism, protein deficiency, disuse of bones due to prolonged periods of immobilization, estrogen deficiencies associated with menopause, a diet lacking vitamins or calcium, and long-term administration of high doses of corticosteroids.

Patients with osteoporosis commonly complain of bone pain, typically in the back, which may be caused by repeated microscopic fractures. Thin areas of porous bone are also evident. Deformity associated with osteoporosis is usually the result of pathological fractures.

Spinal Curvatures

Any persistent, abnormal deviation of the vertebral column from its normal position may cause an abnormal spinal curvature. Three common deviations are **scoliosis, kyphosis,** and **lordosis.** (See Figure 10–11.)

An abnormal lateral curvature of the spine, either to the right or left, is called *scoliosis*. Some rotation of a portion of the vertebral column may also occur. Scoliosis, or ***C**-shaped curvature of the spine,* may be congenital, caused by chronic poor posture during childhood while the vertebrae are still growing, or the result of one leg being longer than the other. Treatment depends on the severity of the curvature and may vary from exercises,

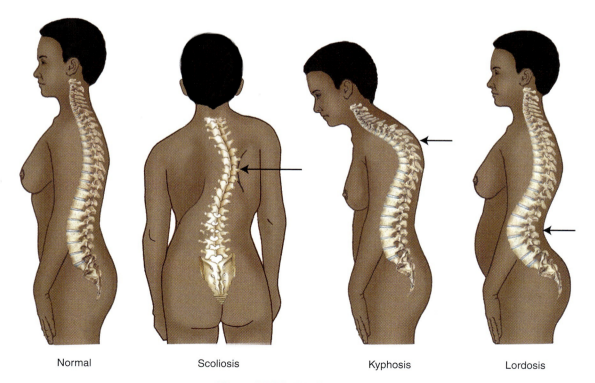

Normal   Scoliosis   Kyphosis   Lordosis

Figure 10-11. Spinal curvatures.

physical therapy, and back braces to surgical intervention. Untreated scoliosis may result in pulmonary insufficiency (curvature may decrease lung capacity), back pain, sciatica, disk disease, or even degenerative arthritis.

An abnormal curvature of the upper portion of the spine is called *kyphosis,* more commonly known as *humpback* or *hunchback.* Rheumatoid arthritis, rickets, poor posture, or chronic respiratory diseases may cause kyphosis. Treatment consists of spine-stretching exercises, sleeping with a board under the mattress, and wearing a brace to straighten the kyphotic curve; surgery is rarely required.

An abnormal, inward curvature of a portion of the lower portion of the spine is called *lordosis,* more commonly known as *swayback.* It may be caused by increased weight of the abdominal contents, resulting from obesity or excessive weight gain during pregnancy. Kyphosis and lordosis also occur in combination with scoliosis.

Joint Disorders

Arthritis, a general term for many joint diseases, is an inflammation of a joint usually accompanied by pain, swelling and, commonly, changes in structure. Because of their location and constant use, joints are prone to stress injuries and inflammation. The main types of arthritis include rheumatoid arthritis, osteoarthritis, and gouty arthritis, or gout.

Rheumatoid arthritis (RA), a systemic disease characterized by inflammatory changes in joints and their related structures, results in crippling deformities. (See Figure 10–12.) This form of arthritis is believed to be caused by an autoimmune reaction of joint tissue. It occurs most commonly in women between ages 23 and 35 but can affect people of any age group. Intensified aggravations (**exacerbations**) of this disease are commonly associated with periods of increased physical or emotional stress. In addition to joint changes, muscles, bones, and skin adjacent to the affected joint atrophy. There is no specific cure, but nonsteroidal anti-inflammatory drugs (NSAIDs), physical therapy, and orthopedic measures are used in treatment of less severe cases.

Osteoarthritis, also called *degenerative joint disease (DJD),* is the most common type of connective tissue disease. Cartilage destruction and new bone formation at the edges of joints (**spurs**) are the most common pathologies seen with osteoarthritis. Even though osteoarthritis is less crippling than rheumatoid arthritis, it may result in fusion of two bone surfaces, thereby completely immobilizing the joint. In addition, small, hard nodules may form at the distal interphalangeal joints of the fingers (**Heberden nodes**).

Gouty arthritis, also called **gout,** is a metabolic disease caused by the accumulation of uric acid crystals in the blood. These crystals may become deposited in joints and soft tissue near joints, causing painful swelling and inflammation. Although the joint chiefly affected is the big toe, any joint may be involved. Sometimes, renal calculi (**nephroliths**) form because of uric acid crystals collecting in the kidney.

Muscle Disorders

Disorders involving the muscles include muscular dystrophy and myasthenia gravis.

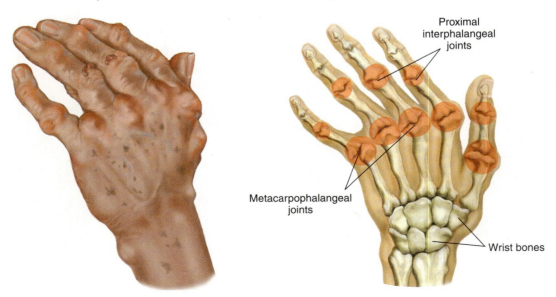

Proximal interphalangeal joints

Metacarpophalangeal joints

Wrist bones

Figure 10-12. Rheumatoid arthritis.

Muscular Dystrophy

Muscular dystrophy, a genetic disease, is characterized by gradual **atrophy** and weakening of muscle tissue. There are several types of muscular dystrophy. The most common type, **Duchenne dystrophy,** affects children; boys more commonly than girls. It is transmitted as a sex-linked disease passed from mother to son. As muscular dystrophy progresses, the loss of muscle function affects not only skeletal muscle but also cardiac muscle. At present, there is no cure for this disease, and most children with muscular dystrophy die before age 30.

Myasthenia Gravis

Myasthenia gravis (MG), a neuromuscular disorder, causes fluctuating weakness of certain skeletal muscle groups (of the eyes, face and, sometimes, limbs). It is characterized by destruction of the receptors in the synaptic region that respond to acetylcholine, a substance that transmits nerve impulses (**neurotransmitter**). As the disease progresses, the muscle becomes increasingly weak and may eventually cease to function altogether. Women tend to be affected more often than men. Initial symptoms include a weakness of the eye muscles and difficulty swallowing (**dysphagia**). Later, the individual has difficulty chewing and talking. Eventually, the muscles of the limbs may become involved. Myasthenia gravis can be controlled, and medical management is the usual form of treatment.

Oncology

The two major types of malignancies that affect bone are those that arise directly from bone or bone tissue, called *primary bone cancer,* and those that arise in another region of the body and spread (**metastasize**) to bone, called *secondary bone cancer.* Primary bone cancers are rare, but secondary bone cancers are quite prevalent. They are usually caused by malignant cells that have metastasized to the bone from the lungs, breast, or prostate.

Malignancies that originate from bone, fat, muscle, cartilage, bone marrow, and cells of the lymphatic system are called *sarcomas.* Three major types of sarcomas include fibrosarcoma, osteosarcoma, and Ewing sarcoma. **Fibrosarcoma** develops in cartilage and generally affects the pelvis, upper legs, and shoulders. Patients with fibrosarcoma are usually between ages 50 and 60. **Osteosarcoma** develops from bone tissue and generally affects the knees, upper arms, and upper legs. Patients with osteosarcoma are usually between ages 20 and 25. **Ewing sarcoma** develops from primitive nerve cells in bone marrow. It usually affects the shaft of long bones but may occur in the pelvis or other bones of the arms or legs. This disease usually affects young boys between ages 10 and 20.

Signs and symptoms of sarcoma include swelling and tenderness, with a tendency toward fractures in the affected area. Magnetic resonance imaging (MRI), bone scan, and computed tomography (CT) scan are diagnostic tests that assist in identifying bone malignancies. All malignancies, including Ewing sarcoma, are staged and graded to determine the extent and degree of malignancy. This staging helps the physician determine an appropriate treatment modality. Generally, combination therapy is used, including chemotherapy for management of metastasis and radiation when the tumor is radiosensitive. In some cases, amputation is required.

Diagnostic, Symptomatic, and Related Terms

This section introduces diagnostic, symptomatic, and related terms and their meanings. Word analyses for selected terms are also provided.

Term	Definition
ankylosis ăng-kĭ-LŌ-sĭs *ankyl:* stiffness, bent, crooked *-osis:* abnormal condition, increase (used primarily with blood cells)	Stiffening and immobility of a joint as a result of disease, trauma, surgery, or abnormal bone fusion
carpal tunnel syndrome (CTS) KĂR-păl	Painful condition resulting from compression of the median nerve within the carpal tunnel (wrist canal through which the flexor tendons and the median nerve pass)

(continued)

Diagnostic, Symptomatic, and Related Terms—cont'd

Term	Definition
claudication klăw-dĭ-KĀ-shŭn	Lameness, limping
contracture kŏn-TRĂK-chūr	Fibrosis of connective tissue in the skin, fascia, muscle, or joint capsule that prevents normal mobility of the related tissue or joint
crepitation krĕp-ĭ-TĀ-shŭn	Dry, grating sound or sensation caused by bone ends rubbing together, indicating a fracture or joint destruction
electromyography ē-lĕk-trō-mī-ŎG-ră-fē *electr/o:* electric *my/o:* muscle *-graphy:* process of recording	Use of electrical stimulation to record the strength of muscle contraction
exacerbation ĕks-ăs-ĕr-BĀ-shŭn	Increase in severity of a disease or any of its symptoms
ganglion cyst GĂNG-lē-ŏn SĬST	Tumor of tendon sheath or joint capsule, commonly found in the wrist *To treat a ganglion cyst, the cyst is aspirated and injected with an anti-inflammatory agent.*
hemarthrosis hĕm-ăr-THRŌ-sĭs *hem:* blood *arthr:* joint *-osis:* abnormal condition; increase (used primarily with blood cells)	Effusion of blood into a joint cavity
hypotonia hī-pō-TŌ-nē-ă *hypo-:* under, below, deficient *ton:* tension *-ia:* conditon	Loss of muscular tone or a diminished resistance to passive stretching
multiple myeloma mī-ĕ-LŌ-mă *myel:* bone marrow; spinal cord *-oma:* tumor	Primary malignant tumor that infiltrates the bone and red bone marrow *Multiple myeloma is a progressive, typically fatal disease that causes multiple tumor masses and bone fractures.*
osteophyte ŎS-tē-ō-fīt	Bony outgrowth that occasionally develops on the vertebra and may exert pressure on the spinal cord also called *bone spur.*
phantom limb FĂN-tŭm	Perceived sensation, following amputation of a limb, that the limb still exists *The sensation that pain exists in the removed part is known as* **phantom limb pain.**
prosthesis prŏs-THĒ-sĭs	Replacement of a missing part by an artificial substitute, such as an artificial extremity
rickets RĬK-ĕts	Form of osteomalacia in children caused by vitamin D deficiency; also called *rachitis*

Diagnostic, Symptomatic, and Related Terms—cont'd

Term	Definition
sequestrum sē-KWĔS-trŭm *sequestr:* separation *-um:* structure, thing	Fragment of necrosed bone that has become separated from surrounding tissue
spondylolisthesis spŏn-dĭ-lō-lĭs-THĒ-sĭs *spondyl/o:* vertebrae (backbone) *-listhesis:* slipping	Any slipping (subluxation) of a vertebra from its normal position in relationship to the one beneath it
spondylosis spŏn-dĭ-LŌ-sĭs *spondyl:* vertebrae (backbone) *-osis:* abnormal condition; increase (used primarily with blood cells)	Degeneration of the cervical, thoracic, and lumbar vertebrae and related tissues *Spondylosis may cause pressure on nerve roots with subsequent pain or paresthesia in the extremities.*
sprain sprăn	Tearing of ligament tissue that may be slight, moderate, or complete *A complete tear of a major ligament is especially painful and disabling. Ligamentous tissue does not heal well because of poor blood supply. Treatment usually consists of surgical reconstruction of the severed ligament.*
strain străn	To exert physical force in a manner that may result in injury, usually muscular
subluxation sŭb-lŭk-SĀ-shŭn	Partial or incomplete dislocation
talipes equinovarus TĂL-ĭ-pēz ē-kwĭ-nō-VĀ-rŭs	Congenital deformity of one or both feet in which the foot is pulled downward and laterally to the side; also called *clubfoot* (See Figure 10–13.) *In talipes, the heel never rests on the ground. Treatment consists of applying casts to progressively straighten the foot and surgical correction for severe cases.*

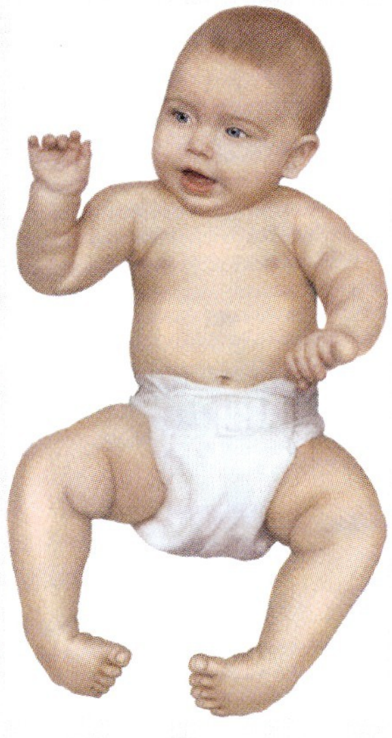

Figure 10-13. Talipes equinovarus.

It is time to review pathological, diagnostic, symptomatic, and related terms by completing Learning Activity 10–5.

Diagnostic and Therapeutic Procedures

This section introduces procedures used to diagnose and treat musculoskeletal disorders. Descriptions are provided as well as pronunciations and word analyses for selected terms.

Procedure	Description
Diagnostic Procedures	
Radiographic	
arthrography ăr-THRŎG-ră-fē *arthr/o:* joint *-graphy:* process of recording	Series of radiographs taken after injection of contrast material into a joint cavity, especially the knee or shoulder, to outline the contour of the joint
bone density tests	Radiographic procedures that use low-energy x-ray absorption to measure bone mineral density (BMD) *Bone density tests are used to determine if demineralization from osteoporosis has occurred. The areas of decreased density indicate osteopenia and osteoporosis. There are two types of bone density tests, dual-energy x-ray absorptiometry (DEXA or DXA) scan, also known as* **bone densitometry,** *and computed tomography (CT).*
computed tomography (CT) kŏm-PŪ-tĕd tō-MŎG-ră-fē *tom/o:* to cut *-graphy:* process of recording	Imaging technique that uses an x-ray beam and a computer to make a series of cross-sectional images of a body part, which together make up a three-dimensional view of the area scanned; formerly called *computerized axial tomography (CAT)* *The CT scan identifies various types of tissue abnormalities, but bony structures appear particularly clear. Thus, CT scan is one of the most sensitive studies for early detection of joint disease.*
discography dĭs-KŎG-ră-fē	Radiological examination of the intervertebral disk structures by injecting a contrast medium *Discography is used to diagnose suspected cases of herniated disk.*
lumbosacral spinal radiography LŬM-bō-sā-krăl SPĪ-năl ră-dē-ŎG-ră-fē *lumb/o:* loins (lower back) *sacr:* sacrum *-al:* pertaining to, relating to *radi/o:* radiation, x-ray, radius (lower arm bone on thumb side) *-graphy:* process of recording	Radiography of the five lumbar vertebrae and the fused sacral vertebrae, including anteroposterior, lateral, and oblique views of the lower spine *The most common indication for lumbosacral (LS) spinal radiography is lower back pain. It is used to identify or differentiate traumatic fractures, spondylosis, spondylolisthesis, and metastatic tumor.*
myelography mī-ĕ-LŎG-ră-fē *myel/o:* bone marrow, spinal cord *-graphy:* process of recording	Radiography of the spinal cord after injection of a contrast medium to identify and study spinal distortions caused by tumors, cysts, herniated intervertebral disks, or other lesions
scintigraphy sĭn-TĬG-ră-fē	Nuclear medicine procedure that visualizes various tissues and organs after administration of a radionuclide *After absorption of the radioactive substance, a scanner detects the radioactive tracer and makes a photographic recording (scintigram) of radionuclide distribution using a gamma camera to detect areas of uptake, called* **hotspots.**

Diagnostic and Therapeutic Procedures—cont'd

Procedure	Description
bone	Scintigraphy procedure in which radionuclide is injected intravenously and taken up into the bone *Bone scintigraphy is used to detect bone disorders, especially arthritis, fractures, osteomyelitis, bone cancers, or areas of bony metastases. Areas of increased uptake (hot spots) are abnormal and may be infection or cancer.*

Therapeutic Procedures

Procedure	Description
reduction	Procedure that restores a bone to its normal position *Following reduction, the bone is immobilized with an external device to maintain proper alignment during the healing process.*
closed	Reduction procedure where fractured bones are realigned by manipulation rather than surgery.
open	Reduction procedure that treats bone fractures by placing the bones in their proper position using surgery *In open reduction of a complicated fracture, an incision is made at the fracture site and the fracture is reduced. Often internal fixation devices such as nails, screws, or plates are required to fix the fracture fragments in their correct anatomical position.*
casting	Application of a solid, stiff dressing formed with plaster of Paris or other material to a body part to immobilize it during the healing process
splinting	Application of an orthopedic device to an injured body part for immobilization, stabilization, and protection during the healing process *A splint is constructed from wood, metal, or plaster of Paris and may be moveable or immovable.*
traction	Use of weights and pulleys to align or immobilize a fracture and facilitate the healing process

Surgical

Procedure	Description
amputation ăm-pŭ-TĀ-shŭn	Partial or complete removal of an extremity due to trauma or circulatory disease *After the extremity is removed, the surgeon cuts a shaped flap from muscle and cutaneous tissue to cover the end of the bone and provide cushion and support for a prosthesis. The most common reason for limb loss is peripheral vascular disease caused by a blood flow blockage from cigarette smoking, physical inactivity, or uncontrolled diabetes mellitus.*
arthrocentesis ăr-thrō-sĕn-TĒ-sĭs *arthr/o:* joint *-centesis:* surgical puncture	Puncture of a joint space using a needle to remove accumulated fluid
arthroclasia ăr-thrō-KLĀ-zē-ă *arthr/o:* joint *-clasia:* to break; surgical fracture	Surgical breaking of an ankylosed joint to provide movement

(continued)

Diagnostic and Therapeutic Procedures—cont'd

Procedure	Description
arthroscopy ăr-THRŎS-kō-pē *arthr/o:* joint *-scopy:* visual examination	Visual examination of the interior of a joint and its structures using a thin, flexible fiberoptic scope called an *arthroscope* that contains a magnifying lens, fiberoptic light, and miniature camera that projects images on a monitor (See Figure 10-14.) *Instruments are introduced into the joint space through a small incision in order to carry out diagnostic and treatment procedures. Arthroscopy is also performed to correct defects, excise tumors, and obtain biopsies.*

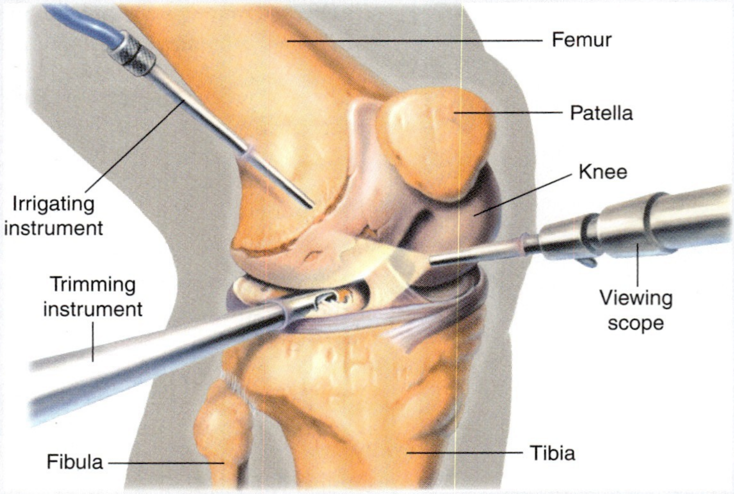

Figure 10-14. Arthroscopy.

Procedure	Description
bone grafting BŌN GRĂFT-ĭng	Implanting or transplanting bone tissue from another part of the body or from another person to serve as replacement for damaged or missing bone tissue
bursectomy bĕr-SĔK-tō-mē	Excision of bursa (padlike sac or cavity found in connective tissue, usually in the vicinity of joints)
laminectomy lăm-ĭ-NĔK-tō-mē *lamin:* lamina (part of vertebral arch) *-ectomy:* excision, removal	Excision of the posterior arch of a vertebra *Laminectomy is most commonly performed to relieve the symptoms of a ruptured intervertebral (slipped) disk.*
revision surgery	Surgery repeated to correct problems of a previously unsuccessful surgery or to replace a worn out prothesis *Revision surgery is usually more complicated than the original surgery.*
bone	Revision surgery are often required to correct bone infection, misalignments of bones, broken prosthesis, and fractures of the bone around the prostheses.

Diagnostic and Therapeutic Procedures—cont'd

Procedure	Description

sequestrectomy
sē-kwĕs-TRĔK-tō-mē
  sequestr: separation
  -ectomy: excision, removal

Excision of a sequestrum (segment of necrosed bone)

synovectomy
sĭn-ō-VĔK-tō-mē
  synov: synovial membrane,
    synovial fluid
  -ectomy: excision, removal

Excision of a synovial membrane

total hip replacement

Surgical procedure to replace a hip joint damaged by a degenerative disease, commonly arthritis (See Figure 10-15.)

In a total hip replacement (THR), the femoral head and the acetabulum are replaced with a metal ball and stem (prosthesis). The acetabulum is plastic coated to avoid metal-to-metal contact on articulating surfaces; the stem is anchored into the central core of the femur to achieve a secure fit.

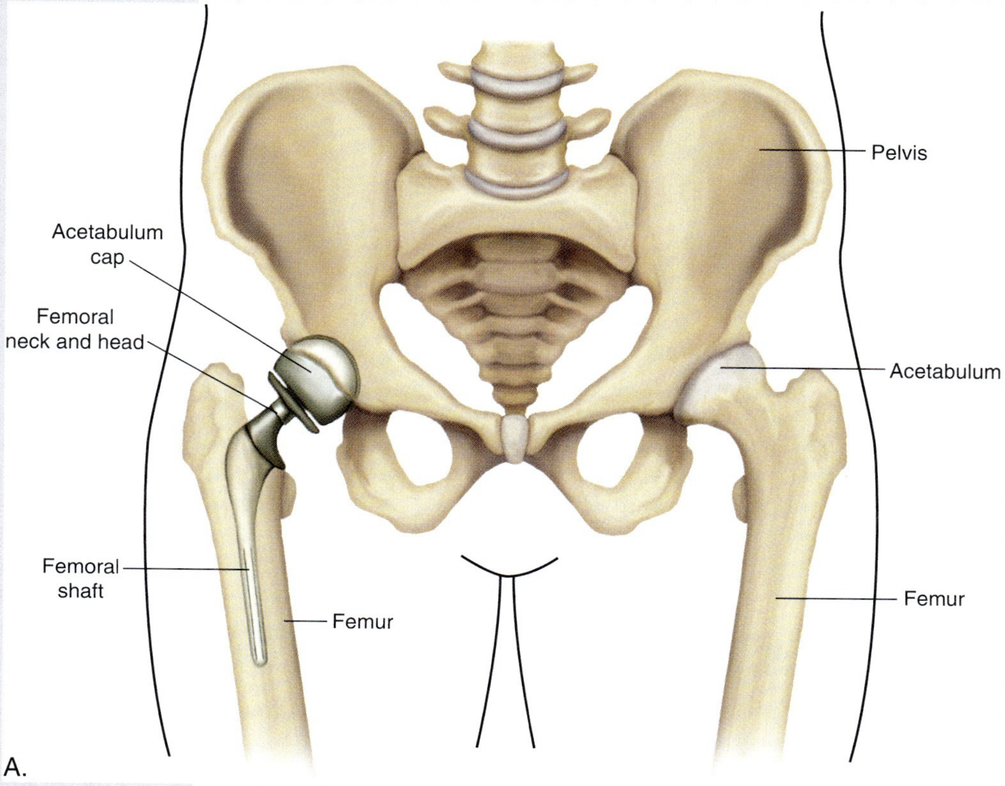

Figure 10-15. Total hip replacement. (A) Right total hip replacement. (B) Radiograph showing total hip replacement of arthritic hip. From McKinnis: *Fundamentals of Musculoskeletal Imaging.* 2nd. Ed. FA Davis, Philadelphia, 2005, p. 314, with permission.

(continued)

Diagnostic and Therapeutic Procedures—cont'd

Procedure	Description

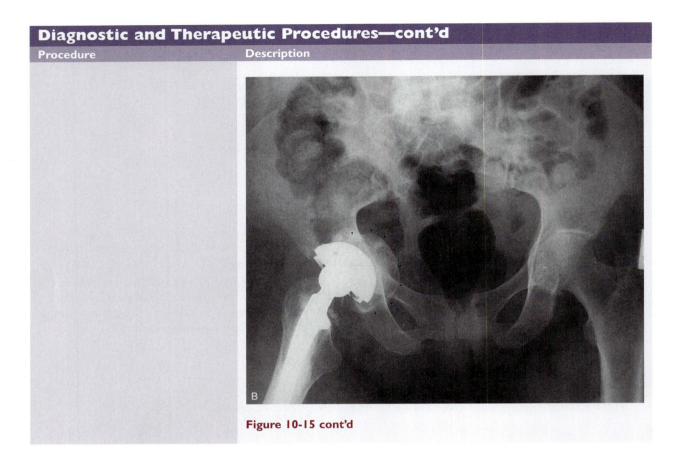

Figure 10-15 cont'd

Pharmacology

Unlike other medications that treat specific disease, most pharmacological agents for musculoskeletal disorders are used to treat symptoms. (See Table 10–3.) Acute musculoskeletal conditions, such as strains, sprains, and "pulled" muscles, are treated with analgesics and anti-inflammatory drugs. Nonsteroidal anti-inflammatory drugs (NSAIDs), salicylates, muscle relaxants, opioid analgesics, or narcotics are commonly used to treat pain by anesthetizing (numbing) the area or decreasing the inflammation. NSAIDs and salicylates are also used to treat arthritis, in addition to gold salts. Calcium supplements are used to treat hypocalcemia.

Table 10-3 Drugs Used to Treat Musculoskeletal Disorders

This table lists common drug classifications used to treat musculoskeletal disorders, their therapeutic actions, and selected generic and trade names.

Classification	Therapeutic Action	Generic and Trade Names
calcium supplements	Treat and prevent hypocalcemia. *Over-the-counter calcium supplements are numerous and are contained in many antacids as a secondary therapeutic effect. They are used to prevent osteoporosis when normal diet is lacking adequate amounts of calcium.*	**calcium carbonate** KĂL-sē-ŭm KĂR-bŏn-āt Calci-Mix, Tums **calcium citrate** KĂL-sē-ŭm SĬT-rāt Cal-Citrate 250, Citracal

Table 10-3	**Drugs Used to Treat Musculoskeletal Disorders—cont'd**		
	Classification	**Therapeutic Action**	**Generic and Trade Names**
	gold salts	Treat rheumatoid arthritis by inhibiting activity within the immune system. *Gold salts contain actual gold in capsules or in solution for injection. This agent prevents further disease progression but cannot reverse past damage.*	**auranofin** aw-RĂN-ŏ-fĭn Ridaura **aurothioglucose** aw-rō-thī-ō-GLOO-kōs Solganal
	nonsteroidal anti-inflammatory drugs	Decrease pain and suppress inflammation *Nonsteroidal anti-inflammatory drugs (NSAIDs) are used to treat acute musculoskeletal conditions, such as sprains and strains, and inflammatory disorders, including rheumatoid arthritis, osteoarthritis, bursitis, gout, and tendinitis.*	**ibuprofen** ī-bū-PRŌ-fĕn Advil, Motrin **naproxen** nă-PRŎK-sĕn Aleve, Naprosyn
	salicylates	Relieve mild to moderate pain and reduce inflammation *Salicylates have anti-inflammatory abilities and alleviate pain. Aspirin (acetylsalicylic acid) is the oldest drug in this classification that is used to treat arthritis.*	**aspirin** ĂS-pĕr-ĭn Acuprin, Aspergum, Bayer Aspirin **magnesium salicylate** măg-NĒ-zē-ŭm să-LĬS-ĭ-lāt Magan, Mobidin
	skeletal muscle relaxants	Relieve muscle spasms and stiffness *These drugs are also prescribed for muscle spasms due to multiple sclerosis, spinal cord injury, cerebral palsy, and stroke.*	**cyclobenzaprine** sī-klō-BĔN-ză-prēn Flexeril **methocarbamol and aspirin** mĕth-ō-KĂR-bă-mōl Robaxin

Abbreviations

This section introduces musculoskeletal–related abbreviations and their meanings.

Abbreviation	Meaning	Abbreviation	Meaning
ACL	anterior cruciate ligament	**Ca**	calcium; cancer
AE	above the elbow	**CDH**	congenital dislocation of the hip
AK	above the knee	**CTS**	carpal tunnel syndrome
BE	barium enema; below the elbow	**CT**	computed tomography
BK	below the knee	**DEXA, DXA**	dual energy x-ray absorptiometry
C1, C2, and so on	first cervical vertebra, second cervical vertebra, and so on	**DJD**	degenerative joint disease

(continued)

Abbreviations—cont'd

Abbreviation	Meaning	Abbreviation	Meaning
EMG	electromyography	MS	musculoskeletal; multiple sclerosis; mental status; mitral stenosis
Fx	fracture	NSAIDs	nonsteroidal anti-inflammatory drugs
MG	myasthenia gravis	ORTH, ortho	orthopedics
HD	hemodialysis; hip disarticulation; hearing distance	P	phosphorus; pulse
HNP	herniated nucleus pulposus (herniated disk)	PCL	posterior cruciate ligament
HP	hemipelvectomy	RA	rheumatoid arthritis; right atrium
IS	intracostal space	RF	rheumatoid factor; radio frequency
IM	intramuscular; infectious mononucleosis	ROM	range of motion
IV	intravenous	SD	shoulder disarticulation
KD	knee disarticulation	THA	total hip arthroplasty
L1, L2, and so on	first lumbar vertebra, second lumbar vertebra, and so on	THR	total hip replacement
LS	lumbosacral spine	TKA	total knee arthroplasty
MG	myasthenia gravis	TKR	total knee replacement
MRI	magnetic resonance imaging	TRAM	transverse rectus abdominis muscle

It is time to review procedures, pharmacology, and abbreviations by completing Learning Activity 10–6.

LEARNING ACTIVITIES

The following activities provide review of the musculoskeletal system terms introduced in this chapter. Complete each activity and review your answers to evaluate your understanding of the chapter.

Learning Activity 10-1
Identifying Muscle Structures

Label the following illustration using the terms listed below.

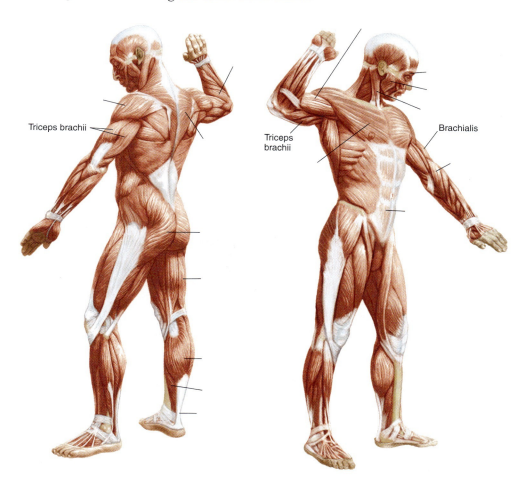

Achilles tendon	*gastrocnemius*	*rectus abdominus*
biceps brachii	*gluteus maximus*	*soleus*
biceps femoris	*masseter*	*sternocleidomastoid*
brachioradialis	*orbicularis oculi*	*trapezius*
deltoid	*pectoralis major*	

 Check your answers by referring to Figure 10–1 on page 267. Review material that you did not answer correctly.

Identifying Sections of a Typical Long Bone (Femur)

Label the following illustration using the terms listed below.

articular cartilage   distal epiphysis   proximal epiphysis

compact bone   medullary cavity   spongy bone

diaphysis   periosteum

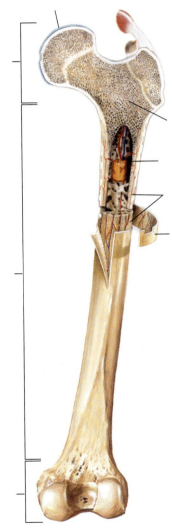

 Check your answers by referring to Figure 10–3 on page 270. Review material that you did not answer correctly.

Identifying Skeletal Structures

Label the following illustration using the terms listed below.

acetabulum	fibula	metatarsals	radius	tarsals
carpals	humerus	pectoral girdle	sacrum	tibia
clavicle	ilium	pelvic girdle	scapula	ulna
coccyx	ischium	phalanges	sternum	
femur	metacarpals	pubis	symphysis pubis	

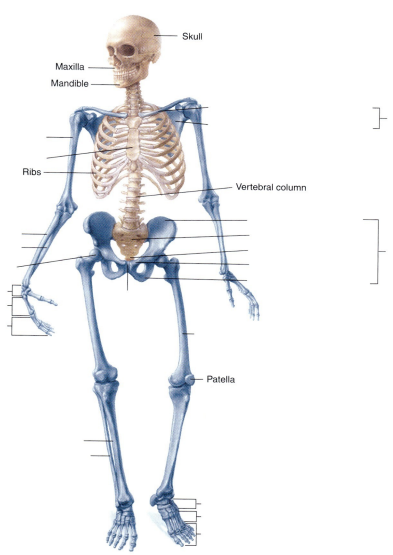

Skull

Maxilla

Mandible

Ribs

Vertebral column

Patella

> Check your answers by referring to Figure 10–4 on page 272. Review material that you did not answer correctly.

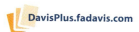

Enhance your study and reinforcement of word elements with the power of DavisPlus. Visit www.davisplus.fadavis.com/gylys/systems for this chapter's flash-card activity. We recommend you complete the flash-card activity before completing activity 10–4 below.

Learning Activity 10-4
Building Medical Words

Use *oste/o* (bone) to build words that mean:

1. bone cells _____

2. pain in bones _____

3. disease of bones and joints _____

4. beginning or formation of bones _____

Use *cervic/o* (neck) to build words that mean:

5. pertaining to the neck _____

6. pertaining to the neck and arm _____

7. pertaining to the neck and face _____

Use *myel/o* (bone marrow; spinal cord) to build words that mean:

8. tumor of bone marrow _____

9. sarcoma of bone marrow (cells) _____

10. bone marrow cell_____

11. resembling bone marrow _____

Use *stern/o* (sternum) to build words that mean:

12. pertaining to above the sternum _____

13. resembling the breastbone _____

Use *arthr/o* (joint) or *chondr/o* (cartilage) to build words that mean:

14. embryonic cell that forms cartilage _____

15. inflammation of a joint _____

16. inflammation of bones and joints _____

Use *pelv/i* (pelvis) to build a word that means:

17. instrument for measuring the pelvis _____

Use *my/o* (muscle) to build words that mean:

18. twitching of a muscle _____

19. any disease of muscle _____

20. rupture of a muscle _____

Build surgical words that mean:

21. excision of one or more of the phalanges (bones of a finger or toe) _____

22. incision of the thorax (chest wall) _____

23. excision of a vertebra _____

24. binding of a joint _____

25. repair of muscle (tissue) _____

✓ *Check your answers in Appendix A. Review material that you did not answer correctly.*

Correct Answers _____ × 4 = _____ % Score

Learning Activity 10-5

Matching Pathological, Diagnostic, Symptomatic, and Related Terms

Match the following terms with the definitions in the numbered list.

ankylosis	ganglion cyst	kyphosis	phantom limb	sequestrum
chondrosarcoma	gout	muscular dystrophy	prosthesis	spondylitis
claudication	greenstick fracture	myasthenia gravis	pyogenic	spondylolisthesis
comminuted fracture	hematopoiesis	necrosis	rickets	subluxation
Ewing sarcoma	hypotonia	osteoporosis	scoliosis	talipes

1. _____ incomplete or partial dislocation
2. _____ softening of the bones caused by vitamin D deficiency
3. _____ slipped vertebrae
4. _____ limping
5. _____ disease causing degeneration of muscles
6. _____ congenital deformity of the foot, which is twisted out of shape or position
7. _____ part of dead or necrosed bone that has become separated from surrounding tissue
8. _____ chronic neuromuscular disorder characterized by weakness manifested in ocular muscles
9. _____ artificial part used for replacement of a missing limb
10. _____ tendon sheath or joint capsule tumor, commonly found in the wrist
11. _____ loss of muscular tonicity; diminished resistance of muscles to passive stretching
12. _____ type of sarcoma that attacks the shafts rather than the ends of long bones
13. _____ bone that is partially bent and partially broken; occurs in children
14. _____ exaggeration of the thoracic curve of the vertebral column; hunpback
15. _____ disease caused by a decrease in bone density; occurs in the elderly
16. _____ deviation of the spine to the right or left
17. _____ cartilaginous sarcoma
18. _____ describes a bone that has splintered into pieces
19. _____ inflammation of the vertebrae
20. _____ metabolic disease caused by accumulation of uric acid, usually in the big toe
21. _____ development and production of blood cells, normally in the bone marrow
22. _____ formation of pus
23. _____ death of cells, tissues, or organs
24. _____ stiffening and immobility of a joint
25. _____ perceived sensation, following amputation, that the limb still exists

Check your answers in Appendix A. Review material that you did not answer correctly.

Correct Answers _____ × 4 = _____ % Score

Learning Activity 10-6
Matching Procedures, Pharmacology, and Abbreviations

Match the following terms with the definitions in the numbered list.

ACL   closed reduction   myelography

amputation   CTS   open reduction

arthrodesis   gold salts   relaxants

arthrography   HNP   salicylates

arthroscopy   laminectomy   sequestrectomy

1. _____ radiograph of spinal cord after injection of a contrast medium
2. _____ treatment of bone fractures by use of surgery to place bones in normal position
3. _____ used to treat rheumatoid arthritis by inhibiting activity with the immune system
4. _____ painful disorder of the wrist and hand due to compression of the median nerve as it passes through the carpal tunnel
5. _____ excision of the posterior arch of a vertebra
6. _____ series of joint radiographs preceded by injection of a radiopaque substance or air into the joint cavity
7. _____ surgical binding or immobilizing of a joint
8. _____ partial or complete removal of a limb
9. _____ herniated nucleus pulposus
10. _____ relieve mild to moderate pain and reduce inflammation
11. _____ visual examination of a joint's interior, especially the knee
12. _____ excising a segment of necrosed bone
13. _____ anterior cruciate ligament
14. _____ relieve muscle spasms and stiffness
15. _____ manipulative treatment of bone fractures by placing the bones in normal position without incision

✓ *Check your answers in Appendix A. Review any material that you did not answer correctly.*

Correct Answers _____ ✕ 6.67 = _____ % Score

MEDICAL RECORD ACTIVITIES

The two medical records included in the activities that follow use common clinical scenarios to show how medical terminology is used to document patient care. Complete the terminology and analysis sections for each activity to help you recognize and understand terms related to the musculoskeletal system.

Medical Record Activity 10-1
Operative Report: Right Knee Arthroscopy and Medial Meniscectomy

Terminology

Terms listed below come from the medical record *Operative Report: Right Knee Arthroscopy and Medial Meniscectomy* that follows. Use a medical dictionary such as *Taber's Cyclopedic Medical Dictionary,* the appendices of this book, or other resources to define each term. Then review the pronunciations for each term and practice by reading the medical record aloud.

Term	Definition
ACL	
arthroscopy ăr-THRŎS-kō-pē	
effusions ĕ-FŪ-zhŭnz	
intracondylar ĭn-tră-KŎN-dĭ-lăr	
Lachman test	
McMurray sign test	
meniscectomy mĕn-ĭ-SĔK-tō-mē	
MRI	
PCL	
synovitis sĭn-ō-VĪ-tĭs	

Listen and Learn Online! *will help you master the pronunciation of selected medical words from this medical record activity. Visit* www.davisplus.com/gylys/systems *to find instructions on completing the* Listen and Learn Online! *exercise for this section and to practice pronunciations.*

OPERATIVE REPORT: RIGHT KNEE ARTHROSCOPY AND MEDIAL MENISCECTOMY

General Hospital

1511 Ninth Avenue ■■ **Sun City, USA 12345** ■■ **(555) 8022-1887**

OPERATIVE REPORT

Date: August 14, 20xx   Physician: Robert L. Mead, MD

Patient: Jay, Elizabeth   Patient ID#: 20798

PREOPERATIVE DIAGNOSIS: Tear, medial meniscus, right knee.

POSTOPERATIVE DIAGNOSIS: Tear, medial meniscus, right knee.

CLINICAL HISTORY: This 42-year-old woman has jogged for the past 10 years, an average of 25 miles each week. She has persistent posteromedial right knee pain with occasional effusions. The patient has MRI-documented medial meniscal tear.

PROCEDURE: Right knee arthroscopy and medial meniscectomy.

ANESTHESIA: General.

COMPLICATIONS: None.

OPERATIVE SUMMARY: Examination of the knee under anesthesia showed a full range of motion, no effusion, no instability, and negative Lachman and negative McMurray sign tests. Arthroscopic evaluation showed a normal patellofemoral groove and normal intracondylar notch with normal ACL and PCL, some anterior synovitis, and a normal lateral meniscus and lateral compartment to the knee. The medial compartment of the knee showed an inferior surface, posterior and mid-medial meniscal tear that was flipped up on top of itself. This was resected, and then the remaining meniscus contoured back to a stable rim. A sterile dressing was applied.

Patient was taken to the post anesthesia care unit in stable condition.

Robert L. Mead, MD
Robert L. Mead, MD

rlm:bg

D: 8-14-20xx
T: 8-14-20xx

Analysis

Review the medical record *Operative report: Right knee arthroscopy and medial meniscectomy* to answer the following questions.

1. Describe the meniscus and identify its location.

_____

2. What is the probable cause of the tear in the patient's meniscus?

_____

3. What does normal ACL and PCL refer to in the report?

_____

4. Explain the McMurray sign test.

_____

5. Because Lachman and McMurray tests were negative (normal), why was the surgery performed?

_____

Radiographic Consultation: Tibial Diaphysis Nuclear Scan

Terminology

Terms listed below come from the medical record *Radiographic Consultation: Tibial Diaphysis Nuclear Scan*. Use a medical dictionary such as *Taber's Cyclopedic Medical Dictionary*, the appendices of this book, or other resources to define each term. Then review the pronunciations for each term and practice by reading the medical record aloud.

Term	Definition
buttressing BŬ-trĕs-ĭng	
cortical KOR-tĭ-kăl	
diaphysis dī-ĂF-ĭ-sĭs	
endosteal ĕn-DŎS-tē-ăl	
focal FŌ-kăl	
fusiform FŪ-zĭ-form	
NSAIDs	
nuclear scan NŪ-klē-ăr	
periosteal pĕr-ē-ŌS-tē-ăl	
resorption rē-SORP-shŭn	
tibial TĬB-ē-ăl	

Listen and Learn Online! *will help you master the pronunciation of selected medical words from this medical record activity. Visit* www.davisplus.com/gylys/systems *to find instructions on completing the Listen and Learn Online! exercise for this section and to practice pronunciations.*

RADIOGRAPHIC CONSULTATION: TIBIAL DIAPHYSIS NUCLEAR SCAN

Physician Center

2422 Rodeo Drive ■■ **Sun City, USA 12345** ■■ **(555)333-2427**

September 3, 20xx

Grant Hammuda, MD
1115 Forest Ave
Sun City, USA 12345

Dear Doctor Hammuda:

We are pleased to provide the following in response to your request for consultation.

This is an 18-year-old male cross-country runner. He complains of pain of more than 1 month's duration, with persistent symptoms over middle one third of left tibia with resting. He finds no relief with NSAIDs.

FINDINGS: Nuclear scan reveals the following: There is focal increased blood flow, blood pool, and delayed radiotracer accumulation within the left mid posterior tibial diaphysis. The delayed spot planar images demonstrate focal fusiform uptake involving 50% to 75% of the tibial diaphysis width.

It is our opinion that with continued excessive, repetitive stress, the rate of resorption will exceed the rate of bone replacement. This will lead to weakened cortical bone with buttressing by periosteal and endosteal new bone deposition. If resorption continues to exceed replacement, a stress fracture will occur.

Please let me know if I can be of any further assistance.

Sincerely yours,

Adrian Jones, MD
Adrian Jones, MD

aj:bg

Analysis

Review the medical record *Radiographic Consultation: Tibial Diaphysis Nuclear Scan* to answer the following questions.

1. Where was the pain located?

_____

2. What medication was the patient taking for pain and did it provide relief?

_____

3. How was the blood flow to the affected area described by the radiologist?

_____

4. How was the radiotracer accumulation described?

_____

5. What will be the probable outcome with continued excessive repetitive stress?

_____

6. What will happen if resorption continues to exceed replacement?

_____

Genitourinary System

Objectives

Upon completion of this chapter, you will be able to:

- Locate and describe the urinary structures as well as the structures of the male reproductive system.
- Describe the functional relationship between the genitourinary system and other body systems.
- Identify, pronounce, spell, and build words related to the genitourinary system.
- Describe pathological conditions, diagnostic and therapeutic procedures, and other terms related to the genitourinary system.
- Explain pharmacology related to the treatment of urinary disorders as well as male reproductive disorders.
- Demonstrate your knowledge of this chapter by completing the learning and medical record activities.

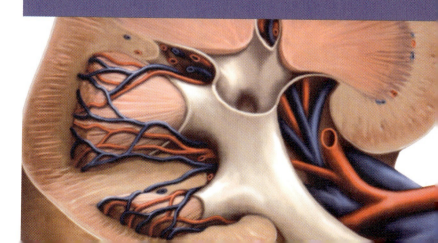

Anatomy and Physiology

The male and female urinary systems have similar structures. In the male, however, some of the urinary structures also have reproductive functions. Thus, the genitourinary system includes the urinary system of both the male and female as well as the reproductive system of the male.

Urinary System

The purpose of the urinary system is to regulate the composition of the extracellular fluids of the body by removing their harmful substances in the form of urine, while retaining beneficial products. Harmful substances, including **nitrogenous wastes** and excess **electrolytes,** are removed by the kidneys and

excreted from the body in urine. Nitrogenous wastes are toxic to the body, and must be continuously eliminated or death will occur. Electrolyte concentration must remain fairly constant for proper functioning of nerves, heart, and muscles. An excess or deficiency of electrolytes can have devastating effects. Besides regulating the composition of extracellular fluids, kidneys also secrete the hormone **erythropoietin.** This hormone acts on bone marrow to stimulate production of red blood cells when blood oxygen levels are low. The macroscopic structures that make up the urinary system include:

- two kidneys
- two ureters
- bladder
- urethra. (See Figure 11–1.)

Anatomy and Physiology Key Terms

This section introduces important genitourinary system terms along with their definitions and pronunciations. Word analyses are provided for selected terms.

Term	Definition
electrolytes ē-LĔK-trō-līts	Mineral salts (sodium, potassium, and calcium) that carry an electrical charge in solution *A proper balance of electrolytes is essential to the normal functioning of the entire body but especially nerves, muscles, and heart.*
filtrate FĬL-trāt	Fluid that passes from the blood through the capillary walls of the glomeruli of the kidney *Filtrate is similar to plasma but with far less protein. Urine is formed from filtrate.*
nitrogenous wastes nī-TRŎJ-ĕn-ŭs	Products of cellular metabolism that contain nitrogen *Nitrogenous wastes include urea, uric acid, creatine, creatinine, and ammonia.*
peristaltic waves pĕr-ĭ-STĂL-tĭk	Sequence of rhythmic contraction of smooth muscles of a hollow organ to force material forward and prevent backflow
peritoneum pĕr-ĭ-tō-NĒ-ŭm	Serous membrane that lines the abdominopelvic cavity and covers most of the organs within the cavity
plasma PLĂZ-mă	Liquid portion of blood, composed primarily of water (90%), and containing dissolved proteins, nutrients, lipids, and various waste products
semen SĒ-mĕn	Fluid containing sperm and secretions from the prostate and other structures of the male reproductive system; also called *seminal fluid*
testosterone tĕs-TŎS-tĕr-ōn	Androgenic hormone responsible for the development of the male sex organs, including the penis, testicles, scrotum, and prostate *Testosterone is also responsible for the development of secondary sex characteristics (musculature, hair patterns, thickened vocal cords, and so forth).*

Pronunciation Help	Long Sound	ā—rate	ē—rebirth	ī—isle	ō—over	ū—unite
	Short Sound	ă—alone	ĕ—ever	ĭ—it	ŏ—not	ŭ—cut

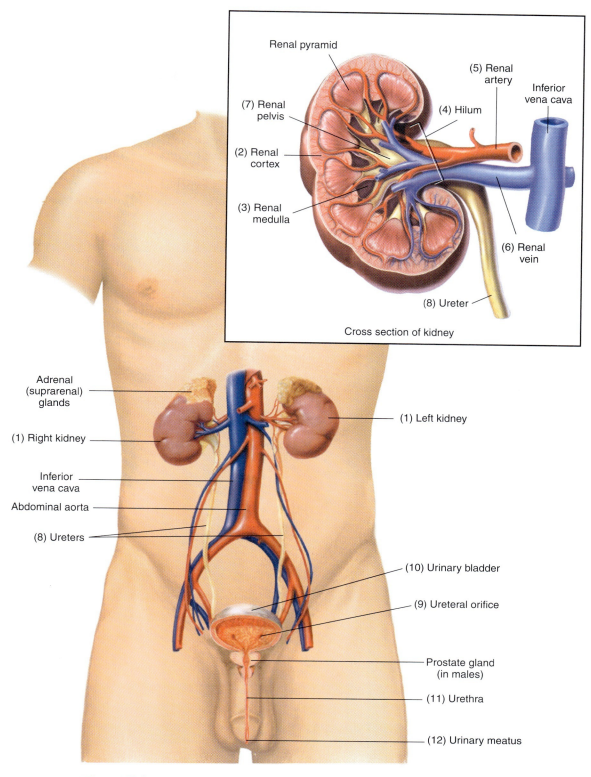

Renal pyramid

(7) Renal pelvis

(2) Renal cortex

(3) Renal medulla

(5) Renal artery

Inferior vena cava

(4) Hilum

(6) Renal vein

(8) Ureter

Cross section of kidney

Adrenal (suprarenal) glands

(1) Right kidney

Inferior vena cava

Abdominal aorta

(8) Ureters

(1) Left kidney

(10) Urinary bladder

(9) Ureteral orifice

Prostate gland (in males)

(11) Urethra

(12) Urinary meatus

Figure 11-1. Urinary structures, including a cross section of the kidney.

The (1) **left and right kidneys,** each about the size of a fist, are located in the abdominal cavity slightly above the waistline. Because they lie outside of the peritoneum, their location is said to be *retroperitoneal.* A concave medial border gives the kidney its beanlike shape. In a frontal section, two distinct areas are visible: an outer section, the (2) **renal cortex,** and a middle area, the (3) **renal medulla,** which contain portions of the microscopic filtering units of the kidney called *nephrons.* Near the medial border is the (4) **hilum** (also called *hilus*), an opening through which the (5) **renal artery** enters and the (6) **renal vein** exits the kidney. The renal artery carries blood that contains waste products to the nephrons for filtering. After waste products are removed, blood leaves the kidney by way of the renal vein.

Waste material, now in the form of urine, passes to a hollow chamber, the (7) **renal pelvis.** This cavity is formed where the (8) **ureter** merges with the kidney. Each ureter is a slender tube about 10 inches to 12 inches long. They each carry urine in peristaltic waves to the bladder. Urine enters the bladder at the (9) **ureteral orifice.** The (10) **urinary bladder,** an expandable hollow organ, acts as a temporary reservoir for urine. The bladder has small folds called *rugae* that expand as the bladder fills. A triangular area at the base of the bladder called the *trigone* is delineated by the openings of the ureters and the urethra.

The base of the trigone forms the (11) **urethra,** a tube that discharges urine from the bladder. The length of the urethra is approximately 1.5 inches in women and about 7 to 8 inches in men. In the male, the urethra passes through the prostate gland and the penis. During urination (**micturition**), urine is expelled from the body through the urethral opening, the (12) **urinary meatus.**

Nephron

Microscopic examination of kidney tissue reveals the presence of approximately 1 million nephrons. (See Figure 11–2.) These microscopic structures are responsible for maintaining homeostasis by continually adjusting and regulating the contents of blood plasma. Substances removed by nephrons are nitrogenous wastes, the end products of protein metabolism, excess electrolytes, and many other products that exceed the amount tolerated by the body.

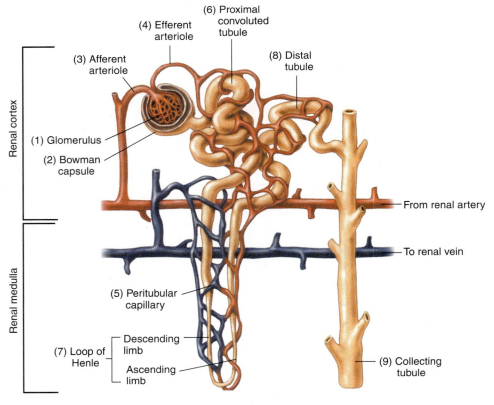

Figure 11-2. Nephron with its associated blood vessels.

Each nephron includes a renal corpuscle and a renal tubule. The **renal corpuscle** is composed of a tuft of capillaries called the (1) **glomerulus** and a modified, enlarged extension of the renal tubule known as (2) **Bowman capsule** that encapsulates the glomerulus. A larger (3) **afferent arteriole** carries blood to the glomerulus, and a smaller (4) **efferent arteriole** carries blood from the glomerulus. The difference in the size of these vessels provides the needed pressure to force blood plasma into Bowman capsule. Once this happens, the fluid is no longer plasma but is called filtrate. As the efferent arteriole passes behind the renal corpuscle, it forms the (5) **peritubular capillaries.** Each renal tubule consists of four sections: the (6) **proximal convoluted tubule,** followed by the narrow (7) **loop of Henle,** then the larger (8) **distal tubule** and, finally, the (9) **collecting tubule.** The collecting tubule transports newly formed urine to the renal pelvis for excretion by the kidneys.

The nephron performs three physiological functions as it produces urine:

- **Filtration** occurs in the renal corpuscle, where plasma containing water, electrolytes, sugar, and other small molecules is forced from the blood within the glomerulus into Bowman capsule to form filtrate.
- **Reabsorption** begins as filtrate travels through the long, twisted pathway of the tubule. Most of the water and some of the electrolytes and amino acids are returned to the peritubular capillaries and reenter the circulating blood.
- **Secretion** is the final stage of urine formation. Substances are actively secreted from the blood in the peritubular capillaries into the filtrate in the renal tubules. Waste products, such as ammonia, uric acid, and metabolic products of medications are secreted into the filtrate to be eliminated in the urine.

Urine leaves the collecting tubule and enters the renal pelvis. From here it passes to the bladder until urination takes place.

 It is time to review urinary system anatomy by completing Learning Activity 11–1.

Male Reproductive System

The purpose of the male reproductive system is to produce, maintain, and transport sperm, the male sex cell required for fertilization of the female egg. It also produces the male hormone testosterone, which is essential to the development of sperm and male secondary sex characteristics. (See Figure 11–3.)

The primary male reproductive organ consists of two (1) **testes** (singular, *testis*) located in an external sac called the (2) **scrotum.** Within the testes are numerous small tubes that twist and coil to form (3) **seminiferous tubules,** which produce sperm. The testes also secrete testosterone, a hormone that develops and maintains secondary sex characteristics. Lying over the superior surface of each testis is a single, tightly coiled tube, the (4) **epididymis.** This structure stores sperm after it leaves the seminiferous tubules. The epididymis is the first duct through which sperm passes after its production in the testes. Tracing the duct upward, the epididymis forms the (5) **vas deferens** (also called the *seminal duct* or *ductus deferens*), a narrow tube that passes through the inguinal canal into the abdominal cavity. The vas deferens extends over the top and down the posterior surface of the bladder, where it joins the (6) **seminal vesicle.**

The union of the vas deferens with the duct from the seminal vesicle forms the (7) **ejaculatory duct.** The seminal vesicle contains nutrients that support sperm viability and produces approximately 60% of the seminal fluid that is ultimately ejaculated during sexual intercourse (**coitus**). The ejaculatory duct passes at an angle through the (8) **prostate gland,** a triple-lobed organ fused to the base of the bladder. The prostate gland secretes a thin, alkaline substance that accounts for about 30% of seminal fluid. Its alkalinity helps protect sperm from the acidic environments of the male urethra and the female vagina. Two pea-shaped structures, the (9) **bulbourethral (Cowper) glands,** are located below the prostate and are connected by a small duct to the urethra. The bulbourethral glands provide the alkaline fluid necessary for sperm viability. The (10) **penis** is the male organ of copulation. It is cylindrical and composed of erectile tissue that encloses the (11) **urethra.** The urethra expels semen and urine from the body. During ejaculation, the sphincter at the base of the bladder closes, which not only stops the urine from being expelled with the semen, but also prevents semen from entering the bladder. The enlarged tip of the penis, the (12) **glans penis,** contains the (13) **urethral orifice (meatus).** A movable hood of skin, called the (14) **prepuce (foreskin)** covers the glans penis.

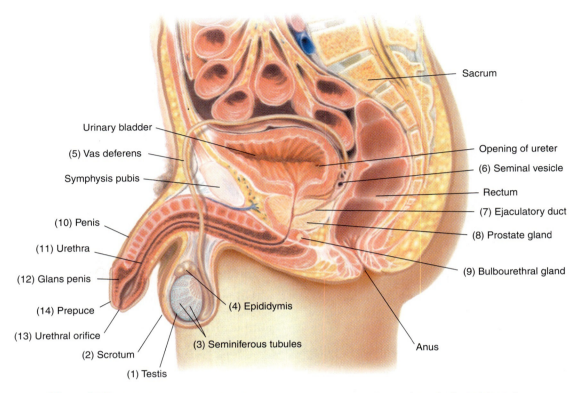

Figure 11-3. Midsagittal section of male reproductive structures shown through the pelvic cavity.

Connecting Body Systems–Genitourinary System

The main function of the genitourinary system is to enable sexual reproduction and to regulate extracellular fluids of the body. Specific functional relationships between the genitourinary system and other body systems are summarized below.

Blood, lymph, and immune
- Male reproductive system transports testosterone throughout the body in blood and lymph.
- Kidneys regulate composition and quality of blood plasma and lymph.
- Kidneys retain needed products and remove those that are excessive or toxic to the body.

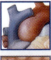
Cardiovascular
- Kidneys help regulate essential electrolytes needed for contraction of the heart.

Digestive
- Kidneys aid in removing glucose from the blood when excessive amounts are consumed.
- Kidneys remove excessive fluids absorbed from the gastrointestinal (GI) tract.

Endocrine
- Kidneys regulate sodium and water balance, which is essential for hormone transport in the blood.
- Kidneys produce erythropoietin, a hormone synthesized mainly in the kidneys and released into the bloodstream.
- Gonads produce hormones that provide feedback to influence pituitary function.

Female reproductive
- Male organs of reproduction work in conjunction with the female reproductive system to enable fertilization of the ovum.
- Kidneys aid in removing waste products produced by the fetus in the pregnant woman.

Connecting Body Systems–Genitourinary System

Integumentary
- Kidneys compensate for extracellular fluid loss due to hyperhidrosis.
- Kidneys adjust electrolytes, especially potassium and sodium, in response to their loss through the dermis.

Musculoskeletal
- Kidneys work in conjunction with bone tissue to maintain a constant calcium level.

Nervous
- Kidneys regulate sodium, potassium, and calcium, which are the electrolytes responsible for the transmission of nervous stimuli.

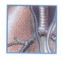

Respiratory
- Kidneys and lungs assist in regulating acid-base balance of the body.

It is time to review male reproductive anatomy by completing Learning Activity 11–2.

Medical Word Elements

This section introduces combining forms, suffixes, and prefixes related to the genitourinary system. Word analyses are also provided.

Element	Meaning	Word Analysis
Combining Forms		
Urinary System		
cyst/o	bladder	**cyst/o**/scope (SĬST-ō-skōp): instrument for examining the bladder *-scope:* instrument for examining
vesic/o		**vesic/o**/cele (VĔS-ĭ-kō-sēl): hernia of the bladder; also called *cystocele* *-cele:* hernia, swelling *With a vesicocele, the bladder herniates into the vaginal wall, which may lead to incomplete emptying of the bladder.*
glomerul/o	glomerulus	**glomerul/o**/pathy (glō-mĕr-ū-LŎP-ă-thē): disease of the glomerulus *-pathy:* disease
lith/o	stone, calculus	**lith/o**/tripsy (LĬTH-ō-trĭp-sē): crushing of a stone *-tripsy:* crushing *The most common method of lithotripsy is extracorporeal shock wave lithotripsy (ESWL). When stones are large or ESWL is not recommended, percutaneous nephrolithotomy or ureteroscopic stone removal are alternate methods of treatment.*
meat/o	opening, meatus	**meat/o**/tomy (mē-ă-TŎT-ō-mē): incision of the meatus *-tomy:* incision *A meatotomy is performed to relieve stenosis of the urethra, which may inhibit the proper passage of urine or semen.*
nephr/o	kidney	**nephr/o**/pexy (NĔF-rō-pĕks-ē): fixation of kidney *-pexy:* fixation (of an organ)
ren/o		**ren**/al (RĒ-năl): pertaining to the kidney *-al:* pertaining to

(continued)

Medical Word Elements—cont'd

Element	Meaning	Word Analysis
pyel/o	renal pelvis	**pyel/o**/plasty (PĪ-ĕ-lō-plăs-tē): surgical repair of the renal pelvis *-plasty:* surgical repair
ur/o	urine, urinary tract	**ur/o**/lith (Ū-rō-lĭth): stone in urinary tract *-lith:* stone, calculus
ureter/o	ureter	**ureter/**ectasis (ū-rē-tĕr-ĔK-tă-sĭs): dilation of the ureter *-ectasis:* dilation, expansion
urethr/o	urethra	**urethr/o**/stenosis (ū-rē-thrō-stĕn-Ō-sĭs): narrowing or stricture of the urethra *-stenosis:* narrowing, stricture
Male Reproductive System		
andr/o	male	**andr/o**/gen/ic (ăn-drō-JĔN-ĭk): pertaining to maleness *gen:* forming, producing, origin *-ic:* pertaining to *Androgenic hormones include all natural or synthetic compounds that stimulate or maintain male characteristics. The most common androgenic hormone is testosterone.*
balan/o	glans penis	**balan/o**/plasty (BĂL-ă-nō-plăs-tē): surgical repair of the glans penis *-plasty:* surgical repair
epididym/o	epididymis	**epididym/o**/tomy (ĕp-ĭ-dĭd-ĭ-MŎT-ō-mē): incision of the epididymis *-tomy:* incision
orch/o	testis (plural, testes)	**orch/**itis (or-KĪ-tĭs): inflammation of testes *-itis:* inflammation *A common cause of orchitis in young boys is a mumps infection.*
orchi/o		**orchi/**algia (or-kē-ĂL-jē-ă): pain in the testes *-algia:* pain
orchid/o		**orchid/o**/ptosis (or-kĭd-ŏp-TŌ-sĭs): downward displacement of the testes *-ptosis:* prolapse, downward displacement
test/o		**test/**ectomy (tĕs-TĔK-tō-mē): excision of a testis *-ectomy:* excision, removal
perine/o	perineum (area between scrotum [or vulva in the female] and anus)	**perine/**al (pĕr-ĭ-NĒ-ăl): pertaining to the perineum *-al:* pertaining to
prostat/o	prostate gland	**prostat/o**/megaly (prŏs-tă-tō-MĔG-ă-lē): enlargement of the prostate gland *-megaly:* enlargement
spermat/o	spermatozoa, sperm cells	**spermat/o**/cele (spĕr-MĂT-ō-sēl): swelling containing spermatozoa *-cele:* hernia, swelling *A spermatocele is usually an epididymal cyst commonly containing sperm.*

Medical Word Elements—cont'd

Element	Meaning	Word Analysis
sperm/o		**sperm**/ic (SPĔR-mĭk): pertaining to sperm cells *-ic:* pertaining to
varic/o	dilated vein	**varic/o**/cele (VĂR-ĭ-kō-sēl): swelling of a dilated vein *-cele:* hernia, swelling *Varicocele is a dilation of the veins of the spermatic cord, the structure that supports the testicles.*
vas/o	vessel; vas deferens; duct	**vas**/ectomy (văs-ĔK-tō-mē): removal of (all or part of) the vas deferens *-ectomy:* excision, removal *Bilateral vasectomy is a surgical procedure to produce sterility in the male.*
vesicul/o	seminal vesicle	**vesicul**/itis (vĕ-sĭk-ū-LĪ-tĭs): inflammation of the seminal vesicle *-itis:* inflammation
Other		
albumin/o	albumin, protein	**albumin**/oid (ăl-BŪ-mĭ-noyd): resembling albumin *-oid:* resembling
azot/o	nitrogenous compounds	**azot**/emia (ăz-ō-TĒ-mē-ă): nitrogenous compounds in the blood *-emia:* blood condition *Nitrogenous products, especially urea, are toxic. If they are not removed from the body, death will result.*
bacteri/o	bacteria (singular, *bacterium*)	**bacteri**/uria (băk-tē-rē-Ū-rē-ă): bacteria in urine *-uria:* urine
crypt/o	hidden	**crypt**/orchid/ism (krĭpt-OR-kĭd-ĭzm): condition of hidden testes; also called *cryptorchism* *orchid:* testis (plural, testes) *-ism:* condition *Cryptorchidism is the failure of the testes to descend into the scrotum; usually a congenital disorder.*
gonad/o	gonads, sex glands	**gonad/o**/pathy (gŏn-ă-DŎP-ă-thē): disease of the sex glands *-pathy:* disease
kal/i	potassium (an electrolyte)	hypo/**kal**/emia (hī-pō-kă-LĒ-mē-ă): abnormally low concentration of potassium in the blood *hypo-:* under, below *-emia:* blood condition *Hypokalemia may result from excessive urination, which depletes potassium from the body.*
keton/o	ketone bodies (acids and acetones)	**keton**/uria (kē-tō-NŪ-rē-ă): presence of ketone bodies in the urine *-uria:* urine *Ketonuria is commonly found in diabetes mellitus, starvation, and excessive dieting.*

(continued)

Medical Word Elements—cont'd

Element	Meaning	Word Analysis
noct/o	night	**noct**/uria (nŏk-TŪ-rē-ă): excessive and frequent urination after going to bed *-uria:* urine *Nocturia is associated with prostate disease, urinary tract infection, and uncontrolled diabetes.*
olig/o	scanty	**olig/o**/sperm/ia (ŏl-ĭ-gō-SPĔR-mē-ă): scanty (decreased production) of sperm *sperm:* spermatozoa, sperm cells *-ia:* condition
py/o	pus	**py/o**/rrhea (pī-ō-RĒ-ă): flow or discharge of pus *-rrhea:* discharge, flow

Suffixes

Element	Meaning	Word Analysis
-cide	killing	sperm/i/**cide** (SPĔR-mĭ-sīd): (agents that) kill sperm; also called *spermaticide* *sperm/i:* spermatozoa, sperm cells
-genesis	forming, producing, origin	lith/o/**genesis** (lĭth-ō-JĔN-ĕ-sĭs): forming or producing stones *lith/o:* stone, calculus
-iasis	abnormal condition (produced by something specified)	lith/**iasis** (lĭth-Ī-ă-sĭs): abnormal condition of stones or calculi *lith/o:* stone, calculus
-ism	condition	an/orch/**ism** (ăn-OR-kĭzm): condition without testes *an-:* without, not *orch:* testis (plural, testes) *Anorchism is the congenital or acquired absence of one or both testes.*
-spadias	slit, fissure	hypo/**spadias** (hī-pō-SPĀ-dē-ăs): a fissure under (the penis) *hypo-:* under, below *Hypospadias is a congenital defect in which the urethra opens on the underside of the glans penis instead of the tip.*
-uria	urine	poly/**uria** (pŏl-ē-Ū-rē-ă): much (excretion of) urine *poly-:* many, much *Polyuria is generally considered to be the excretion of over 2.5 liters per 24 hours.*

Prefixes

Element	Meaning	Word Analysis
dia-	through, across	**dia**/lysis (dī-ĂL-ĭ-sĭs): separation across *-lysis:* separation; destruction; loosening *Renal dialysis is a procedure that uses a membrane to separate and selectively remove waste products from blood when kidneys are unable to complete this function.*
retro-	backward, behind	**retro**/peritone/al (rĕt-rō-pĕr-ĭ-tō-NĒ-ăl): pertaining to (the area) behind the peritoneum *peritone:* peritoneum *-al:* pertaining to

It is time to review medical word elements by completing Learning Activity 11–3. For audio pronunciations of the above-listed key terms, you can visit www.davisplus.fadavis.com/gylys/systems *to download this chapter's* Listen and Learn! *exercises or use the book's audio CD (if included).*

Pathology

Pathology of the urinary system includes a range of disorders from those that are asymptomatic to those that manifest an array of signs and symptoms. Causes for these disorders include congenital anomalies, infectious diseases, trauma, or conditions that secondarily involve the urinary structures. Many times, asymptomatic urinary diseases are first diagnosed when a routine urinalysis shows abnormalities. Forms of glomerulonephritis and chronic urinary tract infection are two such disorders. Symptoms specific to urinary disorders include changes in urination pattern, output, or dysuria. Endoscopic tests, radiological evaluations, and laboratory tests that evaluate renal function are typically employed to diagnose disorders of the urinary system.

Signs and symptoms of male reproductive disorders include pain, swelling, erectile dysfunction, and loss of normal sexual drive (**libido**). Characteristics of infectious diseases, especially those transmitted through sexual activity, commonly include pain, discharge, or lesions as well as a vague feeling of fullness or discomfort in the perineal or rectal area. A complete evaluation of the genitalia, reproductive history, and past and present genitourinary infections and disorders is necessary to identify disorders associated with male reproductive structures.

For diagnosis, treatment, and management of genitourinary disorders, the medical services of a specialist may be warranted. **Urology** is the branch of medicine concerned with male and female urinary disorders and diseases of the male reproductive system. The physician who specializes in diagnoses and treatment of genitourinary disorders is known as a *urologist*. However, the branch of medicine concerned specifically with diseases of the kidney, electrolyte imbalance, renal transplantation, and dialysis therapy is known as *nephrology*. Physicians who practice in this specialty are called *nephrologists*.

Pyelonephritis

One of the most common forms of kidney disease is **pyelonephritis,** (also called *kidney infection* or *complicated urinary tract infection*). In this disorder, bacteria invade the renal pelvis and kidney tissue, commonly as a result of a bladder infection that has ascended to the kidney via the ureters. When the infection is severe, lesions form in the renal pelvis, causing bleeding. The microscopic examination of urine shows large quantities of bacteria (**bacteriuria**), white blood cells (**pyuria**), and, when lesions are present, red blood cells (**hematuria**). The onset of the disease is usually acute, with symptoms including pain around the kidney, dysuria, fatigue, urinary urgency and frequency, chills, fever, nausea, and vomiting. Treatment with antibiotics is usually successful. However, in some cases, organisms may have developed a resistance and alternative antibiotics may be required.

Glomerulonephritis

Any condition that causes the glomerular walls to become inflamed is referred to as *glomerulonephritis*. One of the most common causes of glomerular inflammation is a reaction to the toxins given off by pathogenic bacteria, especially streptococci that have recently infected another part of the body, usually the throat. Glomerulonephritis is also associated with diabetes and autoimmune diseases such as systemic lupus erythematosus, polyarthritis, and scleroderma.

When the glomerular membrane is inflamed, it becomes "leaky" (**permeable**). Red blood cells and protein pass through the glomerulus and enter the tubule.. In some cases, protein solidifies in the nephron tubules and forms solid masses that take the shape of the tubules in which they develop. These masses are called *casts*. They commonly pass out of the kidney by way of the urine and may be visible when urine is examined microscopically. The clinical picture for glomerulonephritis includes blood and protein in the urine (**hematuria** and **proteinuria**) and red cell casts, along with high blood pressure (**hypertension (HTN)**, edema, and impaired renal function. Most patients with acute glomerulonephritis associated with a streptococcal infection recover with no lasting kidney damage.

Nephrolithiasis

Stones (**calculi**) may form in any part of the urinary tract (**urolithiasis**), but most arise in the kidney, a condition called *nephrolithiasis*. (See Figure 11–4.) They commonly form when dissolved urine salts begin to solidify. These stones may increase in size and obstruct urinary structures. If they lodge in the ureters, they cause intense throbbing pain called *colic*. Because urine is hindered from passing into the bladder, it flows backward (**refluxes**) into the renal pelvis and the tubules, causing them to dilate.

In one method of treatment called **extracorporeal shock wave lithotripsy (ESWL)**, calculi are pulverized using concentrated ultrasound waves,

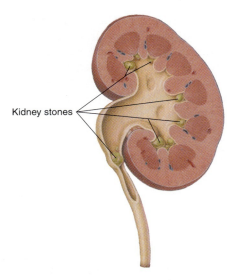

Figure 11-4. Kidney stones in the calices and ureter.

remove the stone. If the stone is large, an ultrasonic or electrohydraulic probe is used to break the stone into smaller fragments, which are then more easily removed. A nephrostomy tube may be inserted and remain in place during healing. For stones that have descended into the ureters, it may be possible to remove them using a specialized ureteroscope fitted with a small basket. The ureteroscope is passed through the urethra and bladder and into the ureter where the basket collects the stone. For larger stones, it may be necessary to break them into smaller pieces using an endoscope fitted with a laser beam before the fragments are removed. This procedure is called *ureteroscopic stone removal*, and no incision is required.

Benign Prostatic Hyperplasia

Benign prostatic hyperplasia (BPH), also called *nodular hyperplasia* or *benign prostatic hypertrophy*, is commonly associated with the aging process. As the prostate gland enlarges, it decreases the urethral lumen, and complete voiding of urine becomes difficult. Urine that remains in the bladder commonly becomes a breeding ground for bacteria. Bladder infection (**cystitis**) and, ultimately, kidney infection (**nephritis**) may result. If medical management of BPH fails, it may be necessary to employ surgical methods. Surgical removal of

called *shock waves,* directed at the stones from a machine outside the body. (See Figure 11–5.) For excessively large stones or patients who have contraindications for ESWL, an alternative treatment is **percutaneous nephrolithotomy (PCNL)**. In this procedure, a small incision is made in the skin, and an opening is formed in the kidney. A nephroscope is inserted into the kidney to locate and

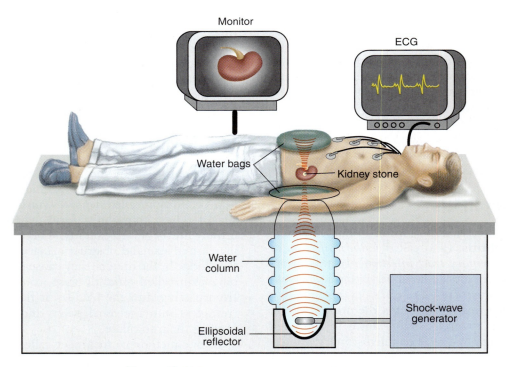

Figure 11-5. Extracorporeal shock wave lithotripsy.

the entire prostate may be done through the perineum (**perineal prostatectomy**) or an abdominal opening above the pubis and directly over the bladder (**suprapubic prostatectomy**). These procedures are invasive and are performed when the entire prostate must be removed, such as when cancer is identified. These methods also enable the removal of lymph nodes for examination. When only a portion of the prostate must be removed, the less invasive **transurethral resection of the prostate (TURP)** is usually performed. In TURP, a resectoscope is inserted through the urethra, and a small loop "chips away" some of the obstructing tissue. At the conclusion of the surgery, the urethra and bladder are irrigated to remove the small chips. (See Figure 11–6.)

Cryptorchidism

Failure of the testes to descend into the scrotal sac prior to birth is called *cryptorchidism.* In many infants born with this condition, the testes descend spontaneously by the end of the first year. If this does not occur, correction of the disorder involves surgical suspension of the testes (**orchiopexy**) in the scrotum. This procedure is usually done before the child reaches age 2. Because an inguinal hernia commonly accompanies cryptorchidism, the hernia may be sutured (**herniorrhaphy**) at the same time.

Acute Tubular Necrosis

In **acute tubular necrosis (ATN)**, the tubular portion of the nephron is injured by a decrease in blood supply (**ischemic ATN**) or after the ingestion of toxic chemicals (**nephrotoxic ATN**). Ischemia may occur because of circulatory collapse, severe hypotension, hemorrhage, dehydration, or other disorders that affect blood supply. ATN does not produce specific signs and symptoms, and diagnosis relies on a positive history of risk factors. General signs and symptoms of ATN include scanty urine production (**oliguria**) fluid retention, mental apathy, nausea, vomiting, and increased blood levels of calcium (**hypercalcemia**). When tubular damage is not severe, the disorder is usually reversible.

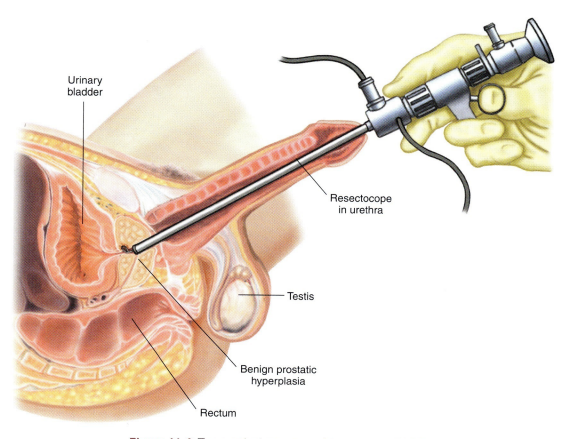

Urinary bladder

Resectocope in urethra

Testis

Benign prostatic hyperplasia

Rectum

Figure 11-6. Transurethral resection of the prostate (TURP).

Oncology

The most common form of cancer in men is carcinoma of the prostate. In the United States, the disease is rarely found in men younger than age 50; however, the incidence dramatically increases with age. Symptoms include difficulty starting urination (**hesitancy**) and stopping the urinary stream, dysuria, urinary frequency, and hematuria. By the time these symptoms develop and the patient seeks treatment, the disease is quite advanced and long-term survival is not likely. Early presymptomatic tests include a blood test for prostate-specific antigen (PSA) and periodic digital rectal examination (DRE). (See Figure 11–7.)

Like other forms of cancer, prostatic carcinomas are staged and graded to determine metastatic potential, response to treatment, chances of survival, and appropriate forms of therapy. Surgery and radiation therapy are usual treatment modalities, but other forms of treatment may also be employed. Surgical treatment includes the removal of the entire prostate (**radical prostatectomy**). Two forms of radiation oncology include brachytherapy and external beam radiation. In **brachytherapy** (also called *internal radiation therapy*), radioactive "seeds" are placed directly in the malignant tissue. They remain in place for long or short periods of time depending on the type of malignancy, its location, and other diagnostic criteria. (See Figure 11–8.) In **external beam radiation (EBR)**, high-energy x-ray beams are generated by a machine and directed at the tumor from outside the body to destroy prostate tissue. Another treatment modality is the application of extreme cold (**cryosurgery**), which results in the destruction of prostate tissue. (See Figure 11–9.) Administering antiandrogenic agents as well as hormones that deplete the body of testicular hormones (**combined hormonal therapy**) has been effective in treatment at the early stages of the disease. Because prostatic cancer is stimulated by testosterone, surgical removal of the testes (**bilateral orchiectomy**) may be necessary.

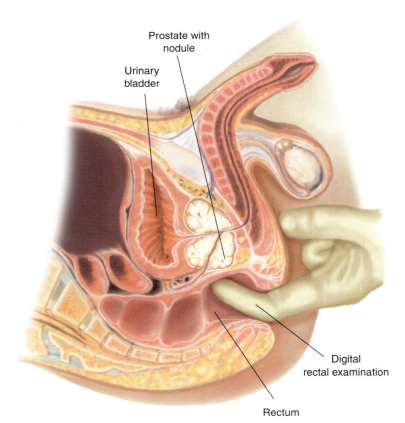

Prostate with nodule

Urinary bladder

Digital rectal examination

Rectum

Figure 11-7. Digital rectal examination.

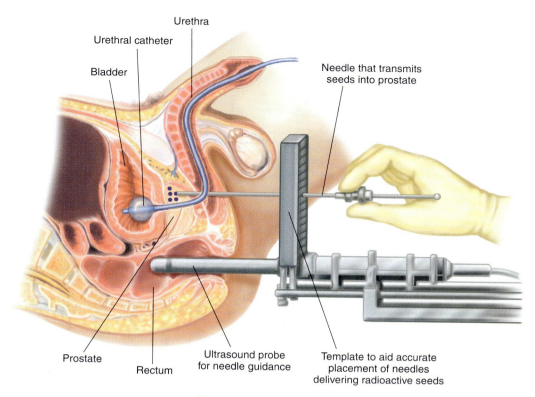

Figure 11-8. Brachytherapy.

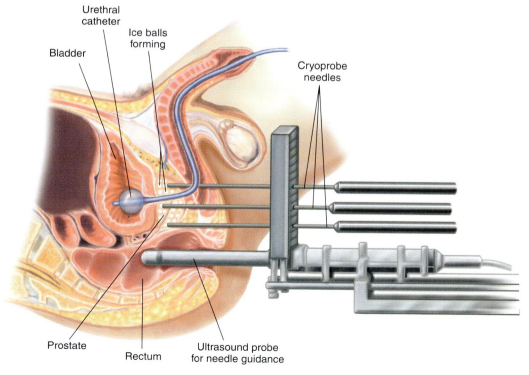

Figure 11-9. Cryosurgery of the prostate.

Diagnostic, Symptomatic, and Related Terms

This section introduces diagnostic, symptomatic, and related terms and their meanings. Word analyses for selected terms are also provided.

Term	Definition
Urinary System	
anuria ăn-Ū-rē-ă *an-:* without, not *uria:* urine	Absence of urine production or urinary output *Anuria may be obstructive, in which there is blockage proximal to the bladder, or unobstructive, which is caused by severe damage to the nephrons of the kidneys.*
azotemia ăz-ō-TĒ-mē-ă *azot:* nitrogenous compounds *-emia:* blood condition	Retention of excessive amounts of nitrogenous compounds (urea, creatinine, and uric acid) in the blood; also called *uremia*
bladder neck obstruction (BNO)	Blockage at base of the bladder that reduces or prevents urine from passing into the urethra *BNO can be caused by benign prostatic hyperplasia, bladder stones, bladder tumors, or tumors in the pelvic cavity.*
chronic renal failure KRŎ-nĭk RĒ-năl	Renal failure that occurs over a period of years, in which the kidneys lose their ability to maintain volume and composition of body fluids with normal dietary intake *Chronic renal failure is the result of decreased numbers of functioning nephrons in the kidneys.*
dysuria dĭs-Ū-rē-ă *dys-:* bad; painful; difficult *uria:* urine	Painful or difficult urination, commonly described as a "burning sensation" while urinating *Dysuria is a symptom of numerous conditions but, most commonly, urinary tract infection (UTI).*
end-stage renal disease (ESRD) dī-ĂL-ĭ-sĭs *dia-:* through, across *-lysis:* separation; destruction; loosening	Condition in which kidney function is permanently lost
enuresis ĕn-ū-RĒ-sĭs *en-:* in, within *ur:* urine *-esis:* condition	Involuntary discharge of urine; also called *incontinence* *Enuresis that occurs during the night is called* **nocturnal enuresis;** *during the day,* **diurnal enuresis.**
fistula FĬS-tū-lă	Abnormal passage from a hollow organ to the surface or from one organ to another *The most common type of urinary fistula is the vesicovaginal fistula where communication occurs between the bladder and vagina. Its causes include previous pelvic surgery such as hysterectomy, difficult and prolonged labor, or reduced blood supply to the area.*
frequency FRĒ-kwĕn-sē	Voiding urine at frequent intervals

Diagnostic, Symptomatic, and Related Terms—cont'd

Term	Definition

hesitancy
HĔZ-ĭ-tĕn-sē

Involuntary delay in initiating urination

hydronephrosis
hī-drō-nĕf-RŌ-sĭs
hydr/o: water
nephr: kidney
-osis: abnormal condition;
   increase (used primarily
   with blood cells)

Abnormal dilation of the renal pelvis and the calyces of one or both kidneys due to pressure from accumulated urine that cannot flow past an obstruction in the urinary tract

The most common causes of hydronephrosis are BPH, urethral strictures, and calculi that lodge in the ureter and cause an obstruction. The pressure impairs, and may eventually interrupt, kidney function. (See Figure 11–10.)

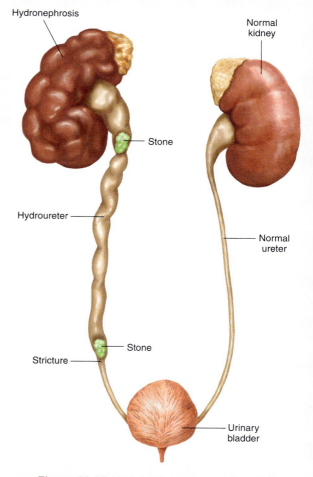

Figure 11-10. Hydronephrosis and hydroureter.

nephrotic syndrome
nĕ-FRŎT-ĭk
nephr/o: kidney
-tic: pertaining to, relating to

Loss of large amounts of plasma protein, usually albumin by way of urine due to increased permeability of the glomerular membrane

Hypoproteinemia, edema, and hyperlipidemia are commonly associated with nephrotic syndrome.

nocturia
nŏk-TŪ-rē-ă
noct: night
-uria: urine

Excessive or frequent urination after going to bed

Nocturia is typically caused by excessive fluid intake, uncontrolled diabetes mellitus, urinary tract infection, prostate disease, impaired renal function, or the use of diuretics.

(continued)

Diagnostic, Symptomatic, and Related Terms—cont'd

Term	Definition
oliguria ōl-ĭg-Ū-rē-ă *olig:* scanty *-uria:* urine	Diminished capacity to form and pass urine, resulting in inefficient excretion of the end products of metabolism *Oliguria is usually caused by fluid and electrolyte imbalances, renal lesions, or urinary tract obstruction.*
polycystic kidney disease (PKD) pŏl-ē-SĬS-tĭk *poly:* many, much *cyst:* bladder *-ic:* pertaining to	Inherited disease in which sacs of fluid called *cysts* develop in the kidneys *If cysts increase in number or size or if they become infected, kidney failure may result. Dialysis or kidney transplant may be necessary for renal failure caused by PKD.*
urgency ŬR-jĕn-sē	Feeling of the need to void immediately *Urinary urgency commonly occurs in urinary tract infection (UTI).*
vesicoureteral reflux (VUR) vĕs-ĭ-kō-ū-RĒ-tĕr-ăl *vesic/o:* bladder *ureter:* ureter *-al:* pertaining to	Disorder caused by the failure of urine to pass through the ureters to the bladder, usually due to impairment of the valve between the ureter and bladder or obstruction in the ureter *VUR may result in the enlargement of the kidney (hydronephrosis) if the obstruction is in the proximal portion of the ureter or enlargement of the ureter (hydroureter) and the kidney if the obstruction is in the distal portion of the ureter.*
Wilms tumor VĬLMZ TOO-mĕr	Rapidly developing malignant neoplasm of the kidney that usually occurs in children *Diagnosis of Wilms tumor is established by an excretory urogram (EU) with tomography. The tumor is well encapsulated in the early stage but may metastasize to other sites, such as lymph nodes and lungs, at later stages.*
Male Reproductive System	
anorchidism ăn-OR-kĭ-dĭzm *an-:* without, not *orchid:* testis (plural, testes) *-ism:* condition	Congenital absence of one or both testes; also called *anorchia* or *anorchism* *Treatment for anorchidism requires replacement of the male hormone testosterone. Boys affected with anorchidism will need testosterone for puberty to occur.*
aspermia ă-SPĔR-mē-ă *a-:* without, not *sperm:* spermatozoa, sperm cells *-ia:* condition	Failure to form or ejaculate semen **Aspermia** *should not be confused with* **azoospermia,** *which is absence of sperm in the ejaculate.*
balanitis băl-ă-NĪ-tĭs *balan:* glans penis *-itis:* inflammation	Inflammation of the skin covering the glans penis *Uncircumcised men with poor personal hygiene are prone to this disorder.*
epispadias ĕp-ĭ-SPĀ-dē-ăs *epi-:* above, upon *-spadias:* slit, fissure	Malformation in which the urethra opens on the dorsum of the penis

Diagnostic, Symptomatic, and Related Terms—cont'd

Term	Definition
erectile dysfunction (ED) ĕ-RĔK-tīl	Repeated inability to initiate or maintain an erection sufficient for sexual intercourse *Any disorder that causes injury to the nerves or impairs blood flow in the penis has the potential to cause ED.*
hydrocele HĪ-drō-sēl *hydr/o:* water *–cele:* hernia, swelling	Accumulation of serous fluid in a saclike cavity, especially the testes and associated structures *Hydrocele is common in male newborns but usually resolves within the first year.*
hypospadias hī-pō-SPĀ-dē-ăs *hypo-:* under, below, deficient *–spadias:* slit, fissure	Developmental anomaly in which the urethra opens on the underside of the penis or, in extreme cases, on the perineum
phimosis fī-MŌ-sĭs *phim:* muzzle *–osis:* abnormal condition; increase (used primarily with blood cells)	Stenosis or narrowing of preputial orifice so that the foreskin cannot be retracted over the glans penis
sterility stĕr-ĬL-ĭ-tē	Inability to produce offspring; in the male, inability to fertilize the ovum
varicocele VĂR-ĭ-kō-sēl *varic/o:* dilated vein *–cele:* hernia, swelling	Swelling and distention of veins of the spermatic cord

It is time to review pathological, diagnostic, symptomatic, and related terms by completing Learning Activity 11–4.

Diagnostic and Therapeutic Procedures

This section introduces procedures used to diagnose and treat genitourinary system disorders. Descriptions are provided as well as pronunciations and word analyses for selected terms.

Procedure	Description
Diagnostic Procedures **Clinical**	
digital rectal examination (DRE)	Screening test that assesses the rectal wall surface for lesions or abnormally firm areas that might indicate cancer *In DRE, the physician inserts a gloved, lubricated finger into the rectum. In males, the physician also evaluates the size and consistency of the prostate. (See Figure 11-7.)*

(continued)

Diagnostic and Therapeutic Procedures—cont'd

Procedure	Description

electromyography (EMG)
ē-lĕk-trō-mī-ŎG-ră-fē
  electr/o: electricity
  my/o: muscle
  -graphy: process of recording
	Measures the contraction of muscles that control urination using electrodes placed in the rectum and urethra
	
	EMG determines whether incontinence is due to weak muscles or other causes.

testicular self-examination (TSE)	Self-examination of the testes for abnormal lumps or swellings in the scrotal sac *TSE is increasingly recommended by physicians to detect abnormalities, especially cancer, when the disease is easily treatable. Testicular cancer is the number one cancer killer in men ages 20 to 30.*
Endoscopic	

cystoscopy (cysto)
sĭs-TŎS-kō-pē
  cyst/o: bladder
  -scopy: examination
	Endoscopy of the urinary bladder for evidence of pathology, obtaining biopsies of tumors or other growths, and removal of polyps
	
	In cystoscopy, a catheter can be inserted thought the hollow channel in the cystoscope to collect tissue samples or introduce contrast media during radiography. (See Figure 11–11.)

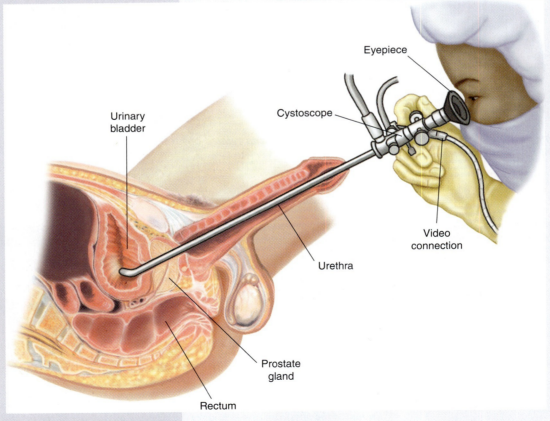

Figure 11-11. Cystoscopy.

Diagnostic and Therapeutic Procedures—cont'd

Procedure	Description
nephroscopy ně-FRŎS-kō-pē *nephr/o:* kidney *-scopy:* examination	Endoscopy of the kidney(s) using a specialized, three-channel endoscope that enables visualization and irrigation of the kidney *The nephroscope is passed through a small incision made in the renal pelvis. Kidney pathology and congenital deformities may be observed.*
urethroscopy ū-rē-THRŎS-kō-pē *urethr/o:* urethra *scopy:* examination	Endoscopy of the urethra using a specialized endoscope, typically for lithotripsy or TURP

Laboratory

Procedure	Description
blood urea nitrogen (BUN) ū-RĒ-ă NĪ-trō-jĕn	Test that determines the amount of urea nitrogen, a waste product of protein metabolism, present in a blood sample *Because urea is cleared from the bloodstream by the kidneys, the BUN test is used as an indicator of kidney function.*
culture and sensitivity (C&S) KŬL-tūr, sĕn-sĭ-TĬ-vĭ-tē	Test that determines the causative organism of a disease and how the organism responds to various antibiotics *C&S tests are performed on urine, blood, and body secretions.*
prostate-specific antigen (PSA) PRŎS-tāt spĕ-SĬF-ĭk ĂN-tĭ-jĕn	Blood test used to detect prostatic disorders, especially prostatic cancer *PSA is a substance produced by the prostate and is normally found in a blood sample in small quantities. The level is elevated in prostatitis, benign prostatic hyperplasia, and tumors of the prostate.*
semen analysis SĒ-mĕn ă-NĂL-ĭ-sĭs	Test that analyzes a semen sample for volume, sperm count, motility, and morphology to evaluate fertility or verify sterilization after a vasectomy
urinalysis (UA) ū-rĭ-NĂL-ĭ-sĭs	Battery of tests performed on a urine specimen, including physical observation, chemical tests, and microscopic evaluation *UA not only provides information on the urinary structures but may also be the first indicator of such system disorders as diabetes and liver and gallbladder disease.*

Radiographic

Procedure	Description
computed tomography (CT) kŏm-PŪ-tĕd tō-MŎG-ră-fē *tom/o:* to cut *-graphy:* process of recording	Imaging technique that rotates an x-ray emitter around the area to be scanned and measures the intensity of transmitted rays from different angles *In the genitourinary system, CTs are used to diagnose tumors, cysts, inflammation, abscesses, perforation, bleeding, and obstructions of the kidneys, ureters, and bladder.)*
cystography sĭs-TŎG-ră-fē *cyst/o:* bladder *-graphy:* process of recording	Radiographic examination of the urinary bladder using a contrast medium *Cystography is used to diagnose tumors or defects in the bladder wall, vesicoureteral reflux, stones, or other pathological conditions of the bladder.*

(continued)

Diagnostic and Therapeutic Procedures—cont'd

Procedure	Description
cystometrography sĭs-tō-mĕ-TRŎG-ră-fē *cyst/o:* bladder *metr/o:* uterus (womb); measure *-graphy:* process of recording	Procedure that assesses volume and pressure in the bladder at various stages of filling using saline and a contrast medium introduced into the bladder through a catheter *Cystometrography is the primary test used to investigate stress incontinence and urge incontinence.*
intravenous pyelography (IVP) ĭn-tră-VĒ-nŭs pī-ĕ-LŎG-ră-fē *intra-:* in, within *ven:* vein *-ous:* pertaining to *pyel/o:* renal pelvis *-graphy:* process of recording	Radiographic examination of the kidneys, and urinary tract after IV injection of a contrast medium; also called *excretory urography (EU)* *IVP detects kidney stones, enlarged prostate, internal injuries after an accident or trauma, and tumors in the kidneys, ureters, and bladder.*
kidney, ureter, bladder (KUB) radiography *radi/o:* radiation, x-ray; radius (lower arm bone on thumb side) *-graphy:* process of recording	Radiographic examination to determine the location, size, and shape of the kidneys in relationship to other organs in the abdominopelvic cavity and to identify abnormalities of the urinary system *KUB radiography identifies stones and calcified areas and does not require a contrast medium.*
nuclear scan renal *ren:* kidney *-al:* pertaining to,	Radiology test in which radioactive materials called *tracers* are introduced into the patient and a specialized camera, which acts as a radiation detector, produces images by recording the emitted tracers Imaging test where a monitor is used to track a radioactive substance as it passes through the kidney
ultrasound (US) ŬL-tră-sownd scrotal SKRŌ-tăl	Radiograph that uses high-frequency sound waves (ultrasound) and displays the reflected echoes on a monitor; also called *sonography, echography,* or *echo* US used to assess scrotal structures and patency of the vas deferens
voiding cystourethrography (VCUG) sĭs-tō-ū-rē-THRŎG-ră-fē *cyst/o:* bladder *urethr/o:* urethra *-graphy:* process of recording	Radiological examination of the bladder and urethra performed before, during, and after voiding using a contrast medium to enhance imaging *VCUG is performed to determine the cause of repeated bladder infections or stress incontinence and to identify congenital or acquired structural abnormalities of the bladder and urethra.*

Therapeutic Procedures

Clinical

dialysis dī-ĂL-ĭ-sĭs *dia-:* through, across *-lysis:* separation; destruction; loosening	Medical procedure used to filter toxic substances from the patient's bloodstream, such as excess electrolytes and nitrogenous wastes *Dialysis provides a means of removing waste products from the blood when kidneys no longer function. Nitrogenous waste products are collected in a solution called dialysate, which is discarded at the end of the procedure. There are two primary methods of dialysis:* hemodialysis *and* peritoneal dialysis.

Diagnostic and Therapeutic Procedures—cont'd

Procedure	Description

hemodialysis
hē-mō-dī-ĂL-ĭ-sĭs
hem/o: blood
dia: through, across
-lysis: separation; destruction; loosening

Method of removing waste substances from the blood by shunting it from the body, passing it through an artificial kidney machine where it is filtered, and then returning the dialyzed blood to the patient's body (See Figure 11–12.)

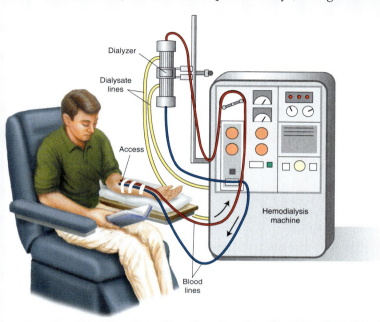

Figure 11-12. Hemodialysis

peritoneal
pĕr-ĭ-tō-NĒ-ăl
peritone: peritoneum
-al: pertaining to

Removal of toxic substances from the body by perfusing the peritoneal cavity with a warm, sterile chemical solution (See Figure 11–13.)

In peritoneal dialysis, the lining of the peritoneal cavity is used as the dialyzing membrane. Dialyzing fluid remains in the peritoneal cavity for 1 to 2 hours and then is removed. The procedure is repeated as often as necessary.

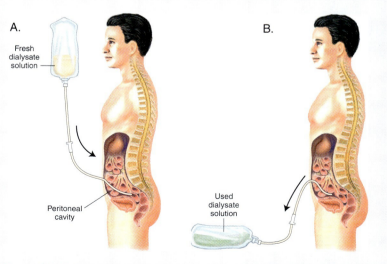

Figure 11-13. Peritoneal dialysis. (A) Introducing dialysis fluid into the peritoneal cavity. (B) Draining dialysate with waste products from the peritoneal cavity.

(continued)

Diagnostic and Therapeutic Procedures—cont'd

Procedure	Description
Surgical	
circumcision sĕr-kŭm-SĬ-zhŭn	Removal of all or part of the foreskin, or *prepuce,* of the penis
nephropexy NĔF-rō-pĕks-ē *nephr/o:* kidney *-pexy:* fixation (of an organ)	Fixation of a floating or mobile kidney
orchidectomy or-kĭ-DĔK-tō-mē *orchid:* testis (plural, testes) *-ectomy:* excision, removal	Removal of one or both testes; also called *orchiectomy* ***Orchidectomy may be indicated for serious disease or injury to the testis or to control cancer of the prostate by removing a source of androgenic hormones.***
transurethral resection of the prostate (TURP) trăns-ū-RĒ-thrăl rē-SĔK-shŭn PRŎS-tāt *trans:* across, through *urethr/o:* urethra *-al:* pertaining to	Surgical procedure that involves inserting a resectoscope into the urethra to "chip away" at the prostate gland to remove the obstruction and flushing out the chips and sending them for analysis to detect possible evidence of cancer ***TURP is used most commonly to relieve obstruction caused by benign prostatic hyperplasia. Because the prostate gland is not completely removed, remaining tissue eventually grows back and may cause obstruction again at a later time.***
urethrotomy ū-rē-THRŎT-ō-mē *urethr/o:* urethra *-tomy:* incision	Incision of a urethral stricture ***Urethrotomy corrects constrictions of the urethra that make voiding difficult.***
vasectomy văs-ĔK-tō-mē *vas:* vessel; vas deferens; duct *-ectomy:* excision, removal	Excision of all or a segment of the vas deferens (See Figure 11–14.) ***Bilateral vasectomy is the most successful method of male contraception. Although the procedure is considered permanent, with advances in microsurgery, vasectomy is sometimes reversible.***

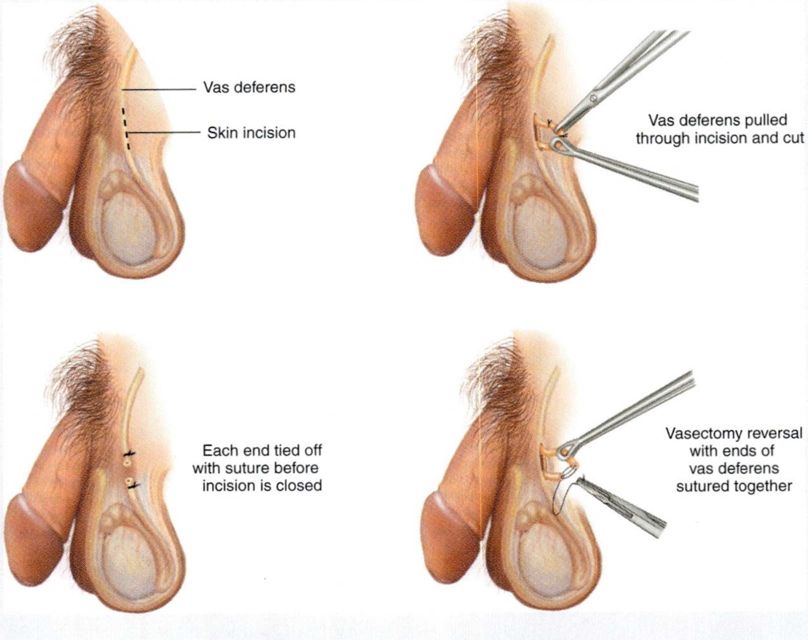
Vas deferens
Skin incision
Vas deferens pulled through incision and cut
Each end tied off with suture before incision is closed
Vasectomy reversal with ends of vas deferens sutured together

Figure 11-14. Vasectomy and reversal.

Pharmacology

Pharmacological agents used to treat urinary tract disorders include antibiotics, diuretics, antidiuretics, urinary antispasmodics, and potassium supplements, which are commonly taken concurrently with many diuretics to counteract potassium depletion. (See Table 11–1.) Pharmacologic agents are used to treat conditions of the male reproductive system including hypogonadism, erectile disfunction, and reproductive concerns and disorders.

Table 11-1	Drugs Used to Treat Genitourinary Disorders

This table lists common drug classifications used to treat urinary and male reproductive disorders, their therapeutic actions, and selected generic and trade names.

Classification	Therapeutic Action	Generic and Trade Names
Urinary System		
antibiotics	Treat bacterial infections of the urinary tract by acting on the bacterial membrane or one of its metabolic processes. *The type of antibiotic prescribed depends on the infecting organism and the type and extent of infection.*	**ciprofloxacin** sĭp-rō-FLŎX-ă-sĭn Cipro **sulfamethoxazole/trimethoprim** sŭl-fă-mĕth-ŎX-ă-zōl trī-MĔTH-ō-prĭm Bactrim
antispasmodics	Decrease spasms in the urethra and bladder by relaxing the smooth muscles lining their walls, thus allowing normal emptying of the bladder. *Bladder spasms can result from such conditions as urinary tract infections and catheterization.*	**oxybutynin** ŏk-sē-BŪ-tĭ-nĭn Ditropan
diuretics	Promote and increase the excretion of urine. *Diuretics are grouped by their action and are used to treat edema, hypertension, heart failure, and various renal and hepatic diseases.*	**furosemide** fū-RŌ-sĕ-mīd Lasix **spironolactone** spī-rō-nō-LĂK-tōn Aldactone
potassium supplements	Replace potassium due to depletion caused by diuretics. *Dietary sources of potassium are usually not sufficient to replace potassium loss caused by diuretics.*	**potassium chloride** pō-TĂS-ē-ŭm KLŌ-rīd K-Tab, Kaon Cl
Male Reproductive System		
androgens	Increase testosterone levels. *Androgens are used to correct hormone deficiency in hypogonadism and treat delayed puberty in males.*	**testosterone base** tĕs-TŎS-tĕr-ōn Androderm, Testim **testosterone cypionate** tĕs-TŎS-tĕr-ōn SĬP-ē-ō-nāt Depo-testosterone

Table 11-1	**Drugs Used to Treat Genitourinary Disorders—cont'd**	
Classification	**Therapeutic Action**	**Generic and Trade Names**
anti-impotence agents	Treat erectile dysfunction (impotence) by increasing blood flow to the penis, resulting in an erection.	**sildenafil citrate** sĭl-DĔN-ă-fĭl SĬT-rāt Viagra
	Anti-impotence drugs should not be used by patients with coronary artery disease or hypertension.	**vardenafil** văr-DĔN-ă-fĭl Levitra

Abbreviations

This section introduces genitourinary–related abbreviations and their meanings.

Abbreviation	Meaning	Abbreviation	Meaning
AGN	acute glomerulonephritis	**ESRD**	end-stage renal disease
ARF	acute renal failure	**ESWL**	extracorporeal shock-wave lithotripsy
ATN	acute tubular necrosis	**EU**	excretory urography
BNO	bladder neck obstruction	**GU**	genitourinary
BPH	benign prostatic hyperplasia; benign prostatic hypertrophy	**HD**	hemodialysis; hip disarticulation; hearing distance
BUN	blood urea nitrogen	**HTN**	hypertension
C&S	culture and sensitivity	**IVP**	intravenous pyelogram, intravenous pyelography
Cath	catheterization; catheter	**K**	potassium (an electrolyte)
CT	computed tomography	**KUB**	kidney, ureter, bladder
cysto	cystoscopy	**Na**	sodium (an electrolyte)
DRE	digital rectal examination	**PCNL**	percutaneous nephrolithotomy
EBT	external beam therapy	**pH**	symbol for degree of acidity or alkalinity
ED	erectile dysfunction; emergency department	**PKD**	polycystic kidney disease
EMG	electromyogram, electromyography	**PSA**	prostate-specific antigen

Abbreviations

Abbreviation	Meaning	Abbreviation	Meaning
RP	retrograde pyelogram, retrograde pyelography	UA	urinalysis
sp. gr.	specific gravity	UTI	urinary tract infection
TSE	testicular self-examination	VCUG	voiding cystourethrography prostate
TURP	transurethral resection of the	VUR	vesicoureteral reflux

It is time to review procedures, pharmacology, and abbreviations by completing Learning Activity 11–5.

LEARNING ACTIVITIES

The activities that follow provide review of the genitourinary system terms introduced in this chapter. Complete each activity and review your answers to evaluate your understanding of the chapter.

Learning Activity 11-1

Identifying Urinary Structures

Label the following illustration using the terms listed below.

hilum	*renal cortex*	*renal vein*	*urethra*	*urinary meatus*
left kidney	*renal medulla*	*right kidney*	*ureteral orifice*	
renal artery	*renal pelvis*	*ureters*	*urinary bladder*	

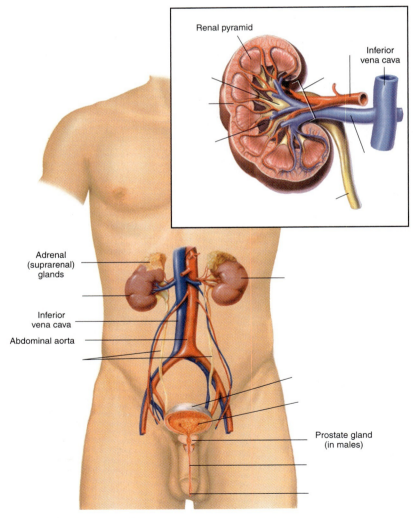

Renal pyramid

Inferior vena cava

Adrenal (suprarenal) glands

Inferior vena cava

Abdominal aorta

Prostate gland (in males)

 Check your answers by referring to Figure 11–1 on page 311. Review material that you did not answer correctly.

Identifying Male Reproductive Structures

Label the following illustration using the terms listed below.

bulbourethral gland	*prepuce*	*testis*
ejaculatory duct	*prostate gland*	*urethra*
epididymis	*scrotum*	*urethral orifice*
glans penis	*seminal vesicle*	*vas deferens*
penis	*seminiferous tubules*	

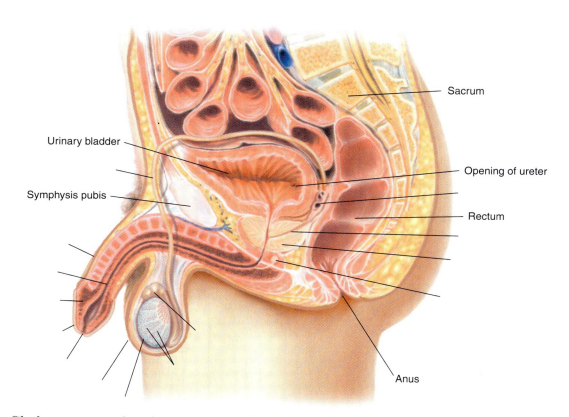

Urinary bladder

Symphysis pubis

Sacrum

Opening of ureter

Rectum

Anus

 Check your answers by referring to Figure 11–3 on page 314. Review material that you did not answer correctly.

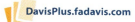 **DavisPlus.fadavis.com**

Enhance your study and reinforcement of word elements with the power of DavisPlus. Visit www.davisplus.fadavis.com/gylys/systems for this chapter's flash-card activity. We recommend you complete the flash-card activity before completing Activity 11–3 below.

Learning Activity 11-3
Building Medical Words

Use *nephr/o* (kidney) to build words that mean:

1. stone in the kidney _____
2. abnormal condition of pus in the kidney _____
3. abnormal condition of water in the kidney _____

Use *pyel/o* (renal pelvis) to build words that mean:

4. dilation of renal pelvis _____
5. disease of renal pelvis _____

Use *ureter/o* (ureter) to build words that mean:

6. dilation of ureter _____
7. calculus in ureter _____

Use *cyst/o* (bladder) to build words that mean:

8. inflammation of bladder _____
9. instrument to view the bladder _____

Use *vesic/o* (bladder) to build words that mean:

10. herniation of bladder _____
11. pertaining to bladder and prostate _____

Use *urethr/o* (urethra) to build words that mean:

12. narrowing or stricture of urethra _____
13. instrument used to incise urethra _____

Use *ur/o* (urine, urinary tract) to build words that mean:

14. radiography of urinary tract _____
15. disease of urinary tract _____

Use the suffix *-uria* (urine) to build words that mean:

16. difficult or painful urination _____
17. scanty urination _____

Use *orchid/o* or *orchi/o* (testes) to build words that mean:

18. disease of testes _____
19. pain in testes _____

Use *balan/o* (glans penis) to build a word that means:

20. discharge from glans penis _____

Build surgical words that mean:

21. excision of testes _____

22. surgical repair of glans penis _____

23. excision of vas deferens _____

24. incision of renal pelvis _____

25. fixation of bladder _____

Check your answers in Appendix A. Review material that you did not answer correctly.

Correct Answers _____ × 4 = _____ % Score

Matching Pathological, Diagnostic, Symptomatic, and Related Terms

Match the following terms with the definitions in the numbered list.

anorchidism	benign prostatic hyperplasia	hesitancy	oliguria
anuria	enuresis	hydrocele	phimosis
aspermia	epispadias	hydronephrosis	pyuria
azotemia	fistula	nephrotic syndrome	sterility
balanitis	herniorrhaphy	nocturia	urgency

1. _____ need to void immediately
2. _____ abnormal passage from a hollow organ to the surface or between organs
3. _____ complete absence of one or both testes
4. _____ absence of urine production
5. _____ nitrogenous wastes in blood
6. _____ dilation of kidneys and calices, usually due to reflux
7. _____ nonmalignant enlargement of the prostate gland
8. _____ difficulty starting urination
9. _____ scanty urine production
10. _____ loss of large amounts of plasma protein, resulting in systemic edema
11. _____ stenosis of the preputial orifice
12. _____ inability to produce offspring
13. _____ malformation in which the urethra opens on the dorsum of the penis
14. _____ lack of or failure to ejaculate semen
15. _____ pus in urine
16. _____ suture of a hernia
17. _____ excessive urination at night
18. _____ involuntary passage of urine
19. _____ accumulation of fluid in a saclike cavity
20. _____ inflammation of skin covering the penis

Check your answers in Appendix A. Review any material that you did not answer correctly.

Correct Answers _____ × 5 = _____ % Score

Matching Procedures, Pharmacology, and Abbreviations

Match the following terms with the definitions in the numbered list.

androgens	*diuretics*	*potassium supplements*
antibiotics	*ESWL*	*PSA*
C&S	*KUB*	*semen analysis*
circumcision	*orchidectomy*	*urethrotomy*
cystoscopy	*peritoneal dialysis*	*vasectomy*

1. _____ radiograph that shows the size, shape, and location of the kidneys
2. _____ test used to verify sterility after vasectomy
3. _____ visual examination of the urinary bladder
4. _____ inhibit or kill bacterial microorganisms
5. _____ laboratory test that evaluates effect of an antibiotic on an organism
6. _____ drugs used to promote the excretion of urine
7. _____ incision of a urethral stricture
8. _____ noninvasive test used to pulverize urinary or bile stones
9. _____ removal of toxic substances by perfusing the peritoneal cavity
10. _____ blood test to detect prostatic disorders, especially cancer
11. _____ most effective form of male contraception
12. _____ surgical removal of the testes
13. _____ surgical removal of all or part of the foreskin
14. _____ used to increase testosterone levels
15. _____ used to treat or prevent the hypokalemia commonly associated with the use of diuretics

✓ *Check your answers in Appendix A. Review material that you did not answer correctly.*

Correct Answers _____ × 6.67 = _____ % Score

MEDICAL RECORD ACTIVITIES

The two medical records included in the following activities use common clinical scenarios to show how medical terminology is used to document patient care. Complete the terminology and analysis sections for each activity to help you recognize and understand terms related to the genitourinary system.

Medical Record Activity 11-1
Operative Report: Ureterocele and Ureterocele Calculus

Terminology

Terms listed in the following table are taken from *Operative report: Ureterocele and ureterocele calculus* that follows. Use a medical dictionary such as *Taber's Cyclopedic Medical Dictionary*, the appendices of this book, or other resources to define each term. Then review the pronunciations for each term and practice by reading the medical record aloud.

Term	Definition
calculus KĂL-kū-lŭs	
cystolithotripsy sĭs-tō-LĬTH-ō-trĭp-sē	
cystoscope SĬST-ō-skōp	
fulguration fŭl-gŭ-RĀ-shŭn	
hematuria hē-mă-TŪ-rē-ă	
resectoscope rē-SĔK-tō-skōp	
transurethral trăns-ū-RĒ-thrăl	
ureterocele ū-RĒ-tĕr-ō-sēl	
urethral sound ū-RĒ-thrăl	

Listen and Learn Online! *will help you master the pronunciation of selected medical words from this medical record activity. Visit* www.davisplus.com/gylys/systems *to find instructions on completing the* Listen and Learn Online! *exercise for this section and to practice pronunciations.*

OPERATIVE REPORT: URETEROCELE AND URETEROCELE CALCULUS

General Hospital

1511 Ninth Avenue ■■ **Sun City, USA 12345** ■■ **(555) 802-1887**

OPERATIVE REPORT

Date: May 14, 20xx   Physician: Elmer Augustino, MD
Patient: Motch, Edwin   Patient: ID#: 48778

PREOPERATIVE DIAGNOSIS: Hematuria with left ureterocele and ureterocele calculus.

POSTOPERATIVE DIAGNOSIS: Hematuria with left ureterocele and ureterocele calculus.

OPERATION: Cystoscopy, transurethral incision of ureterocele, extraction of stone, and cystolithotripsy.

ANESTHESIA: General.

COMPLICATIONS: None.

PROCEDURE: Patient was prepped and draped and placed in the lithotomy position. The urethra was calibrated with ease using a #26 French Van Buren urethral sound. A #24 resectoscope was inserted with ease. The prostate and bladder appeared normal, except for the presence of a left ureterocele, which was incised longitudinally; a large calculus was extracted from the ureterocele. There was minimal bleeding and no need for fulguration. The stone was crushed with the Storz stone-crushing instrument, and the fragments were evacuated. The bladder was emptied and the procedure terminated.

Patient tolerated the procedure well and was transferred to the postanesthesia care unit.

Elmer Augustino, MD
Elmer Augustino, MD

ea:bg

D: 5-14-20xx
T: 5-14-20xx

Analysis

Review the medical record *Operative Report: Ureterocele and Ureterocele Calculus* to answer the following questions.

1. What were the findings from the resectoscopy?

_____

2. What was the name and size of the urethral sound used in the procedure?

_____

3. What is the function of the urethral sound?

_____

4. In what direction was the ureterocele incised?

_____

5. Was fulguration required? Why or why not?

_____

Medical Record Activity 11-2
Operative Report: Extracorporeal Shock-Wave Lithotripsy

Terminology

Terms listed in the following table are taken from the *Operative Report: Extracorporeal Shock-Wave Lithotripsy* that follows. Use a medical dictionary such as *Taber's Cyclopedic Medical Dictionary*, the appendices of this book, or other resources to define each term. Then review the pronunciations for each term and practice by reading the medical record aloud.

Term	Definition
calculus KĂL-kū-lŭs	
calyx KĀ-lĭx	
cystoscope SĬST-ō-skōp	
cystoscopy sĭs-TŎS-kō-pē	
dorsal lithotomy DOR-săl lĭth-ŎT-ō-mē	
ESWL	
extracorporeal ĕks-tră-kor-POR-ē-ăl	
fluoroscopy floo-or-ŎS-kō-pē	

Term	Definition
lithotripsy LĬTH-ō-trĭp-sē	
Lt	
shock-wave	
staghorn calculus STĂG-horn KĂL-kū-lŭs	
stent stĕnt	

 Listen and Learn Online! *will help you master the pronunciation of selected medical words from this medical record activity. Visit* www.davisplus.com/gylys/systems *to find instructions on completing the* Listen and Learn Online! *exercise for this section and to practice pronunciations.*

OPERATIVE REPORT: EXTRACORPOREAL SHOCK-WAVE LITHOTRIPSY

General Hospital

1511 Ninth Avenue ■■ **Sun City, USA 12345** ■■ **(555) 802-1887**

OPERATIVE REPORT

Date: April 1, 20xx
Patient: Marino, Julius

Physician: Elmer Augustino, MD
Room: 7201

PREOPERATIVE DIAGNOSIS: Left renal calculus.

POSTOPERATIVE DIAGNOSIS: Left renal calculus.

PROCEDURE: Extracorporeal shock-wave lithotripsy, cystoscopy with double-J stent removal

INDICATION FOR PROCEDURE: This 69-year-old male had undergone ESWL on 5/15/xx, with double-J stent placement to allow stone fragments to pass from the calyx to the bladder. At that time, approximately 50% of a partial staghorn calculus was fragmented. He now presents for the fragmenting of the remainder of the calculus and removal of the double-J stent.

ANESTHESIA: General.

COMPLICATIONS: None.

OPERATIVE TECHNIQUE: Patient was brought to the Lithotripsy Unit and placed in the supine position on the lithotripsy table. After induction of anesthesia, fluoroscopy was used to position the patient in the focal point of the shock waves. Being well positioned, he was given a total of 4,000 shocks with a maximum power setting of 3.0. After confirming complete fragmentation via fluoroscopy, the patient was transferred to the cystoscopy suite.

Patient was placed in the dorsal lithotomy position and draped and prepped in the usual manner. A cystoscope was inserted into the bladder through the urethra. Once the stent was visualized, it was grasped with the grasping forceps and removed as the scope was withdrawn.

Patient tolerated the procedure well and was transferred to recovery.

Elmer Augustino, MD
Elmer Augustino, MD

ea:bg

D: 5-14-20xx
T: 5-14-20xx

Analysis

Review the medical record *Operative Report: Extracorporeal Shock–Wave Lithotripsy* to answer the following questions.

1. What previous procedures were performed on the patient?

_____

2. Why is this current procedure being performed?

_____

3. What imaging technique was used for positioning the patient to ensure that the shock waves would strike the calculus?

_____

4. In what position was the patient placed in the cystoscopy suite?

_____

5. How was the double-J stent removed?

_____

Female Reproductive System

Chapter Outline

Objectives

Upon completion of this chapter, you will be able to:

- Locate and describe the structures of the female reproductive system.
- Describe the functional relationship between the female reproductive system and other body systems.
- Recognize, pronounce, spell, and build words related to the female reproductive system.
- Describe pathological conditions, diagnostic and therapeutic procedures, and other terms related to the female reproductive system.
- Explain pharmacology related to the treatment of female reproductive disorders.
- Demonstrate your knowledge of this chapter by completing the learning and medical record activities.

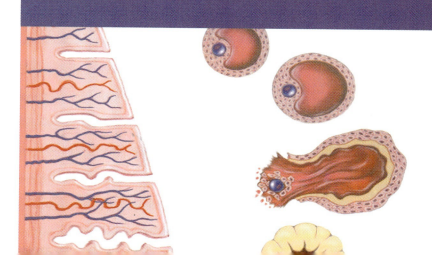

Anatomy and Physiology

The female reproductive system is composed of internal and external organs of reproduction. (See Figure 12–1.) The internal organs include the (1) **ovaries,** (2) **fallopian tubes,** (3) **uterus,** (4) **vagina,** and external genitalia. The external genitalia are collectively known as the *vulva.* Included in these structures are the (5) **labia minora,** (6) **labia majora,** (7) **clitoris,** (8) **Bartholin glands,** and **mons pubis,** an elevation of adipose tissue covered by skin and coarse pubic hair that cushions the **pubis (pubic bone).**

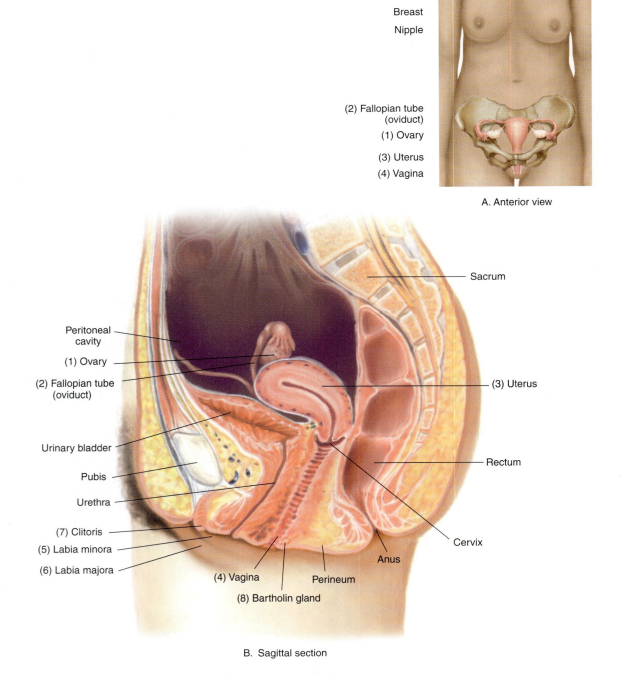

A. Anterior view

B. Sagittal section

Figure 12-1. Female reproductive system. (A) Anterior view. (B) Sagittal section showing organs within the pelvic cavity.

Anatomy and Physiology

This section introduces important female reproductive system terms and their definitions. Word analyses for selected terms are also provided.

Term	Definition
external genitalia jĕn-ĭ-TĀL-ē-ă	The sex, or reproductive, organs visible on the outside of the body; also called *genitals* *The external female genitalia, also known as the* **vulva.** *Male genitalia include the penis, scrotum, and testicles.*
gestation jĕs-TĀ-shŭn *gest:* pregnancy *-ation:* process (of)	Length of time from conception to birth *The human gestational period typically extends approximately 280 days from the last menstrual period. Gestation (pregnancy) of less than 36 weeks is regarded as premature.*
lactation lăk-TĀ-shŭn *lact:* milk *-ation:* process (of)	Production and release of milk by mammary glands
orifice OR-ĭ-fĭs	Mouth; entrance or outlet of any anatomical structure
puerperium pū-ĕr-PĒ-rē-ŭm	Time after childbirth that lasts approximately 6 weeks, during which the anatomical and physiological changes brought about by pregnancy resolve and a woman adjusts to the new or expanded responsibilities of motherhood and nonpregnant life

Pronunciation Help	Long Sound	ā—rate	ē—rebirth	ī—isle	ō—over	ū—unite
	Short Sound	ă—alone	ĕ—ever	ĭ—it	ŏ—not	ŭ—cut

Female Reproductive Organs

The female reproductive organs include the ovaries, fallopian tubes, uterus, and vagina. They are designed to produce **ova** (female reproductive cells), transport the cells to the site of fertilization, provide a favorable environment for a developing fetus through pregnancy and childbirth, and produce female sex hormones. Hormones play an important role in the reproductive process, providing their influence at critical times during preconception, fertilization, and gestation. (See Figure 12–2.)

Ovaries

The (1) **ovaries** are almond-shaped glands located in the pelvic cavity, one on each side of the uterus. Each ovary contains thousands of tiny, saclike structures called (2) **graafian follicles,** each containing an ovum. When an ovum ripens, the (3) **mature follicle** moves to the surface of the ovary, ruptures, and releases the ovum; a process called *ovulation.* After ovulation, the empty follicle is transformed into a structure called the (4) **corpus luteum,** a small yellow mass that secretes estrogen and progesterone. The corpus luteum degenerates at the end of a nonfertile cycle. Estrogen and progesterone influence the menstrual cycle and menopause. They also prepare the uterus for implantation of the fertilized egg, help maintain pregnancy, promote growth of the placenta, and play an important role in development of secondary sex characteristics. (See Chapter 13, Endocrine System.)

Fallopian Tubes

Two (5) **fallopian tubes (oviducts, uterine tubes)** extend laterally from superior angles of the uterus. The (6) **fimbriae** are fingerlike projections that create wavelike currents in fluid surrounding the ovary to move the ovum into the uterine tube. If the egg unites with a spermatozoon, the male reproductive cell, fertilization or conception takes place. If conception does not occur, the ovum disintegrates within 48 hours and is discharged through the vagina.

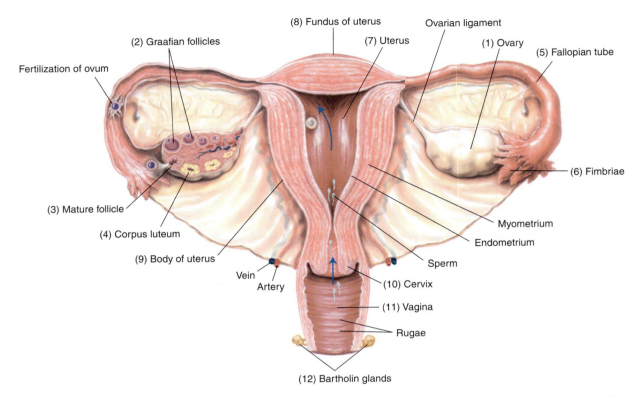

Figure 12-2. Anterior view of the female reproductive system. The developing follicles are shown in the sectioned left cavity.

Uterus and Vagina

The (7) **uterus** contains and nourishes the embryo from the time the fertilized egg is implanted until the fetus is born. It is a muscular, hollow, inverted–pear-shaped structure located in the pelvic area between the bladder and rectum. The uterus is normally in a position of **anteflexion** (bent forward) and consists of three parts: the (8) **fundus,** the upper, rounded part; the (9) **body,** the central part; and the (10) **cervix,** also called the *neck of the uterus* or *cervix uteri,* the inferior constricted portion that opens into the vagina.

The (11) **vagina** is a muscular tube that extends from the cervix to the exterior of the body. Its lining consists of folds of mucous membrane that give the organ an elastic quality. During sexual excitement, the vaginal **orifice** is lubricated by secretions from (12) **Bartholin glands.** In addition to serving as the organ of sexual intercourse and receptor of semen, the vagina discharges menstrual flow. It also acts as a passageway for the delivery of the fetus. The **clitoris,** located anterior to the vaginal orifice, is composed of erectile tissue that is richly innervated with sensory endings. The clitoris is similar in structure to the penis in the

male, but is smaller and has no urethra. The area between the vaginal orifice and the anus is known as the **perineum.** During childbirth, this area may be surgically incised to enlarge the vaginal opening for delivery. If the incision is made, the procedure is called an *episiotomy.*

Mammary Glands

Although mammary glands (breasts) are present in both sexes, they function only in females. (See Figure 12–3.) The breasts are not directly involved in reproduction but become important after delivery. Their biological role is to secrete milk for the nourishment of the newborn; a process called lactation. Breasts begin to develop during puberty as a result of periodic stimulation of the ovarian hormones estrogen and progesterone and are fully developed by age 16. Estrogen is responsible for the development of (1) **adipose tissue,** which enlarges the size of the breasts until they reach full maturity. Breast size is primarily determined by the amount of fat around the glandular tissue but is not indicative of functional ability. Each breast is composed of

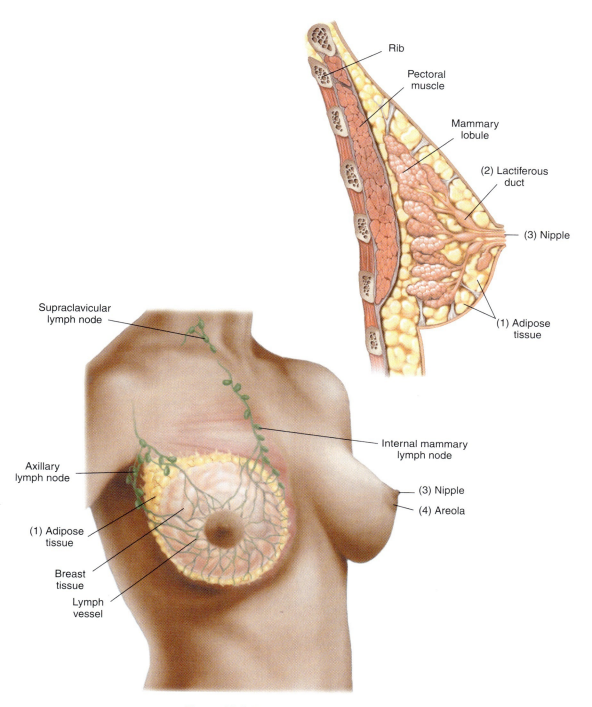

Figure 12-3. Structure of mammary glands.

15 to 20 lobules of milk-producing glands that are drained by a (2) **lactiferous duct,** which opens on the tip of the raised (3) **nipple.** Circling the nipple is a border of slightly darker skin called the (4) **areola.** During pregnancy, the breasts enlarge and remain so until lactation ceases. At menopause, breast tissue begins to atrophy.

Menstrual Cycle

Menarche, the initial menstrual period, occurs at puberty (about age 12) and continues approximately 40 years, except during pregnancy. The duration of the menstrual cycle is approximately 28 days, during which time several phases occur. (See Table 12–1.)

Table 12-1	**Changes in the Menstrual Cycle**

The menstrual cycle consists of a series of phases, during which the uterine endometrium changes as it responds to changing levels of ovarian hormones. These changes are outlined in the table below. In addition, see Figure 12–4 for a graphic representation of these changes.

Phase	Description
Menstrual	
Days 1 to 5	Uterine endometrium sloughs off because of hormonal stimulation; a process that is accompanied by bleeding. The detached tissue and blood are discharged through the vagina as menstrual flow.
Ovulatory	
Days 6 to 14	When menstruation ceases, the endometrium begins to thicken as new tissue is rebuilt. As estrogen level rises, several ova begin to mature in the graafian follicles with only one ovum reaching full maturity. At about the 14th day of the cycle, the graafian follicle ruptures, releasing the egg, a process called *ovulation*. The egg then leaves the ovary and travels down the fallopian tube toward the uterus.
Postovulatory	
Days 15 to 28	The empty graafian follicle fills with a yellow material and is now called the *corpus luteum*. Secretions of estrogen and progesterone by the corpus luteum stimulate the building of the endometrium in preparation for implantation of an embryo. If fertilization does not occur, the corpus luteum begins to degenerate as estrogen and progesterone levels decline.* With decreased hormone levels, the uterine lining begins to shed, the menstrual cycle starts over again, and the first day of menstruation starts.

* Some women experience a loose grouping of symptoms called *premenstrual syndrome (PMS)*. These symptoms usually occur about 5 days after the decline in hormones and include nervous tension, irritability, headaches, breast tenderness, and a feeling of depression.

Pregnancy

During pregnancy, the uterus changes its shape, size, and consistency. It increases greatly in size and muscle mass; houses the growing placenta, which nourishes the embryo-fetus; and expels the fetus after gestation. To prepare and serve as the birth canal at the end of pregnancy, the vaginal canal elongates as the uterus rises in the pelvis. The mucosa thickens, secretions increase, and vascularity and elasticity of the cervix and vagina become more pronounced.

The average pregnancy (**gestation**) lasts approximately 9 months and is followed by childbirth (**parturition**). Up to the third month of pregnancy, the product of conception is referred to as the *embryo*. From the third month to the time of birth, the unborn offspring is referred to as the *fetus*.

Pregnancy also causes enlargement of the breasts, sometimes to the point of pain. Many other changes occur throughout the body to accommodate the development and birth of the fetus. Toward the end of gestation, the myometrium begins to contract weakly at irregular intervals.

At this time, the full-term fetus is usually positioned head down within the uterus.

Labor and Childbirth

Labor is the physiological process by which the fetus is expelled from the uterus. Labor occurs in three stages. The first is the **stage of dilation,** which begins with uterine contractions and terminates when there is complete dilation of the cervix (10 cm). The second is the **stage of expulsion,** the time from complete cervical dilation to birth of the baby. The last stage is the **placental stage,** or **afterbirth.** This stage begins shortly after childbirth when the uterine contractions discharge the placenta from the uterus. (See Figure 12–5.)

Menopause

Menopause is cessation of ovarian activity and diminished hormone production that occurs at about age 50. Menopause is usually diagnosed if absence of menses (**amenorrhea**) has persisted for 1 year. The period in which symptoms of approaching

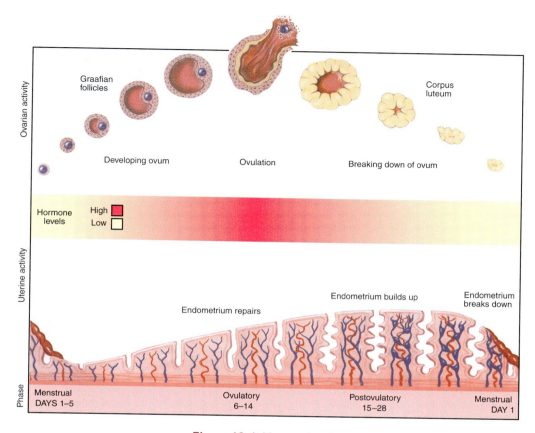

Ovarian activity

Graafian follicles

Developing ovum

Ovulation

Breaking down of ovum

Corpus luteum

Hormone levels

High

Low

Uterine activity

Endometrium repairs

Endometrium builds up

Endometrium breaks down

Phase

Menstrual DAYS 1–5

Ovulatory 6–14

Postovulatory 15–28

Menstrual DAY 1

Figure 12-4. Menstrual cycle.

menopause occur is also known as ***change of life*** or the ***climacteric***.

Many women experience hot flashes and vaginal drying and thinning (**vaginal atrophy**) as estrogen levels fall. Although **hormone replacement therapy (HRT)** has become more controversial, it is still used to treat vaginal atrophy and porous bones (**osteoporosis**), and is believed to play a role in heart attack prevention. Restraint in prescribing estrogens for long periods in all menopausal women arises from concern that there is an increased risk that long-term usage will induce neoplastic changes in estrogen-sensitive aging tissue.

 It is time to review anatomy by completing Learning Activities 12–1 and 12–2.

Pathology

Many female reproductive disorders are caused by infection, injury, or hormonal dysfunction. Although some disorders may be mild and correct themselves over time, others, such as those caused by infection, may require medical attention. Pain, itching, lesions, and discharge are signs and symptoms commonly associated with sexually transmitted diseases and must not be ignored. Other common problems of the female reproductive system are related to hormonal dysfunction that may cause menstrual disorders.

As a preventive measure, a pelvic examination should be performed regularly throughout life. This diagnostic procedure helps identify many pelvic abnormalities and diseases. Cytological and bacteriological specimens are usually obtained at the time of examination.

Gynecology is the branch of medicine concerned with diseases of the female reproductive organs and the breast. **Obstetrics** is the branch of medicine that manages the health of a woman and her fetus during pregnancy, childbirth, and the puerperium. Because of the obvious overlap between gynecology and obstetrics, many practices include both specialties. The physician who simultaneously practices these specialties is called an ***obstetrician/gynecologist***.

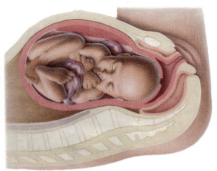

(1) Labor begins, membranes intact

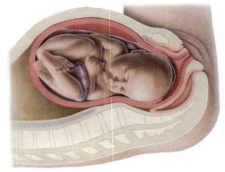

(2) Effacement of cervix,
which is now partially dilated

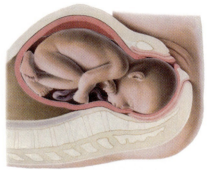

(3) When head reaches floor
of pelvis, it rotates

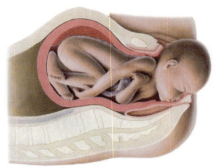

(4) Extension of the cervix allows head
to pass through

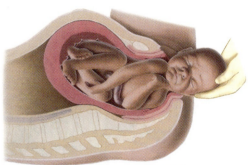

(5) Delivery of head, head rotates to
realign itself with body

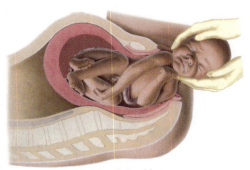

(6) Delivery of shoulders

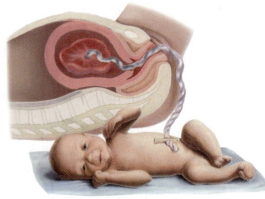

(7) Delivery of infant is complete,
uterus begins to contract

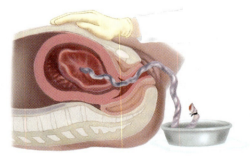

(8) Umbilical cord is cut, external massage
to uterus continues to stimulate
contractions, and placenta is delivered

Figure 12-5. Sequence of labor and childbirth.

Connecting Body Systems–Female Reproductive System

The main function of the female reproductive system is to provide structures that support fertilization and development of offspring. Should these structures be excised, childbearing would no longer be possible and the female production system would lose important functions. Other body systems, however, would continue to function normally. In other words, the female reproductive system depends on the other systems to support its functions, but only provides very limited support to the functions of other body systems. These limited functional relationships are summarized below.

Blood, lymph, and immune
- Female immune system has special mechanisms to inhibit its attack on sperm cells.
- Female reproductive tract secretes enzymes and acids that provide defense against entry of pathogens into the internal reproductive structures.

Cardiovascular
- Estrogens lower blood cholesterol levels and promote cardiovascular health in pre-menopausal women.

Digestive
- Estrogens have an effect on the metabolic rate.

Endocrine
- Estrogens produce hormones that provide a feedback mechanism which influences pituitary function.
- Estrogens assist in the production of human chorion gonadotropin hormone (HCG).

Genitourinary
- The female reproductive system provides the ovum needed to make fertilization by sperm possible.

Integumentary
- Female hormones affect growth and distribution of body hair.
- Female hormones influence the activity of sebaceous glands.
- Female hormones influence skin texture and fat distribution.

Musculoskeletal
- Estrogen influences muscle development and size.
- Estrogen influences bone growth, maintenance, and closure of epiphyseal plates.

Nervous
- Estrogen affects central nervous system development and sexual behavior.
- Estrogens provide antioxidants that have a neuroprotective function.

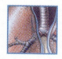

Respiratory
- Sexual arousal and pregnancy produce changes in rate and depth of breathing.
- Estrogen is believed to provide a beneficial effect on alveoli of the lungs.

Menstrual Disorders

Menstrual disorders are usually caused by hormonal dysfunction or pathological conditions of the uterus and may produce a variety of symptoms. Here are commmon disorder:

- Menstrual pain and tension (**dysmenorrhea**) may be the result of uterine contractions, pathological growths, or such chronic disorders as anemia, fatigue, diabetes, and tuberculosis. The female hormone estrogen is used to treat dysmenorrhea and also to regulate menstrual abnormalities.
- Irregular uterine bleeding between menstrual periods (**metrorrhagia**) or after menopause is usually symptomatic of disease, including benign or malignant uterine tumors. Consequently, early diagnosis and treatment are warranted. Metrorrhagia is probably the most significant form of menstrual disorder.

Medical Word Elements

This section introduces combining forms, suffixes, and prefixes related to the female reproductive system. Word analyses are also provided.

Element	Meaning	Word Analysis
Combining Forms		
amni/o	amnion (amniotic sac)	**amni/o**/centesis (ăm-nē-ō-sĕn-TĒ-sĭs): surgical puncture of the amniotic sac -*centesis:* surgical puncture *Amniocentesis is a transabdominal puncture performed under ultrasound guidance using a needle and syringe to remove amniotic fluid.*
cervic/o	neck; cervix uteri (neck of uterus)	**cervic**/itis (sĕr-vĭ-SĪ-tĭs): inflammation of the cervix -*itis:* inflammation
colp/o	vagina	**colp/o**/scopy (kŏl-PŎS-kō-pē): visual examination of the vagina -*scopy:* visual examination
vagin/o		**vagin/o**/cele (VĂJ-ĭn-ō-sēl): vaginal hernia; also called *colpocele* -*cele:* hernia, swelling
galact/o	milk	**galact/o**/poiesis (gă-lăk-tō-poy-Ē-sĭs): production of milk -*poiesis:* formation, production
lact/o		**lact/o**/gen (LĂK-tō-jĕn): forming or producing milk -*gen:* forming, producing, origin *Lactogen refers to any substance that stimulates milk production, such as a hormone.*
gynec/o	woman, female	**gynec/o**/logist (gī-nĕ-KŎL-ō-jĭst): physician specializing in treating disorders of the female reproductive system -*logist:* specialist in study of
hyster/o	uterus (womb)	**hyster**/ectomy (hĭs-tĕr-ĔK-tō-mē): excision of the uterus -*ectomy:* excision, removal

metri/o		endo/**metri**/al (ĕn-dō-MĒ-trē-ăl): pertaining to the lining of the uterus
		  endo-: in, within
		  -*al:* pertaining to, relating to

uter/o		**uter/o**/vagin/al (ū-tĕr-ō-VĂJ-ĭ-năl): relating to the uterus and vagina
		  vagin/o: vagina
		  -*al:* pertaining to

mamm/o	breast	**mamm/o**/gram (MĂM-ō-grăm): radiograph of the breast -*gram:* record, writing
mast/o		**mast/o**/pexy (MĂS-tō-pĕks-ē): surgical fixation of the breast(s) -*pexy:* fixation (of an organ) *Mastopexy is reconstructive, cosmetic surgery performed to affix sagging breasts in a more elevated position, commonly improving their shape.*
men/o	menses, menstruation	**men/o**/rrhagia (mĕn-ō-RĀ-jē-ă): bursting forth of the menses -*rrhagia:* bursting forth (of) *Menorrhagia is an excessive amount of menstrual flow over a longer duration than normal.*

Medical Word Elements—cont'd

Element	Meaning	Word Analysis
metr/o	uterus (womb); measure	**metr/o/ptosis** (mē-trō-TŌ-sĭs): prolapse or downward displacement of the uterus *-ptosis:* prolapse, downward displacement
nat/o	birth	pre/**nat**/al (prē-NĀ-tăl): pertaining to (time period) before birth *pre-:* before, in front *-al:* pertaining to
oophor/o	ovary	**oophor/oma** (ō-ŏf-ō-RŌ-mă): ovarian tumor *-oma:* tumor
ovari/o	ovary	**ovari/o/rrhexis** (ō-vā-rē-ō-RĔK-sĭs): rupture of an ovary *-rrhexis:* rupture
perine/o	perineum	**perine/o/rrhaphy** (pĕr-ĭ-nē-OR-ă-fē): suture of the perineum *-rrhaphy:* suture *Perineorrhaphy is used to repair an episiotomy or a laceration that occurs during delivery of the fetus.*
salping/o	tube (usually fallopian or eustachian [auditory] tubes)	**salping/o/plasty** (săl-PĬNG-gō-plăs-tē): surgical repair of a fallopian tube *-plasty:* surgical repair
Suffixes		
-arche	beginning	men/**arche** (mĕn-ĂR-kē): beginning of menstruation *men:* menses, menstruation
-cyesis	pregnancy	pseudo/**cyesis** (soo-dō-sī-Ē-sĭs): false pregnancy *pseudo-:* false *Pseudocyesis, also called* **false pregnancy,** *is a condition in which a woman develops bodily changes consistent with pregnancy when she is not pregnant.*
-gravida	pregnant woman	multi/**gravida** (mŭl-tĭ-GRĂV-ĭ-dă): woman who has been pregnant more than once *multi-:* many, much
-para	to bear (offspring)	nulli/**para** (nŭl-ĬP-ă-ră): woman who has never produced a viable offspring *nulli-:* none
-salpinx	tube (usually fallopian or eustachian [auditory] tubes)	hem/o/**salpinx** (hē-mō-SĂL-pĭnks): blood in a fallopian tube; also called *hematosalpinx* *hem/o:* blood Hemosalpinx *refers to a collection of blood in a fallopian tube, commonly associated with a tubal pregnancy.*
-tocia	childbirth, labor	dys/**tocia** (dĭs-TŌ-sē-ă): difficult childbirth *dys-:* bad; painful; difficult
-version	turning	retro/**version** (rĕt-rō-VĔR-shŭn): tipping or turning back (of an organ) *retro-:* backward, behind *Retroversion of the uterus occurs in one of every four otherwise healthy women.*

(continued)

Medical Word Elements—c[...]

Element	Meaning	Word A[...]
Prefixes		
ante-	before, in front of	**ante**/version (ăn-tē-VĔR-zhŭn): tipping or turning forward of an organ *-version:* turning
dys-	bad; painful; difficult	**dys**/men/o/rrhea (dĭs-mĕn-ō-RĒ-ă): painful menstruation *men/o:* menses, menstruation *-rrhea:* discharge, flow
endo-	in, within	**endo**/metr/itis (ĕn-dō-mē-TRĪ-tĭs): inflammation of (tissue) within the uterus *metr:* uterus (womb); measure *-itis:* inflammation
multi-	many, much	**multi**/para (mŭl-TĬP-ă-ră): woman who has delivered more than one viable infant *-para:* to bear (offspring)
post-	after	**post**/nat/al (pōst-NĀ-tăl): occurring after birth *nat:* birth *-al:* pertaining to
primi-	first	**primi**/gravida (prī-mĭ-GRĂV-ĭ-dă): woman during her first pregnancy *-gravida:* pregnant woman

It is time to review medical word elements by completing Learning Activity 12–3. For audio pronunciations of the above-listed key terms, you can visit www.davisplus.fadavis.com/gylys/systems to download this chapter's Listen and Learn! exercises or use the book's audio CD (if included).

• Profuse or prolonged bleeding during regular menstruation (**menorrhagia** or **hypermenorrhea**) may, during early life, be caused by endocrine disturbances. However, in later life, it is usually due to inflammatory diseases, fibroids, tumors, or emotional disturbances.

• **Premenstrual syndrome (PMS)** is a disorder with signs and symptoms that range from complaints of headache and fatigue to mood changes, anxiety, depression, uncontrolled crying spells, and water retention. Signs and symptoms involving almost every organ have been attributed to PMS. This syndrome occurs several days before the onset of menstruation and ends when menses begins or a short time after and appears to be related to hormonal changes. The reason most individuals with PMS seek medical assistance is related to mood change. Simple changes in behavior, such as an increase in exercise and a reduction in caffeine, salt, and alcohol use, may be beneficial.

Endometriosis

Endometriosis is the presence of functional endometrial tissue in areas outside the uterus. (See Figure 12–6.) The endometrial tissue develops into what are called **implants, lesions,** or **growths** and can cause pain, infertility, and other problems. The ectopic tissue is usually confined to the pelvic area but may appear anywhere in the abdominopelvic cavity. Like normal endometrial tissue, the ectopic endometrium responds to hormonal fluctuations of the menstrual cycle.

Pelvic and Vaginal Infections

Pelvic inflammatory disease (PID) is a general term for inflammation of the uterus, fallopian tubes, ovaries, and adjacent pelvic structures and is usually caused by bacterial infection. The infection may be confined to a single organ or it may involve all the internal reproductive organs. The disease-producing organisms (**pathogens**) generally enter through the vagina during coitus, induced

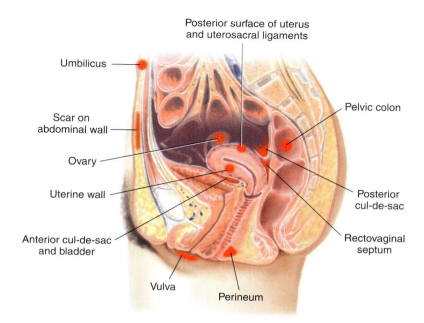

Figure 12-6. Endometriosis.

abortion, childbirth, or the postpartum period. As an ascending infection, the pathogens spread from the vagina and cervix to the upper structures of the female reproductive tract. Two of the most common causes of PID are gonorrhea and chlamydial infection, which are sexually transmitted diseases (STDs). Unless treated promptly, PID may result in scarring of the narrow fallopian tubes and the ovaries, causing sterility. The widespread infection of the reproductive structures can also lead to fatal septicemia. Because regions of the uterine tubes have an internal diameter slightly larger than the width of a human hair, the scarring and closure of the tubes is one of the major causes of female infertility.

Vaginitis

The vagina is generally resistant to infection because of the acidity of vaginal secretions. Occasionally, however, localized infections and inflammations occur from viruses, bacteria, or yeast. If confined to the vagina, these infections are called *vaginitis.* Although symptoms may be numerous and varied, the most common symptoms are genital itching, painful intercourse, and foul-smelling vaginal discharge. It is not uncommon for vaginitis to be accompanied by urethral inflammation (**urethritis**) because of the proximity of the urethra to the vagina. Two of the most common types of vaginitis are candidiasis and trichomoniasis.

Candidiasis, also called *moniliasis,* is caused by *Candida albicans,* a yeast that is present as part of the normal flora of the vagina. Steroid therapy, diabetes, or pregnancy may cause a change in the vaginal environment that disrupts the normal flora and promotes the overgrowth of this organism, resulting in a yeast (**fungal**) infection. The use of antibiotics may also disrupt the normal balance of microorganisms in the vagina by destroying "friendly bacteria," thus allowing the overpopulation of yeast. Antifungal agents (**mycostatics**) that suppress the growth of fungi are used to treat this disease.

Trichomoniasis, caused by the protozoan *Trichomonas vaginalis,* is now known to be one of the most common causes of sexually transmitted lower genital tract infections. Trichomoniasis is discussed more fully in the sexually transmitted disease section below.

Sexually Transmitted Disease

Sexually transmitted disease (STD), also called *venereal disease,* is any of several contagious diseases acquired as a result of sexual activity with an infected partner. As many as 20 different STDs have been identified, of which the newest and most serious is acquired immune deficiency syndrome (AIDS). (For a full description of AIDS, see Chapter 9, Blood, Lymph, and Immune Systems.) In the United States, the widespread occurrence of STDs is regarded as an epidemic. As a group, STDs are the single most important cause of reproductive disorders. Until recently, gonorrhea and syphilis were the most common STDs. However, over the past few decades, chlamydia has become the most widespread STD. Viral diseases, such as genital herpes and genital warts, are also increasing in prevalence. The current STDs of medical concern include gonorrhea, syphilis, chlamydia, genital herpes, genital warts, and trichomoniasis.

Gonorrhea

Gonorrhea is caused by the bacterium *Neisseria gonorrhoeae*. It involves the mucosal surface of the genitourinary tract and, possibly, the rectum and pharynx. This disease may be acquired through sexual intercourse and through orogenital and anogenital contact. Some women do not experience pain or manifest overt clinical symptoms (**asymptomatic**) until the disease has spread to the ovaries (**oophoritis**) and fallopian tubes (**salpingitis**), causing PID. The most common symptom of gonorrhea in women is a greenish yellow cervical discharge. The organism may infect the eyes of the newborn during vaginal delivery, which may result in blindness. As a precaution, silver nitrate is instilled in the eyes of newborns immediately after delivery as a preventive measure to ensure that this infection does not occur. The most common sign of gonorrhea in males is a discharge of pus from the penis. Other signs and symptoms include inflammation of the urethra (**urethritis**), which may cause painful urination (**dysuria**). If left untreated, the disease may infect the bladder (**cystitis**) and inflame the joints (**arthritis**). In addition, sterility may result from formation of scars that close the reproductive tubes of both sexes. Both sex partners must be treated because the infection can recur.

Syphilis

Although less common than gonorrhea, syphilis is the more serious of the two diseases. It is caused by infection with the bacterium *Treponema pallidum*. If left untreated, syphilis may become a chronic, infectious, multisystemic disease. Syphilis is characterized by three distinct phases. In the first phase, a primary sore (**chancre**) develops at the point where the organism enters the body. The chancre is an ulcerated sore with hard edges that contains contagious organisms. The second phase produces a variety of symptoms that make diagnosis of the disease difficult. The third phase is the latent phase whereby the disease may remain dormant for years.

Although there may be no symptoms of the disease during this time, the patient is nevertheless infectious. Symptoms may include blindness, insanity, and eventual death. Treatment with antibiotic therapy is effective.

Chlamydia

Chlamydia, caused by infection with the bacterium *Chlamydia trachomatis*, is the most prevalent and one of the most damaging STDs in the United States. In women, chlamydial infections are associated with mucopurulent discharge and inflammation of the cervix uteri (**cervicitis**) that may lead to PID. Chlamydia can be transmitted to the newborn baby during the birth process and cause a form of conjunctivitis or pneumonia. In men, chlamydial infections are associated with a whitish discharge from the penis that may lead to urethritis or epididymitis. Chlamydia in men, women, and babies can be successfully treated with antibiotics. However, many cases are asymptomatic, especially in women, and the disease commonly remains untreated until irreversible damage to the reproductive structures has occurred.

Genital Herpes

Genital herpes causes red, blisterlike, painful lesions that closely resemble the common fever blister or cold sore that appears on the lips and around the mouth. Although both diseases are caused by the herpes simplex virus (HSV), genital herpes is associated with type 2 (HSV-2), and oral herpes is associated with type 1 (HSV-1). Regardless, both forms can cause oral and genital infections through oral-genital sexual activity. Fluid in the blisters is highly infectious and contains the active virus. However, this disease is associated with a phenomenon called *viral shedding*. During viral shedding, the virus is present on the skin of the infected patient, and can be transmitted to sexual partners, even when no lesions are present. Individuals with herpes infection may have only one episode or may have repeated attacks that usually lessen in severity over the years. The disease may be transmitted to a baby during the birth process and, although rare, may lead to death of the infant. In females, lesions appear in the vaginal area, buttocks, and thighs. In men, lesions appear on the glans, foreskin, or penile shaft.

Genital Warts

Genital warts (**condylomas**) are caused by the human papillomavirus (HPV). Of the 100 identified types of HPV, only about 30 are spread through sexual contact. The warts may be very small and almost unnoticeable or may be large and appear in clusters. In females, the lesions may be found on the vulva, in the vagina, or on the cervix. In males, the lesions commonly appear on the penis or around the rectum. Many warts disappear without treatment, but there is no way to determine which ones will resolve. When treatment is required, surgical excision or freezing the wart is the usual method. HPV infection has been found to increase the risk of certain cancers, including penile, vaginal, cervical, and anal cancer. The virus is linked to 80% of all cases of invasive cervical cancer. Thus, women who have been diagnosed with HPV infection are urged to have Papanicolaou (Pap) tests every 6 months after diagnosis. There is also a much greater incidence of miscarriages in individuals with HPV disease.

Trichomoniasis

Trichomoniasis, caused by the protozoan *Trichomonas vaginalis*, affects males and females, but symptoms are more common in females. In women, it causes vaginitis, urethritis, and cystitis. Signs and symptoms include a frothy, yellow-green vaginal discharge with a strong odor. The infection may also cause discomfort during intercourse and urination. Irritation and itching in the female genital area and, in rare cases, lower abdominal pain can also occur. When symptoms are present in males, they include irritation inside the penis, mild discharge, or slight burning after urination or ejaculation. Treatment is generally very effective but reinfection is common if sexual partners are not treated simultaneously.

Uterine Fibroids

About 30% to 40% of all women develop benign tumors called *fibroids* (also called *leiomyomas* or, more commonly, *myomas*). These benign tumors develop slowly between ages 25 and 40 and commonly enlarge in response to fluctuating endocrine stimulation after this period. Although some individuals are asymptomatic with these types of tumors, when present they include menorrhagia, backache, constipation, and urinary symptoms. In addition, such tumors commonly cause metrorrhagia and even sterility.

Treatment of uterine fibroid tumors depends on their size and location. If the patient plans to have children, treatment is as conservative as possible. As a rule, large tumors that produce symptoms, such as pelvic pain and pressure accompanied by heavy menstrual periods (**menorrhagia**) or bleeding in between periods (**metrorrhagia**), should be removed. Usually, the uterus is removed (**hysterectomy**), but the ovaries are preserved. If the tumor is small, a myomectomy may be performed. However, when the tumor is producing excessive bleeding, the uterus and the tumor are excised.

Oncology

The two most common forms of cancer (CA) involving the female reproductive system are breast cancer and cervical cancer.

Breast Cancer

Breast cancer, also called *carcinoma of the breast,* is the most common malignancy of women in the United States. This disease appears to be associated with ovarian hormonal function. In addition, a diet high in fats appears to increase the incidence of breast cancer. Other contributing factors include a family history of the disease and, possibly, the use of hormone replacement therapy (HRT). Women who have not borne children (**nulliparous**) or those who have had an early onset of menstruation (**menarche**) or late onset of menopause are also more likely to develop breast cancer. Because this type of malignancy is highly responsive to treatment when detected early, women are urged to practice breast self-examination monthly and to receive periodic mammograms after age 40. Many breast malignancies are detected by the patient.

Cervical Cancer

Cancer of the cervix most commonly affects women between ages 40 and 49. Statistics indicate that infection associated with sexual activity has some relationship to the incidence of cervical cancer. First coitus at a young age, large number of sex partners, infection with certain sexually transmitted viruses, and frequent intercourse with men whose previous partners had cervical cancer are all associated with increased risk of developing cervical cancer.

The Pap test, a cytological examination, can detect cervical cancer before the disease becomes clinically evident. Abnormal cervical cytology routinely calls for colposcopy, which can detect the presence and extent of preclinical lesions requiring biopsy and histological examination. Treatment of cervical cancer consists of surgery, radiation, and chemotherapy. If left untreated, the cancer will eventually metastasize and lead to death.

Diagnostic, Symptomatic, and Related Terms

This section introduces diagnostic, symptomatic, and related terms and their meanings. Word analyses for selected terms are also provided.

Term	Definition
Female Reproductive System	
adnexa ăd-NĔK-să	Accessory parts of a structure *Adnexa uteri are the ovaries and fallopian tubes.*
atresia ă-TRĒ-zē-ă	Congenital absence or closure of a normal body opening, such as the vagina
choriocarcinoma kō-rē-ō-kăr-sĭ-NŌ-mă *chori/o:* chorion *carcin:* cancer *–oma:* tumor	Malignant neoplasm of the uterus or at the site of an ectopic pregnancy *Although its actual cause is unknown, choriocarcinoma is a rare tumor that may occur after pregnancy or abortion.*
contraceptive diaphragm kŏn-tră-SĔP-tĭv DĪ-ă-frăm	Contraceptive device consisting of a hemisphere of thin rubber bonded to a flexible ring; inserted into the vagina together with spermicidal jelly or cream up to 2 hours before coitus so that spermatozoa cannot enter the uterus, thus preventing conception
corpus luteum KOR-pŭs LŪ-tē-ŭm	Ovarian scar tissue that results from rupturing of a follicle during ovulation and becomes a small yellow body that produces progesterone after ovulation
dyspareunia dĭs-pă-RŪ-nē-ă	Occurrence of pain during sexual intercourse
endocervicitis ĕn-dō-sĕr-vĭ-SĪ-tĭs *endo–:* in, within *cervic:* neck; cervix uteri (neck of the uterus) *–itis:* inflammation	Inflammation of the mucous lining of the cervix uteri *Endocervicitis is usually chronic, commonly due to infection, and accompanied by cervical erosion.*
fibroids FĪ-broyds *fibr:* fiber, fibrous tissue *–oids:* resembling	Benign uterine tumors composed of muscle and fibrous tissue; also called *leiomyomas (myomas)* and *fibromyomata uteri* *Myomectomy or hysterectomy may be indicated if the fibroids grow too large, causing such symptoms as metrorrhagia, pelvic pain, and menorrhagia.*
infertility ĭn-fĕr-TĬL-ĭ-tē	Inability or diminished ability to produce offspring
hormonal contraception hor-MŌ-năl kŏn-tră-SĔP-shŭn	Use of hormones to suppress ovulation and prevent conception
oral contraceptive pills OR-ăl kŏn-tră-SĔP-tĭv	Birth control pills containing estrogen and progesterone in varying proportions *When taken according to schedule, oral contraceptive pills (OCPs) are about 98% effective.*

Diagnostic, Symptomatic, and Related Terms—cont'd

Term	Definition
menarche mĕn-ĂR-kē *men:* menses, menstruation *-arche:* beginning	Beginning of menstrual function
oligomenorrhea ŏl-ĭ-gō-mĕn-ō-RĒ-ă *olig/o:* scanty *men/o:* menses, menstruation *-rrhea:* discharge, flow	Scanty or infrequent menstrual flow
perineum pĕr-ĭ-NĒ-ŭm	Region between the vulva and anus that constitutes the pelvic floor
puberty PŪ-bĕr-tē	Period during which secondary sex characteristics begin to develop and the capability of sexual reproduction is attained
pyosalpinx pī-ō-SĂL-pĭnks *py/o:* pus *-salpinx:* tube (usually fallopian or eustachian [auditory] tubes)	Pus in the fallopian tube
retroversion rĕt-rō-VĔR-shŭn *retro-:* backward, behind *-version:* turning	Turning or state of being turned back, especially an entire organ, such as the uterus, being tipped from its normal position
sterility stĕr-ĬL-ĭ-tē	Inability of the female to become pregnant or the male to impregnate the female
vaginismus văj-ĭn-ĬZ-mŭs	Painful spasm of the vagina from contraction of its surrounding muscles
viable VĪ-ă-bl	Capable of sustaining life; denotes a fetus sufficiently developed to live outside of the uterus *A viable infant is one who at birth weighs at least 500 g or is 24 weeks or more of gestational age. Because an infant is determined viable does not mean the baby is born alive.*

Obstetrics

Term	Definition
abortion ă-BOR-shŭn	Termination of pregnancy before the embryo or fetus is capable of surviving outside the uterus
abruptio placentae ă-BRŬP-shē-ō plă-SĔN-tē	Premature separation of a normally situated placenta

(continued)

Diagnostic, Symptomatic, and Related Terms—cont'd

Term	Definition
amnion ĂM-nē-ŏn	Membrane, continuous with and covering the fetal side of the placenta, that forms the outer surface of the umbilical cord *The fetus is suspended in amniotic fluid.*
breech presentation	Common abnormality of delivery in which the fetal buttocks or feet present first rather than the head
Down syndrome, trisomy 21 SĬN-drŏm, TRĪ-sō-mē	Congenital condition characterized by physical malformations and some degree of mental retardation *Trisomy 21 is the occurrence of three copies of chromosome 21 rather than two copies and occurs in about 1 of 700 live births. The terms* **Down syndrome** *and* **trisomy 21** *are preferred to the term* **mongolism.**
dystocia dĭs-TŌ-sē-ă *dys-:* bad; painful; difficult *-tocia:* childbirth, labor	Difficult labor, which may be produced by the large size of the fetus or the small size of the pelvic outlet
eclampsia ĕ-KLĂMP-sē-ă	Most serious form of toxemia during pregnancy *Signs of eclampsia include high blood pressure, edema, convulsions, renal dysfunction, proteinuria, and, in severe cases, coma.*
ectopic pregnancy ĕk-TŎP-ĭk PRĔG-năn-sē	Pregnancy in which the fertilized ovum does not reach the uterine cavity but becomes implanted on any tissue other than the lining of the uterine cavity, such as a fallopian tube, an ovary, the abdomen, or even the cervix uteri *Kinds of ectopic pregnancy include* **abdominal pregnancy, ovarian pregnancy,** *and* **tubal pregnancy.** (See Figure 12–7.)
gravida GRĂV-ĭ-dă	Pregnant woman *The term* **gravida** *may be followed by numbers, indicating number of pregnancies, such as* **gravida** *1, 2, 3, 4 or I, II, III, IV, and so forth.*
multigravida mŭl-tĭ-GRĂV-ĭ-dă *multi-:* many, much *-gravida:* pregnant woman	Woman who has been pregnant more than once
multipara mŭl-TĬP-ă-ră *multi-:* many, much *-para:* to bear (offspring)	Woman who has delivered more than one viable infant
para PĂR-ă	Woman who has given birth to one or more viable infants *Para followed by a Roman numeral or preceded by a Latin prefix* (primi-, quadri-, *and so forth) designates the number of times a pregnancy has culminated in a single or multiple birth. For example,* **para** *I and* **primipara** *refer to a woman who has given birth for the first time.* **Para** *II refers to a woman who has given birth a second time. Whether the births were multiple (twins, triplets) is irrelevant.*

Diagnostic, Symptomatic, and Related Terms—cont'd

Term	Definition

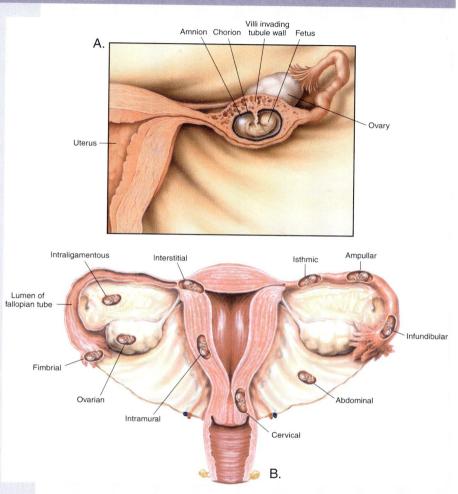

Figure 12-7. Ectopic pregnancy (A) and sites of ectopic pregnancy (B).

Term	Definition
parturition păr-tū-RĬSH-ŭn	Process of giving birth
pelvimetry pĕl-VĬM-ĕ-trē *pelv/i:* pelvis *-metry:* act of measuring	Measurement of pelvic dimensions to determine whether the head of the fetus will be able to pass through the bony pelvis during the delivery process *Measurement of the pelvis is usually determined by ultrasound during the early part of pregnancy. X-ray pelvimetry may be performed late in the pregnancy or during labor if more precise measurements are needed. The size of the pelvic outlet determines whether or not the baby is delivered vaginally or by cesarean section.*
placenta previa plă-SĔN-tă PRĒ-vē-ă	Condition in which the placenta is attached near the cervix and ruptures prematurely, with spotting as the early symptom *Prevention of hemorrhage may necessitate a cesarean delivery.*

(Continued)

Diagnostic, Symptomatic, and Related Terms—cont'd

Term	Definition
primigravida prī-mĭ-GRĂV-ĭ-dă *primi-:* first *-gravida:* pregnant woman	Woman pregnant for the first time
primipara prī-MĬP-ă-ră *primi-:* first *-para:* to bear (offspring)	Woman who has given birth to one viable infant, her first child, indicated by the notation *para I* on the patient's chart
puerperium pū-ĕr-PĒ-rē-ŭm	Period of 42 days after childbirth and expulsion of the placenta and membranes, during which the reproductive organs usually return to normal

 It is time to review pathological, diagnostic, symptomatic, and related terms by completing Learning Activity 12—4.

Diagnostic and Therapeutic Procedures

This section introduces procedures used to diagnose and treat female reproductive disorders. Descriptions are provided as well as pronunciations and word analyses for selected terms.

Procedure	Description
Diagnostic Procedures	
Clinical	
amniocentesis ăm-nē-ō-sĕn-TĒ-sĭs *amni/o:* amnion (amniotic sac) *-centesis:* surgical puncture	Transabdominal puncture of the amniotic sac under ultrasound guidance using a needle and syringe to remove amniotic fluid (See Figure 12—8.) *The sample obtained in amniocentesis is chemically and cytologically studied to detect genetic and biochemical disorders and fetal maturity. The procedure also enables transfusion of platelets or blood to the fetus and instillation of drugs for treating the fetus.*
insufflation ĭn-sŭ-FLĀ-shŭn	Delivery of pressurized air or gas into a cavity, chamber, or organ to allow visual examination, remove an obstruction, or apply medication *Insufflation is performed to increase the distance between structures so the physician can see more clearly and better diagnose possible disorders.*
tubal TŪ-băl	Test for patency of the uterine tubes made by transuterine insufflation with carbon dioxide; also called *Rubin test*
Endoscopic	
colposcopy kŏl-PŎS-kō-pē *colp/o:* vagina *-scopy:* visual examination	Visual examination of the vagina and cervix with an optical magnifying instrument (colposcope) *Colposcopy is used chiefly to identify areas of cervical dysplasia in women with abnormal Papanicolaou tests and as an aid in biopsy or excision procedures, including cautery, cryotherapy, and loop electrosurgical excision.*

Diagnostic and Therapeutic Procedures—cont'd

Procedure	Description

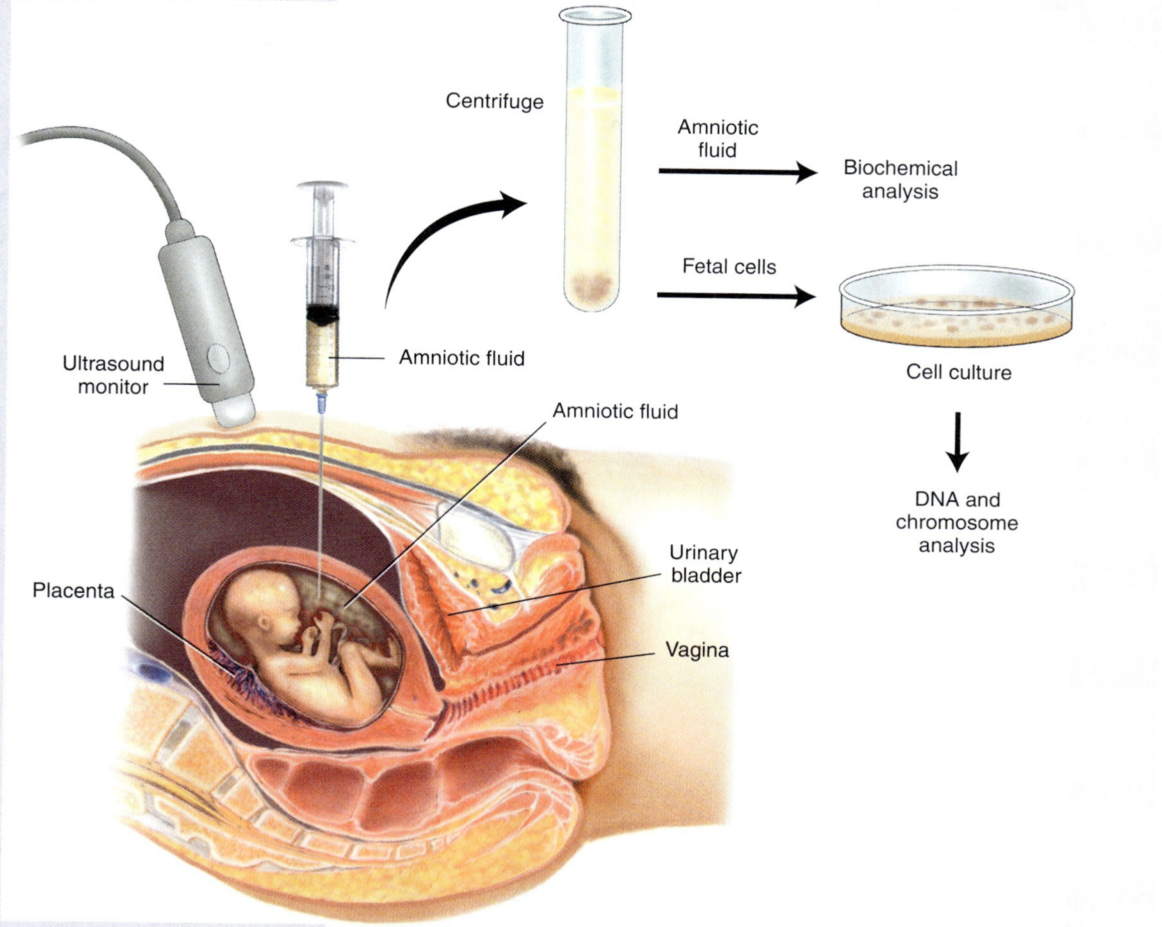

Figure 12-8. Amniocentesis.

laparoscopy
lăp-ăr-ŎS-kō-pē
lapar/o: abdomen
-scopy: visual examination

Visual examination of the abdominal cavity with a laparoscope through one or more small incisions in the abdominal wall, usually at the umbilicus (See Figure 12–9.)

Laparoscopy has become a standard technique for many routine surgical procedures, including gynecological sterilization by fulguration of the oviducts and tubal ligation.

Laboratory

chorionic villus sampling (CVS)
kor-ē-ŎN-ĭk VĬL-ŭs SĂM-plĭng

Sampling of placental tissues for prenatal diagnosis of potential genetic defects

In CVS, the sample is obtained through a catheter inserted into the uterus. The advantage of CVS over amniocentesis is that it can be undertaken in the first trimester of pregnancy.

(continued)

Diagnostic and Therapeutic Procedures—cont'd

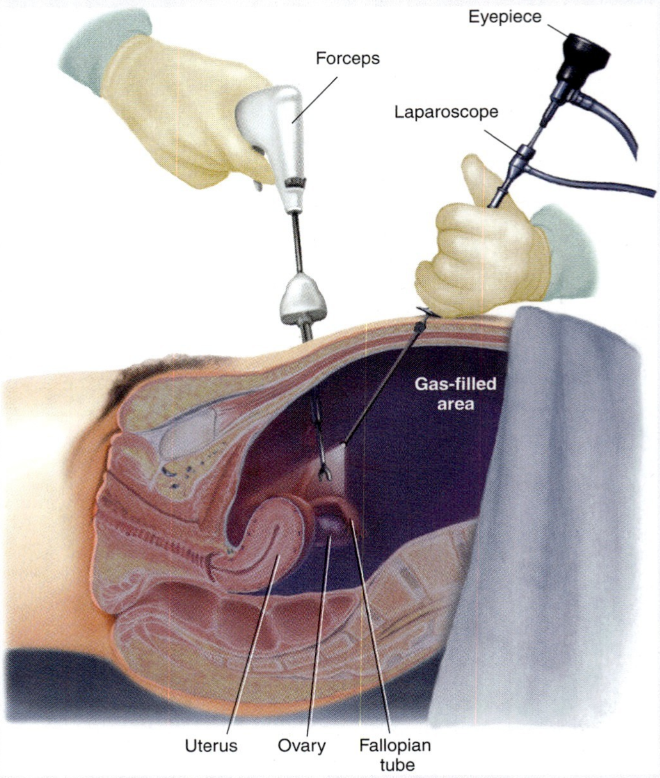

Procedure	Description

Figure 12-9. Laparoscopy.

Procedure	Description
endometrial biopsy ĕn-dō-MĒ-trē-ăl BĪ-ŏp-sē *endo-:* in, within *metri:* uterus (womb); measure *-al:* pertaining to, relating to	Removal of a sample of uterine endometrium for microscopic study *Endometrial biopsy is commonly used in fertility assessment to confirm ovulation and as a diagnostic tool to determine the cause of dysfunctional and postmenopausal bleeding.*
Papanicolaou (Pap) test pă-pă-NĬ-kō-lă-oo	Cytological study used to detect abnormal cells sloughed from the cervix and vagina, usually obtained during routine pelvic examination *A Pap test is commonly used to screen for and diagnose cervical cancer. It may also be used to evaluate cells from any organ, such as the pleura and peritoneum, to detect changes that indicate malignancy.*
Radiographic	
mammography măm-ŎG-ră-fē *mamm/o:* breast *-graphy:* process of recording	Radiographic examination of the breast to screen for breast cancer *Mammography is used to detect tumors, cysts, and microcalcifictions and may help locate a malignant lesion.*

Diagnostic and Therapeutic Procedures—cont'd

Procedure	Description
hysterosalpingography hĭs-tĕr-ō-săl-pĭn-GŎG-ră-fē *hyster/o:* uterus (womb) *salping/o:* tube (usually fallopian or eustachian [auditory] tube) *-graphy:* process of recording	Radiography of the uterus and uterine tubes (oviducts) following injection of a contrast medium *Hysterosalpingography is used to determine pathology in the uterine cavity, evaluate tubal patency, and determine the cause of infertility.*
ultrasonography (US) ŭl-tră-sŏn-ŎG-ră-fē *ultra-:* excess, beyond *son/o:* sound *-graphy:* process of recording	Process by which high-frequency sound waves (ultrasound) produce and display an image from reflected "echoes" on a monitor; also called *ultrasound, sonography,* and *echo*
pelvic PĔL-vĭk	US of the pelvic region used to evaluate abnormalities in the female reproductive system as well as the fetus in the obstetric patient
transvaginal trănz-VĂJ-ĭ-năl *trans-:* through, across *vagin:* vagina *-al:* pertaining to	US of the pelvic area performed with a probe inserted into the vagina, which provides sharper images of pathological and normal structures within the pelvis

Therapeutic Procedures

Surgical

Procedure	Description
breast implant revision	Surgery designed to correct an unsuccessful procedure that has created a cosmetic problem or poses a health risk *Breast implant revision is commonly performed to replace older silicone implants with new saline-filled implants.*
cerclage sĕr-KLĂZH	Suturing the cervix to prevent it from dilating prematurely during pregnancy, thus decreasing the chance of a spontaneous abortion. The sutures are removed prior to delivery *Cerclage is sometimes referred to as a "purse-string" procedure.*
cesarean birth sē-SĀR-ē-ăn	Incision of the abdomen and uterus to remove the fetus; also called *C-section* *Cesarean birth is most commonly used in the event of cephalopelvic disproportion, presence of sexually transmitted disease, fetal distress, and breech presentation.*
colpocleisis kŏl-pō-KLĪ-sĭs *colp/o:* vagina *-cleisis:* closure	Surgical closure of the vaginal canal
conization kŏn-ĭ-ZĀ-shŭn	Excision of a cone-shaped piece of tissue, such as mucosa of the cervix, for histological examination
cordocentesis kor-dō-sĕn-TĒ-sĭs	Sampling of fetal blood drawn from the umbilical vein and performed under ultrasound guidance *Cord blood is evaluated in the laboratory to identify hemolytic diseases or genetic abnormalities.*

(continued)

Diagnostic and Therapeutic Procedures—cont'd

Procedure	Description
cryosurgery krī-ō-SĔR-jĕr-ē	Process of freezing tissue to destroy cells; also called *cryocautery* *Cryosurgery is used for chronic cervical infections and erosions because offending organisms may be entrenched in cervical cells and glands. The process destroys these infected areas and, in the healing process, normal cells are replenished.*
dilatation and curettage (D&C) dĭl-ă-TĀ-shŭn, kū-rĕ-TĂZH	Widening of the cervical canal with a dilator and scraping of the uterine endometrium with a curette *D&C is used to obtain a sample for cytological examination of tissue, control abnormal uterine bleeding, and treat incomplete abortion.* (See Figure 12-10.)

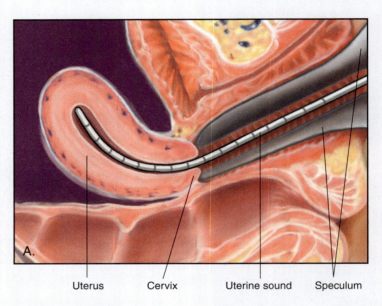

A.

| Uterus | Cervix | Uterine sound | Speculum |

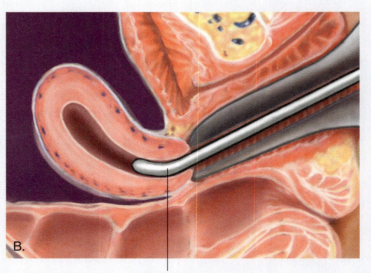

B.

Cervical dilator

Diagnostic and Therapeutic Procedures—cont'd

Procedure	Description

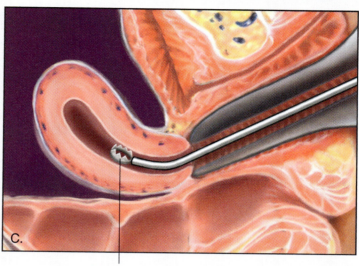

Serrated curet

Figure 12-10. Dilatation and curettage. (A) Examination of the uterine cavity with a uterine sound. (B) Dilatation of the cervix with a series of cervical dilators. (C) Curettage (scraping) of the uterine lining with a serrated uterine curet.

episiorrhaphy
ĕ-pĭs-ē-OR-ă-fē
episi/o: vulva
-rrhaphy: suture

Repair of a lacerated vulva or an episiotomy

episiotomy
ĕ-pĭs-ē-ŎT-ō-mē
episi/o: vulva
-tomy: incision

Incision of the perineum from the vaginal orifice usually done to prevent tearing of the tissue and to facilitate childbirth

hysterectomy
hĭs-tĕr-ĔK-tō-mē
hyster: uterus (womb)
-ectomy: excision, removal

Excision of the uterus (See Figure 12–11.)

Indications for hysterectomy include abnormalities of the uterus and cervix (cancer, severe dysfunctional bleeding, large or bleeding fibroid tumors, prolapse of the uterus, or severe endometriosis). The approach to excision may be abdominal or vaginal.

subtotal

Hysterectomy where the cervix, ovaries, and fallopian tubes remain

total

Hysterectomy where the cervix is removed but the ovaries and fallopian tubes remain; also called *complete hysterectomy*

total plus bilateral salpingo-oophorectomy
bī-LĂT-ĕr-ăl săl-pĭng-gō-ō-ŏf-ō-RĔK-tō-mē

Total (complete) hysterectomy, including uterus, cervix, fallopian tubes, and ovaries

intrauterine device
ĭn-tră-Ū-tĕr-ĭn

Plastic or metal object placed inside the uterus to prevent implantation of a fertilized egg in the uterine lining

(continued)

Diagnostic and Therapeutic Procedures—cont'd

Procedure	Description

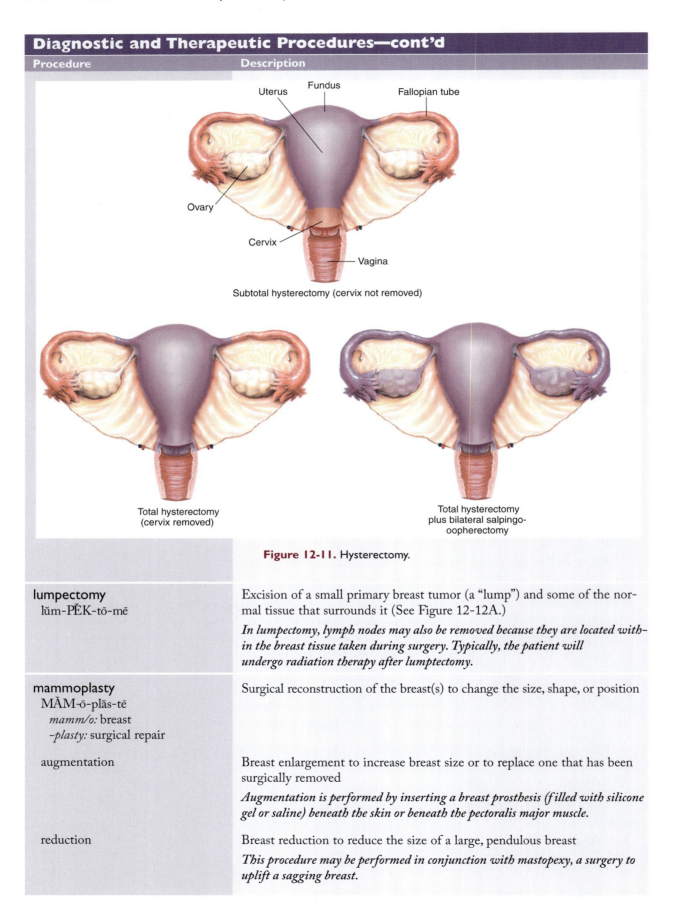

Subtotal hysterectomy (cervix not removed)

Total hysterectomy
(cervix removed)

Total hysterectomy
plus bilateral salpingo-
oopherectomy

Figure 12-11. Hysterectomy.

Procedure	Description
lumpectomy lŭm-PĔK-tō-mē	Excision of a small primary breast tumor (a "lump") and some of the normal tissue that surrounds it (See Figure 12-12A.) *In lumpectomy, lymph nodes may also be removed because they are located within the breast tissue taken during surgery. Typically, the patient will undergo radiation therapy after lumpectomy.*

mammoplasty
MĂM-ō-plăs-tē
  mamm/o: breast
  -plasty: surgical repair
	Surgical reconstruction of the breast(s) to change the size, shape, or position

augmentation	Breast enlargement to increase breast size or to replace one that has been surgically removed *Augmentation is performed by inserting a breast prosthesis (filled with silicone gel or saline) beneath the skin or beneath the pectoralis major muscle.*
reduction	Breast reduction to reduce the size of a large, pendulous breast *This procedure may be performed in conjunction with mastopexy, a surgery to uplift a sagging breast.*

Diagnostic and Therapeutic Procedures—cont'd

Procedure	Description
mastectomy măs-TĔK-tō-mē *mast:* breast *-ectomy:* excision, removal	Excision of the entire breast
total (simple)	Excision of the entire breast, nipple, areola, and the involved overlying skin; also called *simple mastectomy* *In total mastectomy, lymph nodes are removed only if they are included in the breast tissue being removed.*
modified radical	Excision of the entire breast, including the lymph nodes in the underarm (axillary dissection) (See Figure 12–12B.) *Most women who have mastectomies today have modified radical mastectomies.*
radical	Excision of the entire breast, all underarm lymph nodes, and chest wall muscles under the breast

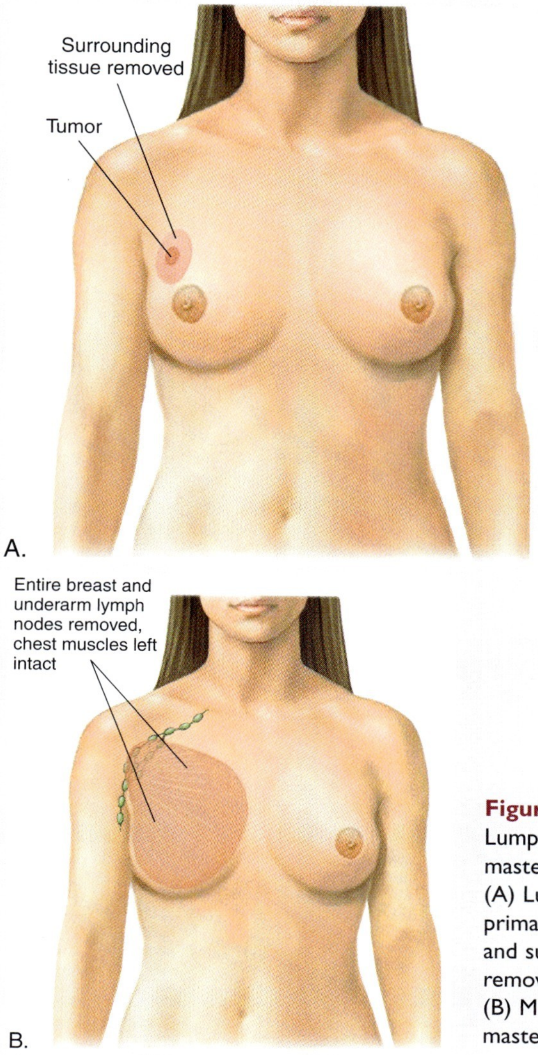

Surrounding tissue removed

Tumor

A.

Entire breast and underarm lymph nodes removed, chest muscles left intact

B.

Figure 12-12.
Lumpectomy and mastectomy.
(A) Lumpectomy with primary tumor in red and surrounding tissue removed in pink.
(B) Modified radical mastectomy.

(continued)

Diagnostic and Therapeutic Procedures—cont'd

Procedure	Description

myomectomy
mī-ō-MĔK-tō-mē
  my/o: muscle
  -ectomy: excision, removal
	Excision of a myomatous tumor, generally uterine

reconstructive breast surgery	Reconstruction of a breast that has been removed because of cancer or other disease *Reconstruction is commonly possible immediately following mastectomy so the patient awakes from anesthesia with a breast mound already in place.*
tissue (skin) expansion	Common breast reconstruction technique in which a balloon expander is inserted beneath the skin and chest muscle, saline solution is gradually injected to increase size, and the expander is then replaced with a more permanent implant (See Figure 12–13.)

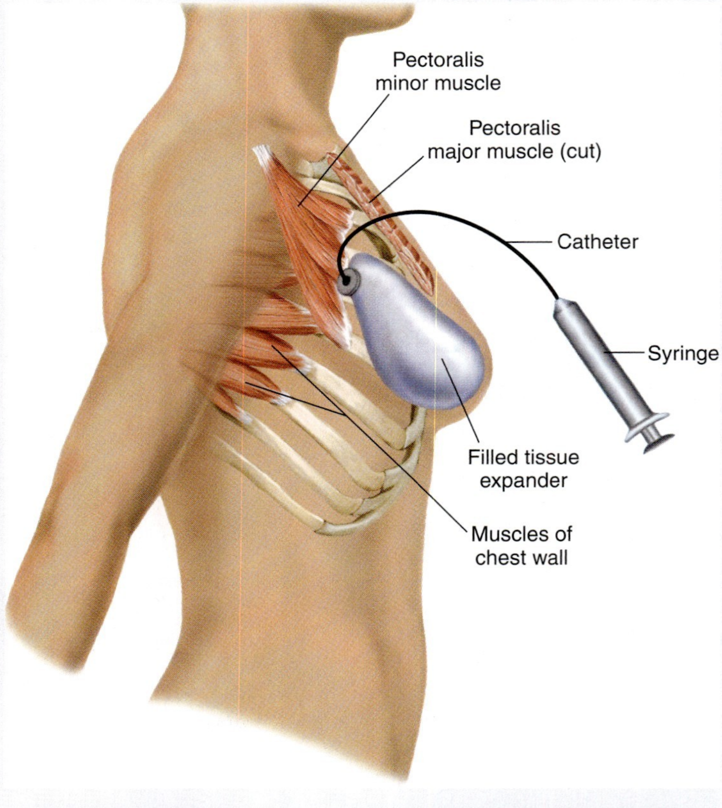

Figure 12-13. Tissue expander for breast reconstruction.

Diagnostic and Therapeutic Procedures—cont'd

Procedure	Description

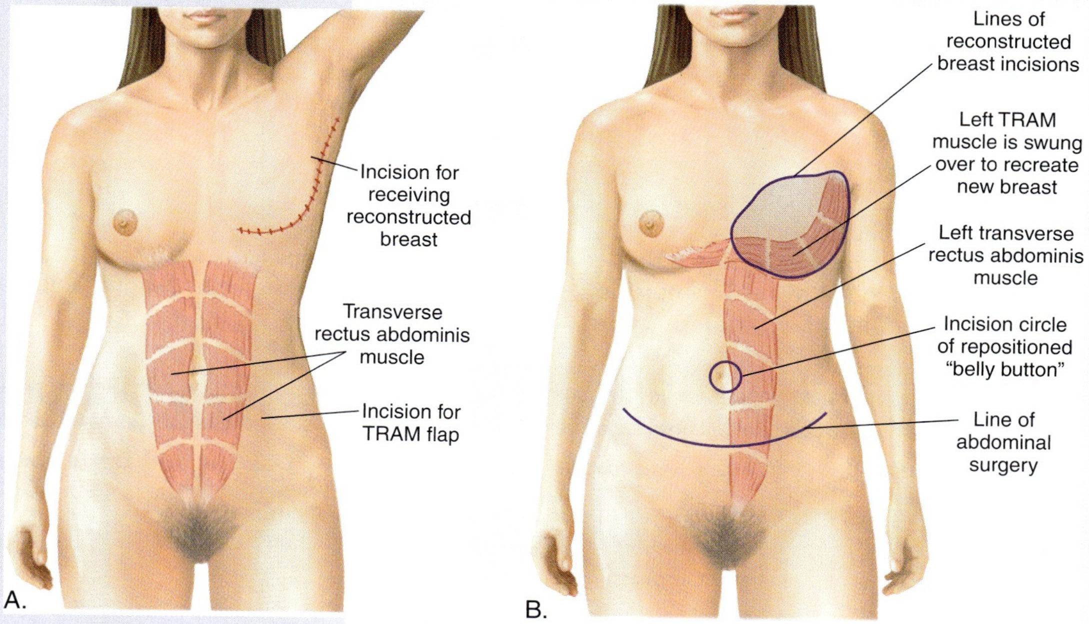

Figure 12-14. TRAM flap. (A) After mastectomy. (B) Process of TRAM reconstruction.

transverse rectus abdominis muscle (TRAM) flap	Surgical creation of a skin flap using skin and fat from the lower half of the abdomen which is passed under the skin to the breast area. The abdominal tissue (flap) is shaped into a natural-looking breast and sutured into place (See Figure 12–4.) *The TRAM flap procedure is a popular reconstruction option.*
salpingo-oophorectomy săl-pĭng-gō-ō-ŏf-ō-RĔK-tō-mē *salping/o:* tube (usually fallopian or eustachian [auditory] tubes) *oophor:* ovary *-ectomy:* excision, removal	Excision of an ovary and fallopian tube *A salpingo-oophorectomy is usually identified as* right, left, *or* bilateral.
tubal ligation TŪ-băl lī-GĀ-shŭn	Procedure that ties (ligates) the fallopian tubes to prevent pregnancy *Tubal ligation is a form of sterilization surgery that is usually performed during laparoscopy.*

Pharmacology

Hormones perform a vital role in reproduction and sexual development of the female. Hormone replacement therapy (HRT) is the use of synthetic or natural estrogens or a combination of estrogen and progestin to replace the decline or lack of natural hormones, a condition that accompanies hysterectomy and menopause. (See Table 12–2.) Such symptoms as vaginal dryness, hot flashes, and fatigue are commonly relieved or lessened using HRT. The medical profession is currently rethinking the use of hormone replacement in menopause because of an apparent increased risk of some disorders with extended use of the combination therapy. Use of estrogen alone for HRT is still in clinical trials but has not exhibited the strong contraindications of the combination form of HRT. Estrogen may be administered orally, transdermally, by injection, or as a topical cream (to treat vaginal symptoms only). Other hormones, including oxytocins and prostaglandins, are used for obstetrical applications. In addition, pharmacological agents are available for birth control and family planning. These include oral contraceptives, implants, morning-after pills (**abortifacients**), and spermicides.

Table 12-2	**Drugs Used to Treat Obstetrical and Gynecological Disorders**	
Classification	**Therapeutic Action**	**Generic and Trade Names**
antifungals	Treat vaginal yeast infection by altering the yeast cell membrane or interfering with a metabolic process.	**miconazole** mī-KŎN-ă-zōl Monistat
	Most antifungals used to treat yeast infections are applied topically as ointments, suppositories, or vaginal tablets.	**nystatin** NĬS-tă-tĭn Mycostatin, Nilstat
estrogens	Treat symptoms of menopause (hot flashes, vaginal dryness, fatigue) through hormone replacement therapy (HRT).	**conjugated estrogens** KŎN-jū-gā-tĕd ĔS-trō-jĕnz Cenestin, Premarin
	Long-term use of estrogen has been linked with an increased risk of thrombophlebitis and breast and endometrial cancer.	
oral contraceptives	Prevent ovulation.	**desogestrel/ethinyl estradiol** dĕz-ō-JĔS-trăl/ĔTH-ĭ-nĭl ĕs-tră-DĪ-ŏl Desogen, Ortho-Cept
	Oral contraceptives, or birth control pills, contain a combination of estrogen and progestin and are highly effective in preventing pregnancy if taken as directed.	**ethinyl estradiol/norgestrel** ĔTH-ĭ-nĭl ĕs-tră-DĪ-ŏl/nor-JĔS-trĕl Lo/Ovral-28
oxytocics	Induce labor at term by increasing the strength and frequency of uterine contractions.	**oxytocin** ŏk-sē-TŌ-sĭn Pitocin
	Oxytocics are also used during the postpartum period to control bleeding after the expulsion of the placenta.	
prostaglandins	Terminate pregnancy.	**dinoprostone** dī-nō-PRŎS-tōn Prostin E2, Cervidil
	Large doses of certain prostaglandins can cause the uterus to contract strongly enough to spontaneously abort a fetus.	**mifepristone** mī-fĕ-PRĬS-tōn Mifeprex

Table 12-2	Drugs Used to Treat Obstetrical and Gynecological Disorders—cont'd		
Classification	**Therapeutic Action**		**Generic and Trade Names**
spermicides	Chemically destroy sperm by creating a highly acidic environment in the uterus.		**nonoxynol 9, octoxynol 9** nŏn-ŎK-sĭ-nŏl, ŏk-TŎK-sĭ-nŏl
	Spermicides are available in foam, jelly, gel, and suppositories. They are used within the female vagina for contraception. Spermicides have a higher failure rate than other methods of birth control.		Semicid, Koromex, Ortho-Gynol

Abbreviations

This section introduces female reproductive-related abbreviations and their meanings.

Abbreviation	Meaning	Abbreviation	Meaning
Gynecologic			
AB; Ab, ab	antibody; abortion	**LH**	luteinizing hormone
AI	artificial insemination	**LMP**	last menstrual period
BSE	breast self-examination	**LSO**	left salpingo-oophorectomy
CA	cancer; chronological age; cardiac arrest	**OCPs**	oral contraceptive pills
D&C	dilatation (dilation) and curettage	**Pap**	Papanicolaou (test)
DUB	dysfunctional uterine bleeding	**PID**	pelvic inflammatory disease
FSH	follicle-stimulating hormone	**PMP**	previous menstrual period
G	gravida (pregnant)	**PMS**	premenstrual syndrome
GC	gonococcus *(Neisseria gonorrhoeae)*	**RSO**	right salpingo-oophorectomy
GYN	gynecology	**STD**	sexually transmitted disease
HRT	hormone replacement therapy	**TAH**	total abdominal hysterectomy
HSG	hysterosalpingography	**TRAM**	transverse rectus abdominis muscle
HSV	herpes simplex virus	**TVH**	total vaginal hysterectomy
IUD	intrauterine device	**VD**	venereal disease
Fetal-Obstetrical			
CPD	cephalopelvic disproportion	**CVS**	chorionic villus sampling
CS, C-section	cesarean section	**CWP**	childbirth without pain

(continued)

Abbreviations—cont'd

Abbreviation	Meaning	Abbreviation	Meaning
FECG, FEKG	fetal electrocardiogram	**LBW**	low birth weight
FHR	fetal heart rate	**NB**	newborn
FHT	fetal heart tone	**OB**	obstetrics
FTND	full-term normal delivery	**para 1, 2, 3 and so on**	unipara, bipara, tripara (number of viable births)
IUGR	intrauterine growth rate; intrauterine growth retardation	**UC**	uterine contractions
IVF-ET	*in vitro* fertilization and embryo transfer		

It is time to review procedures, pharmacology, and abbreviations by completing Learning Activity 12–5.

LEARNING ACTIVITIES

The activities that follow provide review of the female reproductive system terms introduced in this chapter. Complete each activity and review your answers to evaluate your understanding of the chapter.

Learning Activity 12-1
Identifying Female Reproductive Structures (Lateral View)

Label the following illustration using the terms listed below.

Bartholin gland	*labia majora*	*uterus*
clitoris	*labia minora*	*vagina*
fallopian tube	*ovary*	

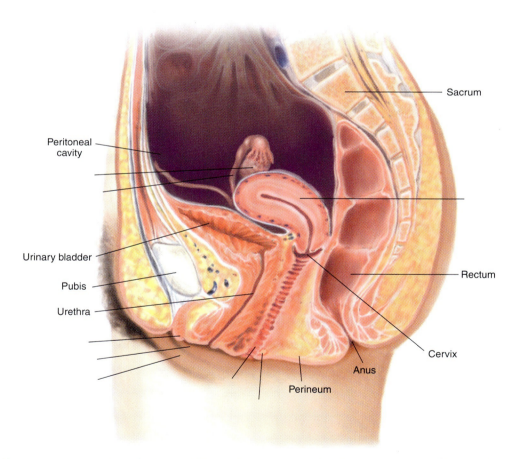

 Check your answers by referring to Figure 12–1 on page 350. Review material that you did not answer correctly.

Learning Activity 12-2

Identifying Female Reproductive Structures (Anterior View)

Label the following illustration using the terms listed below.

Bartholin glands	*fertilization of ovum*	*ovarian ligament*
body of the uterus	*fimbriae*	*ovary*
cervix	*fundus of uterus*	*uterus*
corpus luteum	*graafian follicles*	*vagina*
fallopian tube	*mature follicle*	

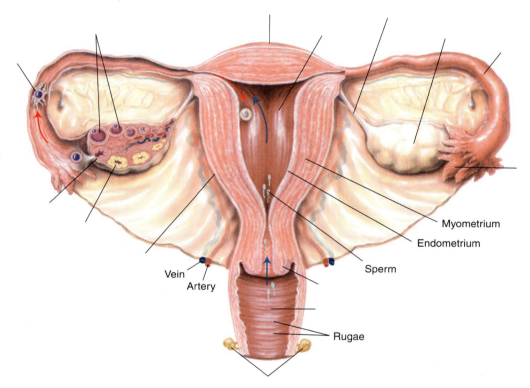

 Check your answers by referring to Figure 12–2 on page 352. Review material that you did not answer correctly.

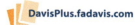 **DavisPlus.fadavis.com**

Enhance your study and reinforcement of word elements with the power of DavisPlus. Visit www.davisplus.fadavis.com/gylys/systems for this chapter's flash-card activity. We recommend you complete the flash-card activity before completing Activity 12–3 below.

Learning Activity 12-3
Building Medical Words

Use *gynec/o* (woman, female) to build words that mean:

1. disease (specific to) women _____
2. physician who specializes in diseases of the female _____

Use *cervic/o* (neck; cervix uteri) to build words that mean:

3. inflammation of cervix uteri and vagina _____
4. pertaining to cervix uteri and bladder _____

Use *colp/o* (vagina) to build words that mean:

5. instrument used to examine the vagina _____
6. visual examination of the vagina _____

Use *vagin/o* (vagina) to build words that mean:

7. inflammation of the vagina _____
8. herniation of the vagina _____

Use *hyster/o* (uterus) to build words that mean:

9. myoma of uterus _____
10. disease of uterus _____
11. radiography of uterus and oviducts _____

Use *metr/o* (uterus) to build words that mean:

12. hemorrhage from uterus _____
13. inflammation around the uterus _____

Use *uter/o* (uterus) to build words that mean:

14. herniation of the uterus _____
15. relating to uterus and cervix _____
16. pertaining to uterus and bladder _____

Use *oophor/o* (ovary) to build words that mean:

17. inflammation of an ovary _____
18. inflammation of an ovary and oviduct _____

Use *salping/o* (fallopian tube) to build words that mean:

19. herniation of a fallopian tube _____
20. radiography of uterine tubes _____

Build surgical words that mean:

21. fixation of (a displaced) ovary _____

22. excision of uterus and ovaries _____

23. suturing the perineum _____

24. excision of uterus, oviducts, and ovaries _____

25. puncture of the amnion (amniotic sac) _____

✓ *Check your answers in Appendix A. Review material that you did not answer correctly.*

Correct Answers _____ ✕ 4 = _____ % Score

Matching Pathological, Diagnostic, Symptomatic, and Related Terms

Match the following terms with the definitions in the numbered list.

asymptomatic	congenital	gestation	oligomenorrhea	pruritus vulvae
atresia	Down syndrome	leiomyoma	parturition	pyosalpinx
candidiasis	dystocia	menarche	primigravida	retroversion
chancre	eclampsia	metrorrhagia	primipara	viable
condylomas				

1. _____ accumulation of pus in a uterine tube
2. _____ woman who has had one pregnancy that has resulted in a viable offspring
3. _____ pregnancy; 40 weeks in human beings
4. _____ primary syphilitic sore
5. _____ entire organ, such as the uterus, that is tipped backward from its normal position
6. _____ present at birth
7. _____ difficult labor or childbirth
8. _____ congenital absence of a normal body opening, such as the vagina
9. _____ trisomy 21
10. _____ intense itching of the external female genitalia
11. _____ without symptoms
12. _____ irregular uterine bleeding between menstrual periods
13. _____ beginning of menstrual function
14. _____ benign uterine tumor composed of muscle and fibrous tissue
15. _____ infrequent menstrual flow
16. _____ process of giving birth
17. _____ most serious form of toxemia during pregnancy
18. _____ capable of living outside the uterus
19. _____ genital warts
20. _____ woman during her first pregnancy

✓ *Check your answers in Appendix A. Review material that you did not answer correctly.*

Correct Answers _____ × 5 = _____ % Score

Learning Activity 12-5

Matching Procedures, Pharmacology, and Abbreviations

Match the following terms with the definitions in the numbered list.

amniocentesis	cordocentesis	estrogens	lumpectomy	prostaglandins
antifungals	cryocautery	hysterosalpingogra-phy	OCPs	TAH
chorionic villus sampling	D&C		oxytocins	tubal ligation
	episiotomy	IUD		ultrasonography
colpocleisis		laparoscopy	Pap test	

1. _____ cytological study to detect cancer in cells that an organ has shed

2. _____ radiography of uterus and oviducts after injection of a contrast medium

3. _____ transabdominal puncture of the amniotic sac to remove amniotic fluid for biochemical and cytological study

4. _____ class of drugs used to treat vaginal yeast infections

5. _____ surgical closure of the vaginal canal

6. _____ procedure that widens the cervical canal with a dilator and scrapes the uterine endometrium with a curette

7. _____ excision of entire uterus, including the cervix, through an abdominal incision

8. _____ tying uterine tubes to prevent pregnancy

9. _____ birth control pills taken orally

10. _____ examination of the abdominal cavity using an endoscope

11. _____ incision of the perineum to facilitate childbirth

12. _____ noninvasive technique using echoes to produce images of internal structures in the body

13. _____ test to detect chromosomal abnormalities that can be done earlier than amniocentesis

14. _____ hormone replacement to reduce adverse symptoms of menopause

15. _____ agents used to induce labor and to rid the uterus of an unexpelled placenta or a fetus that has died

16. _____ freezing tissue to destroy cells

17. _____ birth control method in which an object is placed inside the uterus to prevent pregnancy

18. _____ sampling of fetal blood drawn from the umbilical vein

19. _____ excision of a small primary breast tumor

20. _____ agents used to terminate pregnancy

✔ *Check your answers in Appendix A. Review any material that you did not answer correctly.*

Correct Answers _____ × 5 = _____ % Score

MEDICAL RECORD ACTIVITIES

The two medical records included in the activities that follow use common clinical scenarios to show how medical terminology is used to document patient care. Complete the terminology and analysis sections for each activity to help you recognize and understand terms related to the female reproductive system.

Medical Record Activity 12-1

SOAP Note: Primary Herpes 1 Infection

Terminology

Terms listed below come from *SOAP Note: Primary Herpes 1 Infection* that follows. Use a medical dictionary such as *Taber's Cyclopedic Medical Dictionary,* the appendices of this book, or other resources to define each term. Then review the pronunciations for each term and practice by reading the medical record aloud.

Term	Definition
adenopathy ăd-ĕ-NŎP-ă-thē	
chlamydia klă-MĬD-ē-ă	
GC screen	
herpes lesions HĔR-pēz LĔ-zhŭnz	
introitus ĭn-TRŌ-ĭ-tŭs	
labia LĀ-bē-ă	
LMP	
monilial mō-NĬL-ē-ăl	
OCPs	
pruritus proo-RĪ-tŭs	
R/O	
vulvar VŬL-văr	
Wet prep WĔT PRĔP	

Listen and Learn Online! *will help you master the pronunciation of selected medical words from this medical record activity.* Visit www.davisplus.com/gylys/systems *to find instructions on completing the* Listen and Learn Online! *exercise for this section and to practice pronunciations.*

SOAP NOTE: PRIMARY HERPES 1 INFECTION

PROGRESS NOTES

O'Malley, Roberta

09/01/xx

S: This 24-year-old patient started having some sore areas around the labia, both rt and lt side. She stated that the last few days she started having a brownish discharge. She has pruritus and pain of her vulvar area with adenopathy, p.m. fever, and blisters. Apparently, her partner had a cold sore and they had oral-genital sex. Patient has been using condoms since last seen in April. She has not missed any OCPs. LMP 5/15/xx.

O: Patient has what looks like herpes lesions and ulcers all over vulva and introitus area. Rt labia appears as an ulcerlike lesion; it appears to be almost like an infected follicle. Speculum inserted, a brown discharge noted. GC screen, chlamydia screen, and genital culture obtained from that. Wet prep revealed monilial forms. Viral culture obtained from the ulcerlike lesion on the right labia.

A: Primary herpes 1 infection; will rule out other infectious etiologies.

P: Patient advised to return next week for consultation with Dr. Abdu.

Joanna Masters, MD
Joanna Masters, MD

JM:st

Analysis

Review the medical record *SOAP Note: Primary Herpes 1 Infection* to answer the following questions.

1. Did the patient have any discharge? If so, describe it.

2. What type of discomfort did the patient experience around the vulvar area?

3. Has the patient been taking her oral contraceptive pills regularly?

4. Where was the viral culture obtained?

5. Even though the patient's partner used a condom, how do you think the patient became infected with herpes?

Preoperative Consultation: Menometrorrhagia

Terminology

Terms listed below come from *Preoperative Consultation: Menometrorrhagia* that follows. Use a medical dictionary such as *Taber's Cyclopedic Medical Dictionary,* the appendices of this book, or other resources to define each term. Then review the pronunciations for each term and practice by reading the medical record aloud.

Term	Definition
ablation ăb-LĀ-shŭn	
benign bē-NĪN	
cesarean section sē-SĀR-ē-ăn	
cholecystectomy kō-lē-sĭs-TĔK-tō-mē	
dysmenorrhea dĭs-mĕn-ō-RĒ-ă	
endometrial biopsy ĕn-dō-MĒ-trē-ăl BĪ-ŏp-sē	
fibroids FĪ-broyds	
gravida 2 GRĂV-ĭ-dă	
hysterectomy hĭs-tĕr-ĔK-tō-mē	
laparoscopic lăp-ă-rō-SKŎP-ĭk	
mammogram MĂM-ō-grăm	
menometrorrhagia mĕn-ō-mĕt-rō-RĀ-jē-ă	
palliative PĂL-ē-ā-tĭv	
para I PĂR-ă	
postoperative pōst-ŎP-ĕr-ă-tĭv	

Term	Definition
Premarin PRĔM-ă-rĭn	
salpingo-oophorectomy săl-pĭng-gō-ō-ŏf-ō-RĔK- tō-mē	
therapeutic abortion thĕr-ă-PŪ-tĭk ă-BOR-shŭn	
thyroid function test THĪ-royd FŬNG-shŭn	

 Listen and Learn Online! *will help you master the pronunciation of selected medical words from this medical record activity. Visit* www.davisplus.com/gylys/systems *to find instructions on completing the* Listen and Learn Online! *exercise for this section and to practice pronunciations.*

PREOPERATIVE CONSULTATION: MENOMETRORRHAGIA

Physician Center
2422 Rodeo Drive   ■■   Sun City, USA 12345   ■■   (555)7888-2427

PREOPERATIVE CONSULTATION

July 2, 20xx
Mazza, Rosemary

CHIEF COMPLAINT: Dysmenorrhea and night sweats

HISTORY OF PRESENT ILLNESS: Patient is a 43-year-old gravida 2, para 1 with multiple small uterine fibroids, irregular menses twice a month, family history of ovarian cancer, benign endometrial biopsy, normal Pap, normal mammogram, and normal thyroid function tests. Negative cervical cultures. She has completed childbearing and desires definitive treatment of endometrial ablation, hormonal regulation.

SURGICAL HISTORY: Cesarean section, therapeutic abortion, and cholecystectomy.

ASSESSMENT: This is a patient with menometrorrhagia who declines palliative treatment and desires definitive treatment in the form of a hysterectomy.

PLAN: The plan is to perform a laparoscopic-assisted vaginal hysterectomy, as the patient has essentially no uterine prolapse, and she desires her ovaries to be taken out. She desires to be started on Premarin in the postoperative period. She has been counseled concerning the risks of surgery, including injury to bowel or bladder, infection, and bleeding. She voices understanding and agrees to the plan to perform a laparoscopic-assisted vaginal hysterectomy and bilateral salpingo-oophorectomy.

Julia Masters, MD
Julia Masters, MD

JM:st

Analysis

Review the medical record *Preoperative consultation: Menometrorrhagia* to answer the following questions.

1. How many pregnancies did this patient have? How many viable infants did she deliver?

_____

2. What is a therapeutic abortion?

_____

3. Why did the physician propose to perform a hysterectomy?

_____

4. What is a vaginal hysterectomy?

_____

5. Does the surgeon plan to remove one or both ovaries and fallopian tubes?

_____

6. Why do you think the physician will use the laparoscope to perform the hysterectomy?

_____

Endocrine System

CHAPTER

13

Chapter Outline

Objectives

Upon completion of this chapter, you will be able to:

- Locate and describe the structures of the endocrine system.
- Describe the functional relationship between the endocrine system and other body systems.
- Recognize, pronounce, spell, and build words related to the endocrine system.
- Describe pathological conditions, diagnostic and therapeutic procedures, and other terms related to the endocrine system.
- Explain pharmacology related to the treatment of endocrine disorders.
- Demonstrate your knowledge of this chapter by completing the learning and medical record activities.

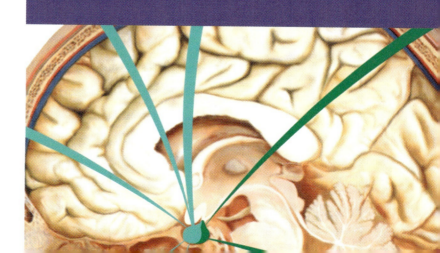

Anatomy and Physiology

The primary function of the endocrine system is to keep the body in **homeostasis,** the body's internal state of equilibrium that is maintained so all body systems can function most effectively. Thus, the endocrine system comprises a network of ductless glands, which have a rich blood supply that enables the **hormones** they produce to enter the bloodstream and influence body functions.

Hormones are chemicals produced by glands that cause a specific effect at a **target.** A target, also known as a *target cell,* is programmed with receptors to respond to a unique hormone. Although hormones travel throughout the entire body in blood and lymph, they affect only targets that have specific receptors for the hormone. Once bound to the receptor, the hormone initiates a specific biological effect. Hormones control diverse activities. such as growth, metabolism, reproduction, energy level, and sexual characteristics.

Although the nervous system provides many of the same functions as the endocrine system, it is designed to act instantaneously by transmitting electrical impulses to specific body locations. It is one of the most complicated systems of the body. Nonetheless, the endocrine and nervous systems work together like an interlocking supersystem to control many intricate activities of the body.

This chapter discusses the structure and functions of hormones and the **pituitary, thyroid, parathyroid, adrenal, pancreatic,** and **pineal glands.** (See Figure 13–1.) (See Chapter 9, Blood, Lymph, and Immune Systems, for information on the function of the **thymus;** Chapter 11, Genitourinary System, for information on the **testes;** and Chapter 12, Female Reproductive System, for information on the **ovaries.**)

Endocrine System

The **endocrine** system includes glands that secrete hormones directly into the bloodstream rather than though a duct (**exocrine glands**).

Although a given hormone travels anywhere in the body that blood does, it affects only a specific target. Hormones influence their target cells by chemically binding to specific receptors. Only the target cells for a given hormone have receptors that bind and recognize that hormone. The receptors initiate specific biological effects when the hormones bind to them. For example, thyroid-stimulating hormone (TSH) binds to receptors on cells of the thyroid gland, but it does not bind to cells of the ovaries because ovarian cells do not have TSH receptors.

The release of a hormone by an endocrine gland to a target is determined by the body's need for the hormone at any given time and is regulated to avoid overproduction (**hypersecretion**) or underproduction (**hyposecretion**). Unfortunately, there are times when the body's regulating mechanism does not operate properly and hormone levels become excessive or deficient, causing various disorders.

Pituitary Gland

The (1) **pituitary gland,** or **hypophysis,** is a pea-sized organ located at the base of the brain. It is known as the *master gland* because it regulates many body activities and stimulates other glands to secrete their own specific hormones. (See Figure 13–2.) The pituitary gland consists of two distinct portions, an anterior lobe (**adenohypophysis**) and a posterior lobe (**neurohypophysis**). The anterior lobe, triggered by the action of the hypothalamus, produces at least six hormones. The posterior lobe stores and secretes two hormones produced by the hypothalamus: antidiuretic hormone (ADH) and oxytocin. These hormones are released into the bloodstream as needed. (See Table 13–1.)

Thyroid Gland

The (2) **thyroid gland** is the largest gland of the endocrine system. An H-shaped organ located in the neck just below the larynx, this gland is composed of two large lobes that are separated by a strip of tissue called an **isthmus.** Thyroid hormone (TH) is the body's major metabolic hormone. TH increases the rate of oxygen consumption and thus the rate at which carbohydrates, proteins, and fats are metabolized. TH is actually two active iodine-containing hormones, **thyroxine (T_4)** and **triiodothyronine (T_3).** Thyroxine is the major hormone secreted by the thyroid; most triiodothyronine is formed at the target tissues by conversion of T_4 to T_3. Except for the adult brain, spleen, testes, uterus, and the thyroid gland itself, thyroid hormone affects virtually every cell in the body. TH also influences growth hormone and plays an important role in maintaining blood pressure. (See Table 13–2.)

Parathyroid Glands

The (3) **parathyroid glands** consist of at least four separate glands located on the posterior surface of the lobes of the thyroid gland. The only hormone known to be secreted by the parathyroid

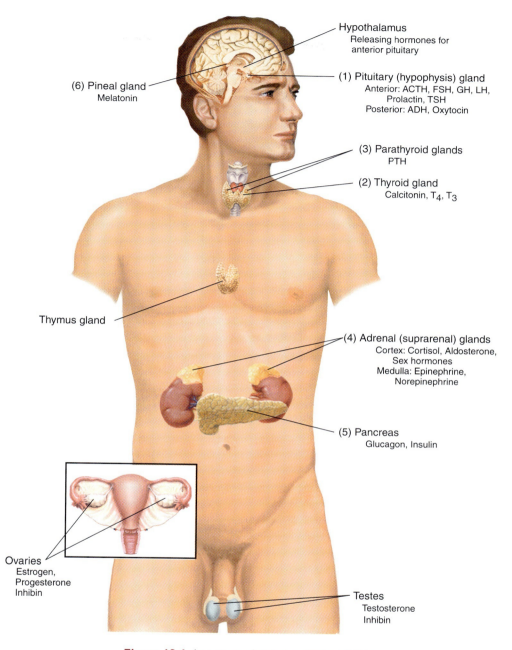

Hypothalamus
Releasing hormones for
anterior pituitary

(6) Pineal gland
Melatonin

(1) Pituitary (hypophysis) gland
Anterior: ACTH, FSH, GH, LH,
Prolactin, TSH
Posterior: ADH, Oxytocin

(3) Parathyroid glands
PTH

(2) Thyroid gland
Calcitonin, T_4, T_3

Thymus gland

(4) Adrenal (suprarenal) glands
Cortex: Cortisol, Aldosterone,
Sex hormones
Medulla: Epinephrine,
Norepinephrine

(5) Pancreas
Glucagon, Insulin

Ovaries
Estrogen,
Progesterone
Inhibin

Testes
Testosterone
Inhibin

Figure 13-1. Locations of major endocrine glands.

glands is parathyroid hormone (PTH). PTH helps to regulate calcium balance by stimulating three target organs: bones, kidneys, and intestines. (See Table 13–3.) Because of PTH stimulation, calcium and phosphates are released from bones, increasing concentration of these substances in blood. Thus, calcium that is necessary for the proper functioning of body tissues is available in the bloodstream. At the same time, PTH enhances the absorption of calcium and phosphates from foods in the intestine, causing a

rise in blood levels of calcium and phosphates. PTH causes the kidneys to conserve blood calcium and to increase the excretion of phosphates in the urine.

Adrenal Glands

The (4) **adrenal glands** are paired organs covering the superior surface of the kidneys. Because of their location, the adrenal glands are also known as *suprarenal glands.* Each adrenal gland is divided

Anatomy and Physiology Key Terms

This section introduces important endocrine system terms and their definitions. Word analyses for selected terms are also provided.

Term	Definition
antagonistic ăn-tăg-ō-NĬST-ĭk	Acting in opposition; mutually opposing
electrolytes ē-LĔK-trō-līts	Mineral salts (sodium, potassium, and calcium) that carry an electrical charge in solution *A proper balance of electrolytes is essential to the normal functioning of the entire body.*
glucagon GLOO-kă-gŏn	Hormone produced by pancreatic alpha cells that increases the blood glucose level by stimulating the liver to change stored glycogen (a starch form of sugar) to glucose *Glucagon opposes the action of insulin and is used to reverse hypoglycemic reactions in insulin shock.*
glucose GLOO-kōs	Simple sugar that is the end product of carbohydrate digestion *Glucose is the primary source of energy for living organisms.*
homeostasis hō-mē-ō-STĀ-sĭs *homeo-:* same, alike *-stasis:* standing still	Relative constancy or balance in the internal environment of the body, maintained by processes of feedback and adjustment in response to external or internal changes
hormones HOR-mōnz	Chemical substances produced by specialized cells of the body that are released slowly in minute amounts directly into the bloodstream *Hormones are produced primarily by endocrine glands and are carried through the bloodstream to the target organ.*
insulin ĬN-sŭ-lĭn	Hormone produced by pancreatic beta cells that acts to remove sugar (glucose) from the blood by promoting its storage in tissues as carbohydrates (glycogen)
sympathomimetic sĭm-pă-thō-mĭm-ĔT-ĭk	Agent that mimics the effects of the sympathetic nervous system *Epinephrine and norepinephrine are sympathomimetic hormones because they produce effects that mimic those brought about by the sympathetic nervous system.*
target	Structure, organ, or tissue to which something is directed *In the endocrine system, a target is the structure, organ, or tissue on which a hormone exerts its specific effect.*

Pronunciation Help	Long Sound	ā—rate	ē—rebirth	ī—isle	ō—over	ū—unite
	Short Sound	ă—alone	ĕ—ever	ĭ—it	ŏ—not	ŭ—cut

into two sections, each of which has its own structure and function. The outer adrenal cortex makes up the bulk of the gland and the adrenal medulla makes up the inner portion. Although these regions are not sharply divided, they represent distinct glands that secrete different hormones.

Adrenal Cortex

The adrenal cortex secretes three types of steroid hormones:

1. **Mineralocorticoids,** mainly aldosterone, are essential to life. These hormones act mainly through the kidneys to maintain the balance

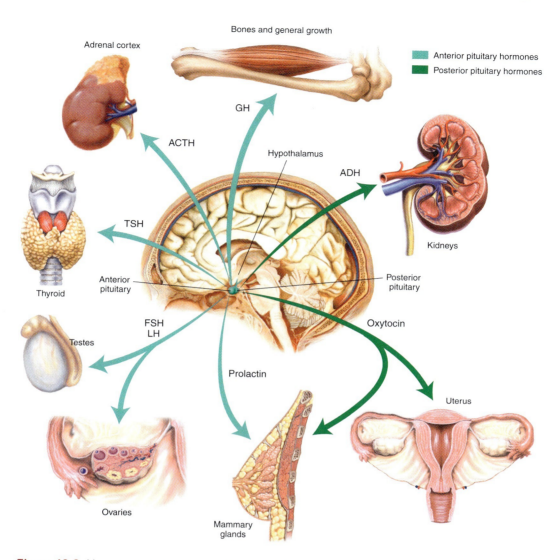

Figure 13-2. Hormones secreted by the anterior and posterior pituitary gland, along with target organs.

Table 13-1	**Pituitary Hormones**

This table identifies pituitary hormones, their target organs and functions, and associated disorders.

Hormone	Target Organ and Functions	Disorders
Anterior Pituitary Hormones (Adenohypophysis)		
Adrenocorticotropic hormone (ACTH)	• Adrenal cortex—promotes secretions of some hormones by adrenal cortex, especially cortisol	• Hyposecretion is rare. • Hypersecretion causes Cushing disease.
Follicle-stimulating hormone (FSH)	• Ovaries—in females, stimulates egg production; increases secretion of estrogen	• Hyposecretion causes failure of sexual maturation.
	• Testes—in males, stimulates sperm production	• Hypersecretion has no known significant effects.

(continued)

Table 13-1	Pituitary Hormones—cont'd	
Hormone	**Target Organ and Functions**	**Disorders**
Growth hormone (GH) or somatotropin	• Bone, cartilage, liver, muscle, and other tissues—stimulates somatic growth; increases use of fats for energy	• Hyposecretion in children causes pituitary dwarfism. • Hypersecretion in children causes gigantism; hypersecretion in adults causes acromegaly.
Luteinizing hormone (LH)	• Ovaries—in females, promotes ovulation; stimulates production of estrogen and progesterone • Testes—in males, promotes secretion of testosterone	• Hyposecretion causes failure of sexual maturation. • Hypersecretion has no known significant effects.
Prolactin	• Breast—in conjunction with other hormones, promotes lactation	• Hyposecretion in nursing mothers causes poor lactation. • Hypersecretion in nursing mothers causes galactorrhea.
Thyroid-stimulating hormone (TSH)	• Thyroid gland—stimulates secretion of thyroid hormone	• Hyposecretion in infants causes cretinism; hyposecretion in adults causes myxedema. • Hypersecretion causes Graves disease, indicated by exophthalmos. (See Figure 13–3.

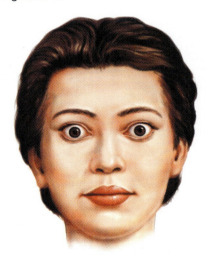

Figure 13-3. Exophthalmos caused by Graves disease.

Posterior Pituitary Hormones (Neurohypophysis)		
Antidiuretic hormone (ADH)	• Kidney—increases water reabsorption (water returns to the blood)	• Hyposecretion causes diabetes insipidus. • Hypersecretion causes syndrome of inappropriate antidiuretic hormone (SIADH).
Oxytocin	• Uterus—stimulates uterine contractions; initiates labor • Breast—promotes milk secretion from the mammary glands	• Unknown

Table 13-2	**Thyroid Hormones**

This table identifies thyroid hormones, their functions, and associated disorders.

Hormone	Functions	Disorders
Calcitonin	• Regulates calcium levels in the blood in conjunction with parathyroid hormone • Secreted when calcium levels in the blood are high in order to maintain homeostasis	• The most significant effects are exerted in childhood when bones are growing and changing dramatically in mass, size, and shape. • At best, calcitonin is a weak hypocalcemic agent in adults.
Thyroxine (T_4) and triiodothyronine (T_3)	• Increases energy production from all food types • Increases rate of protein synthesis	• Hyposecretion in infants causes cretinism; hyposecretion in adults causes myxedema. • Hypersecretion causes Graves disease, indicated by exophthalmos. (See Figure 13–3.)

Table 13-3	**Parathyroid Hormones**

This table identifies parathyroid hormones, their target organs and functions, and associated disorders.

Hormone	Target Organ and Functions	Disorders
Parathyroid hormone (PTH)	• Bones—increases the reabsorption of calcium and phosphate from bone to blood • Kidneys—increases calcium absorption and phosphate excretion • Small intestine—increases absorption of calcium and phosphate	• Hyposecretion causes tetany. • Hypersecretion causes osteitis fibrosa cystica

of sodium and potassium (**electrolytes**) in the body. More specifically, aldosterone causes the kidneys to conserve sodium and excrete potassium. At the same time, it promotes water conservation and reduces urine output.

2. **Glucocorticoids,** mainly cortisol, influence the metabolism of carbohydrates, fats, and proteins. The glucocorticoid with the greatest activity is cortisol. It helps regulate the concentration of glucose in the blood, protecting against low blood sugar levels between meals. Cortisol also stimulates the breakdown of fats in adipose tissue and releases fatty acids into the blood. The increase in fatty acids causes many cells to use relatively less glucose.

3. **Sex hormones,** including androgens, estrogens, and progestins, help maintain secondary sex characteristics, such as development of the breasts and adult distribution of hair.

Adrenal Medulla

The adrenal medulla cells secrete two closely related hormones, epinephrine (**adrenaline**) and norepinephrine (**noradrenaline**). Both hormones are activated when the body responds to crisis situations, and are considered **sympathomimetic** agents because they produce effects that mimic those brought about by the sympathetic nervous system. Because hormones of the adrenal medulla merely intensify activities set into motion by the sympathetic nervous system, their deficiency is not a problem.

Of the two hormones, epinephrine is secreted in larger amounts. In the physiological response to stress, epinephrine is responsible for maintaining blood pressure and cardiac output, keeping airways open wide, and raising blood glucose levels. All these functions are useful for frightened, traumatized, injured, or sick persons. Norepinephrine reduces the diameter of blood vessels in the periphery (vasoconstriction), thereby raising blood pressure. (See Table 13–4.)

Table 13-4 Adrenal Hormones

This table identifies adrenal hormones, their target organs and functions, and associated disorders.

Hormone	Target Organ and Functions	Disorders
Adrenal Cortex Hormones Glucocorticoids (mainly cortisol)	• Body cells—promote gluconeogenesis; regulate metabolism of carbohydrates, proteins, and fats; and help depress inflammatory and immune responses	• Hyposecretion causes Addison disease. • Hypersecretion causes Cushing syndrome. (See Figure 13–4.)

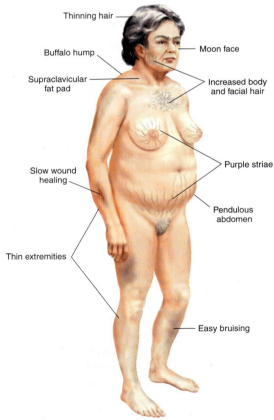

Thinning hair
Buffalo hump
Supraclavicular fat pad
Moon face
Increased body and facial hair
Slow wound healing
Purple striae
Pendulous abdomen
Thin extremities
Easy bruising

Figure 13-4. Physical manifestations of Cushing syndrome.

Hormone	Target Organ and Functions	Disorders
Mineralocorticoids (mainly aldosterone)	• Kidneys—increase blood levels of sodium and decrease blood levels of potassium in the kidneys	• Hyposecretion causes Addison disease. • Hypersecretion causes aldosteronism.

Table 13-4	**Adrenal Hormones—cont'd**		
Hormone	**Target Organ and Functions**		**Disorders**
Sex hormones (any of the androgens, estrogens, or related steroid hormones) produced by the ovaries, testes, and adrenal cortices	• In females, possibly responsible for female libido and source of estrogen after menopause (Otherwise, effects in adults are insignificant.)		• Hypersecretion of adrenal androgen in females leads to virilism (development of male characteristics). • Hypersecretion of adrenal estrogen and progestin secretion in males leads to feminization (development of feminine characteristics). • Hyposecretion has no known significant effects.
Adrenal Medullary Hormones			
Epinephrine and norepinephrine	• Sympathetic nervous system target organs—hormone effects mimic sympathetic nervous system activation (sympathomimetic), increase metabolic rate and heart rate, and raise blood pressure by promoting vasoconstriction		• Hyposecretion has no known significant effects. • Hypersecretion causes prolonged "fight-or-flight" reaction and hypertension.

Table 13-5	**Pancreatic Hormones**		
This table identifies pancreatic hormones, their target organs and functions, and associated disorders.			
Hormone	**Target Organ and Functions**		**Disorders**
Glucagon	• Liver and blood—raises blood glucose level by accelerating conversion of glycogen into glucose in the liver (glycogenolysis) and other nutrients into glucose in the liver (gluconeogenesis) and releasing glucose into blood (glycogen to glucose)		• Persistently low blood glucose levels (hypoglycemia) may be caused by deficiency in glucagon.
Insulin	• Tissue cells—lowers blood glucose level by accelerating glucose transport into cells and the use of that glucose for energy production (glucose to glycogen)		• Hyposecretion of insulin causes diabetes mellitus. • Hypersecretion of insulin causes hyperinsulinism.

Pancreas

The (5) **pancreas** lies inferior to the stomach in a bend of the duodenum. It functions as an exocrine and endocrine gland. A large pancreatic duct runs through the gland, carrying enzymes and other exocrine digestive secretions from the pancreas to the small intestine. The endocrine portion of the pancreas consists of groups of cells called *islets of Langerhans*. The islets secrete two distinct types of hormones: alpha cells that produce **glucagon** and beta cells that produce **insulin.** Both hormones play important roles in carbohydrate metabolism.

When blood **glucose** levels are low (**hypoglycemia**), glucagon stimulates the release of glucose from storage sites in the liver. Because the liver converts stored glycogen to glucose (**glycogenolysis**), the blood glucose level rises. The overall effect, therefore, is a rise in the blood glucose level. When blood glucose levels are high (**hyperglycemia**), the pancreatic beta cells are stimulated to produce insulin. This insulin production causes glucose to enter body cells to be used for energy and acts to clear glucose from the blood by promoting its storage as glycogen. Insulin and glucagon function **antagonistically** so that normal secretion of both hormones ensures a blood glucose level that fluctuates within normal limits. (See Table 13–5.)

Pineal Gland

The (6) **pineal gland,** which is shaped like a pine cone, is attached to the posterior part of the third ventricle of the brain. Although the exact functions of this gland have not been established, there is evidence that it secretes the hormone melatonin. It is believed that melatonin may inhibit the activities of the ovaries. When melatonin production is high, ovulation is blocked, and there may be a delay in puberty.

Connecting Body Systems–Endocrine System

The main function of the endocrine system is to secrete hormones that have a diverse effect on cells, tissues, organs, and organ systems. Specific functional relationships between the endocrine system and other body systems are summarized below.

Blood, lymph, and immune
- Hormones from the thymus stimulate lymphocyte production.
- Glucocorticoids depress the immune response and inflammation.

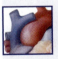

Cardiovascular
- Hormones influence heart rate, contraction strength, blood volume, and blood pressure.
- Estrogen helps maintain vascular health in women.

Digestive
- Hormones help control digestive system activity.
- Hormones influence motility and glandular activity of the digestive tract, gallbladder secretion, and secretion of enzymes from the pancreas.
- Insulin and glucagon adjust glucose metabolism in the liver.

Female reproductive
- Hormones play a major role in the development and function of the reproductive organs.
- Hormones influence the menstrual cycle, pregnancy, parturition, and lactation.
- Sex hormones play a major role in the development of secondary sex characteristics.
- Hormone oxytocin triggers contraction of the pregnant uterus and then later stimulates the release of breast milk.

Genitourinary
- Hormones play a major role in the development and function of the reproductive organs.
- Hormones play a role in sexual development, sex drive, and gamete production.

Integumentary
- Hormones regulate activity of the sebaceous glands, distribution of subcutaneous tissue, and growth of hair.
- Hormones stimulate melanocytes to produce skin pigment.
- Estrogen hormone increases skin hydration.

Musculoskeletal
- Hormone secretions influence blood flow to muscles during exercise.
- Hormones influence muscle metabolism, mass, and strength.
- Hormones from the pituitary and thyroid glands and the gonads stimulate bone growth.
- Hormones govern blood calcium balance.

Nervous
- Several hormones play an important role in the normal maturation and function of the nervous system.

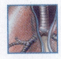

Respiratory
- Hormones stimulate red blood cell production when the body experiences a decrease in oxygen.
- Epinephrine influences ventilation by dilating the bronchioles; epinephrine and thyroxine stimulate cell respiration.

 It is time to review anatomy by completing Learning Activity 13–1.

Medical Word Elements

This section introduces combining forms, suffixes, and prefixes related to the endocrine system. Word analyses are also provided.

Element	Meaning	Word Analysis
Combining Forms		
adren/o	adrenal glands	**adren/o**/megaly (ăd-rēn-ō-MĔG-ă-lē): enlargement of adrenal glands *-megaly:* enlargement
adrenal/o		**adrenal**/ectomy (ăd-rē-năl-ĔK-tō-mē): excision of (one or both) adrenal glands *-ectomy:* excision, removal
calc/o	calcium	hyper/**calc**/emia (hī-pĕr-kăl-SĒ-mē-ă): excessive calcium in the blood *hyper-:* excessive, above normal *-emia:* blood condition
crin/o	secrete	endo/**crin/o**/logy (ĕn-dō-krĭn-ŎL-ō-jē): study of endocrine glands (and their functions) *endo-:* in, within *-logy:* study of
gluc/o	sugar, sweetness	**gluc/o**/genesis (gloo-kō-JĔN-ĕ-sĭs): forming or producing glucose *-genesis:* forming, producing, origin
glyc/o		hypo/**glyc**/emia (hī-pō-glī-SĒ-mē-ă): abnormally low level of glucose in the blood *hypo-:* under, below *-emia:* blood condition *Hypoglycemia is usually caused by administration of too much insulin, excessive secretion of insulin by the islet cells of the pancreas, or dietary deficiency.*
glycos/o		**glycos**/uria (glī-kō-SŪ-rē-ă): abnormal amount of glucose, in the urine *-uria:* urine
home/o	same, alike	**home/o**/stasis (hō-mē-ō-STĀ-sĭs): state of equilibrium in the internal environment of the body *-stasis:* standing still
kal/i	potassium (an electrolyte)	**kal**/emia (kă-LĒ-mē-ă): potassium in the blood *-emia:* blood condition
pancreat/o	pancreas	**pancreat/o**/tomy (păn-krē-ă-TŎT-ō-mē): incision of the pancreas *-tomy:* incision
parathyroid/o	parathyroid glands	**parathyroid**/ectomy (păr-ă-thī-royd-ĔK-tō-mē): excision of (one or more of the) parathyroid glands *-ectomy:* excision, removal
thym/o	thymus gland	**thym**/oma (thī-MŌ-mă): tumor of the thymus gland *-oma:* tumor *A thymoma is a rare neoplasm of the thymus gland. Treatment includes surgical removal, radiation therapy, or chemotherapy.*

(continued)

Medical Word Elements—cont'd

Element	Meaning	Word Analysis
thyr/o	thyroid gland	**thyr/o**/megaly (thī-rō-MĔG-ă-lē): enlargement of the thyroid gland *-megaly:* enlargement

thyroid/o		hyper/**thyroid**/ism (hī-pĕr-THĪ-royd-ĭzm): condition of excessive thyroid gland (function)
		   hyper-: excessive, above normal
		   -ism: condition

toxic/o	poison	**toxic/o**/logist (tŏks-ĭ-KŎL-ō-jĭst): specialist in the study of poisons *-logist:* specialist in study of *Toxicologists also study the effects of toxins and antidotes used for treatment of toxic disorders.*
Suffixes		
-crine	secrete	endo/**crine** (ĔN-dō-krĭn): secrete internally or within *endo-:* in, within
-dipsia	thirst	poly/**dipsia** (pŏl-ē-DĬP-sē-ă): excessive thirst *poly-:* many, much *Polydipsia is one of the three "polys" (polyphagia and polyuria) associated with diabetes.*
-gen	forming, producing, origin	andr/o/**gen** (ĂN-drō-jĕn): any steroid hormone that increases masculinization *andr/o:* male
-toxic	poison	thyr/o/**toxic** (thī-rō-TŎKS-ĭk): pertaining to toxic activity of the thyroid gland *thyr/o:* thyroid gland
-uria	urine	glycos/**uria** (glī-kō-SŪ-rē-ă): glucose in the urine *glycos:* sugar, sweetness
Prefixes		

eu-	good, normal	**eu**/thyr/oid (ū-THĪ-royd): resembling a normal thyroid gland
		   thyr/o: thyroid gland
		   -oid: resembling

exo-	outside, outward	**exo**/crine (ĔKS-ō-krĭn): secrete outwardly *-crine:* secrete *Exocrine glands secrete their products outwardly through excretory ducts*

hyper-	excessive, above normal	**hyper**/glyc/emia (hī-pĕr-glī-SĒ-mē-ă): excessive glucose in the blood
		   glyc: sugar, sweetness
		   -emia: blood condition
		Abnormally high blood glucose levels are found in patients with diabetes mellitus or those treated with drugs such as prednisone.

Medical Word Elements—cont'd

Element	Meaning	Word Analysis
hypo-	under, below	**hypo**/insulin/ism (hī-pō-ĬN-sŭ-lĭn-ĭzm): condition of deficiency of insulin *-ism:* condition *Hypoinsulinism is a characteristic of type 1 diabetes mellitus.*
poly-	many, much	**poly**/uria (pŏl-ē-Ū-rē-ă): excessive urination *-uria:* urine *Some causes of polyuria are diabetes, use of diuretics, excessive fluid intake, and hypercalcemia.*

 It is time to review medical word elements by completing Learning Activity 13–2. For audio pronunciations of the above-listed key terms, you can visit www.davisplus.fadavis.com/gylys/systems to download this chapter's Listen and Learn! exercises or use the book's audio CD (if included).

Pathology

Disorders of the endocrine system are caused by underproduction (**hyposecretion**) or overproduction (**hypersecretion**) of hormones. In general, hyposecretion is treated with drug therapy in the form of hormone replacement. Hypersecretion is generally treated by surgery. Most hormone deficiencies result from genetic defects in the glands, surgical removal of the glands, or production of poor-quality hormones.

Pituitary Disorders

Pituitary disorders are related to hypersecretion or hyposecretion of growth hormone, which leads to body-size abnormalities. Abnormal variations of ADH secretion lead to disorders in the composition of blood and marked electrolyte imbalance.

Thyroid Disorders

Thyroid gland disorders are common and may develop at any time during life. They may be the result of a developmental problem, injury, disease, or dietary deficiency. One form of hypothyroidism that develops in infants is called *cretinism.* If not treated, this disorder leads to mental retardation, impaired growth, low body temperatures, and abnormal bone formation. Usually these symptoms do not appear at birth because the infant has received thyroid hormones from the mother's blood during fetal development. When hypothyroidism develops during adulthood, it is known as

myxedema. The characteristics of this disease are edema, low blood levels of T_3 and T_4, weight gain, cold intolerance, fatigue, depression, muscle or joint pain, and sluggishness.

Hyperthyroidism results from excessive secretions of T_3, T_4, or both. Two of the most common disorders of hyperthyroidism are Graves disease and toxic goiter. **Graves disease** is considerably more prevalent and is characterized by an elevated metabolic rate, abnormal weight loss, excessive perspiration, muscle weakness, and emotional instability. Also, the eyes are likely to protrude (**exophthalmos**) because of edematous swelling in the tissues behind them. (See Figure 13–3.) At the same time, the thyroid gland is likely to enlarge, producing **goiter.** (See Figure 13–5.)

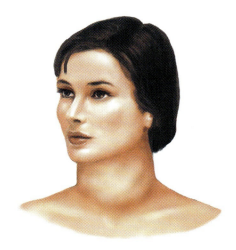

Figure 13-5. Enlargement of the thyroid gland in goiter.

It is believed that **toxic goiter** may occur because of excessive release of thyroid-stimulating hormone (TSH) from the anterior lobe of the pituitary gland. Overstimulation by TSH causes thyroid cells to enlarge and secrete extra amounts of hormones. Treatment for **hyperthyroidism** may involve drug therapy to block the production of thyroid hormones or surgical removal of all or part of the thyroid gland. Another method for treating this disorder is to administer a sufficient amount of radioactive iodine to destroy the thyroid secretory cells.

Parathyroid Disorders

As with the thyroid gland, dysfunction of the parathyroids is usually characterized by inadequate or excessive hormone secretion.

Insufficient production of parathyroid hormone (PTH), called *hypoparathyroidism,* can be caused by primary parathyroid dysfunction or elevated blood calcium levels. This condition can result from an injury or from surgical removal of the glands, sometimes in conjunction with thyroid surgery. The primary effect of hypoparathyroidism is a decreased blood calcium level (**hypocalcemia**). Decreased calcium lowers the electrical threshold, causing neurons to depolarize more easily, and increases the number of nerve impulses, resulting in muscle twitches and spasms (**tetany**).

Excessive production of PTH, called *hyperparathyroidism,* is commonly caused by a benign tumor. The increase in PTH secretion leads to demineralization of bones (**osteitis fibrosa cystica**), making them porous (**osteoporosis**) and highly susceptible to fracture and deformity. When this condition is the result of a benign glandular tumor (**adenoma**) of the parathyroid, the tumor is removed. Treatment may also include orthopedic surgery to correct severe bone deformities. Excess PTH also causes calcium to be deposited in the kidneys. When the disease is generalized and all bones are affected, this disorder is known as **von Recklinghausen disease.** Renal symptoms and kidney stones (**nephrolithiasis**) may also develop.

Disorders of the Adrenal Glands

As discussed, the adrenal glands consist of the adrenal cortex and adrenal medulla. Each has its own structure and function as well as its own set of associated disorders.

Adrenal Cortex

The adrenal cortex is mainly associated with Addison disease and Cushing syndrome.

Addison disease

Addison disease, a relatively uncommon chronic disorder caused by a deficiency of cortical hormones, results when the adrenal cortex is damaged or atrophied. Atrophy of the adrenal glands is probably the result of an autoimmune process in which circulating adrenal antibodies slowly destroy the gland. The gland usually suffers 90% destruction before clinical signs of adrenal insufficiency appear. Hypofunction of the adrenal cortex interferes with the body's ability to handle internal and external stress. In severe cases, the disturbance of sodium and potassium metabolism may be marked by depletion of sodium and water through urination, resulting in severe chronic dehydration. Other clinical manifestations include muscle weakness, anorexia, gastrointestinal symptoms, fatigue, hypoglycemia, hypotension, low blood sodium (**hyponatremia**), and high serum potassium (**hyperkalemia**). If treatment for this condition begins early, usually with adrenocortical hormone therapy, the prognosis is excellent. If untreated, the disease will continue a chronic course with progressive but relatively slow deterioration. In some patients, the deterioration may be rapid.

Cushing syndrome

Cushing syndrome is a cluster of symptoms produced by excessive amounts of cortisol, adrenocorticotropic hormone (ACTH), or both circulating in the blood. (See Figure 13–4.) Causes of this excess secretion include:

- long-term administration of steroid drugs (glucocorticoids) in treating such diseases as rheumatoid arthritis, lupus erythematosus, and asthma
- adrenal tumor resulting in excessive production of cortisol
- Cushing disease, a pituitary disorder caused by hypersecretion of ACTH from an adenoma in the anterior pituitary gland

Regardless of the cause, Cushing syndrome alters carbohydrate and protein metabolism and electrolyte balance. Overproduction of mineralocorticoids and glucocorticoids causes blood glucose concentration to remain high, depleting tissue protein. In addition, sodium retention causes increased fluid in tissue that leads to edema. These metabolic changes produce weight gain and may cause structural changes, such as a moon-shaped face, grossly exaggerated head and trunk, and pencil-thin arms and legs. Other symptoms include fatigue, high blood pressure, and excessive hair growth in unusual places (**hirsutism**), especially in women. The treatment goal for this disease is to restore serum cortisol to normal levels. Nevertheless, treatment varies with the cause and may necessitate radiation, drug therapy, surgery, or a combination of these methods.

Adrenal Medulla

No specific diseases can be traced directly to a deficiency of hormones from the adrenal medulla. However, medullary tumors sometimes cause excess secretions. The most common disorder is a neoplasm known as *pheochromocytoma,* which produces excessive amounts of epinephrine and norepinephrine. Most of these tumors are encapsulated and benign. These hypersecretions produce high blood pressure, rapid heart rate, stress, fear, palpitations, headaches, visual blurring, muscle spasms, and sweating. Typical treatment consists of antihypertensive drugs and surgery.

Pancreatic Disorders

Diabetes is a general term that, when used alone, refers to diabetes mellitus (DM). It is by far the most common pancreatic disorder. DM is a chronic metabolic disorder of impaired carbohydrate, protein, and fat metabolism due to insufficient production of insulin or the body's inability to utilize insulin properly. When body cells are deprived of glucose, their principal energy fuel, they begin to metabolize proteins and fats. As fat is metabolized, ketones are produced and enter the blood, causing a condition called *ketosis.* Hyperglycemia and ketosis are responsible for the host of troubling and commonly life-threatening symptoms of diabetes mellitus. Insulin is an essential hormone that prepares body cells to absorb and use glucose as an energy source. When insulin is lacking, sugar does not enter cells but returns to the bloodstream with a subsequent rise in its concentration in the blood (hyperglycemia). When blood glucose levels reach a certain concentration, sugar "spills" into the urine and is expelled from the body (glucosuria), along with electrolytes, particularly sodium. Sodium and potassium losses result in muscle weakness and fatigue. Because glucose is unavailable to cells, cellular starvation results and leads to hunger and an increased appetite (polyphagia.)

Although genetics and environmental factors, such as obesity and lack of exercise, seem significant in the development of this disease, the cause

of diabetes is not always clear. (See Table 13–5.) Diabetes mellitus occurs in two primary forms:

- *Type 1 diabetes* is usually diagnosed in children and young adults and was previously called *juvenile diabetes.* In type 1 diabetes, the body does not produce sufficient insulin. Treatment includes injection of insulin to maintain a normal level of glucose in the blood. (See Table 13–6.)
- *Type 2 diabetes* is the most common form and is distinctively different from type 1. Its onset was typically later in life but it has become more prevalent in children as the incidence of obesity has increased. Risk factors include a family history of diabetes and obesity. In type 2 diabetes, the body is deficient in producing sufficient insulin or the body's cells are resistant to insulin action in target tissues. Hyperglycemia that results may cause cell starvation and, over time, may damage the kidneys, eyes, nerves, or heart. Treatment for type 2 diabetes includes exercise, diet, weight loss, and, if needed, insulin or oral antidiabetic agents. Oral antidiabetic agents activate the release of pancreatic insulin and improve the body's sensitivity to insulin. (See Table 13–6.)

Complications

Diabetes is associated with a number of primary and secondary complications. Patients with type 1 diabetes usually report rapidly developing symptoms. With type 2 diabetes, the patient's symptoms are usually vague, long standing, and develop gradually.

Primary complications of type 1 diabetes include **diabetic ketoacidosis (DKA).** DKA, also referred to as *diabetic acidosis* or *diabetic coma,* may develop over several days or weeks. It can be caused by too little insulin, failure to follow a prescribed diet, physical or emotional stress, or undiagnosed diabetes.

Secondary complications due to long-standing diabetes emerge years after the initial diagnosis (Dx). Common chronic complications include diabetic retinopathy and diabetic nephropathy. In diabetic retinopathy, the retina's blood vessels are destroyed, causing visual loss and, eventually, blindness. In diabetic nephropathy, destruction of the kidneys causes renal insufficiency and commonly requires hemodialysis or renal transplantation.

Gestational diabetes may occur in women who are not diabetic, but develop diabetes during pregnancy. That is, they develop an inability to metabolize carbohydrates (glucose intolerance) with resultant hyperglycemia. Gestational diabetes most

Table 13-6	Clinical Manifestations of Diabetes

According to the American Diabetes Association, the following signs and symptoms are manifestations of type 1 and type 2 diabetes.

Type 1 Diabetes

Type 1 diabetes may be suspected if any one of the associated signs and symptoms appears. Children usually exhibit dramatic, sudden symptoms and must receive prompt treatment. Signs and symptoms that signal type 1 diabetes can be remembered using the mnemonic **CAUTION.** Type 1 diabetes is characterized by the sudden appearance of:

• **C**onstant urination (polyuria) and glycosuria
• **A**bnormal thirst (polydipsia)
• **U**nusual hunger (polyphagia)
• **T**he rapid loss of weight
• **I**rritability
• **O**bvious weakness and fatigue
• **N**ausea and vomiting.

Type 2 Diabetes

Many adults may have type 2 diabetes with none of the associated signs or symptoms. The disease is commonly discovered during a routine physical examination. In addition to any of the signs and symptoms associated with type 1 diabetes, those for type 2 diabetes can be remembered using the acronym **DIABETES:**

• **D**rowsiness
• **I**tching
• **A** family history of diabetes
• **B**lurred vision
• **E**xcessive weight
• **T**ingling, numbness, and pain in the extremities
• **E**asily fatigued
• **S**kin infections and slow healing of cuts and scratches, especially of the feet.

---

often resolves after childbirth (**parturition**); however, this places women at risk of the development of type 2 diabetes later in life.

Oncology

Oncological disorders of the endocrine system vary based on the organ involved and include pancreatic cancer, pituitary tumors, and thyroid carcinoma.

Pancreatic Cancer

Most carcinomas of the pancreas arise as epithelial tumors (**adenocarcinomas**) and make their presence known by obstruction and local invasion. Because the pancreas is richly supplied with nerves, pain is a prominent feature of pancreatic cancer, whether it arises in the head, body, or tail of the organ.

The prognosis in pancreatic cancer is poor, with only a 2% survival rate in 5 years. Pancreatic cancer is the fourth leading cause of cancer death in the United States. The highest incidence is among people ages 60 to 70. The etiology is unknown, but cigarette smoking, exposure to occupational chemicals, a diet high in fats, and heavy coffee intake are associated with an increased incidence of pancreatic cancer.

Pituitary Tumors

Pituitary tumors are generally not malignant; however, because their growth is invasive, they are considered neoplastic and are usually treated as such. Initial signs and symptoms include weight changes, intolerance to heat or cold, headache, blurred vision, and, commonly, personality changes, dementia, and seizures. Tomography, skull radiographs, pneumoencephalography, angiography, and computed tomography scans assist in diagnosis. Depending on the size of the tumor and its location, different treatment modalities are employed. Treatments include surgical removal, radiation, or both.

Thyroid Carcinoma

Cancer of the thyroid gland, or *thyroid carcinoma*, is classified according to the specific tissue that is affected. In general, however, all types share many predisposing factors, including radiation, prolonged TSH stimulation, familial disposition, and chronic goiter. The malignancy usually begins with a painless, commonly hard nodule or a nodule in the adjacent lymph nodes accompanied with an enlarged thyroid. When the tumor is large, it typically destroys thyroid tissue, which results in symptoms of hypothyroidism. Sometimes the tumor stimulates the production of thyroid hormone, resulting in symptoms of hyperthyroidism. Treatment includes surgical removal, radiation, or both.

Diagnostic, Symptomatic, and Related Terms

This section introduces diagnostic, symptomatic, and related terms and their meanings. Word analyses for selected terms are also provided.

Term	Definition
acromegaly ăk-rō-MĔG-ă-lē *acr/o:* extremity *-megaly:* enlargement	Chronic metabolic disorder characterized by a gradual, marked enlargement and thickening of the bones of the face and jaw *Acromegaly afflicts middle-aged and older persons and is caused by overproduction of growth hormone (GH). Treatment includes radiation, pharmacological agents, or surgery, which commonly involves partial resection of the pituitary gland.*
diuresis dī-ū-RĒ-sĭs *di-:* double *ur:* urine *-esis:* condition	Increased formation and secretion of urine *Diuresis occurs in such conditions as diabetes mellitus, diabetes insipidus, and acute renal failure. Alcohol and coffee are common diuretics that increase formation and secretion of urine.*
glucagon GLOO-kă-gŏn	Hormone secreted by the pancreatic alpha cells *Glucagon increases the blood glucose level by stimulating the liver to change stored glycogen to glucose. Glucagon opposes the action of insulin. It is used as an injection in diabetes to reverse hypoglycemic reactions and insulin shock.*
glucose GLOO-kōs	Simple sugar that is the end product of carbohydrate digestion *Glucose is found in many foods, especially fruits, and is a major source of energy. The determination of blood glucose levels is an important diagnostic test in diabetes and other disorders.*
glycosuria glī-kō-SŪ-rē-ă *glycos:* sugar, sweetness *-uria:* urine	Presence of glucose in the urine or abnormal amount of sugar in the urine
Graves disease	Multisystem autoimmune disorder characterized by pronounced hyperthyroidism usually associated with enlarged thyroid gland and exophthalmos (abnormal protrusion of the eyeball) (See Figure 13-3.)
hirsutism HĔR-soot-ĭzm	Excessive distribution of body hair, especially in women *Hirsutism in women is usually caused by abnormalities of androgen production or metabolism.*

(continued)

Diagnostic, Symptomatic, and Related Terms—cont'd

Term	Definition
hypercalcemia hī-pĕr-kăl-SĒ-mē-ă *hyper-:* excessive, above normal *calc:* calcium *-emia:* blood	Excessive amount of calcium in the blood
hyperkalemia hī-pĕr-kă-LĒ-mē-ă *hyper-:* excessive, above normal *kal:* potassium (an electrolyte) *-emia:* blood	Excessive amount of potassium in the blood *Hyperkalemia is most commonly a result of defective renal excretion of potassium.*
hypervolemia hī-pĕr-vŏl-Ē-mē-ă *hyper-:* excessive, above normal *vol:* volume *-emia:* blood	Abnormal increase in the volume of circulating fluid (plasma) in the body *Hypervolemia commonly results from retention of large amounts of sodium and water by the kidneys. Signs and symptoms of hypervolemia include weight gain, edema, dyspnea, tachycardia, and pulmonary congestion.*
hyponatremia hī-pō-nă-TRĒ-mē-ă *hypo-:* under, below, deficient *natr:* sodium (an electrolyte) *-emia:* blood	Abnormal condition of low sodium in the blood
insulinoma ĭn-sū-lĭn-Ō-mă *insulin:* insulin *-oma:* tumor	Tumor of the islets of Langerhans of the pancreas
obesity ō-BĒ-sĭ-tē	Excessive accumulation of fat that exceeds the body's skeletal and physical standards, usually an increase of 20 percent or more above ideal body weight *Obesity may be due to excessive intake of food (exogenous) or metabolic or endocrine abnormalities (endogenous).*
morbid obesity ō-BĒ-sĭ-tē	Body mass index (BMI) of 40 or greater, which is generally 100 or more pounds over ideal body weight *Morbid obesity is a disease with serious psychological, social, and medical ramifications and one that threatens necessary body functions such as respiration.*
panhypopituitarism păn-hī-pō-pĭ-TŪ-ĭ-tăr-ĭzm *pan-:* all *hyp/o:* under, below, deficient *pituitar:* pituitary gland *-ism:* condition	Total pituitary impairment that brings about a progressive and general loss of hormonal activity
pheochromocytoma fē-ō-krō-mō-sī-TŌ-mă	Small chromaffin cell tumor, usually located in the adrenal medulla

Diagnostic, Symptomatic, and Related Terms—cont'd

Term	Definition
thyroid storm THĬ-royd *thyr:* thyroid gland *-oid:* resembling	Crisis of uncontrolled hyperthyroidism caused by the release into the bloodstream of increased amount of thyroid hormone; also called *thyroid crisis* or *thyrotoxic crisis* *Thyroid storm may occur spontaneously or be precipitated by infection, stress, or thyroidectomy performed on a patient who is inadequately prepared with antithyroid drugs. Thyroid storm is considered a medical emergency and, if left untreated, may be fatal.*
virile VĬR-ĭl	Masculine or having characteristics of a man
virilism VĬR-ĭl-ĭzm	Masculinization in a woman or development of male secondary sex characteristics in the woman

 It is time to review pathological, diagnostic, symptomatic, and related terms by completing Learning Activity 13–3.

Diagnostic and Therapeutic Procedures

This section introduces procedures used to diagnose and treat endocrine disorders. Descriptions are provided as well as pronunciations and word analyses for selected terms.

Procedure	Description
Diagnostic Procedures	
Clinical	
exophthalmometry ĕk-sŏf-thăl-MŎM-ĕ-trē *ex-:* out, out from *ophthalm/o:* eye *-metry:* act of measuring	Test that measures the degree of forward displacement of the eyeball (exophthalmos) as seen in Graves disease (See Figure 13-3.) *The test is administered with an instrument called an exophthalmometer, which allows measurement of the distance from the center of the cornea to the lateral orbital rim.*
Laboratory	
fasting blood glucose GLOO-kōs	Test that measures blood glucose levels after a 12-hour fast
glucose tolerance test (GTT) GLOO-kōs	Test that measures the body's ability to metabolize carbohydrates by administering a standard dose of glucose and measuring glucose levels in the blood and urine at regular intervals *GTT is commonly used to help diagnose diabetes or other disorders that affect carbohydrate metabolism.*
insulin tolerance test ĬN-sŭ-lĭn	Test that determines insulin levels in serum (blood) by administering insulin and measuring blood glucose levels in blood at regular intervals *In hypoglycemia, glucose levels may be lower and return to normal more slowly.*

(continued)

Diagnostic and Therapeutic Procedures—cont'd

Procedure	Description
protein-bound iodine (PBI) Ī-ō-dīn	Test that measures the concentration of thyroxine in a blood sample *The PBI test provides an index of thyroid activity.*
thyroid function test (TFT) THĪ-royd	Test that detects an increase or decrease in thyroid function *The TFT measures levels of thyroid-stimulating hormone (TSH), triiodothyronine (T_3), and thyroxine (T_4).*
total calcium KĂL-sē-ŭm	Test that measures calcium to detect bone and parathyroid disorders *Hypercalcemia can indicate primary hyperparathyroidism; hypocalcemia can indicate hypoparathyroidism.*

Radiographic

computed tomography (CT) kŏm-PŪ-tĕd tō-MŎG-ră-fē *tom/o:* to cut *-graphy:* process of recording	Imaging technique that rotates an x-ray emitter around the area to be scanned and measures the intensity of transmitted rays from different angles *In a CT scan, the computer generates a detailed cross-sectional image that appears as a slice. CT scan is used to detect disease and tumors in soft body tissues, such as the pancreas, thyroid, and adrenal glands, and may be used with or without a contrast medium.*
magnetic resonance imaging (MRI) măg-NĔT-ĭk RĔZ-ĕn-ăns ĬM-ĭj-ĭng	Noninvasive imaging technique that uses radio waves and a strong magnetic field rather than an x-ray beam to produce multiplanar cross-sectional images *MRI is the method of choice for diagnosing a growing number of diseases because it provides superior soft-tissue contrast, allows multiple plane views, and avoids the hazards of ionizing radiation. MRI is used to identify abnormalities of pituitary, pancreatic, adrenal, and thyroid glands.*
radioactive iodine uptake (RAIU) rā-dē-ō-ĂK-tĭv Ī-ō-dīn	Administration of radioactive iodine (RAI) orally or intravenously (IV) as a tracer to test how quickly the thyroid gland takes up (uptake) iodine from the blood *Results of the radioactive iodine uptake (RAIU) test are used to determine thyroid function.*
thyroid scan THĪ-royd *thyr:* thyroid gland *-oid:* resembling	After injection of a radioactive substance, a scanner detects radioactivity and visualizes the thyroid gland *Thyroid scanning is used to identify pathological formations such as nodules and tumors.*

Therapeutic Procedures
Surgical

microneurosurgery of the pituitary gland mī-krō-nū-rō-SĔR-jĕr-ē, pĭ-TŪ-ĭ-tār-ē	Microdissection of a tumor using a binocular surgical microscope for magnification
parathyroidectomy păr-ă-thī-royd-ĔK-tō-mē *para-:* near, beside; beyond *thyroid:* thyroid gland *-ectomy:* excision, removal	Excision of one or more of the parathyroid glands, usually to control hyperparathyroidism

Diagnostic and Therapeutic Procedures—cont'd

Procedure	Description
pinealectomy pĭn-ē-ăl-ĔK-tō-mē	Removal of the pineal body
thymectomy thī-MĔK-tō-mē *thym:* thymus gland *-ectomy:* excision, removal	Excision of the thymus gland
thyroidectomy thī-royd-ĔK-tō-mē *thyroid:* thyroid gland *-ectomy:* excision, removal	Excision of the thyroid gland *Thyroidectomy is performed for goiter, tumors, or hyperthyroidism that does not respond to iodine therapy and antithyroid drugs.*
partial	Method of choice for removing a fibrous, nodular thyroid
subtotal	Removal of most of the thyroid to relieve hyperthyroidism

Pharmacology

Common disorders associated with endocrine glands include hyposecretion and hypersecretion of hormones. When deficiencies of this type occur, natural and synthetic hormones, such as insulin and thyroid agents, are prescribed. These agents normalize hormone levels to maintain proper functioning and homeostasis. Therapeutic agents are also available to regulate various substances in the body, such as glucose levels in diabetic patients. Hormone replacement therapy (HRT), such as synthetic thyroid and estrogen, treat these hormonal deficiencies. Although specific drugs are not covered in this section, hormonal chemotherapy drugs are used to treat certain cancers, such as testicular, ovarian, breast, and endometrial cancer. (See Table 13–7.)

Table 13-7 Drugs Used to Treat Endocrine Disorders

This table lists common drug classifications used to treat endocrine disorders, their therapeutic actions, and selected generic and trade names.

Classification	Therapeutic Action	Generic and Trade Names
antidiuretics	Reduce or control excretion of urine.	**vasopressin** văs-ō-PRĔS-ĭn Pitressin, Pressyn
antithyroids	Treat hyperthyroidism by impeding the formation of T_3 and T_4 hormone. *Antithyroids are administered in preparation for a thyroidectomy and in thyrotoxic crisis.*	**methimazole** mĕth-ĬM-ă-zōl Tapazole **strong iodine solution** Ī-ō-dīn Lugol's solution

(continued)

Table 13-7	Drugs Used to Treat Endocrine Disorders—cont'd	
Classification	**Therapeutic Action**	**Generic and Trade Names**

corticosteroids	Replace hormones lost in adrenal insufficiency (Addison disease).
	
	Corticosteroids are also widely used to suppress inflammation, control allergic reactions, reduce rejection in transplantation, and treat some cancer.
		cortisone
		KOR-tĭ-sōn
		  Cortisone acetate
		hydrocortisone
		hī-drō-KOR-tĭ-sōn
		  A-Hydrocort, Cortef

growth hormone replacements	Increase skeletal growth in children and growth hormone deficiencies in adults *Growth hormones increase spinal bone density and help manage growth failure in children.*	**somatropin (recombinant)** sō-mă-TRŌ-pĭn Humatrope, Norditropin

insulins	Lower blood glucose by promoting its entrance into body cells and converting glucose to glycogen (a starch-storage form of glucose).
	
	Insulin links with an insulin receptor on the cell membrane, and transports glucose inside the cell where it is metabolized. Type 1 diabetes must always be treated with insulin. Insulin can also be administered through an implanted pump which infuses the drug continuously. Type 2 diabetes that cannot be controlled with oral antidiabetics may require insulin to maintain a normal level of glucose in the blood.
		regular insulin
		ĬN-sŭ-lĭn
		  Humulin R*, Novolin R
		NPH insulin
		ĬN-sŭ-lĭn
		  Humulin N, Novolin N, Humulin

oral antidiabetics	Treat type 2 diabetes mellitus by stimulating the pancreas to produce more insulin and decrease peripheral resistance to insulin.
	
	Antidiabetic drugs are not insulin and they are not used in treating type 1 diabetes mellitus.
		glipizide
		GLĬP-ĭ-zīd
		  Glucotrol, Glucotrol XL
		glyburide
		GLĪ-bū-rīd
		  DiaBeta, Glynase

thyroid supplements	Replace or supplement thyroid hormones
	
	Each thyroid supplement contains T_3, T_4, or a combination of both. Thyroid supplements are also used to treat some types of thyroid cancer.
		levothyroxine
		lē-vō-thī-RŎK-sēn
		  Levo-T, Levoxyl, Synthroid
		liothyronine
		lī-ō-THĪ-rō-nēn
		  Cytomel, Triostat

*The trade name for all human genetically produced insulins is *Humulin*. Traditionally, insulin has been derived from beef or pork pancreas. Human insulin is genetically produced using recombinant DNA techniques to avoid the potential for allergic reaction.

Abbreviations

This section introduces endocrine-related abbreviations and their meanings.

Abbreviation	Meaning	Abbreviation	Meaning
ACTH	adrenocorticotropic hormone	MSH	melanocyte-stimulating hormone
ADH	antidiuretic hormone (vasopressin)	NPH	neutral protamine Hagedorn (insulin)
BMI	body mass index	PBI	protein-bound iodine
BMR	basal metabolic rate	PRL	prolactin
DI	diabetes insipidus; diagnostic imaging	PGH	pituitary growth hormone
DKA	diabetic ketoacidosis	PTH	parathyroid hormone; also called *parathormone*
DM	diabetes mellitus	RAI	radioactive iodine
FSH	follicle-stimulating hormone	RAIU	radioactive iodine uptake
GH	growth hormone	T_3	triiodothyronine (thyroid hormone)
HRT	hormone replacement therapy	T_4	thyroxine (thyroid hormone)
K	potassium (an electrolyte)	TFT	thyroid function test
LH	luteinizing hormone	TSH	thyroid-stimulating hormone
mg/dl, mg/dL	milligrams per deciliter		

It is time to review procedures, pharmacology, and abbreviations by completing Learning Activity 13–4.

LEARNING ACTIVITIES

The activities that follow provide review of the endocrine system terms introduced in this chapter. Complete each activity and review your answers to evaluate your understanding of the chapter.

Learning Activity 13-1
Identifying Endocrine Structures

Label the following illustration using the terms listed below.

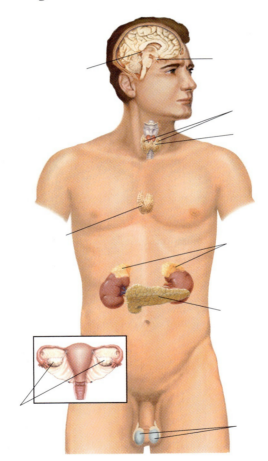

adrenal (suprarenal) glands	*parathyroid glands*	*testes*
ovaries	*pineal gland*	*thymus gland*
pancreas	*pituitary (hypophysis) gland*	*thyroid gland*

 Check your answers by referring to Figure 13–1 on page 395. Review material that you did not answer correctly.

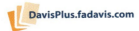 **DavisPlus.fadavis.com**

Enhance your study and reinforcement of word elements with the power of Davis Plus. Visit **www.davisplus.fadavis.com/gylys/systems** *for this chapter's flash-card activity. We recommend you complete the flash-card activity before completing activity 13–2 below.*

Learning Activity 13-2
Building Medical Words

Use *glyc/o* (sugar) to build words that mean:

1. blood condition of excessive glucose _____

2. blood condition of deficiency of glucose _____

3. formation of glycogen _____

Use *pancreat/o* (pancreas) to build words that mean:

4. inflammation of the pancreas _____

5. destruction of the pancreas _____

6. disease of the pancreas _____

Use *thyr/o* or *thyroid/o* (thyroid gland) to build words that mean:

7. inflammation of the thyroid gland _____

8. enlargement of the thyroid _____

Build surgical words that mean:

9. excision of a parathyroid gland _____

10. removal of the adrenal gland _____

Check your answers in Appendix A. Review material that you did not answer correctly.

Correct Answers _____ × 10 = _____ Score

Learning Activity 13-3

Matching Pathological, Diagnostic, Symptomatic, and Related Terms

Match the following terms with the definitions in the numbered list.

Addison disease	glycosuria	myxedema
cretinism	hirsutism	pheochromocytoma
Cushing syndrome	hyperkalemia	type 1 diabetes
diuresis	hyponatremia	type 2 diabetes
exophthalmic goiter	insulin	virile

1. _____ having characteristics of a man; masculine

2. _____ hypothyroidism acquired in adulthood

3. _____ increased excretion of urine

4. _____ excessive growth of hair in unusual places, especially in women

5. _____ hypothyroidism that appears as a congenital condition and is commonly associated with other endocrine abnormalities

6. _____ hormone produced by beta cells of the pancreas

7. _____ caused by deficiency in the secretion of adrenocortical hormones

8. _____ characterized by protrusion of the eyeballs, increased heart action, enlargement of the thyroid gland, weight loss, and nervousness

9. _____ excessive amount of potassium in the blood

10. _____ small chromaffin cell tumor, usually located in the adrenal medulla

11. _____ insulin-dependent diabetes mellitus; occurs most commonly in children and adolescents (juvenile onset)

12. _____ decreased concentration of sodium in the blood

13. _____ abnormal presence of glucose in the urine

14. _____ metabolic disorder caused by hypersecretion of the adrenal cortex resulting in excessive production of glucocorticoids, mainly cortisol

15. _____ non-insulin-dependent diabetes mellitus; occurs later in life (maturity onset)

✔ *Check your answers in Appendix A. Review material that you did not answer correctly.*

Correct Answers _____ × 6.67 = _____ Score

Learning Activity 13-4
Matching Procedures, Pharmacology, and Abbreviations

Match the following terms with the definitions in the numbered list.

antithyroids	*growth hormone*	*protein-bound iodine*
CT scan	*GTT*	*RAIU*
corticosteroids	*Humulin*	T_3
exophthalmometry	*MRI*	T_4
FBS	*oral antidiabetics*	*thyroid scan*

1. _____ measures circulating glucose level after a 12-hour fast

2. _____ measures thyroid function and monitors how quickly ingested iodine is taken into the thyroid gland

3. _____ replacement hormones for adrenal insufficiency (Addison disease)

4. _____ increases skeletal growth in children

5. _____ radioactive compound is administered and localizes in the thyroid gland; used to detect thyroid abnormalities

6. _____ thyroxine

7. _____ used to treat type 2 diabetes

8. _____ diagnostic test used to determine hypoglycemia, hyperglycemia, and adjustments in insulin dosage

9. _____ used to treat hyperthyroidism by impeding the formation of T_3 and T_4 hormone

10. _____ test to measure the concentration of thyroxine in a blood sample

11. _____ triiodothyronine

12. _____ noninvasive imaging technique that uses radio waves and a strong magnetic field to produce multiplanar cross-sectional images

13. _____ test that measures the degree of forward displacement of the eyeball as seen in Graves disease

14. _____ imaging technique achieved by rotating an x-ray emitter around the area to be scanned and measuring the intensity of transmitted rays from different angles; used to detect disease in soft body tissues, such as the pancreas, thyroid, and adrenal glands

15. _____ trade name for all human genetically produced insulins

Check your answers in Appendix A. Review any material that you did not answer correctly.

Correct Answers _____ × 6.67 = _____ **Score**

MEDICAL RECORD ACTIVITIES

The two medical records included in the activities that follow use common clinical scenarios to show how medical terminology is used to document patient care. Complete the terminology and analysis sections for each activity to help you recognize and understand terms related to the endocrine system.

Medical Record Activity 13-1
Consultation Note: Hyperparathyroidism

Terminology

Terms listed below come from *Consultation Note: Hyperparathyroidism* that follows. Use a medical dictionary such as *Taber's Cyclopedic Medical Dictionary,* the appendices of this book, or other resources to define each term. Then review the pronunciations for each term and practice by reading the medical record aloud.

Term	Definition
adenoma ăd-ĕ-NŌ-mă	
claudication klăw-dĭ-KĀ-shŭn	
diabetes mellitus dī-ă-BĒ-tēz MĔ-lĭ-tŭs	
endocrinologist ĕn-dō-krĭn-ŎL-ō-jĭst	
hypercalciuria hī-pĕr-kăl-sē-Ū-rē-ă	
hyperparathyroidism hī-pĕr-păr-ă-THĪ-roy-dĭzm	
impression ĭm-PRĔSH-ŭn	
osteoarthritis ŏs-tē-ō-ăr-THRĪ-tĭs	
parathyroid păr-ă-THĪ-royd	
peripheral vascular disease pĕr-ĬF-ĕr-ăl VĂS-kū-lăr	

Listen and Learn Online! *will help you master the pronunciation of selected medical words from this medical record activity. Visit* www.davisplus.com/gylys/systems *to find instructions on completing the* Listen and Learn Online! *exercise for this section and to practice pronunciations.*

CONSULTATION NOTE: HYPERPARATHYROID

Consultation Note

Day, Phyllis   5/25/xx
Med Record: P25882

HISTORY OF PRESENT ILLNESS: This 66-year-old former blackjack dealer is under evaluation for hyperparathyroidism. Surgery evidently has been recommended, but there is confusion as to how urgent this is. She has a 13-year history of type 1 diabetes mellitus, a history of shoulder pain, osteoarthritis of the spine, and peripheral vascular disease with claudication. She states her 548-pack/year smoking history ended 3-1/2 years ago. Her first knowledge of parathyroid disease was about 3 years ago when laboratory findings revealed an elevated calcium level. This subsequently led to the diagnosis of hyperparathyroidism. She was further evaluated by an endocrinologist in the Lake Tahoe area, who determined that she also had hypercalciuria, although there is nothing to suggest a history of kidney stones.

IMPRESSION: Hyperparathyroidism and hypercalciuria, probably a parathyroid adenoma

PLAN: Patient advised to make a follow-up appointment with her endocrinologist.

Juan Perez, MD
Juan Perez, MD

D: 05-25-xx
T: 05-25-xx
jp:lg

Analysis

Review the medical record *Consultation Note: Hyperparathyroidism* to answer the following questions.

1. What is an adenoma?

_____

2. What does the physician suspect caused the patient's hyperparathyroidism?

_____

3. What type of laboratory findings revealed parathyroid disease?

_____

4. What is hypercalciuria?

_____

5. If the patient smoked 548 packs of cigarettes per year, how many packs did she smoke in an average day?

_____

Medical Record Activity 13-2

SOAP Note: Diabetes Mellitus

Terminology

Terms listed below come from *SOAP Note: Diabetes Mellitus* that follows. Use a medical dictionary such as *Taber's Cyclopedic Medical Dictionary,* the appendices of this book, or other resources to define each term. Then review the pronunciations for each term and practice by reading the medical record aloud.

Term	Definition
Accu-chek ĂK-ū-chĕk	
morbid obesity MOR-bĭd ō-BĒ-sĭ-tē	
obesity, exogenous ō-BĒ-sĭ-tē, ĕks-ŎJ-ĕ-nŭs	
polydipsia pŏl-ē-DĬP-sē-ă	
polyphagia pŏl-ē-FĀ-jē-ă	
polyuria pŏl-ē-Ū-rē-ă	

 Listen and Learn Online! *will help you master the pronunciation of selected medical words from this medical record activity. Visit* www.davisplus.com/gylys/systems *to find instructions on completing the* Listen and Learn Online! *exercise for this section and to practice pronunciations.*

SOAP NOTE: DIABETES MELLITUS

Emergency Department Record

Date: 2/4/xx
Patient: Pleume, Roberta
Age: 68

Time Registered: 1445 hours
Physician: Samara Batichara, MD
Patient ID#: 22258

Chief Complaint: Frequent urination, increased hunger and thirst.

S: This 200-pound patient was admitted to the hospital because of a 10-day history of polyuria, polydipsia, and polyphagia. She has been very nervous, irritable, and very sensitive emotionally and cries easily. During this period, she has had headaches and has become very sleepy and tired after eating. On admission, her Accu-Chek was 540 mg/dL. Family history is significant in that both parents and two sisters have type 1 diabetes.

O: Physical examination was essentially negative. The abdomen was difficult to evaluate because of morbid obesity.

A: Diabetes mellitus; obesity, exogenous.

P: Patient admitted to the hospital for further evaluation.

Samara Batichara, MD
Samara Batichara, MD

D: 02-04-xx
T: 02-04-xx

sb:lb

Analysis

Review the medical record *SOAP Note: Diabetes Mellitus* to answer the following questions.

1. How long has this patient been experiencing voracious eating?

_____

2. Was the patient's obesity due to overeating or metabolic imbalance?

_____

3. Why did the doctor experience difficulty in examining the patient's abdomen?

_____

4. Was the patient's blood glucose above or below normal on admission?

_____

5. What is the reference range for fasting blood glucose?

_____

Nervous System

CHAPTER

14

Chapter Outline

Objectives

Upon completion of this chapter, you will be able to:

- Locate and describe the structures of the nervous system.
- Describe the functional relationship between the nervous system and other body systems.
- Recognize, pronounce, spell, and build words related to the nervous system.
- Describe pathological conditions, diagnostic and therapeutic procedures, and other terms related to the nervous system.
- Explain pharmacology related to the treatment of nervous disorders.
- Demonstrate your knowledge of this chapter by completing the learning and medical record activities.

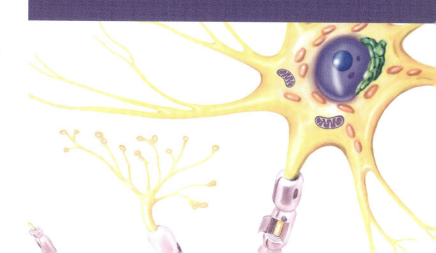

Anatomy and Physiology

The nervous system is one of the most complicated systems of the body in both structure and function. It senses physical and chemical changes in the internal and external environments, processes them, and then responds to maintain homeostasis. Voluntary activities, such as walking and talking, and involuntary activities, such as digestion and circulation, are coordinated, regulated, and integrated by the nervous system. The entire neural network of the body relies on the transmission of nervous impulses. **Nervous impulses** are electrochemical stimuli that travel from cell to cell as they send information from one area of the body to another. The speed at which this occurs is almost instantaneous, thus providing an immediate response to change.

Cellular Structure of the Nervous System

Despite its complexity, the nervous system is composed of only two principal types of cells: neurons and neuroglia. **Neurons** are cells that transmit impulses. They are commonly identified by the direction the impulse travels as **afferent** when the direction is toward the brain or spinal cord or **efferent** when the direction is away from the brain or spinal cord. **Neuroglia** are cells that support neurons and bind them to other neurons or other tissues of the body. Although they do not transmit impulses, they provide a variety activities essential to the proper functioning of neurons. Along with neurons, neuroglia contitute the nervous tissue of the body.

Anatomy and Physiology Key Terms

This section introduces important nervous system terms and their definitions. Word analyses for selected terms are also provided.

Term	Definition
afferent ĂF-ĕr-ĕnt	Carry or move inward or toward a central structure *The term **afferent** refers to certain arteries, veins, lymphatic vessels, and nerves.*
blood-brain barrier	Protective mechanism that blocks specific substances found in the bloodstream from entering delicate brain tissue
central nervous system (CNS) NĔR-vĕs	Network of nervous tissue found in the brain and spinal cord
efferent ĔF-ĕ-rĕnt	Carry or move away from a central structure *The term **efferent** refers to certain arteries, veins, lymphatic vessels, and nerves.*
nerve fiber	Projection of a neuron, especially the axon that transmits impulses
neurilemma nū-rĭ-LĔM-ă	Additional sheath external to myelin that is formed by Schwann cells and found only on axons in the peripheral nervous system *Because neurilemma does not disintegrate after injury to the axon, its enclosed hollow tube provides an avenue for regeneration of injured axons.*
ventricle VĔN-trĭk-l 　*ventr:* belly, belly side 　*-ical:* pertaining to	Chamber or cavity of an organ that receives or holds a fluid

Pronunciation Help	Long Sound	ā—rate	ē—rebirth	ī—isle	ō—over	ū—unite
	Short Sound	ă—alone	ĕ—ever	ĭ—it	ŏ—not	ŭ—cut

Neurons

The three major structures of the neuron are the cell body, axon, and dendrites. (See Figure 14–1.) The (1) **cell body** is the enlarged structure of the neuron that contains the (2) **nucleus** of the cell and various organelles. Its branching cytoplasmic projections are (3) **dendrites** that carry impulses to the cell body and (4) **axons** that carry impulses from the cell body. Dendrites resemble tiny branches on a tree, providing additional surface area for receiving impulses from other neurons. Axons are long, single projections ranging from a few millimeters to more than a meter in length. Axons transmit impulses to dendrites of other neurons as well as muscles and glands.

Axons in the **peripheral nervous system** and the **central nervous system** possess a white, lipoid covering called (5) **myelin sheath.** This covering acts as an electrical insulator that reduces the possibility

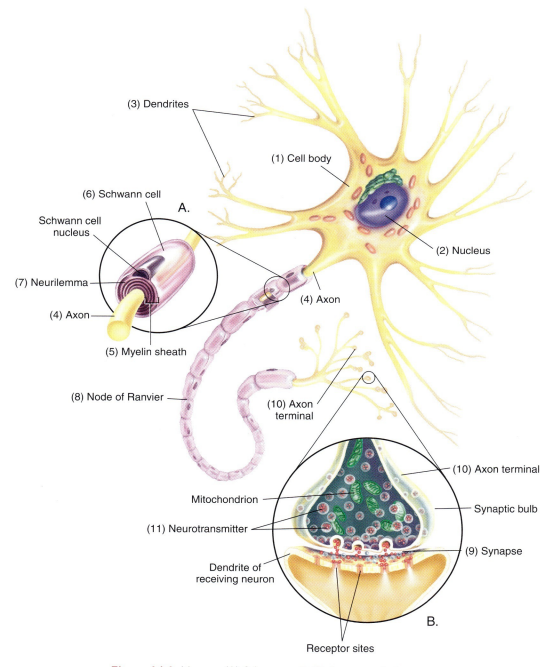

Figure 14-1. Neuron. (A) Schwann cell. (B) Axon terminal synapse.

of an impulse stimulating adjacent nerves. It also accelerates impulse transmission through the axon. On nerves in the peripheral nervous system, myelin sheath is formed by a neuroglial cell called a (6) **Schwann cell** that wraps tightly around the axon. Its exterior surface forms a thin tube called (7) neurilemma, or **neurolemma.** The neurilemma does not disintegrate after an axon has been crushed or severed, as does the axon and myelin sheath, but remains intact. This intact sheath provides a pathway for possible neuron regeneration after injury.

The myelin sheath covering the axons in the central nervous system is formed by oligodendrocytes rather than Schwann cells. Oligodendrocytes do not produce neurilemma, thus injury or damage to neurons located in the central nervous system is irreparable. The short unmyelinated spaces between adjacent segments of myelin sheath are called (8) **nodes of Ranvier.** These nodes help speed the transmission of impulses down the axon because an impulse jumps across the nodes at a faster rate than it is able to travel through the myelinated axon.

The functional connection between two neurons or between a neuron and its target (muscle or gland) is a gap or space called a (9) **synapse.** Impulses must travel from the (10) **axon terminal** of one neuron to the dendrite of the next neuron or to its target by crossing this synapse. The impulse within the transmitting axon causes a chemical substance called a (11) **neurotransmitter** to be released at the end of its axon. The neurotransmitter diffuses across the synapse and attaches to the receiving neuron at specialized receptor sites. When sufficient receptor sites are occupied, it signals an acceptance "message" and the impulse passes to the receiving neuron. The receiving neuron immediately inactivates the neurotransmitter, and prepares the site for receiving another stimulus.

Neuroglia

The term **neuroglia** literally means *nerve glue* because these cells were originally believed to serve only one function: to bind neurons to each other and to other structures. They are now known to supply nutrients and oxygen to neurons and assist in other metabolic activities. They also play an important role when the nervous system suffers injury or infection. The four major types of neuroglia include astrocytes, oligodendrocytes, microglia, and ependyma. (See Figure 14–2.)

Astrocytes, as their name suggests, are star-shaped neuroglia. They provide three-dimensional mechanical support for neurons and form tight sheaths around the capillaries of the brain. These

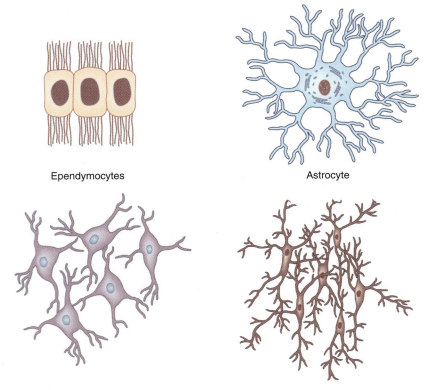

Ependymocytes

Astrocyte

Oligodendrocytes

Microglia

Figure 14-2. Four types of neuroglia.

sheaths provide an obstruction, called the **blood-brain barrier,** that keeps large molecular substances from entering the delicate tissue of the brain. Even so, small molecules, such as water, carbon dioxide, oxygen, and alcohol, readily pass from blood vessels through the barrier and enter the interstitial spaces of the brain. Researchers must take the blood-brain barrier into consideration when developing drugs for treatment of brain disorders. Astrocytes also perform mildly phagocytic functions in the brain and spinal cord. **Oligodendrocytes,** also called *oligodendroglia,* are responsible for developing myelin on neurons of the central nervous system. **Microglia,** the smallest of the neuroglia, possess phagocytic properties and may become very active during times of infection. **Ependyma** are ciliated cells that line fluid-filled cavities of the central nervous system, especially the ventricles of the brain. They assist in the circulation of cerebrospinal fluid (CSF).

Nervous System Divisions

The nervous system consists of two main divisions: the central nervous system and the peripheral nervous system. The **central nervous system (CNS)** consists of the brain and spinal cord. The **peripheral nervous system (PNS)** includes all other nervous tissues of the body. (See Table 14–1.)

Central Nervous System

The **central nervous system (CNS)** consists of the brain and spinal cord. Its nervous tissue is classified as *white matter* or *gray matter*. Bundles of axons with their white lipoid myelin sheath constitutes white matter and unmyelinated fibers, dendrites, and nerve cell bodies make up gray matter

of the brain and spinal cord. The brain is protected by the bony skull and the spinal cord is protected by vertebrae.

Brain

In addition to being one of the largest organs of the body, the brain is highly complex in structure and function. (See Figure 14–3.) It integrates almost every physical and mental activity of the body and is the center for memory, emotion, thought, judgment, reasoning, and consciousness. The four major structures of the brain are:

* cerebrum
* cerebellum
* diencephalon
* brainstem.

Cerebrum

The (1) **cerebrum** is the largest and uppermost portion of the brain. It consists of two hemispheres divided by a deep longitudinal fissure, or groove. The fissure does not completely separate the hemispheres. A structure called the (2) **corpus callosum** joins these hemispheres, permitting communication between the right and left sides of the brain. Each hemisphere is divided into five lobes. Four of these lobes are named for the bones that lie directly above them: (3) **frontal**, (4) **parietal**, (5) **temporal**, and (6) **occipital**. The fifth lobe, the **insula** (not shown in Figure 14–3), is hidden from view and can be seen only upon dissection.

The cerebral surface consists of numerous folds, or convolutions, called *gyri.* The gyri are separated by furrows or fissures called *sulci.* A thin layer called the *cerebral cortex* covers the entire cerebrum and is composed of gray matter.

Table 14-1	**Nervous System Structures and Functions**	
	This table lists the structures of the nervous system along with their functions.	
Structures	**Function**	
Central		
Brain	Center for thought and emotion, interpretation of sensory stimuli, and coordination of body functions	
Spinal cord	Main pathway for transmission of information between the brain and body	
Peripheral		
Cranial nerves	Includes 12 pairs of nerves that emerge from the base of the skull and may act in either a motor capacity, sensory capacity, or both	
Spinal nerves	Includes 31 pairs of nerves that emerge from the spine and act in both motor and sensory capacities	

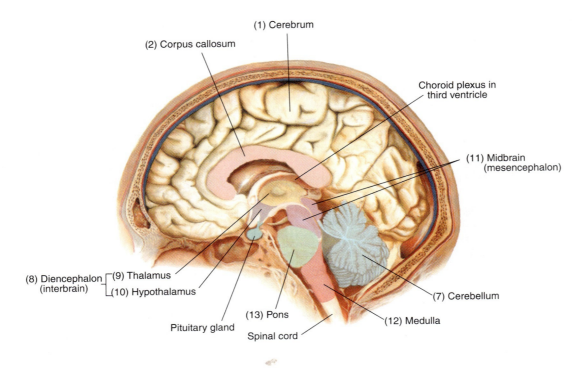

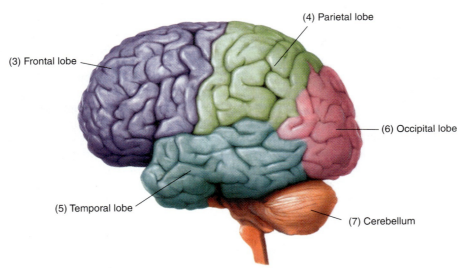

Figure 14-3. Brain structures.

The remainder of the cerebrum is primarily composed of white matter (myelinated axons). Major functions of the cerebrum include sensory perception and interpretation, language, voluntary movement, memory, and the emotional aspects of behavior.

Cerebellum

The second largest structure of the brain, the (7) **cerebellum,** occupies the posterior portion of the skull. All functions of the cerebellum involve movement. When the cerebrum initiates muscular movement, the cerebellum coordinates and refines it. The cerebellum also aids in maintaining equilibrium and balance.

Diencephalon

The (8) **diencephalon** (also called *interbrain*) is composed of many smaller structures, including the thalamus and the hypothalamus. The (9) **thalamus** receives all sensory stimuli except olfactory and processes and transmits them to the appropriate centers in the cerebral cortex. In addition, the thalamus receives impulses from the cerebrum and relays them to efferent nerves. The (10) **hypothalamus** regulates activities of the **autonomic nervous system (ANS),** including impulses that regulate heartbeat, body temperature, and fluid balance. It also controls many endocrine functions.

Brainstem

The brainstem completes the last major section of the brain. It is composed of three structures: the (11) **midbrain** (also called *mesencephalon*), separating the cerebrum from the brainstem; the (12) **medulla,** which attaches to the spinal cord; and (13) the **pons,** or "bridge," connecting the midbrain to the medulla. In general, the brainstem is a pathway for impulse conduction between the brain and spinal cord. The brainstem is the origin of 10 of the 12 pairs of cranial nerves and controls respiration, blood pressure, and heart rate. Because the brainstem is the site that controls the beginning of life (the initiation of the beating heart in a fetus) and the end of life (the cessation of respiration and heart activity) it is sometimes called the *primary brain.*

Spinal cord

The **spinal cord** transmits sensory impulses from the body to the brain and motor impulses from the brain to muscles and organs of the body. The sensory nerve tracts are called *ascending tracts* because the direction of the impulse is upward. Conversely, motor nerve tracts are called *descending tracts* because they carry impulses in a downward direction to muscles and organs. A cross-section of the spinal cord reveals an inner gray matter composed of cell bodies and dendrites and an outer white matter area composed of myelinated tissue of the ascending and descending tracts.

The entire spinal cord is located within the spinal cavity of the vertebral column, with spinal nerves exiting between the intervertebral spaces throughout almost the entire length of the spinal column. Unlike the cranial nerves, which have specific names, the spinal nerves are identified by the region of the vertebral column from which they exit.

Meninges

The brain and spinal cord receive limited protection from three coverings called *meninges* (singular, *meninx*). These coverings include the dura mater, arachnoid, and pia mater.

The **dura mater** is the outermost covering of the brain and spinal cord. It is tough, fibrous, and dense, and composed primarily of connective tissue. Because of its thickness, this membrane is also called the *pachymeninges.* Beneath the dura mater is a cavity called the *subdural space,* which is filled with serous fluid.

The **arachnoid** is the middle covering and, as its name suggests, has a spider-web appearance. It fits loosely over the underlying structures. A **subarachnoid space** contains **cerebrospinal fluid,** a colorless fluid that contains proteins, glucose, urea, salts, and some white blood cells. This fluid circulates around the spinal cord and brain and through ventricles located within the inner portion of the brain. It provides nutritive substances to the central nervous system and adds additional protection for the brain and spinal cord by acting as a shock absorber. Normally, cerebrospinal fluid is absorbed as rapidly as it is formed, maintaining a constant fluid volume. Any interference with its absorption results in a collection of fluid in the brain; a condition called *hydrocephalus.*

The **pia mater** is the innermost meninx. This membrane directly adheres to the brain and spinal cord. As it passes over the brain, it follows the contours of the gyri and sulci. It contains numerous blood vessels and lymphatics that nourish the underlying tissues. Because of the thinness and delicacy of the arachnoid and pia mater, these two meninges are collectively called the *leptomeninges.*

Peripheral Nervous System

The **peripheral nervous system (PNS)** is composed of all nervous tissue located outside of the spinal column and skull. Its anatomical structures consists of 12 pairs of cranial nerves and 31 pairs of spinal nerves. Functionally, the PNS is subdivided into the somatic nervous system(SNS) and the autonomic nervous system (ANS).

The **somatic nervous system** consists of nerve fibers that transmit sensory information to the brain and spinal cord, and nerve fibers that transmit impulses from the brain and spinal cord to muscles under conscious or voluntary control, such as those required for walking and talking. The **autonomic nervous system** consists of nerves that control involuntary movement, such as digestion, heart contraction, and vasoconstriction. It also regulates secretion by glands.

The ANS is subdivided into the sympathetic and parasympathetic divisions. To a large extent, these subdivisions oppose the action of the other, although in certain instances, they may exhibit independent or complimentary action. In general, the **sympathetic** subdivision produces responses evident in "fight-or-flight" situations. It responds when immediate actions are required. Blood flow increases in skeletal muscles to prepare an individual to either fight or retreat from a threatening situation. The **parasympathetic** subdivision generally responds when immediate action is not required or a threatening situation subsides. This subdivision is sometimes called the "rest and relax" or "rest and digest" condition. (See Table 14–2.)

Cranial Nerves

The cranial nerves originate in the base of the brain and emerge though openings in the base of the skull. They are designated by name or number. (See Figure 14–4.) Cranial nerves may be sensory, motor, or a mixture of both. **Sensory nerves** are afferent, and receive impulses from the sense organs, including the eyes, ears, nose, tongue, and skin and transmit them to the CNS. **Motor nerves** conduct impulses to muscles and glands. Some cranial nerves are composed of both sensory and motor fibers. They are called *mixed nerves.* An example of a mixed nerve is the facial nerve. It acts in a motor capacity by transmitting impulses for smiling or frowning. However, it also acts in a sensory capacity by transmitting taste impulses from the tongue to the brain.

Spinal Nerves

The spinal nerves emerge from the intervertebral spaces in the spinal column. All 31 pairs of spinal nerves are mixed nerves. (See Figure 14–5.) They exit from the spinal canal between the vertebrae and extend to various parts of the body. Each of them is identified according to the vertebra from which they exit. Each of them has two points of attachment to the spinal cord: an anterior (ventral) root and a posterior (dorsal) root. The **anterior root** contains motor fibers and the **posterior root** contains sensory fibers. These two roots unite to form the spinal nerve that has both afferent and efferent qualities.

Table 14-2	Actions Regulated by Sympathetic and Parasympathetic Systems

This table summarizes some of the responses regulated by the sympathetic and parasympathetic divisions of the peripheral nervous system.

Sympathetic Division	Parasympathetic Division
Dilates pupils	Constricts pupils
Inhibits the flow of saliva	Increases the flow of saliva
Relaxes bronchi	Constricts bronchi
Accelerates heart rate	Slows heart rate
Slows digestive activities	Accelerates digestive activities
Constricts visceral blood vessels	Dilates visceral blood vessels

Connecting Body Systems–Nervous System

The main function of the nervous system is to identify and respond to internal and external changes in the environment to maintain homeostasis. Specific functional relationships between the nervous system and other body systems are discussed below.

Blood, Lymph, and Immune
- Nervous system identifies changes in blood and lymph composition and provides the stimuli to maintain homeostasis.
- Nervous system identifies pathologically altered tissue and assists the immune system in containing injury and promoting healing.

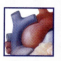

Cardiovascular
- Nervous tissue, especially the conduction system of the heart, transmits a contraction impulse.
- Nervous system identifies pressure changes on vascular walls and responds to regulate blood pressure.

Digestive
- Nervous stimuli of digestive organs propel food by peristalsis.
- Nerve receptors in the lower colon identify the need to defecate.

Endocrine
- The hypothalamus regulates hormone production.

Female reproductive
- Nervous system transmits contraction impulses needed for delivery of a fetus.
- Nervous system provides stimuli needed for lactation.
- Nervous system regulates hormones needed for the menstrual cycle.

Genitourinary
- Nervous tissue in reproductive organs receives pleasure responses.
- Nervous system responds to pressure changes in bladder walls that indicate the need to void.
- Nervous system stimulates the thirst reflex when body fluid levels are low.

Integumentary
- Sensory nervous system supplies receptors in the skin that respond to environmental stimuli.
- Autonomic nervous system regulates body temperature by controlling shivering and sweating.

Musculoskeletal
- Nervous system provides impulses for contraction resulting in voluntary and involuntary movement of muscles.
- Autonomic nervous tissue responds to positional changes.

Respiratory
- Nervous system stimulates muscle contractions that create pressure changes necessary for ventilation.
- Nervous system regulates rate and depth of breathing.

 It is time to review nervous system structures by completing Learning Activity 14–1.

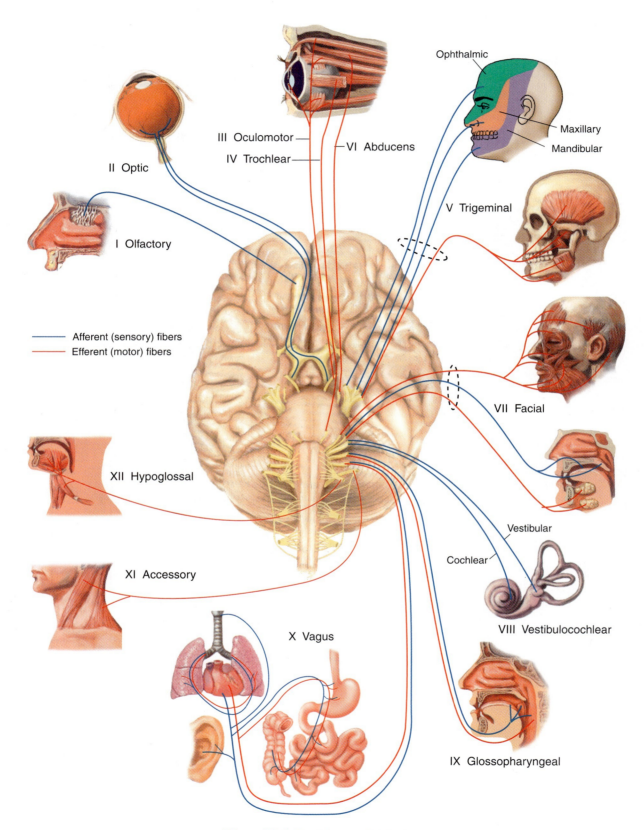

II Optic

III Oculomotor

IV Trochlear

VI Abducens

I Olfactory

Ophthalmic

Maxillary

Mandibular

V Trigeminal

Afferent (sensory) fibers
Efferent (motor) fibers

VII Facial

XII Hypoglossal

Vestibular

Cochlear

XI Accessory

VIII Vestibulocochlear

X Vagus

IX Glossopharyngeal

Figure 14-4. Cranial nerve distribution.

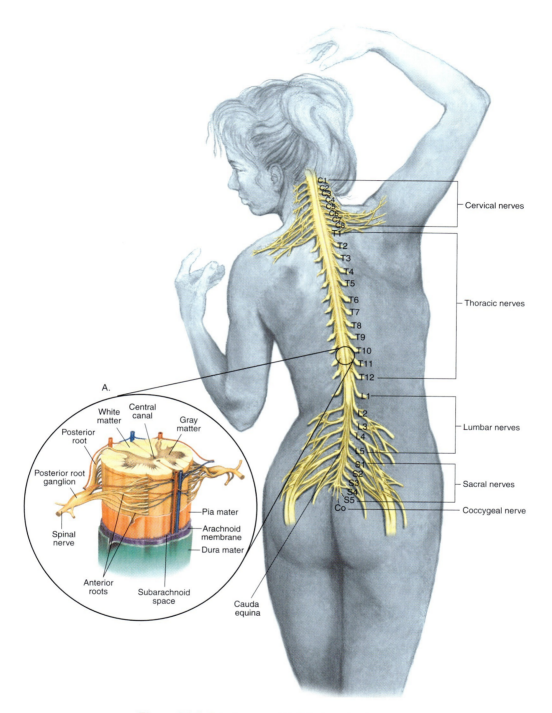

Cervical nerves

Thoracic nerves

Lumbar nerves

Sacral nerves

Coccygeal nerve

C1
C2
C3
C4
C5
C6
C7
C8
T1
T2
T3
T4
T5
T6
T7
T8
T9
T10
T11
T12
L1
L2
L3
L4
L5
S1
S2
S3
S4
S5
Co

A.

White
matter

Central
canal

Gray
matter

Posterior
root

Posterior root
ganglion

Spinal
nerve

Pia mater

Arachnoid
membrane

Dura mater

Anterior
roots

Subarachnoid
space

Cauda
equina

Figure 14-5. Spinal nerves. (A) Spinal cord enlargement.

Medical Word Elements

This section introduces combining forms, suffixes, and prefixes related to the nervous system. Word analyses are also provided.

Element	Meaning	Word Analysis
Combining Forms		
cerebr/o	cerebrum	**cerebr/o/tomy** (sĕr-ĕ-BRŎT-ō-mē): incision of the cerebrum *-tomy:* incision
crani/o	cranium (skull)	**crani/o/malacia** (krā-nē-ō-mă-LĀ-shē-ă): softening of the cranium *-malacia:* softening
dendr/o	tree	**dendr/oid** (DĔN-droyd): resembling a (branching) tree *-oid:* resembling *Dendrons, the highly branched portion of the neuron, conduct nerve impulses toward the cell body.*
encephal/o	brain	**encephal/o/cele** (ĕn-SĔF-ă-lō-sēl): herniation of the brain *-cele:* hernia, swelling *Encephalocele is a condition in which portions of the brain and meninges protrude through a bony midline defect in the skull. It is usually associated with a neural tube defect.*
gangli/o	ganglion (knot or knotlike mass)	**gangli/ectomy** (găng-glē-ĔK-tō-mē): excision of a ganglion *-ectomy:* excision, removal *A ganglion is a mass of nerve cell bodies (gray matter) in the peripheral nervous system.*
gli/o	glue; neuroglial tissue	**gli/oma** (glī-Ō-mă): tumor (composed of) neuroglial tissue *-oma:* tumor *A glioma is a tumor composed of neuroglial or supporting tissue of the nervous system.*
kinesi/o	movement	brady/**kines**/ia (brăd-ē-kĭ-NĒ-sē-ă): condition of slow movement *brady-:* slow *-ia:* condition
lept/o	thin, slender	**lept/o/mening/o/pathy** (lĕp-tō-mĕn-ĭn-GŎP-ă-thē): disease of the meninges *-mening/o:* meninges (membranes covering brain and spinal cord) *-pathy:* disease *The leptomeninges include the pia mater and arachnoid, both of which are thin and delicate in structure, as opposed to the dura mater.*
lex/o	word, phrase	dys/**lex**/ia (dĭs-LĔK-sē-ă): difficulty using words *dys-:* bad; painful; difficult *-ia:* condition *Dyslexia is difficulty or inability with reading, including the tendency to reverse letters or words when reading or writing.*

Element	Meaning	Word Analysis
mening/o	meninges (membranes covering brain and spinal cord)	**mening/o/cele** (měn-ĬN-gō-sēl): herniation of the meninges *-cele:* hernia, swelling
meningi/o		**meningi/oma** (měn-ĭn-jē-Ō-mă): tumor in the meninges *-oma:* tumor

myel/o	bone marrow; spinal cord	poli/o/**myel**/itis (pōl-ē-ō-mī-ĕl-Ī-tĭs): inflammation of the gray matter of the spinal cord
		  poli/o: gray; gray matter (of brain or spinal cord)
		  -itis: inflammation

narc/o	stupor; numb-ness; sleep	**narc/o/tic** (năr-KŎT-ĭk): relating to sleep *-tic:* pertaining to *Narcotics depress the central nervous system, thus relieving pain and producing sleep.*
neur/o	nerve	**neur/o/lysis** (nū-RŎL-ĭs-ĭs): destruction of a nerve *-lysis:* separation; destruction; loosening *Neurolysis is sometimes performed using cryoablation or radio-frequency techniques to relieve intractable pain as a temporary or permanent measure.*
radicul/o	nerve root	**radicul**/algia (ră-dĭk-ū-LĂL-jē-ă): pain in the nerve root *-algia:* pain

sthen/o	strength	hyper/**sthen**/ia (hī-pĕr-STHĒ-nē-ă): condition of excessive strength
		  hyper-: excessive, above normal
		  -ia: condition
		Hypersthenia is a condition of excessive strength or tonicity of the body or a body part.

thalam/o	thalamus	**thalam/o/tomy** (thăl-ă-MŎT-ō-mē): incision of the thalamus *-tomy:* vincision *Thalamotomy is performed to treat intractable pain or psychoses.*

thec/o	sheath (usually refers to meninges)	intra/**thec**/al (ĭn-tră-THĒ-kăl): pertaining to the space within a sheath
		  intra-: in, within
		  -al: pertaining to

ton/o	tension	dys/**ton**/ia (dĭs-TŌ-nē-ă): bad or poor (muscle) tone
		  dys-: bad; painful; difficult
		  -ia: condition
		Dystonia usually refers to a movement disorder characterized by sustained muscle contractions resulting in a persistently abnormal posture.

ventricul/o	ventricle (of heart or brain)	**ventricul/o/metry** (věn-trĭk-ū-LŎM-ě-trē): measurement of ventricle (pressure) *-metry:* act of measuring
Suffixes		
-algesia	pain	an/**algesia** (ăn-ăl-JĒ-zē-ă): absence of (a normal sense of) pain *an-:* without, not
-algia		syn/**algia** (sĭn-ĂL-jē-ă): joined (referred) pain *syn-:* union, together, joined *Synalgia is pain experienced in a part of the body other than the place of pathology. For example, right shoulder pain is commonly associated with gallstones.*

(continued)

Medical Word Elements—cont'd

Element	Meaning	Word Analysis
-asthenia	weakness, debility	my/**asthenia** (mī-ăs-THĒ-nē-ă): muscle weakness *my:* muscle
-esthesia	feeling	hyper/**esthesia** (hī-pĕr-ĕs-THĒ-zē-ă): increased feeling *hyper-:* excessive, above normal *Hyperesthesia involves a marked sensitivity to touch, pain, or other sensory stimuli.*
-kinesia	movement	hyper/**kinesia** (hī-pĕr-kǐ-NĒ-zē-ă): excessive movement; also called *hyperactivity* *hyper-:* excessive, above normal
-lepsy	seizure	narc/o/**lepsy** (NĂR-kō-lĕp-sē): seizure of sleep *narc/o:* sleep *In narcolepsy, the individual has a sudden and uncontrollable urge to sleep at an inappropriate time, such as when driving.*
-paresis	partial paralysis	hemi/**paresis** (hĕm-ē-PĂR-ĕ-sĭs): paralysis of one-half (of the body); also called *hemiplegia* *hemi-:* one-half *When used alone, the term* **paresis** *means partial paralysis or motor weakness.*
-phasia	speech	a/**phasia** (ă-FĀ-zē-ă): without speech *a-:* without, not
-plegia	paralysis	quadri/**plegia** (kwŏd-rǐ-PLĒ-jē-ă): paralysis of four (extremities) *quadri-:* four
-taxia	order, coordination	a/**taxia** (ă-TĂK-sē-ă): without coordination *a-:* without, not *Ataxia refers to poor muscle coordination, especially when voluntary movements are attempted.*
Prefixes		
pachy-	thick	**pachy**/mening/itis (păk-ē-mĕn-ĭn-JĪ-tĭs): inflammation of the dura mater *mening:* meninges (membranes covering brain and spinal cord) *–itis:* inflammation *The dura mater is a thick membrane that provides protection for the brain and spinal cord.*
para-	near, beside; beyond	**para**/plegia (păr-ă-PLĒ-jē-ă): paralysis of lower body and limbs *–plegia:* paralysis *Paraplegia is the paralysis of the lower limbs of the body.*
syn-	union, together, joined	**syn**/algia (sǐn-ĂL-jē-ă): referred pain *algia:* pain *Pain in a deteriorated hip commonly causes referred pain in a healthy knee.*

uni-	one	**uni**/later/al (ū-nǐ-LĂT-ĕr-ăl): pertaining to one side
		  later: side, to one side
		  -al: pertaining to

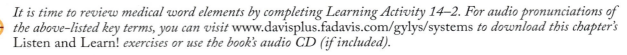

It is time to review medical word elements by completing Learning Activity 14–2. For audio pronunciations of the above-listed key terms, you can visit www.davisplus.fadavis.com/gylys/systems to download this chapter's
Listen and Learn! *exercises or use the book's audio CD (if included).*

Pathology

Damage to the brain and spinal cord invariably causes signs and symptoms in other parts of the body. Common signs and symptoms for many neurological disorders include headache, insomnia, back or neck pain, weakness, and involuntary movement (**dyskinesia**). Careful observation of the patient during the history and physical examination may provide valuable clues about mental status and cognitive and motor ability. Muscle strength, coordination, gait, balance, and reflexes provide additional diagnostic clues. Lumbar puncture provides a sample of CSF for analysis and helps identify various types of meningitis and encephalitis. Radiology—especially computed tomography (CT) and magnetic resonance imaging (MRI) scans—provide detailed images that can locate cerebrovascular irregularities, lesions, and tumors.

Radiculopathy

Radiculopathy, also called *radiculitis,* is an inflammation of the nerve root associated with the spinal column. Spinal nerves exit the spinal column at each level along the length of the spine. When pressure is applied to the nerve root (**compression**), the patient experiences tingling, numbness, weakness, or a radiating pain starting in the spine and moving outward. Pressure can be the result of a herniated disc, degenerative changes, arthritis, fractures, bone spurs, or tumors. The areas most commonly affected are the neck (**cervical radiculopathy**) and the lower back (**lumbar radiculopathy, sciatica**). The offending nerve root is commonly identified during the history and physical examination by evaluating the area of the skin known to be served by a specific nerve. MRIs and CT scans help to localize the site and nature of compression. Rest and anti-inflammatory medications are usually recommended. However, for disabling pain that lasts for several months or is accompanied by loss of bowel or bladder control, surgery to remove the cause of the pressure (**decompression surgery**) may be the only option.

Cerebrovascular Disease

Cerebrovascular disease refers to any functional abnormality of the cerebrum caused by disorders of the blood vessels of the brain. It is most commonly associated with a **stroke,** also called *cerebrovascular accident (CVA)*. The three major types of strokes are ischemic stroke, intracerebral hemorrhage, and subarachnoid hemorrhage. The most common type, which accounts for about 80% of all strokes, is ischemic stroke. **Ischemic stroke** is caused by a narrowing of the arteries of the brain or the arteries of the neck (**carotid**), generally due to atherosclerosis. (See Chapter 8, Figure 8–5.) This narrowing causes insufficient oxygen delivery to the brain tissue and, within a few minutes, the tissue begins to die. Occasionally, pieces of plaque break loose and travel to the narrower vessels of the brain, causing occlusion, also resulting in ischemia. An **intracerebral hemorrhage** is caused by the sudden rupture of an artery within the brain. After the rupture, released blood compresses brain structures and destroys them. In a **subarachnoid hemorrhage**, blood is released into the space surrounding the brain. This condition is commonly caused by a ruptured aneurysm and is usually fatal.

Signs and symptoms of stroke include weakness in one half of the body (**hemiparesis**), paralysis in one half of the body (**hemiplegia**), inability to speak (**aphasia**), lack of muscle coordination (**ataxia**), stupor, loss of consciousness (LOC), coma, or even death. If the CVA is mild, the patient may experience a brief "blackout," blurred vision, or dizziness and may be unaware of the "minor stroke." Stroke symptoms that resolve within 24 hours are known as a *transient ischemic attack (TIA)*. About one third of all strokes are preceded by a TIA. A family history of cerebrovascular disease and high blood pressure appears to be a contributing factor to stroke. Computed tomography (CT) is usually performed to determine the type of stroke. "Clot buster" (**thrombolytic**) medication is usually administered within 3 hours of symptom onset when ischemic stroke is diagnosed. Antihypertensives may also be administered to control blood pressure. Treatment involves speech, physical, and occupational therapy and various medications, depending on the type of stroke

Seizure Disorders

Seizure disorders include any medical condition characterized by sudden changes in behavior or consciousness as a result of uncontrolled electrical activity in the brain. However, chronic or recurring seizure disorders are called *epilepsies.* Causes of epilepsy include brain injury, congenital anomalies, metabolic disorders, brain tumors, vascular disturbances, and genetic disorders.

Seizures are characterized by sudden bursts of abnormal electrical activity in neurons, resulting in temporary changes in brain function. Two major types of seizures are partial and generalized.

In **partial seizures,** only a portion of the brain is involved. There is a short alteration of consciousness of about 10 to 30 seconds with repetitive, unusual movements and confusion. In a **generalized seizure,** the entire brain is involved. The most common type of generalized seizure is the **tonic-clonic seizure;** also called *grand mal seizure.* In the **tonic phase** of a tonic-clonic seizure, the entire body becomes rigid; in the **clonic phase** there is uncontrolled jerking. Recovery may take minutes to hours and usually leaves the patient weak. In **status epilepticus,** tonic-clonic seizures follow one after another without an intervening period of recovery. It is a life-threatening emergency that involves the whole cortex and emergency medical attention is essential. Diagnosis and evaluation commonly rely on electroencephalography and magnetoencephalography to locate the affected area of the brain. Epilepsy can usually be controlled by antiepileptic medications.

Parkinson Disease

Parkinson disease, also called *shaking palsy,* is a progressive neurological disorder affecting the portion of the brain responsible for controlling movement. As neurons degenerate, the patient develops uncontrollable nodding of the head, decreased speed of movement (**bradykinesia, hypokinesia**), tremors, large joint stiffness, and a shuffling gait. Muscle rigidity causes facial expressions to appear fixed and masklike with unblinking eyes. Sometimes the patient exhibits "pill rolling," in which he or she inadvertently rubs the thumb against the index finger.

In patients with Parkinson disease, dopamine (a neurotransmitter that facilitates the transmission of impulses at synapses) is lacking in the brain. Management involves the administration of L-dopa, which can cross the blood-brain barrier. L-dopa is converted in the brain to dopamine. Even so, this treatment only reduces symptoms; it is not a cure for Parkinson disease.

Multiple Sclerosis

Multiple sclerosis (MS) is a progressive, degenerative disease of the central nervous system. MS is characterized by inflammation, hardening and, finally, loss of myelin (**demyelination**) throughout the spinal cord and brain. As myelin deteriorates, the transmission of electrical impulses from one neuron to another is impeded. In effect, the conduction pathway develops "short circuits."

Signs and symptoms of MS include tremors, muscle weakness, and bradykinesia. Occasionally, visual disturbances exist. During remissions, symptoms temporarily disappear, but progressive hardening of myelin areas leads to other attacks. Ultimately, most voluntary motor control is lost and the patient becomes bedridden. Death occurs anywhere from 7 to 30 years after the onset of the disease. Young adults, usually women, between ages 20 and 40 are the most common victims of MS. The etiology of the disease is unclear, but autoimmune disease or a slow viral infection is believed to be the most probable cause.

Alzheimer Disease

Alzheimer disease (AD) is a progressive neurological disorder that causes memory loss and serious mental deterioration. Small lesions called *plaques* develop in the cerebral cortex and disrupt the passage of electrochemical signals between cells. The clinical manifestations of Alzheimer disease include memory loss and cognitive decline. There is also a decline in social skills and ability to carry out activities of daily living. Most patients undergo personality, emotional, and behavioral changes. As the disease progresses, loss of concentration and increased fatigue, restlessness, and anxiety are common. Alzheimer disease was once considered rare but is now identified as a leading cause of senile dementia. Although there is no specific treatment, moderate relief has been associated with medications that prevent a breakdown of brain chemicals required for neurotransmission.

Mental Illness

Mental illness includes an array of psychological disorders, syndromes, and behavioral patterns that cause alterations in mood, behavior, and thinking. (See Table 14-3.) Its forms range from mild to serious. For example, anxiety may manifest as a slight apprehension or uneasiness lasting a few days to a more severe form involving intense fears lasting for months and even years.

Psychosis refers to a serious mental disorder commonly characterized by false beliefs despite overwhelming evidence to the contrary (**delusions**). The psychotic patient typically "hears voices" and "sees visions" in the absence of an actual stimulus (**hallucinations**). The patient's speech is usually incoherent and disorganized and behavior is erratic.

Neurosis is a mental disorder caused by an emotion experienced in the past that overwhelmingly interferes or affects a present emotion. For example,

Table 14-3	**Common Terms Associated with Mental Illness**

This table lists common terms or disorders associated with mental illness along with their definitions.

Term	Definition
affective disorder	Psychological disorder in which the major characteristic is an abnormal mood, usually mania or depression
anorexia nervosa	Eating disorder characterized by a refusal to maintain adequate weight for age and height and an all-consuming desire to remain thin
anxiety	Psychological "worry" disorder characterized by excessive pondering or thinking "what if...." *Feelings of worry, dread, lack of energy, and a loss of interest in life are common signs associated with anxiety.*
attention deficit hyperactivity disorder **(ADHD)**	Disorder affecting children and adults characterized by impulsiveness, overactivity, and the inability to remain focused on a task *Behavioral modification, medical management, or a combination of both are commonly used in the treatment of ADHD.*
bipolar disorder	Mental disorder that causes unusual shifts in mood, emotion, energy, and ability to function; also called *manic-depressive illness*
bulimia nervosa	Eating disorder characterized by binging (overeating) and purging (vomiting or use of laxatives)
depression	Mood disorder associated with sadness, despair, discouragement, and, commonly, feelings of low self-esteem, guilt, and withdrawal
mania	Mood disorder characterized by mental and physical hyperactivity, disorganized behavior, and excessively elevated mood
panic attack	Sudden, intense, overwhelming feeling of fear that comes without warning and is not attributable to any immediate danger *A key symptom of a panic attack is the fear of its recurrence.*

a child bitten by a dog may show irrational fear of animals as an adult. Many mental disorders are forms of neuroses, including irrational fears (**phobias**), exaggerated emotional and reflexive behaviors (**hysterias**), or irrational, uncontrolled performance of ritualistic actions for fear of a dire consequence (**obsessive compulsive disorders**).

Research and education have removed much of the stigma attached to mental illness. Today, mental illness is becoming a more recognizable and treatable disorder. Many psychological disorders can be effectively treated or managed by family physicians, school psychologists, marriage counselors, family counselors, and even support groups such as grief support groups and Alcoholics Anonymous.

Diagnosis and treatment of serious mental disorders usually require the skills of a medical specialist called a *psychiatrist*. In the capacity of a physician, the psychiatrist is licensed to prescribe medications and perform medical procedures not available to those who do not hold a medical license. Psychiatrists commonly work in association with **clinical psychologists,** who are individuals trained in evaluating human behavior, intelligence, and personality.

Oncology

Intracranial tumors that originate directly in brain tissue are called *primary intracranial tumors.* They are commonly classified according to histological type and include those that originate in neurons and those that develop in glial tissue. Signs and symptoms of intracranial tumors include headaches, especially upon arising in the morning, during coughing episodes, and upon bending or sudden movement. Occasionally, the optic disc in the back of the eyeball swells (**papilledema**) because of increased intracranial pressure. Personality changes are common and include depression, anxiety, and irritability.

Intracranial tumors can arise from any structure within the cranial cavity, including the pituitary and pineal glands, cranial nerves, and the arachnoid and pia mater (**leptomeninges**). In addition, all of these tissues may be the sites of metastatic spread from primary malignancies that occur outside of the nervous system. Metastatic tumors of the cranial cavity tend to exhibit growth characteristics similar to those of the primary malignancy but tend to grow more slowly than the parent tumor. Metastatic tumors of the cranial cavity are usually easier to remove than primary intracranial tumors.

Computed tomography (CT) scans and magnetic resonance imaging (MRI) help establish a diagnosis but are not definitive. Surgical removal relieves pressure and confirms or rules out malignancy. Even after surgery, most intracranial tumors require radiation therapy as a second line of treatment. Chemotherapy combined with radiation therapy usually provides the best chance for survival and quality of life.

Diagnostic, Symptomatic, and Related Terms

This section introduces diagnostic, symptomatic, and related terms and their meanings. Word analyses for selected terms are also provided.

Term	Definition
agnosia ăg-NŌ-zē-ă *a-:* without, not *gnos:* knowing *-ia:* condition	Inability to comprehend auditory, visual, spatial, olfactory, or other sensations even though the sensory sphere is intact *The type of agnosia is usually identified by the sense or senses affected, such as visual agnosia. Agnosia is common in parietal lobe tumors.*
asthenia ăs-THĒ-nē-ă *a-:* without, not *sthen:* strength *-ia:* condition	Weakness, debility, or loss of strength *Asthenia is a characteristic of multiple sclerosis (MS).*
ataxia ă-TĂK-sē-ă *a-:* without, not *tax:* order, coordination *-ia:* condition	Lack of muscle coordination in the execution of voluntary movement *Ataxia may be the result of head injury, stroke, MS, alcoholism, or a variety of hereditary disorders.*
aura AW-ră	Premonitory awareness of an approaching physical or mental disorder; peculiar sensation that precedes seizures
autism AW-tĭzm	Developmental disorder characterized by extreme withdrawal and an abnormal absorption in fantasy, usually accompanied by an inability to communicate even on a basic level *A person with autism may engage in repetitive behavior, such as rocking or repeating words.*
closed head trauma TRAW-mă	Injury to the head in which the dura mater remains intact and brain tissue is not exposed *In closed head trauma, the injury site may occur at the impact site, where the brain hits the inside of the skull (coup) or at the rebound site, where the opposite side of the brain strikes the skull (contrecoup).*

Diagnostic, Symptomatic, and Related Terms—cont'd

Term	Definition
coma KŌ-mă	Abnormally deep unconsciousness with absence of voluntary response to stimuli
concussion kŏn-KŬSH-ŭn	Injury to the brain, occasionally with transient loss of consciousness as a result of injury or trauma to the head *Delayed symptoms of concussion may include headache, nausea, vomiting, and blurred vision.*
convulsion kŏn-VŬL-shŭn	Any sudden and violent contraction of one or more muscles
dementia dĭ-MĔN-shē-ă *de-:* cessation *ment:* mind *-ia:* condition	Broad term that refers to cognitive deficit, including memory impairment
dyslexia dĭs-LĔK-sē-ă *dys-:* bad; painful; difficult *lex:* word, phrase *-ia:* condition	Inability to learn and process written language despite adequate intelligence, sensory ability, and exposure
Guillain-Barré syndrome gē-YĂ băr-RĀ SĬN-drōm	Autoimmune condition that causes acute inflammation of the peripheral nerves in which myelin sheaths on the axons are destroyed, resulting in decreased nerve impulses, loss of reflex response, and sudden muscle weakness *This disease usually follows a viral gastrointestinal or respiratory infection, stress, or trauma. The muscle weakness involves the entire body and the patient may temporarily require respiratory support until the inflammation subsides.*
herpes zoster HĔR-pēz ZŎS-tĕr	Painful, acute infectious disease of the posterior root ganglia of only a few segments of the spinal or cranial nerves; also called *shingles* *Herpes zoster is caused by the same organism (varicella-zoster) that causes chickenpox in children. The disease is self-limiting and usually resolves in 10 days to 5 weeks.*
Huntington chorea HŬNT-ĭng-tŭn kō-RĒ-ă	Inherited disease of the CNS characterized by quick, involuntary movements, speech disturbances, and mental deterioration. *Onset of Huntington chorea is commonly between ages 30 and 50.*
hydrocephalus hī-drō-SĔF-ă-lŭs	Accumulation of fluid in the ventricles of the brain, causing increased intracranial pressure (ICP), thinning of brain tissue, and separation of cranial bones
lethargy LĔTH-ăr-jē	Abnormal inactivity or lack of response to normal stimuli; also called sluggishness
neurosis nū-RŌ-sĭs *neur:* nerve *-osis:* abnormal condition; increase (used primarily with blood cells)	Nonpsychotic mental illness that triggers feelings of distress and anxiety and impairs normal behavior *A child who has been consistently been warned of "germs" by an over protective parent may later develop an irrational fear of using public restrooms, for example, or touching doorknobs or phones.*

(continued)

Diagnostic, Symptomatic, and Related Terms—cont'd

Term	Definition
palsy PAWL-zē	Paralysis, usually partial, and commonly characterized by weakness and shaking or uncontrolled tremor
Bell	Facial paralysis caused by a functional disorder of the seventh cranial nerve, associated with herpes virus *Bell palsy is self-limiting and usually spontaneously resolves in 3 to 5 weeks.*
cerebral sĕ-RĒ-brăl *cerebr:* cerebrum *-al:* pertaining to	Type of paralysis that affects movement and body position and, sometimes, speech and learning ability *Cerebral palsy (CP) commonly occurs as a result of trauma to the brain during the birthing process.*
paralysis pă-RĂL-ĭ-sĭs *para-:* near, beside; beyond *-lysis:* separation, destruction, loosening	Loss of voluntary motion in one or more muscle groups with or without loss of sensation *Strokes and spinal cord injuries are the common causes of paralysis. Strokes usually affect only one side of the body. Spinal cord injuries result in paralysis below the site of the injury. (See Figure 14-6.)*
hemiplegia hĕm-ē-PLĒ-jē-ă *hemi-:* one-half *-plegia:* paralysis	Paralysis of one side of the body, typically as the result of a stroke; also called *unilateral paralysis*
paraplegia păr-ă-PLĒ-jē-ă *para-:* near, beside; beyond *-plegia:* paralysis	Paralysis of both lower limbs, typically as a result of trauma or disease of the lower spinal cord
quadriplegia kwŏd-rĭ-PLĒ-jē-ă *quadri-:* four *-plegia:* paralysis	Paralysis of both arms and legs, typically as a result of trauma or disease of the upper spinal cord
psychosis sī-KŌ-sĭs *psych:* mind *-osis:* abnormal condition; increase (used primarily with blood cells)	Major emotional disorder in which contact with reality is lost to the point that the individual is incapable of meeting challenges of daily life
spina bifida SPĪ-nă BĬ-fĭ-dă	Defect in which the neural tube (tissue that forms the brain and spinal cord in the fetus) fails to close during embryogenesis *Spina bifida is a birth defect that includes meningocele, meningomyelocele, and occulta. (See Figure 14–7.)*
meningocele mĕn-ĬN-gō-sēl *mening/o:* meninges (membranes covering brain and spinal cord) *-cele:* hernia, swelling	Form of spina bifida in which the spinal cord develops properly but the meninges protrude through the spine

Diagnostic, Symptomatic, and Related Terms—cont'd

Term	Definition

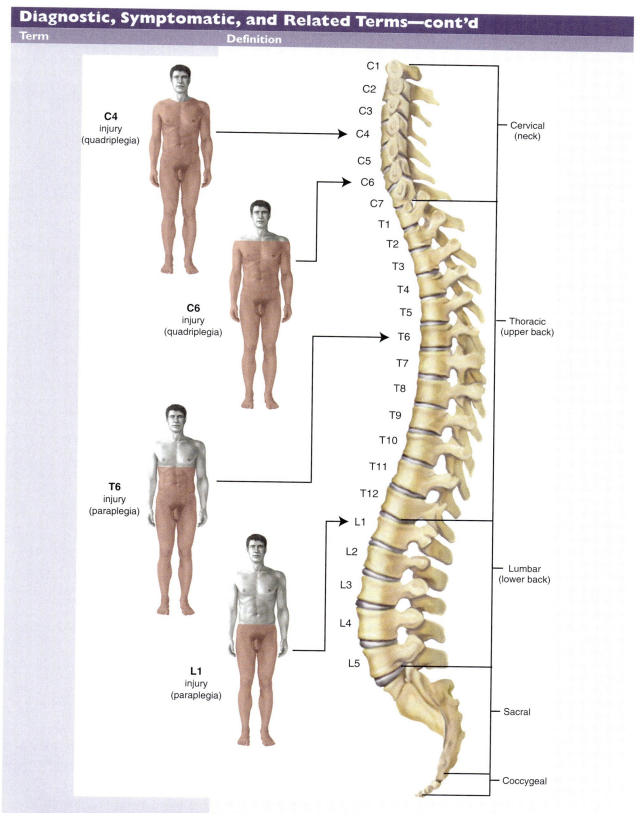

C4
injury
(quadriplegia)

C6
injury
(quadriplegia)

T6
injury
(paraplegia)

L1
injury
(paraplegia)

C1
C2
C3
C4
C5
C6
C7 — Cervical (neck)
T1
T2
T3
T4
T5
T6
T7
T8
T9
T10
T11 — Thoracic (upper back)
T12
L1
L2
L3
L4 — Lumbar (lower back)
L5
— Sacral
— Coccygeal

Figure 14-6. Spinal cord injuries showing extent of paralysis.

(continued)

Diagnostic, Symptomatic, and Related Terms—cont'd

Term	Definition
myelomeningocele mī-ĕ-lō-mĕn-ĬN-gō-sēl *myel/o:* bone marrow; spinal cord *mening/o:* meninges (membranes covering brain and spinal cord) *-cele:* hernia, swelling	Most severe form of spina bifida in which the spinal cord and meninges protrude through the spine
occulta ŏ-KŬL-tă	Form of spina bifida in which one or more vertebrae are malformed and the spinal cord is covered with a layer of skin

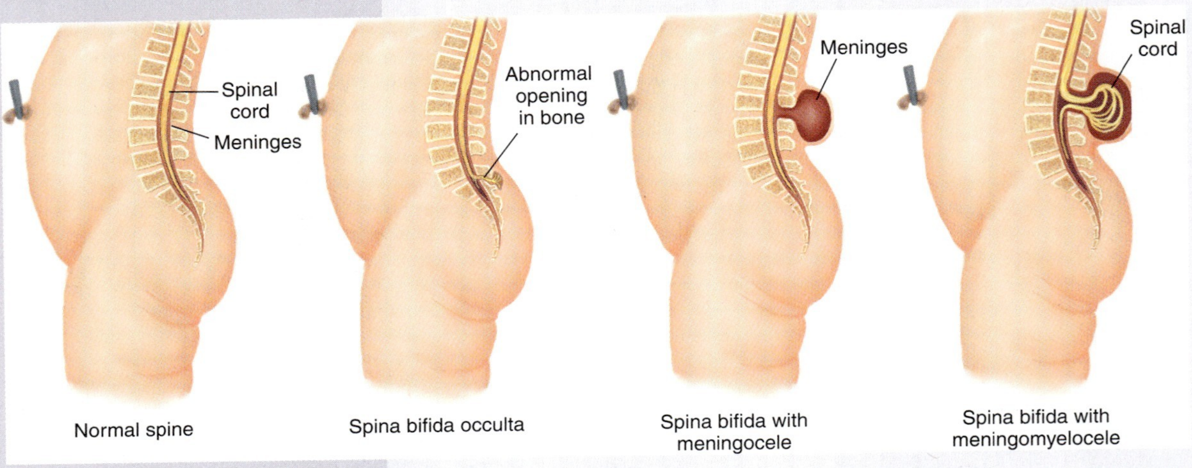

Figure 14-7. Spina bifida.

paresthesia păr-ĕs-THĒ-zē-ă	Sensation of numbness, prickling, tingling, or heightened sensitivity *Paresthesia can be caused by disorders affecting the central nervous system, such as stroke, transient ischemic attack, multiple sclerosis, transverse myelitis, and encephalitis.*
poliomyelitis pōl-ē-ō-mī-ĕl-Ī-tĭs *poli/o:* gray; gray matter (of brain or spinal cord) *myel:* bone marrow; spinal cord *-itis:* inflammation	Inflammation of the gray matter of the spinal cord caused by a virus, commonly resulting in spinal and muscle deformity and paralysis *Polio is preventable with standard vaccinations administered to children.*
Reye syndrome RĪ SĬN-drōm	Acute encephalopathy and fatty infiltration of the brain, liver and, possibly, the pancreas, heart, kidney, spleen, and lymph nodes *Reye syndrome is usually seen in children younger than age 15 who had an acute viral infection. Mortality in Reye syndrome may be as high as 80%. The use of aspirin by children experiencing chickenpox or influenza may induce Reye syndrome.*
sciatica sī-ĂT-ĭ-kă	Severe pain in the leg along the course of the sciatic nerve felt at the base of the spine, down the thigh, and radiating down the leg due to a compressed nerve

Diagnostic, Symptomatic, and Related Terms—cont'd

Term	Definition
syncope SĬN-kō-pē	Temporary loss of consciousness due to the sudden decline of blood flow to the brain; *also called fainting*
vasovagal văs-ō-VĀ-găl	Syncope due to a drop in blood pressure brought on by the response of the nervous system to abrupt emotional stress, pain, or trauma
tonic-clonic seizure	General type of seizure characterized by the loss of consciousness and stiffening of the body (tonic phase) followed by rhythmic, jerking movements (clonic phase)
transient ischemic attack (TIA) TRĂN-zē-ĕnt ĭs-KĒ-mĭk	Temporary interference with blood supply to the brain lasting from a few minutes to a few hours *Symptoms of TIA may include numbness or weakness in the extremities, especially on one side of the body; confusion or difficulty in talking or understanding speech; visual impairment; dizziness; loss of balance; and difficulty walking.*

 It is time to review pathological, diagnostic, symptomatic, and related terms by completing Learning Activity 14–3.

Diagnostic and Therapeutic Procedures

This section introduces procedures used to diagnose and treat nervous disorders. Descriptions are provided as well as pronunciations and word analyses for selected terms.

Procedure	Description
Diagnostic Procedures	
Clinical	
electroencephalography (EEG) ē-lĕk-trō-ĕn-sĕf-ă-LŎG-ră-fē *electr/o:* electricity *encephal/o:* brain *-graphy:* process of recording	Recording of electrical activity in the brain, whose cells emit distinct patterns of rhythmic electrical impulses *Different wave patterns in the EEG are associated with normal and abnormal waking and sleeping states. They help diagnose such conditions as tumors, infections, and seizure disorders.*
electromyography (EMG) ē-lĕk-trō-mī-ŎG-ră-fē *electr/o:* electricity *my/o:* muscle *-graphy:* process of recording	Recording of electrical signals (action potentials) that occur in a muscle when it is at rest and during contraction to assess nerve damage *In the EMG, an electrode inserted into a muscle records impulses and displays them on a monitor called an oscilloscope.*
lumbar puncture LŬM-băr PŬNK-chūr	Needle puncture of the spinal cavity to extract spinal fluid for diagnostic purposes, introduce anesthetic agents into the spinal canal, or remove fluid to allow other fluids (such as radiopaque substances) to be injected; also called *spinal puncture* and *spinal tap* (See Figure 14–8.)

(continued)

Diagnostic and Therapeutic Procedures—cont'd

Procedure	Description

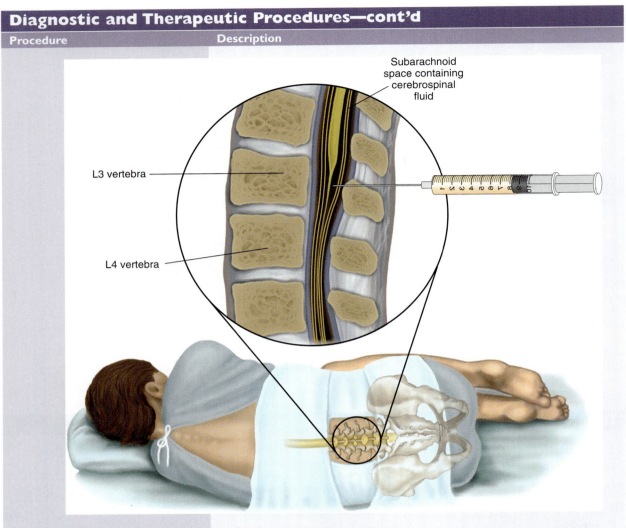

Subarachnoid space containing cerebrospinal fluid

L3 vertebra

L4 vertebra

Figure 14-8. Lumbar puncture.

nerve conduction velocity (NCV) NĔRV kŏn-DŬK-shŭn vĕ-LŎ-sĭ-tē	Test that measures the speed at which impulses travel through a nerve *In NCV, one electrode stimulates a nerve while other electrodes, placed over different areas of the nerve record an electrical signal (action potential) as it travels through the nerve. This test is used for diagnosing muscular dystrophy and neurological disorders that destroy myelin.*

Laboratory

cerebrospinal fluid (CSF) analysis sĕr-ē-brō-SPĪ-năl, ă-NĂL-ĭ-sĭs *cerebr/o:* cerebrum *spin:* spine *-al:* pertaining to	Series of chemical, microscopic, and microbial tests used to diagnose disorders of the central nervous system, including viral and bacterial infections, tumors, and hemorrhage

Diagnostic and Therapeutic Procedures—cont'd

Procedure	Description

Radiographic

angiography
ăn-jē-ŎG-ră-fē

angi/o: vessel (usually blood or lymph)
-graphy: process of recording

Radiography of the blood vessels after introduction of a contrast medium

Angiography is used to visualize vascular abnormalities. The contrast medium may be injected into an artery or vein or administered through a catheter inserted in a peripheral artery, run through the vessel, and positioned at a visceral site.

cerebral
sĕr-Ē-brăl

cerebr/o: cerebrum
-al: pertaining to

Angiography of blood vessels of the brain after injection of a contrast medium; also called *cerebral arteriography*

Vascular tumors, aneurysms, and occlusions are identified using cerebral angiography, which is usually performed when intracranial procedures are being considered.

computed tomography (CT)
kŏm-PŪ-tĕd tō-MŎG-ră-fē

tom/o: to cut
-graphy: process of recording

Imaging technique achieved by rotating an x-ray emitter around the area to be scanned and measuring the intensity of transmitted rays from different angles

CT of the brain can be performed with or without contrast media. It is effective in visualizing tumors, abscesses, hemorrhage, trauma and fractures.

myelography
mī-ĕ-LŎG-ră-fē

myel/o: bone marrow; spinal cord
-graphy: process of recording

Diagnostic radiological examination of the spinal canal, nerve roots, and spinal cord after injection of contrast medium into the spinal canal

Myelography is usually performed in conjunction with CT and when an MRI is not possible because the patient has a pacemaker or other implantable device.

positron emission tomography (PET)
PŎZ-ĭ-trŏn ē-MĬSH-ŭn tō-MŎG-ră-fē

Scan using computed tomography to record the positrons (positively charged particles) emitted from a radiopharmaceutical and produce a cross-sectional image of metabolic activity in body tissues to determine the presence of disease

PET is especially useful in scanning the brain and nervous system to diagnose disorders that involve abnormal tissue metabolism, such as schizophrenia, brain tumors, epilepsy, stroke, and Alzheimer disease.

ultrasonography (US)
ŭl-tră-sŏn-ŎG-ră-fē

ultra-: excess, beyond
son/o: sound
-graphy: process of recording

Imaging procedure using high-frequency sound waves (ultrasound) that display the reflected "echoes" on a monitor; also called *ultrasound, sonography, echo,* and *echogram*

echoencephalography
ĕk-ō-ĕn-sĕf-ă-LŎG-ră-fē

echo-: repeated sound
encephal/o: brain
-graphy: process of recording

Ultrasound technique used to study intracranial structures of the brain and, especially, diagnose conditions that cause a shift in the midline structures of the brain

Therapeutic Procedures

Surgical

cryosurgery
krī-ō-SĔR-jĕr-ē

Technique that exposes abnormal tissue to extreme cold to destroy it

Cryosurgery is sometimes used to destroy malignant tumors of the brain.

(continued)

Diagnostic and Therapeutic Procedures—cont'd

Procedure	Description
stereotaxic radiosurgery stĕr-ē-ō-TĂK-sĭk rā-dē-ō-SŬR-jĕr-ē	Precise method of locating and destroying sharply circumscribed lesions on specific, tiny areas of pathological tissue in deep-seated structures of the central nervous system; also called *stereotaxy* or *stereotactic surgery* *Stereotaxic radiosurgery is used in the treatment of seizure disorders, aneurysms, brain tumors, and many other neuropathological conditions and is performed without a surgical incision. The pathological site is localized with three-dimensional coordinates, and high doses of radiation are used to destroy it.*
thalamotomy thăl-ă-MŎT-ō-mē *thalam/o:* thalamus *-tomy:* incision	Partial destruction of the thalamus to treat intractable pain, involuntary movements, or emotional disturbances *Thalamotomy produces few neurological deficits or changes in personality.*
tractotomy trăk-TŎT-ō-mē	Transection of a nerve tract in the brainstem or spinal cord *Tractotomy is sometimes used to relieve intractable pain.*
trephination trĕf-ĭn-Ā-shŭn	Technique that cuts a circular opening into the skull to reveal brain tissue and decrease intracranial pressure
vagotomy vā-GŎT-ō-mē	Interruption of the function of the vagus nerve to relieve peptic ulcer *Vagotomy is performed when ulcers in the stomach and duodenum do not respond to medication or changes in diet.*

Pharmacology

Neurological agents are used to relieve or eliminate pain, suppress seizures, control tremors, and reduce muscle rigidity. (See Table 14–4.) Hypnotics, a class of drugs used as sedatives, depress CNS function to relieve agitation and induce sleep. Anesthetics are capable of producing a complete or partial loss of feeling and are used for surgery. Psychotherapeutic agents alter brain chemistry to treat mental illness. These drugs are used as mood stabilizers in various mental disorders. They also reduce symptoms of depression and treat ADHD and narcolepsy.

Table 14-4   Drugs Used to Treat Neurological and Psychiatric Disorders

This table lists common drug classifications used to treat neurological and psychiatric disorders, their therapeutic actions, and selected generic and trade names.

Classification	Therapeutic Action	Generic and Trade Names
Neurological anesthetics	Produce partial or complete loss of sensation, with or without loss of consciousness. *Anesthetics may be classified as general or local.*	
general	Act upon the brain to produce complete loss of feeling with loss of consciousness. *General anesthetics are delivered by the blood stream to all areas of the body, including the brain. Since they suppress all reflexes including coughing, and swallowing, breathing tubes are usually required.*	**propofol** PRŎ-pō-fŏl Diprivan

Table 14-4 Drugs Used to Treat Neurological and Psychiatric Disorders—cont'd

Classification	Therapeutic Action	Generic and Trade Names
local	Act upon nerves or nerve tracts to affect a local area only. *Local anesthetics are injected directly into the area involved in the local surgery. Patients may remain fully alert unless additional medications to induce sleep are given.*	**procaine** PRŌ-kān Novocain **lidocaine** LĪ-dō-kān Xylocaine
anticonvulsants	Prevent uncontrolled neuron activity associated with seizures by altering electrical transmission along neurons or altering the chemical composition of neurotransmitters; also called *antiepileptics* *Many anticonvulsants are also used as mood stabilizers.*	**carbamazepine** kăr-bă-MĂZ-ĕ-pēn Tegretol **valproate** văl-PRŌ-āt Depacon
antiparkinsonian agents	Control tremors and muscle rigidity associated with Parkinson disease by increasing dopamine in the brain	**levodopa** lē-vō-DŌ-pă L-dopa, Larodopa **levodopa/carbidopa** kăr-bĭ-DŌ-pă Sinemet, Sinemet CR
Psychiatric		
antipsychotics	Treat psychosis, paranoia, and schizophrenia by altering chemicals in the brain, including the limbic system (group of brain structures), which controls emotions	**clozapine** CLŌ-ză-pēn Clozaril **risperidone** rĭs-PĔR-ĭ-dōn Risperdal
antidepressants	Treat multiple symptoms of depression by increasing levels of specific neurotransmitters *Antidepressants fall under different classifications and some are also used to treat anxiety and pain.*	**paroxetine** pă-RŎK-sĕ-tēn Paxil **fluoxetine** floo-ŎK-sĕ-tēn Prozac
hypnotics	Depress central nervous system (CNS) functions, promote sedation and sleep, and relieve agitation, anxiousness, and restlessness *Hypnotics may be nonbarbiturates or barbiturates. Barbiturate hypnotics carry a risk of addiction.*	**secobarbital** sē-kō-BĂR-bĭ-tŏl Seconal **temazepam** tĕ-MĂZ-ĕ-păm Restoril
psychostimulants	Reduce impulsive behavior by increasing the level of neurotransmitters *Psychostimulants have a calming effect on people with attention deficit hyperactivity disorder (ADHD) and are also used to treat narcolepsy.*	**dextroamphetamine** dĕks-trō-ăm-FĔT-ă-mēn Dexedrine **methylphenidate** mĕth-ĭl-FĔN-ĭ-dāt Ritalin

Abbreviations

This section introduces nervous system–related abbreviations and their meanings.

Abbreviation	Meaning	Abbreviation	Meaning
ADAD	Alzheimer disease	ICP	intracranial pressure
ADHD	attention-deficit hyperactivity disorder	LOC	loss of consciousness
ALS	amyotrophic lateral sclerosis; also called *Lou Gehrig disease*	LP	lumbar puncture
ANS	autonomic nervous system	MRA	magnetic resonance angiogram; magnetic resonance angiography
BEAM	brain electrical activity mapping	MRI	magnetic resonance imaging
CNS	central nervous system	MS	musculoskeletal; multiple sclerosis; mental status; mitral stenosis
CP	cerebral palsy	NCV	nerve conduction velocity
CSF	cerebrospinal fluid	PET	positron emission tomography
CT	computed tomography	PNS	peripheral nervous system
CVA	cerebrovascular accident	SNS	sympathetic nervous system; somatic nervous system
EEG	ectroencephalography	TIA	transient ischemic attack
EMG	electromyography		

It is time to review procedures, pharmacology, and abbreviations by completing Learning Activity 14–4.

The activities that follow provide a review of the nervous system terms introduced in this chapter. Complete each activity and review your answers to evaluate your understanding of the chapter.

Learning Activity 14-1
Identifying Structures of the Brain

Label the following illustration using the terms listed below.

cerebellum   diencephalon (interbrain)   hypothalamus   occipital lobe   temporal lobe

cerebrum   medulla   parietal lobe   thalamus

       frontal lobe

corpus callosum   midbrain (mesencephalon)   pons

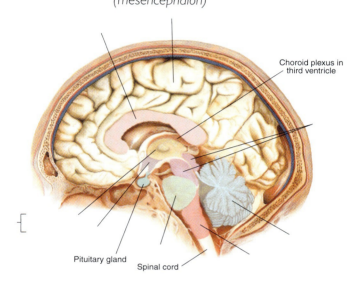

Choroid plexus in third ventricle

Pituitary gland

Spinal cord

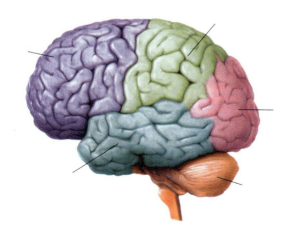

Check your answers by referring to Figure 14–3 on page 430. Review material that you did not answer correctly.

 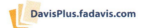

Enhance your study and reinforcement of word elements with the power of DavisPlus. Visit www.davisplus.fadavis.com/gylys/systems for this chapter's flash-card activity. We recommend you complete the flash-card activity before completing activity 14–2 below.

Learning Activity 14-2
Building Medical Words

Use *encephal/o* (brain) to build words that mean:

1. disease of the brain _____
2. herniation of the brain _____
3. radiography of the brain _____

Use *cerebr/o* (cerebrum) to build words that mean:

4. disease of the cerebrum _____
5. inflammation of the cerebrum _____

Use *crani/o* (cranium [skull]) to build words that mean:

6. herniation (through the) cranium _____
7. instrument for measuring the skull _____

Use *neur/o* (nerve) to build words that mean:

8. pain in a nerve _____
9. specialist in the study of the nervous system _____
10. crushing a nerve _____

Use *myel/o* (bone marrow; spinal cord) to build words that mean:

11. herniation of the spinal cord _____
12. paralysis of the spinal cord _____

Use *psych/o* (mind) to build words that mean:

13. pertaining to the mind _____
14. abnormal condition of the mind _____

Use the suffix *–kinesia* (movement) to build words that mean:

15. movement that is slow _____
16. painful or difficult movement _____

Use the suffix *–plegia* (paralysis) to build words that mean:

17. paralysis of one half (of the body) _____
18. paralysis of four (limbs) _____

Use the suffix *–phasia* (speech) to build words that mean:

19. difficult speech _____
20. lacking or without speech _____

Build surgical terms that mean:

21. destruction of a nerve _____

22. incision of the skull _____

23. surgical repair of the skull _____

24. suture of a nerve _____

25. incision of the brain _____

 ✓ *Check your answers in Appendix A. Review material that you did not answer correctly.*

Correct Answers _____ × 4 = _____ % Score

Learning Activity 14-3
Learning Activity 14-3
Matching Pathological, Diagnostic, Symptomatic, and Related Terms

Match the following terms with the definitions in the numbered list.

Alzheimer disease	bulimia nervosa	Guillain-Barré syndrome	multiple sclerosis	phobias
aphasia	clonic phase	hemiparesis	myelomeningocele	poliomyelitis
autism	concussion	ischemic stroke	paraplegia	radiculopathy
bipolar disorder	epilepsies	lethargy	Parkinson disease	shingles

1. _____ weakness in one half of the body

2. _____ inability to speak

3. _____ pathological condition associated with formation of small plaques in the cerebral cortex

4. _____ eating disorder characterized by binging and purging

5. _____ part of the grand mal seizure characterized by uncontrolled jerking of the body

6. _____ autoimmune condition that causes acute inflammation of peripheral nerves

7. _____ type of neurosis characterized by irrational fears

8. _____ mental disorder that causes unusual shifts in mood, emotion, and energy

9. _____ chronic or recurring seizure disorders

10. _____ commonly caused by narrowing of the carotid arteries

11. _____ disease caused by the same organism that causes chickenpox in children

12. _____ disease of the nerve root associated with the spinal cord

13. _____ paralysis of the lower portion of the trunk and both legs

14. _____ disease that causes inflammation of the gray matter of the spinal cord

15. _____ abnormal inactivity or lack of response to normal stimuli

16. _____ most severe form of spina bifida where the spinal cord and meninges protrude though the spine

17. _____ mental disorder characterized by extreme withdrawal and abnormal absorption in fantasy

18. _____ disease characterized by head nodding, bradykinesia, tremors, and shuffling gait

19. _____ disease characterized by demyelination in the spinal cord and brain

20. _____ loss of consciousness caused by trauma to the head

✔ *Check your answers in Appendix A. Review any material that you did not answer correctly.*

Correct Answers _____ × 5 = _____ % Score

Learning Activity 14-4

Matching Procedures, Pharmacology, and Abbreviations

Match the following terms with the definitions in the numbered list.

antipsychotics	CSF analysis	general anesthetics	myelography	psychostimulants
cerebral angiography	echoencephalography	hypnotics	NCV	tractotomy
cryosurgery	electromyography	lumbar puncture	PET	trephination

1. _____ tests the speed at which impulses travel through a nerve

2. _____ reduce impulsive behavior by increasing the level of neurotransmitters; treat ADHD and narcolepsy

3. _____ treat psychosis, paranoia, and schizophrenia by altering chemicals in the brain, including the limbic system, which controls emotions

4. _____ act upon the brain to produce complete loss of feeling with loss of consciousness

5. _____ ultrasound technique used to study the intracranial structures of the brain

6. _____ technique that employs extreme cold to destroy tissue

7. _____ radiological examination of the spinal canal, nerve roots, and spinal cord

8. _____ visualization of the cerebrovascular system after injection of radiopaque dye

9. _____ laboratory test used to diagnose viral and bacterial infections, tumors, and hemorrhage

10. _____ recording of electrical signals when a muscle is at rest and during contraction to assess nerve damage

11. _____ procedure to extract spinal fluid for diagnostic purposes, introduce anesthetic agents, or remove fluid to allow other fluids to be injected

12. _____ scan using computed tomography to record the positrons emitted from a radiopharmaceutical

13. _____ transection of a nerve tract in the brainstem or spinal cord

14. _____ agents that depress central nervous system (CNS) functions, promote sedation and sleep, and relieve agitation, anxiousness, and restlessness

15. _____ cutting a circular opening into the skull to reveal brain tissue and decrease intracranial pressure

✔ *Check your answers in Appendix A. Review any material that you did not answer correctly.*

Correct Answers _____ × 6.67 = _____ % Score

MEDICAL RECORD ACTIVITIES

The two medical records included in the following activities use common clinical scenarios to show how medical terminology is used to document patient care. Complete the terminology and analysis sections for each activity to help you recognize and understand terms related to the nervous system.

Medical Record Activity 14-1
Discharge Summary: Subarachnoid Hemorrhage

Terminology

Terms listed below come from *Discharge Summary: Subarachnoid Hemorrhage* that follows. Use a medical dictionary such as *Taber's Cyclopedic Medical Dictionary*, the appendices of this book, or other resources to define each term. Then review the pronunciations for each term and practice by reading the medical record aloud.

Term	Definition
aneurysm ĂN-ū-rĭzm	
cerebral MRI	
cisterna subarach- noidalis sĭs-TĔR-nă sŭb-ă-răk- NOYD-ă-lĭs	
CSF	
CT	
hydrocephalus hī-drŏ-SĔF-ă-lŭs	
lumbar puncture LŬM-băr PŬNK-chūr	
meningismus mĕn-ĭn-JĬS-mŭs	
occipital ŏk-SĬP-ĭ-tăl	
R/O	
subarachnoid sŭb-ă-RĂK-noyd	

Listen and Learn Online! *will help you master the pronunciation of selected medical words from this medical record activity. Visit* www.davisplus.com/gylys/systems *to find instructions on completing the* Listen and Learn Online! *exercise for this section and to practice pronunciations.*

DISCHARGE SUMMARY: SUBARACHNOID HEMORRHAGE

General Hospital

1511 Ninth Avenue ■■ **Sun City, USA 12345** ■■ **(555) 8022-1887**

DISCHARGE SUMMARY

ADMISSION DATE: July 5, 20xx   DISCHARGE DATE: July 16, 20xx

ADMITTING DIAGNOSIS: Severe headaches associated with nausea and vomiting.

DISCHARGE DIAGNOSIS: Subarachnoid hemorrhage.

HISTORY OF PRESENT ILLNESS: Patient is a 61-year-old woman who presents at this time complaining of an "extreme severe headache while swimming." She also complains of associated neck pain, occipital pain, nausea, and vomiting.

A CT scan was obtained that showed blood in the cisterna subarachnoidalis consistent with subarachnoid hemorrhage. The patient also had mild acute hydrocephalus. Neurologically, the patient was found to be within normal limits. A cerebral MRI was performed and no aneurysm was noted.

HOSPITAL COURSE: The patient was hospitalized on 7/5/xx. On 7/7/xx, she had sudden worsening of her headache, associated with nausea and vomiting. Also, she was noted to have meningismus on examination. A lumbar puncture was performed to R/O possible rebleed. At the time of the lumbar puncture, CSF in four tubes was read as consistent with recurrent subarachnoid hemorrhage. A repeat MRI was performed without evidence of an aneurysm.

PROCEDURE: On 7/9/xx, the patient underwent repeat MRI, which again showed no aneurysm. The patient was deemed stable for discharge on 7/10/xx.

ACTIVITY: Patient instructed to avoid any type of activity that could result in raised pressure in the head. The patient was advised that she should undergo no activity more vigorous than walking.

Michael R. Saadi, MD
Michael R. Saadi, MD

MRS:dp

D: 7-16-20xx
T: 7-16-20xx

Patient: Gomez, Anna   Physician: Michael R. Saadi, MD
Room #: 609 P   Patient ID#: 920276

Analysis

Review the medical record *Discharge Summary: Subarachnoid Hemorrhage* to answer the following questions.

1. In what part of the head did the patient feel pain?

_____

2. What imaging tests were performed, and what was the finding in each test?

_____

3. What was the result of the lumbar puncture?

_____

4. What was the result of the repeat MRI?

_____

5. Regarding activity, what limitations were placed upon the patient?

_____

Medical Record Activity 14-2

Consultation Report: Acute Onset Paraplegia

Terminology

Terms listed below come from *Consultation Report: Acute Onset Paraplegia* that follows. Use a medical dictionary such as *Taber's Cyclopedic Medical Dictionary*, the appendices of this book, or other resources to define each term. Then review the pronunciations for each term and practice by reading the medical record aloud.

Term	Definition
abscess ĂB-sĕs	
acute ă-KŪT	
clonidine KLŌ-nĭ-dēn	
epidural ĕp-ĭ-DOO-răl	
fluoroscopy floo-or-ŎS-kō-pē	
infarct ĬN-fărkt	

Term	Definition
L2–3	
lumbar LŬM-băr	
methadone MĚTH-ă-dōn	
myelitis mī-ĕ-LĪ-tĭs	
paraplegia păr-ă-PLĒ-jē-ă	
paresthesia păr-ĕs-THĒ-zē-ă	
subarachnoid sŭb-ă-RĂK-noyd	
T10–11	
transverse trăns-VĔRS	

Listen and Learn Online! *will help you master the pronunciation of selected medical words from this medical record activity. Visit* www.davisplus.com/gylys/systems *to find instructions on completing the* Listen and Learn Online! *exercise for this section and to practice pronunciations.*

CONSULTATION REPORT: ACUTE ONSET PARAPLEGIA

Physician Center

2422 Rodeo Drive   ■■   **Sun City, USA 12345**   ■■   **(555)788-2427**

CONSULTATION

August 15, 20xx
Jacobs, Elaine

CHIEF COMPLAINT: Low back pain and lower extremity weakness.

HISTORY OF PRESENT ILLNESS: This is a 41-year-old right-handed white female with a history of low back pain for the past 15 to 20 years after falling at work. She has had four subsequent lumbar surgeries, with the most recent in 7/20/xx. She was admitted to the hospital for pain management. The patient had a subarachnoid catheter placement for pain control and management on 7/28/xx, at the L10–11 level. This was followed by trials of clonidine for hypertension and methadone for pain control, with bladder retention noted after clonidine administration. Upon catheter removal, the patient noted the subacute onset of paresis, paresthesias, and pain in the legs approximately 2 ½ to 3 hours later. We were consulted neurologically for assessment of the lower extremity weakness.

IMPRESSION: Patient has symptoms of acute-onset paraplegia. Differential diagnoses include a subarachnoid hemorrhage, epidural abscess, and transverse myelitis.

PLAN: Patient will be placed on IV steroids with compression stockings for lymphedema should physical therapy be cleared by cardiology for manipulation of that region. Documentation of spinal fluid will be obtained under fluoroscopy. Her glucose and blood pressures must be carefully monitored.

Jake S. Domer, MD
Jake S. Domer, MD

JSD:st

Analysis

Review the medical record *Consultation report: acute onset paraplegia* to answer the following questions.

1. What was the original cause of the patient's current problems and what treatments were provided?

2. Why was the patient admitted to the hospital?

3. What medications did the patient receive and why was each given?

4. What was the cause of bladder retention?

5. What occurred after the catheter was removed?

6. What three disorders were listed in the differential diagnosis?

7. How will lymphedema be controlled should physical therapy be undertaken?

Special Senses

CHAPTER

15

Chapter Outline

Objectives

Upon completion of this chapter, you will be able to:

- Locate and describe the main structures of the eye and ear.

- Recognize, pronounce, spell, and build words related to the special senses.

- Describe pathological conditions, diagnostic and therapeutic procedures, and other terms related to the special senses.

- Explain pharmacology related to the treatment of eye and ear disorders.

- Demonstrate your knowledge of this chapter by completing the learning and medical record activities.

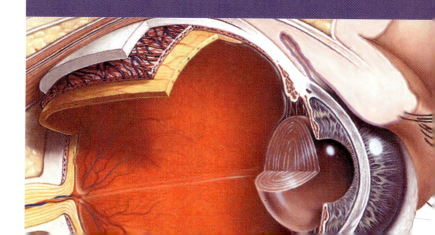

Anatomy and Physiology

General sensations perceived by the body include touch, pressure, pain, and temperature. These sensations are not identified with any specific site of the body. Specific sensations include smell (**olfaction**), taste (**gustation**), vision, hearing (**audition**), and equilibrium. Each specific sensation is connected to a specific organ or structure in the body. (For a discussion of olfaction, see Chapter 7, Respiratory System; for a discussion of gustation, see Chapter 6, Digestive System.) This chapter presents information on the sense of vision provided by the eye and senses of hearing and equilibrium provided by the ear.

Eye

The eye is a globe-shaped organ composed of three distinct **tunics,** or layers: the fibrous tunic, the vascular tunic, and the sensory tunic. (See Figure 15–1.)

Anatomy and Physiology Key Terms

This section introduces important terms associated with the special senses and their definitions. Word analyses for selected terms are also provided.

Term	Definition
accommodation ă-kŏm-ō-DĀ-shŭn	Adjustment of the eye for various distances so that images fall on the retina of the eye
acuity ă-KŪ-ĭ-tē	Clearness or sharpness of a sensory function
adnexa ăd-NĔK-să	Tissues or structures in the body adjacent to or near a related structure *The adnexa of the eye include the extraocular muscles, orbits, eyelids, conjunctiva, and lacrimal apparatus.*
articulating ăr-TĬK-ū-lāt-ing	Being loosely joined or connected together to allow motion between the parts
humor	Any fluid or semifluid of the body
labyrinth LĂB-ĭ-rĭnth	Series of intricate communicating passages *The labyrinth of the ear includes the cochlea, semicircular canals, and vestibule.*
opaque ō-PĀK	Substance that does not allow the passage of light; not transparent
perilymph PĔR-ĭ-lĭmf	Fluid that very closely resembles spinal fluid but found in the cochlea
photopigment fō-tō-PĬG-mĕnt	Light-sensitive pigment in the retinal cones and rods that absorbs light and initiates the visual process; also called *visual pigment*
refractive rĭ-FRĂK-tĭv	Ability to bend light rays as they pass from one medium to another
tunic TŪ-nĭk	Layer or coat of tissue; also called *membrane layer* *The fibrous, vascular, and sensory tunics are the three tunics of the eyeball.*

Pronunciation Help	Long Sound	ā—rate	ē—rebirth	ī—isle	ō—over	ū—unite
	Short Sound	ă—alone	ĕ—ever	ĭ—it	ŏ—not	ŭ—cut

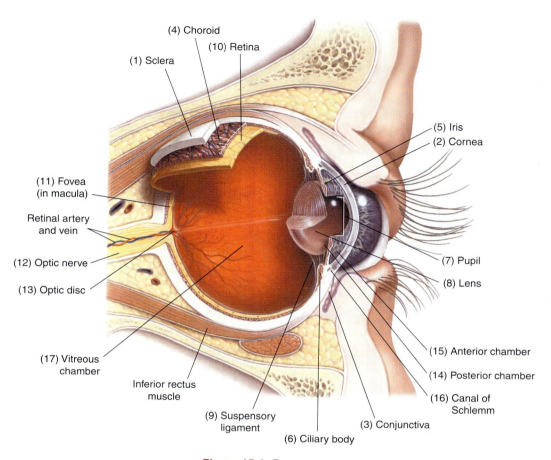

(4) Choroid
(10) Retina
(1) Sclera
(5) Iris
(2) Cornea
(11) Fovea
(in macula)
Retinal artery
and vein
(12) Optic nerve
(13) Optic disc
(7) Pupil
(8) Lens
(17) Vitreous
chamber
Inferior rectus
muscle
(15) Anterior chamber
(14) Posterior chamber
(16) Canal of
Schlemm
(9) Suspensory
ligament
(6) Ciliary body
(3) Conjunctiva

Figure 15-1. Eye structures.

Fibrous Tunic

The outermost layer of the eyeball, the **fibrous tunic,** serves as a protective coat for the more sensitive structures beneath. It includes the (1) **sclera** and the (2) **cornea.** The sclera, or "white of the eye," provides strength, shape, and structure to the eye. As the sclera passes in front of the eye, it bulges forward to become the cornea. Rather than being opaque, the cornea is transparent, allowing light to enter the interior of the eye. The cornea is one of the few body structures that does not contain capillaries and must rely on eye fluids for nourishment. A thin membrane, the (3) **conjunctiva,** covers the outer surface of the eye and lines the eyelids.

Vascular Tunic

The middle layer of the eyeball, the **vascular tunic,** is also known as the *uvea.* The **uvea** consists of the choroid, iris, and ciliary body. The (4) **choroid** provides the blood supply for the entire eye. It contains pigmented cells that prevent extraneous light from entering the inside of the eye. An opening in the

choroid allows the optic nerve to enter the inside of the eyeball. The anterior portion of the choroid contains two modified structures, the (5) **iris** and the (6) **ciliary body.** The iris is a colored, contractile membrane whose perforated center is called the (7) **pupil.** The iris regulates the amount of light passing through the pupil to the interior of the eye. As environmental light increases, the pupil constricts; as light decreases, the pupil dilates. The ciliary body is a circular muscle that produces aqueous humor. The ciliary body is attached to a capsular bag that holds the (8) **lens** between the (9) **suspensory ligaments.** As the ciliary muscle contracts and relaxes, it alters the shape of the lens making it thicker or thinner. These changes in shape allow the eye to focus on an image, a process called accommodation.

Sensory Tunic

The innermost **sensory tunic** is the delicate, double-layered (10) **retina.** It consists of a thin, outer **pigmented layer** lying over the choroid and a thick, inner **nervous layer,** or visual portion. The retina is responsible for the reception and transmission of visual impulses to the brain. It has two types of visual receptors: rods and cones. **Rods** function in dim light and produce black-and-white vision. **Cones** function in bright light and produce color vision. In the central portion of the retina is a highly sensitive structure called the *macula.* In the center of the macula is the (11) **fovea.** When the eye focuses on an object, light rays from that object are directed to the fovea. Because the fovea is composed of only cones that lie very close to each other, it provides the greatest acuity for color vision.

Other Structures

Rods and cones contain a chemical called *photopigment,* or *visual pigment.* As light strikes the photopigment, a chemical change occurs that stimulates rods and cones. The chemical changes produce impulses that are transmitted through the (12) **optic nerve** to the brain, where they are interpreted as vision. The optic nerve and blood vessels of the eye enter at the (13) **optic disc.** Its center is referred to as the **blind spot** because the area has neither rods nor cones for vision.

One of two major fluids (**humors**) of the eye is **aqueous humor.** It is found in the (14) **posterior chamber** and (15) **anterior chamber** of the anterior segment and provides nourishment for the lens and the cornea. Aqueous humor is continually produced by the ciliary body and is drained from the eye through a small opening called the (16) **canal of Schlemm.** If aqueous humor fails to drain from the eye at the rate at which it is produced, a condition called *glaucoma* results. The second major humor of the eye is **vitreous humor,** a jellylike substance that fills the interior of eye, the (17) **vitreous chamber.**

The vitreous humor, lens, and aqueous humor are the refractive structures of the eye, focusing light rays sharply on the retina. If any one of these structures does not function properly, vision is impaired.

The adnexa of the eye include all supporting structures of the eye globe. Six extraocular muscles control the movement of the eye: the superior, inferior, lateral, and medial rectus muscles and the superior and inferior oblique muscles. These muscles coordinate the eyes so that they move in a synchronized manner.

Two movable folds of skin constitute the eyelids, each with eyelashes that protect the front of the eye. (See Figure 15–2.) The (1) **conjunctiva** lines the inner surface of the eyelids and the cornea. Lying superior and to the outer edge of each eye are the (2) **lacrimal glands,** which produce tears that bathe and lubricate the eyes. The tears collect at the inner edges of the eyes, the **canthi** (singular, *canthus*), and pass through pinpoint openings, the (3) **lacrimal canals,** to the mucous membranes that line the inside of the (4) **nasal cavity.**

Ear

The ear is the sense receptor organ for hearing and equilibrium. Hearing is a function of the cochlea; the semicircular canals and vestibule control equilibrium.

Hearing

The ear consists of three major sections: the outer ear, or **external ear;** the middle ear, or **tympanic cavity;** and the inner ear, or labyrinth. (See Figure 15–3.) The external ear conducts sound waves through air; the middle ear, through bone; and the

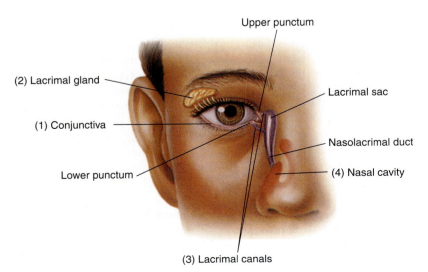

Upper punctum

(2) Lacrimal gland

Lacrimal sac

(1) Conjunctiva

Nasolacrimal duct

Lower punctum

(4) Nasal cavity

(3) Lacrimal canals

Figure 15-2. Lacrimal apparatus.

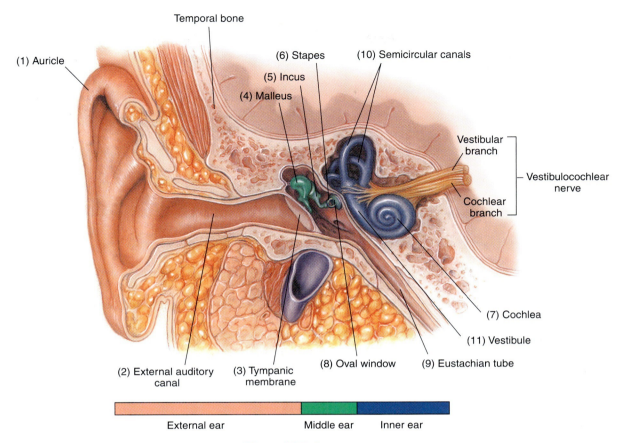

Temporal bone

(1) Auricle

(6) Stapes (10) Semicircular canals

(5) Incus

(4) Malleus

Vestibular branch

Vestibulocochlear nerve

Cochlear branch

(7) Cochlea

(11) Vestibule

(2) External auditory canal

(3) Tympanic membrane

(8) Oval window (9) Eustachian tube

External ear Middle ear Inner ear

Figure 15-3. Ear structures.

inner ear, through fluid. This series of transmissions ultimately generates impulses that are sent to the brain and interpreted as sound.

An (1) **auricle** (or *pinna*) collects waves traveling through air and channels them to the (2) **external auditory canal,** also called the *ear canal.* The ear canal is a slender tube lined with glands that produce a waxy secretion called *cerumen.* Its stickiness traps tiny foreign particles and prevents them from entering the deeper areas of the canal. The (3) **tympanic membrane** (also called the *tympanum* or *eardrum*) is a flat, membranous structure drawn over the end of the ear canal. Sound waves entering the ear canal strike against the tympanic membrane, causing it to vibrate. These vibrations cause movement of the three smallest bones of the body, collectively called the *ossicles.* These tiny articulating bones, the (4) **malleus** (or *hammer*), the (5) **incus** (or *anvil*), and the (6) **stapes** (or *stirrups*), are located within the tympanic cavity and form a coupling between the tympanic membrane and the (7) **cochlea,** the first structure of the inner ear. The cochlea is a snail-shaped structure filled with a fluid

called *perilymph.* Its inner surfaces are lined with a highly sensitive hearing structure called the **organ of Corti,** which contains tiny nerve endings called the **hair cells.** A membrane-covered opening on the external surface of the cochlea called the (8) **oval window** provides a place for attachment of the stapes. The movement of the ossicles in the middle ear causes the stapes to exert a gentle pumping action against the oval window. The pumping action forces the perilymph to disturb the hair cells, generating impulses that are transmitted to the brain by way of the auditory nerve, where they are interpreted as sound. The (9) **eustachian tube** connects the middle ear to the pharynx. It equalizes pressure on the outer and inner surfaces of the eardrum. When sudden pressure changes occur, pressure can be equalized on either side of the tympanic membrane by a deliberate swallow.

Equilibrium

The inner ear consists of a system of fluid-filled tubes and sacs as well as nerves that connect these structures to the brain. Because of its mazelike design, it is referred to as the *labyrinth*. The labyrinth, which rests inside the skull bones, includes not only the cochlea (the organ devoted to hearing) but also the vestibular system, which is devoted to the control of balance and eye movements. The vestibular system contains the (10) **semicircular canals** and the (11) **vestibule.** The vestibule joins the cochlea and the semicircu- lar canals. Many complex structures located in this maze are responsible for maintaining both static and dynamic equilibrium. **Static equilibrium** refers to the orientation of the body relative to gravity. It allows an individual to maintain posture and orientation while at rest. **Dynamic equilibri- um** refers to maintaining body position in response to movement.

 It is time to review eye and ear anatomy by completing Learning Activities 15–1 and 15–2.

Medical Word Elements

This section introduces combining forms, suffixes, and prefixes related to the special senses. Word analyses are also provided.

Element	Meaning	Word Analysis
Combining Forms		
Eye		
ambly/o	dull, dim	**ambly**/opia (ăm-blē-Ō-pē-ă): dimness of vision -*opia:* vision *In amblyopia, visual stimulation through the optic nerve of one eye (lazy eye) is impaired, thus resulting in poor or dim vision.*
aque/o	water	**aque**/ous (Ā-kwē-ŭs): pertaining to water -*ous:* pertaining to
blephar/o	eyelid	**blephar/o**/ptosis (blĕf-ă-rō-TŌ-sĭs): prolapse or downward displacement of the eyelid -*ptosis:* prolapse, downward displacement
choroid/o	choroid	**choroid/o**/pathy (kō-roy-DŎP-ă-thē): disease of the choroid -*pathy:* disease
conjunctiv/o	conjunctiva	**conjunctiv**/al (kŏn-jŭnk-TĪ-văl): pertaining to the conjunctiva -*al: pertaining to*
core/o	pupil	**core/o**/meter (kō-rē-ŎM-ĕ-tĕr): instrument for measuring the pupil -*meter:* instrument for measuring
pupill/o		**pupill/o**/graphy (pū-pĭ-LŎG-ră-fē): process of recording (movement of) the pupil -*graphy:* process of recording
corne/o	cornea	**corne**/al (KOR-nē-ăl): pertaining to the cornea -*al:* pertaining to
cycl/o	ciliary body of eye; circular; cycle	**cycl/o**/plegia (sī-klō-PLĒ-jē-ă): paralysis of the ciliary body -*plegia:* paralysis
dacry/o	tear; lacrimal apparatus (duct, sac, or gland)	**dacry**/oma (dăk-rē-Ō-mă): tumorlike swelling of the lacrimal duct -*oma:* tumor

Medical Word Elements—cont'd

Element	Meaning	Word Analysis
lacrim/o		**lacrim/o**/tomy (lăk-rĭ-MŎT-ō-mē): incision of the lacrimal duct or sac *-tomy:* incision
dacryocyst/o	lacrimal sac	**dacryocyst/o**/ptosis (dăk-rē-ō-sĭs-tŏp-TŌ-sĭs): prolapse of the lacrimal sac *-ptosis:* prolapse, downward displacement
glauc/o	gray	**glauc/**oma (glaw-KŌ-mă): gray tumor *-oma:* tumor *If not treated, glaucoma results in increased intraocular pressure (IOP) that destroys the retina and optic nerve. Because of diminished blood flow to the back of the eye, the optic nerve appears pale gray, hence the name glaucoma.*
goni/o	angle	**goni/o**/scopy (gŏ-nē-ŎS-kŏ-pē): visual examination of the irideocorneal angle *-scopy:* visual examination *Gonioscopy is used to differentiate the two forms of glaucoma (open- and closed-angle).*
irid/o	iris	**irid/o**/plegia (ĭr-ĭd-ō-PLĒ-jē-ă): paralysis of (the sphincter of) the iris *-plegia:* paralysis
kerat/o	horny tissue; hard; cornea	**kerat/o**/tomy (kĕr-ă-TŎT-ō-mē): incision of the cornea *-tomy:* incision
ocul/o	eye	**ocul/o**/myc/osis (ŏk-ū-lō-mī-KŌ-sĭs): fungal infection of the eye (or its parts) *myc:* fungus *-osis:* abnormal condition; increase (used primarily with blood cells)
ophthalm/o		**opthalm/o**/logist (ŏf-thăl-MŎL-ō-jĭst): specialist in the study of the eye *-logist:* specialist in study of *Ophthalmologists are physicians who specialize in the medical and surgical management of diseases and disorders of the eyes.*
opt/o	eye, vision	**opt/o**/metry (ŏp-TŎM-ĕ-trē): act of measuring vision *-metry:* act of measuring *Optometry is the science of diagnosing, managing, and treating nonsurgical conditions and diseases of the eye and visual system.*
optic/o		**optic/**al (ŎP-tĭ-kăl): pertaining to the eye or vision *-al:* pertaining to
phac/o	lens	**phac/o**/cele (FĀK-ō-sēl): herniation (displacement) of the lens into the interior chamber of the eye *-cele:* hernia, swelling *The usual cause of phacocele is blunt trauma to the eye.*
phot/o	light	**phot/o**/phobia (fō-tō-FŌ-bē-ă): abnormal fear of (intolerance to) light *-phobia:* fear *Intolerance to light is associated with people who suffer from migraines or have light-colored eyes or glaucoma. Some medications also cause a marked intolerance to light.*
presby/o	old age	**presby/**opia (prĕz-bē-Ō-pē-ă): (poor) vision (associated with) old age *-opia:* vision *Presbyopia is the loss of accommodation due to weakening of the ciliary muscles as a result of the aging process.*

(continued)

Medical Word Elements—cont'd

Element	Meaning	Word Analysis
retin/o	retina	**retin/o**/sis (rĕt-ĭ-NŌ-sĭs): abnormal condition of the retina *-osis:* abnormal condition; increase (used primarily with blood cells) *Retinosis includes any degenerative process of the retina not associated with inflammation.*
scler/o	hardening; sclera (white of eye)	**scler/o**/malacia (sklĕ-rō-mă-LĀ-shē-ă): softening of the sclera *-malacia:* softening
scot/o	darkness	**scot/o**/ma (skō-TŌ-mă): dark, tumorlike spot *-oma:* tumor *Scotoma is an area of diminished vision in the visual field.*
vitr/o	vitreous body (of eye)	**vitr/**ectomy (vĭ-TRĔK-tō-mē): removal of the (contents of the) vitreous chamber *-ectomy:* excision, removal *The removal of the vitreous allows surgical procedures that would otherwise be impossible, including repair of macular holes and tears in the retina.*
Ear		
audi/o	hearing	**audi/o**/meter (aw-dē-ŎM-ĕ-tĕr): instrument to measure hearing *-meter:* instrument for measuring
labyrinth/o	labyrinth (inner ear)	**labyrinth/o**/tomy (lăb-ĭ-rĭn-THŎT-ō-mē): incision of the labyrinth *-tomy:* incision
mastoid/o	mastoid process	**mastoid/**ectomy (măs-toyd-ĔK-tō-mē): removal of the mastoid process *-ectomy:* excision, removal
ot/o	ear	**ot/o**/py/o/rrhea (ō-tō-pī-ō-RĒ-ă): discharge of pus from the ear *py/o:* pus *-rrhea:* discharge, flow
salping/o	tubes (usually fallopian or eustachian [auditory] tubes)	**salping/o**/scope (săl-PĬNG-gō-skōp): instrument to examine the eustachian tubes *-scope:* instrument to view or examine
staped/o	stapes	**staped/**ectomy (stā-pĕ-DĔK-tō-mē): excision of the stapes *-ectomy:* excision, removal *Stapedectomy is performed to improve hearing, especially in cases of otosclerosis.*
myring/o	tympanic membrane (eardrum)	**myring/o**/myc/osis (mĭr-ĭn-gō-mī-KŌ-sĭs): abnormal condition due to fungal infection of the tympanic membrane *myc:* fungus *-osis:* abnormal condition; increase (used primarily with blood cells)
tympan/o		**tympan/o**/stomy (tĭm-pă-NŎS-tō-mē): forming an opening in the tympanic membrane *-stomy:* forming an opening (mouth) *This procedure is usually performed to insert small pressure-equalizing (PE) tubes through the tympanum.*

Medical Word Elements—cont'd

Element	Meaning	Word Analysis
Suffixes		
-acusia	hearing	an/**acusia** (ăn-ă-KŪ-sē-ă): not hearing (deafness) *an-:* without, not
-cusis		presby/**cusis** (prĕz-bĭ-KŪ-sĭs): hearing (loss) associated with old age *presby:* old age ***Presbycusis generally occurs in both ears and primarily affects high-pitched tones.***
-opia	vision	dipl/**opia** (dĭp-LŌ-pē-ă): double vision *dipl-:* double, twofold
-opsia		heter/**opsia** (hĕt-ĕr-ŎP-sē-ă): inequality of vision (in the two eyes) *heter-:* different
-tropia	turning	eso/**tropia** (ĕs-ō-TRŌ-pē-ă): turning inward (of the eyes); also called *convergent strabismus* or *crossed eyes* *eso-:* inward
Prefixes		
exo-	outside, outward	**exo**/tropia (ĕks-ō-TRŌ-pē-ă): abnormal turning outward of (one or both eyes); also called *divergent strabismus* *-tropia:* turning
hyper-	excessive, above normal	**hyper**/opia (hī-pĕr-Ō-pē-ă): excess (farsighted) vision *-opia:* vision

It is time to review medical word elements by completing Learning Activity 15–3. For audio pronunciations of the above-listed key terms, you can visit www.davisplus.fadavis.com/gylys/systems *to download this chapter's* Listen and Learn! *exercises or use the book's audio CD (if included).*

Pathology

Common signs and symptoms of eye disorders include decrease in visual acuity, headaches, and pain in the eye or adnexa. However, many disorders of the eye are serious but asymptomatic; therefore, regular eye checkups are necessary. For diagnosis, treatment, and management of visual disorders, the medical services of a specialist may be warranted. **Ophthalmology** is the medical specialty concerned with disorders of the eye. The physician who treats these disorders is called an *ophthalmologist.* Optometrists work with ophthalmologists in a medical practice or practice independently. **Optometrists** are not medical doctors, but are doctors of optometry (OD). They diagnose vision problems and eye disease, prescribe eyeglasses and contact lenses, and prescribe drugs to treat eye disorders. Although they cannot perform surgery, they commonly provide preoperative and postoperative care.

Common signs and symptoms of ear disorders include hearing impairment, ringing in the ears, pain or drainage from the ears, loss of balance, dizziness, or nausea. Young children are especially vulnerable to middle ear infections that, if not treated, may cause hearing loss. For diagnosis, treatment, and management of hearing disorders, the medical services of a specialist may be warranted. **Otolaryngology** is the medical specialty concerned with disorders of the ear, nose, and throat. The physician who treats these disorders is called an *otolaryngologist.* Many otolaryngologists employ audiologists. **Audiologists** are allied health-care professionals who work with patients with hearing, balance, and related problems. They perform hearing examinations, evaluate hearing loss, clean and irrigate the ear canal, fit and dispense hearing aids or other assistive devices, and provide audiological rehabilitation, including auditory training and instruction in speech or lip reading.

Eye Disorders

Eye disorders include not only visual deficiencies associated with refractive errors, but also disorders of associated structures, such as the eye muscles, nerves, and blood vessels. A complete examination of the eye and its adnexa is necessary to identify the source of any disorder. Most ocular examinations begin by recording visual acuity (VA) and visual field (VF). Then the eyelids, pupils, cornea, and lacrimal structures are examined and intraocular pressure is assessed as well. If infection is detected, it must be located and identified by culturing eye and nasal discharges and performing computed tomography (CT) of the sinuses. Occasionally, the patient may be referred for dental examination to determine if abscesses in the mouth are the source of infection. Family history is important because many eye disorders have a genetic predisposition, including glaucoma. Common eye disorders include errors of refraction, cataracts, glaucoma, strabismus, and macular degeneration.

Errors of Refraction

An error of refraction (**ametropia**) exists when light rays fail to focus sharply on the retina. This may be due to a defect in the lens, cornea, or the shape of the eyeball. If the eyeball is too long, the image falls in front of the retina, causing nearsightedness. (See Figure 15–4.) In farsightedness (**hyperopia, hypermetropia**), the opposite of myopia, the eyeball is too short and the image falls behind the retina. A form of farsightedness is **presbyopia,** a defect associated with the aging process. The onset of presbyopia usually occurs between ages 40 and 45. Distant objects are seen clearly, but near objects are not in proper focus. In another form of ametropia called *astigmatism (Ast),* the cornea or lens has a defective curvature. This curvature causes light rays to diffuse over a large area of the retina rather than being sharply focused.

Corrective lenses usually compensate for the various types of ametropia. An alternative to corrective lenses is **laser-assisted in situ keratomileusis (LASIK)** surgery. This procedure changes the shape of the cornea and, in most instances, the change is permanent. A small incision is made in the cornea to produce a flap. The flap is lifted to the side while a laser reshapes the underlying corneal tissue. At the completion of the procedure, the corneal flap is replaced. The procedure usually takes less than 15 minutes. However, not all people are candidates for this surgery. Some medical conditions, certain medications, or the shape and structure of the eye may preclude this procedure as a viable alternative to corrective lenses.

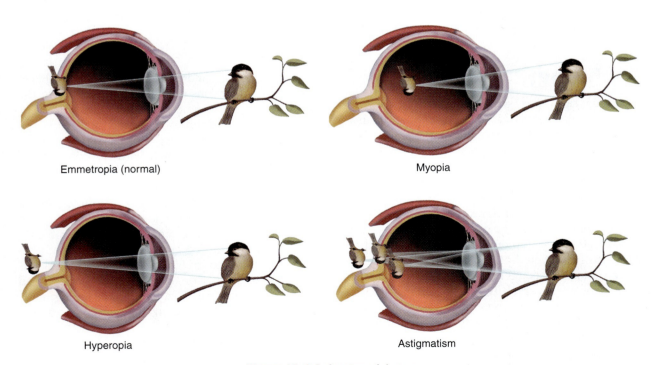

Emmetropia (normal)

Myopia

Hyperopia

Astigmatism

Figure 15-4. Refraction of the eye.

Cataracts

Cataracts are opacities that form on the lens and impair vision. These opacities are commonly produced by protein that slowly builds up over time until vision is affected. The most common form of cataract is age related. More than one half of Americans older than age 65 have cataracts to a greater or lesser extent. Congenital cataracts found in children are usually a result of genetic defects or maternal rubella during the first trimester of pregnancy. This rare form of cataract is treated in the same manner as age-related cataract. The usual treatment is removal of the clouded lens by emulsifying it using ultrasound or a laser probe (**phacoemulsification**). This method is typically referred to as *small incision cataract surgery* (**SICS**) because the cataract is broken into very small particles that can be removed through the tiny incision. (See Figure 15–5.) An artificial, bendable intraocular lens (IOL) is then inserted into the capsule. Once in position, the lens unfolds. The surgery is usually performed using a topical anesthetic, and the incision normally does not require stitches. This is one of the safest and most effective surgical procedures performed in medicine.

Glaucoma

Glaucoma is characterized by increased intraocular pressure (IOP) caused by the failure of aqueous humor to drain from the eye through a tiny duct called the *canal of Schlemm.* (See Fig. 15–6.) The increased pressure on the optic nerve destroys it, and vision is permanently lost.

Although there are various forms of glaucoma, all of them eventually lead to blindness unless the condition is detected and treated in its early stages. Glaucoma may occur as a primary or congenital disease or secondary to other causes, such as injury, infection, surgery, or prolonged topical corticosteroid use. Primary glaucoma can be chronic or acute. The **chronic form** is also called **open-angle,** *simple* or *wide-angle glaucoma.* The **acute form** is called *angle-closure* or *narrow-angle glaucoma.* Chronic glaucoma may produce no symptoms except gradual loss of peripheral vision over a period of years. Headaches, blurred vision, and dull pain in the eye may also be present. Cupping of the optic discs may be noted on ophthalmoscopic examination. Acute glaucoma is accompanied by extreme ocular pain, blurred vision, redness of the eye, and dilation of the pupil. Nausea and vomiting may also occur. If untreated, acute glaucoma causes complete and permanent blindness within 2 to 5 days.

Glaucoma is diagnosed by **tonometry,** a screening test that measures intraocular pressure by determining the resistance of the eyeball to indentation by an applied force. A slit lamp examination (SLE) with a high-intensity beam is used to assess the external surface and internal segments of the eye after administration of a local anesthetic. Devices such as a **tonometer,** which measures intraocular pressure, and a **gonioscope,** which visualizes the anterior chamber angle, expand the scope of the examination. Several methods of tonometry are available, but the one that is considered most accurate is **applanation tonometry.** (See Figure 15–7.) Numbing drops are used and the test is pain free. Treatment for glaucoma includes medications that cause the pupils to constrict (**miotics**), which permits aqueous humor to

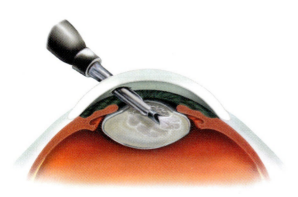

Cataract removal

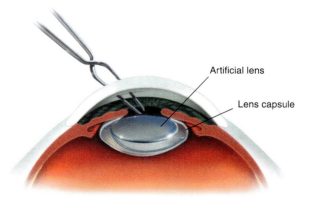

Artificial lens

Lens capsule

Artificial lens insertion

Figure 15-5. Phacoemulsification.

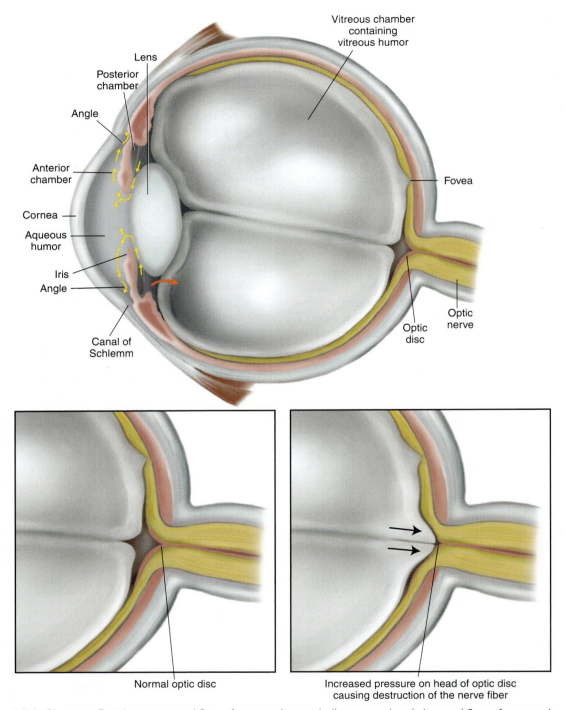

Figure 15-6. Glaucoma. Eye showing normal flow of aqueous humor (yellow arrows) and abnormal flow of aqueous humor (red arrow) causing destruction of optic nerve.

escape from the eye, thereby relieving pressure. If miotics are ineffective, surgery may be necessary.

Strabismus

Strabismus, also called *heterotropia* or *tropia*, is a condition in which one eye is misaligned with the other and the eyes do not focus simultaneously when viewing an object. This misalignment may be in any direction—inward (**esotropia**), outward (**exotropia**), up, down, or a combination. The deviation may be a constant condition or may arise intermittently with stress, exhaustion, or illness. (See Figure 15–8.) In normal vision, each eye views an image from a somewhat different vantage point,

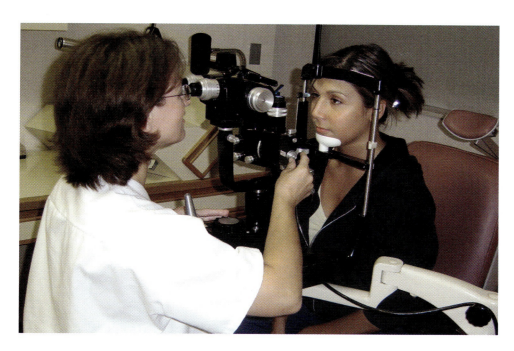

Figure 15-7. Applanation tonometry using a slit lamp to measure intraocular pressure (courtesy of Richard H. Koop, MD).

thus transmitting a slightly different image to the brain. The result is binocular perception of depth or three-dimensional space, a phenomenon known as *stereopsis*. Strabismus commonly causes a loss of stereopsis. In children, strabismus is commonly, but not always, associated with "lazy-eye syndrome" (**amblyopia**). Vision is suppressed in the "lazy" eye so that the child uses only the "good" eye for vision. The vision pathway fails to develop in the "lazy" eye.

There is a critical period during which amblyopia must be corrected, usually before age 6. If not detected and treated early in life, amblyopia can cause a permanent loss of vision in the affected eye, with associated loss of stereopsis. Treatment for strabismus depends on the cause. It commonly consists of covering the normal eye, forcing the child to use the deviated, or lazy, eye. Eye exercises and corrective lenses may be prescribed, or surgical correction may be necessary.

Macular Degeneration

Macular degeneration is a deterioration of the macula, the most sensitive portion of the retina. The macula is responsible for central, or "straight-ahead," vision required for reading, driving, detail work, and recognizing faces. (See Figure 15–9.) Although deterioration of the macula is associated with toxic effects of some drugs, the most common type is **age-related macular degeneration (ARMD, AMD)**. ARMD is a leading cause of visual loss in the United States. The disease is unpredictable and progresses differently in each individual.

So far, two forms of ARMD have been identified: wet and dry. The less common, but more severe, form is **wet,** or *neovascular ARMD.* It affects about 10% of those afflicted with the disease. Small blood vessels form under the macula. Blood and other fluids leak from these vessels and destroy the visual cells, leading to severe loss of central vision and permanent visual impairment. If identified in its early stages, laser surgery can be employed to destroy the newly forming vessels. This treatment is called *laser photocoagulation.* It is successful in about one half of the patients with wet ARMD. However, the effects of the procedure commonly do not last and new vessels begin to form.

The more common form of the macular degeneration is **dry ARMD.** Small yellowish deposits called *drusen* develop on the macula and interfere with central vision. Drusen are dried retinal pigment epithelial cells that form granules on the macula. Although some vision is lost, this form of the disease rarely leads to total blindness. Patients with dry ARMD are encouraged to see their ophthalmologist frequently and perform a simple at-home test that identifies visual changes that may indicate the development of the more serious neovascular ARMD.

Ear Disorders

Common signs and symptoms of ear disorders include hearing loss, earache, vertigo, and tinnitus. Hearing tests are important in diagnosing hearing loss as well as aiding in localizing the source and nature of the hearing deficiency. In addition, many infections of the nose and throat refer pain (**synalgia**)

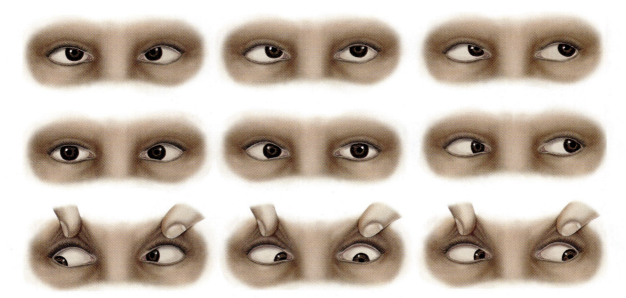

Figure 15-8. Types of strabismus.

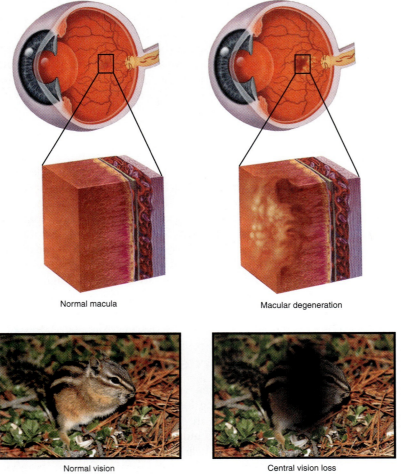

Normal macula

Macular degeneration

Normal vision

Central vision loss

Figure 15-9. Macular degeneration.

to the ear. Therefore, an examination of the nose and throat is usually essential in identifying the cause of ear pain. Common ear disorders include otitis media and otosclerosis.

Otitis Media

Otitis media (OM) is an inflammation of the middle ear. This infection may be caused by a virus or bacterium. However, the most common culprit is *Streptococcus pneumoniae.* Otitis media is found most commonly in infants and young children, especially in the presence of an upper respiratory infection (URI). Symptoms may include earache and draining of pus from the ear (**otopyorrhea**). In its most severe form, otitis media may lead to infection of the mastoid process (**mastoiditis**) or inflammation of brain tissue near the middle ear (**otoencephalitis**). Recurrent episodes of otitis media may cause scarring of the tympanic membrane, leading to hearing loss. Treatment consists of bed rest, medications to relieve pain (**analgesics**), and antibiotics. Occasionally, an incision of the eardrum (**myringotomy, tympanotomy**) may be necessary to relieve pressure and promote drainage.

The usual treatment for children with recurrent infection is the use of **pressure-equalizing tubes** (**PE tubes**) that are passed through the tympanic membrane. These tubes help drain fluid from the middle ear. (See Figure 15–10.)

Otosclerosis

Otosclerosis is a disorder characterized by an abnormal hardening (**ankylosis**) of bones of the middle ear that causes hearing loss. The ossicle most commonly affected is the stapes, the bone that attaches to the oval window of the cochlea. The formation of a spongy growth at the footplate of the stapes decreases its ability to move the oval window, resulting in hearing loss. Occasionally, the patient perceives a ringing sound (**tinnitus**) within the ear, along with dizziness and a progressive loss of hearing, especially of low tones. Development of otosclerosis is typically closely tied to genetic factors; if one or both parents have the disorder, the child is at high risk for developing the disease. Surgical correction involves removing part of the stapes (**stapedectomy** or, more commonly, **stapedotomy**) and implanting a prosthetic device that allows sound waves to pass to the inner ear. The procedure requires only a local anesthetic and usually lasts only 45 minutes. Hearing is immediately restored.

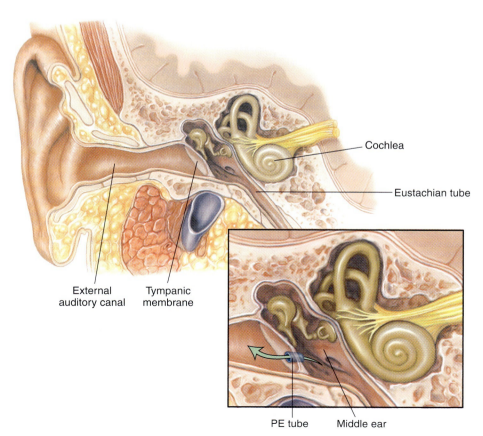

External auditory canal   Tympanic membrane

Cochlea

Eustachian tube

PE tube   Middle ear

Figure 15-10. Placement of pressure-equalizing (PE) tube.

Oncology

Two major **neoplastic diseases** account for more than 90% of all primary intraocular diseases: **retinoblastoma**, found primarily in children, and **melanoma**, found primarily in adults. Most retinoblastomas tend to be familial. The cell involved is the retinal neuron. Vision is impaired and, in about 30% of patients, the disease is found in both eyes (**bilateral**). Melanoma may occur in the orbit, the bony cavity of the eyeball, the iris, or the ciliary body, but it arises most commonly in the pigmented cells of the choroid. The disease is usually asymptomatic until there is a hemorrhage into the anterior chamber. Any discrete, fleshy mass on the iris should be examined by an ophthalmologist. If malignancy occurs in the choroid, it usually appears as a brown or gray mushroom-shaped lesion.

Treatment for retinoblastoma usually involves the removal of the affected eye(s) (**enucleation**), followed by radiation. In melanoma where the lesion is on the iris, an iridectomy is performed. For melanoma of the choroid, enucleation is necessary. Many eye tumors are noninvasive and are not necessarily life threatening.

Both malignant and nonmalignant tumors can arise in the external ear, the canal, or the middle ear. Malignant tumors of the ear include basal cell carcinoma and squamous cell tumors. The most common ear malignancy is basal cell carcinoma, which usually occurs on the top of the pinna as the result of sun exposure. It is found more commonly in elderly patients or those with fair skin. Small, craterlike ulcers form as the disease progresses. Basal cell carcinoma does not readily metastasize; however, failure to treat it in a timely manner may result in the need for extensive surgery to remove the tumor. Squamous cell carcinoma, on the other hand, is much more invasive. However, it is a very rare type of ear tumor. In appearance, it closely resembles basal cell carcinoma, and biopsy is required to make a definitive diagnosis. Squamous cell carcinoma grows more slowly than basal cell carcinoma; however, because of its tendency to metastasize to the surrounding nodes and the nodes of the neck, it must be removed. Surgery combined with radiation therapy is the most effective treatment for squamous cell carcinoma.

Diagnostic, Symptomatic, and Related Terms

This section introduces diagnostic, symptomatic, and related terms and their meanings. Word analyses for selected terms are also provided.

Term	Definition
Eye	
achromatopsia ă-krō-mă-TŎP-sĕ-ă *a-: without, not* *chromat: color* *-opsia: vision*	Severe congenital deficiency in color perception; also called *complete color blindness*
chalazion kă-LĀ-zē-ōn	Small, hard tumor developing on the eyelid, somewhat similar to a sebaceous cyst
conjunctivitis kŏn-jŭnk-tĭ-VĪ-tĭs *conjunctiv: conjunctiva* *-itis: inflammation*	Inflammation of the conjunctiva with vascular congestion, producing a red or pink eye; may be secondary to viral, bacterial, or fungal infections or allergy
convergence kŏn-VĔR-jĕnts	Medial movement of the two eyeballs so that they are both directed at the object being viewed
diopter (D) dī-ŎP-tĕr	Measurement of refractive error *When the D value is negative, it signifies an eye with myopia. When the D value is positive, it signifies an eye with hyperopia.*

Diagnostic, Symptomatic, and Related Terms—cont'd

Term	Definition
ectropion ĕk-TRŌ-pē-ŏn	Eversion, or outward turning, of the edge of the lower eyelid
emmetropia (Em) ĕm-ĕ-TRŌ-pē-ă	State of normal vision *In emmetropia, when the eye is at rest, the image is focused directly on the retina.*
entropion ĕn-TRŌ-pē-ŏn	Inversion or inward turning of the edge of the lower eyelid
epiphora ĕ-PĬF-ō-ră	Abnormal overflow of tears *Epiphora is sometimes caused by obstruction of the tear ducts.*
exophthalmos ĕks-ŏf-THĂL-mŏs	Protrusion of one or both eyeballs *Common causes of exophthalmos include hyperactive thyroid, trauma, and tumor.*
hordeolum hor-DĒ-ō-lŭm	Localized, circumscribed, inflammatory swelling of one of the several sebaceous glands of the eyelid, generally caused by a bacterial infection; also called *stye*
metamorphopsia mĕt-ă-mor-FŎP-sē-ă *meta-:* change; beyond *morph:* form, shape, structure *-opsia:* vision	Visual distortion of objects *Metamorphopsia is commonly associated with errors of refraction, retinal disease, choroiditis, detachment of the retina, and tumors of the retina or choroid.*
nyctalopia nĭk-tă-LŌ-pē-ă *nyctal:* night *-opia:* vision	Impaired vision in dim light; also called *night blindness* *Common causes of nyctalopia include cataracts, vitamin A deficiency, certain medications, and hereditary causes.*
nystagmus nĭs-TĂG-mŭs	Involuntary eye movements that appear jerky and may reduce vision or be associated with other, more serious conditions that limit vision
papilledema păp-ĭl-ĕ-DĒ-mă	Edema and hyperemia of the optic disc usually associated with increased intracranial pressure; also called *choked disc*
photophobia fō-tō-FŌ-bē-ă *phot/o:* light *-phobia:* fear	Unusual intolerance and sensitivity to light *Photophobia commonly occurs in such diseases as meningitis, inflammation of the eyes, measles, and rubella.*
presbyopia prĕz-bē-Ō-pē-ă *presby:* old age *-opia:* vision	Loss of accommodation of the crystalline lens associated with the aging process *During the aging process, proteins in the lens become harder and less elastic and muscle fibers surrounding the lens lose strength. These changes cause a decreased ability to focus, especially at close range.*
retinopathy rĕt-ĭn-ŎP-ă-thē *retin/o:* retina *-pathy:* disease	Any disorder of retinal blood vessels
diabetic dī-ă-BĔT-ĭk	Disorder that occurs in patients with diabetes and is manifested by small hemorrhages, edema, and formation of new vessels on the retina, leading to scarring and eventual loss of vision

(continued)

Diagnostic, Symptomatic, and Related Terms—cont'd

Term	Definition
trachoma trā-KŌ-mă	Chronic, contagious form of conjunctivitis common in the southwestern United States that typically leads to blindness
visual field	Area within which objects may be seen when the eye is in a fixed position
Ear	
anacusis ăn-ă-KŪ-sĭs *an-:* without, not *-acusis:* hearing	Complete deafness; also called *anacusia* *Anacusis may be unilateral or bilateral. Anacusis should not be confused with hearing loss. Hearing loss refers to impairment in hearing and the individual may be able to respond to auditory stimuli including speech.*
conduction impairment kŏn-DŬK-shŭn	Blocking of sound waves as they pass through the external and middle ear (conduction pathway)
labyrinthitis lăb-ĭ-rĭn-THĪ-tĭs *labyrinth:* labyrinth (inner ear) *-itis:* inflammation	Inflammation of the inner ear that usually results from an acute febrile process *Labyrinthitis may lead to progressive vertigo.*
Ménière disease měn-ē-ĀR	Disorder of the labyrinth that leads to progressive loss of hearing *Ménière disease is characterized by vertigo, sensorineural hearing loss, and tinnitus.*
noise-induced hearing loss (NIHL)	Condition caused by the destruction of hair cells, the organs responsible for hearing, caused by sounds that are "too long, too loud, or too close" *Target shooting, leaf blowing, motorcycle engines, rock concerts, woodworking, and other such environmental noises all produce sounds that may, over time, cause NIHL.*
otitis externa ō-TĪ-tĭs ĕks-TĔR-nă *ot:* ear *-itis:* inflammation	Infection of the external auditory canal *Common causes of otitis externa include exposure to water when swimming (swimmer's ear), bacterial or fungal infections, seborrhea, eczema, and chronic conditions such as allergies.*
presbyacusis prěz-bē-ă-KŪ-sĭs *presby:* old age *-acusis:* hearing	Impairment of hearing resulting from old age; also called *presbyacusia* *In presbyacusis, patients are generally able to hear low tones but lose the ability to hear higher tones. This condition usually affects speech perception, especially in the presence of background noise, as in a restaurant or a large crowd. This type of hearing loss is irreversible.*
pressure-equalizing (PE) tubes	Tubes that are inserted through the tympanic membrane, commonly to treat chronic otitis media; also called *tympanostomy tubes* or *ventilation tubes* *PE tubes remain in the ear several months, and then fall out on their own or are removed surgically. (See Figure 15–10.)*

Diagnostic, Symptomatic, and Related Terms—cont'd

Term	Definition
tinnitus tĭn-Ī-tŭs	Perception of ringing, hissing, or other sounds in the ears or head when no external sound is present *Tinnitus may be caused by a blow to the head, ingestion of large doses of aspirin, anemia, noise exposure, stress, impacted wax, hypertension, and certain types of medications and tumors.*
vertigo VĔR-tĭ-gō	Hallucination of movement, or a feeling of spinning or dizziness *Vertigo may be caused by a variety of disorders, including Ménière disease and labyrinthitis.*

 It is time to review pathological, diagnostic, symptomatic, and related terms by completing Learning Activity 15–4.

Diagnostic and Therapeutic Procedures

This section introduces procedures used to diagnose and treat eye and ear disorders. Descriptions are provided as well as pronunciations and word analyses for selected terms.

Procedure	Description
Diagnostic Procedures	
Clinical	
audiometry aw-dē-ŎM-ĕ-trē *audi/o:* hearing *-metry:* act of measuring	Measurement of hearing acuity at various sound wave frequencies *In audiometry, pure tones of controlled intensity are delivered through earphones to one ear at a time while the patient indicates if the tone was heard. The minimum intensity (volume) required to hear each tone is graphed.*
caloric stimulation test	Test that uses different water temperatures to assess the vestibular portion of the nerve of the inner ear (acoustic nerve) to determine if nerve damage is the cause of vertigo *In the caloric stimulation test, cold and warm water are separately introduced into each ear while electrodes placed around the eye record nystagmus. Eyes move in a predictable pattern when the water is introduced, except with acoustic nerve damage.*
electronystagmography (ENG) ē-lĕk-trō-nĭs-tăg-MŎG-ră-fē	Method of assessing and recording eye movements by measuring the electrical activity of the extraocular muscles *In ENG, electrodes are placed above, below, and to the side of each eye. A ground electrode is placed on the forehead. The electrodes record eye movement relative to the position of the ground electrode.*
ophthalmodynamometry ŏf-thăl-mō-dī-nă-MŎM-ĕ-trē	Measurement of the blood pressure of the retinal vessels *Ophthalmodynamometry is a screening test used to determine reduction of blood flow in the carotid artery.*
tonometry tōn-ŎM-ĕ-trē *ton/o:* tension *-metry:* act of measuring	Evaluation of intraocular pressure by measuring the resistance of the eyeball to indentation by an applied force *Tonometry is used to detect glaucoma. Several kinds of tonometers can be used. The applanation method of tonometry uses a sensor to depress the cornea and is considered the most accurate method of tonometry. (See Figure 15-7.)*

(continued)

Diagnostic and Therapeutic Procedures—cont'd

Procedure	Description
visual acuity (VA) test ă-KŪ-ĭ-tē	Part of an eye examination that determines the smallest letters that can be read on a standardized chart at a distance of 20 feet *Visual acuity (VA) is expressed as a fraction. The top number refers to the distance from the chart and the bottom number indicates the distance at which a person with normal eyesight could read the same line. For example 20/40 indicates that the patient correctly read letters at 20 feet that could be read by a person with normal vision at 40 feet.*
Endoscopic	
gonioscopy gō-nē-ŎS-kō-pē *goni/o:* angle *-scopy:* visual examination	Examination of the angle of the anterior chamber of the eye to determine ocular motility and rotation and diagnose and manage glaucoma
ophthalmoscopy ŏf-thăl-MŎS-kō-pē *ophthalm/o:* eye *-scopy:* visual examination	Visual examination of the interior of the eye using a hand-held instrument called an *ophthalmoscope,* which has various adjustable lenses for magnification and a light source to illuminate the interior of the eye *Ophthalmoscopy is used to detect eye disorders as well as other disorders that cause changes in the eye.*
otoscopy ō-TŎS-kō-pē *ot/o:* ear *-scopy:* visual examination	Visual examination of the external auditory canal and the tympanic membrane using an otoscope
pneumatic nū-MĂT-ĭk	Procedure that assesses the ability of the tympanic membrane to move in response to a change in air pressure *In pneumatic otoscopy, a tight seal is created in the ear canal and then a very slight positive pressure and then a negative pressure is applied by squeezing and releasing a rubber bulb attached to the pneumatic otoscope. The fluctuation in air pressure causes movement of a normal tympanic membrane.*
retinoscopy rĕt-ĭn-ŎS-kō-pē *retin/o:* retina *-scopy:* visual examination	Evaluation of refractive errors of the eye by projecting a light into the eyes and determining the movement of reflected light rays *Retinoscopy is especially important in determining errors of refraction in babies and small children who cannot be refracted by traditional methods.*
Radiographic	
dacryocystography dăk-rē-ō-sĭs-TŎG-ră-fē *dacryocyst/o:* lacrimal sac *-graphy:* process of recording	Radiographic imaging procedures of the nasolacrimal (tear) glands and ducts *Dacryocystography is performed for excessive tearing (epiphora) to determine the cause of hypersecretion of the lacrimal gland or obstruction in the lacrimal passages.*
fluorescein angiography floo-RĔS-ēn ăn-jē-ŎG-ră-fē *angio:* vessel (usually blood or lymph) *-graphy:* process of recording	Assesses blood vessels and their leakage in and beneath the retina after injection of fluorescein dye. The dye circulates while photographs of the vessels within the eye are obtained. *Fluorescein angiography facilitates the* in vivo *study of the retinal blood flow circulation and is particularly useful in the management of diabetic retinopathy and macular degeneration, two leading causes of blindness.*

Diagnostic and Therapeutic Procedures—cont'd

Procedure	Description
Therapeutic Procedures	

Clinical

orthoptic training or-THŎP-tĭk TRĀ-nĭng *orth:* straight *opt:* eye, vision *-ic:* pertaining to	Exercises intended to improve eye movements or visual tracking that use training glasses, prism glasses, or tinted or colored lenses

Surgical

blepharoplasty BLĔF-ă-rō-plăs-tē *blephar/o:* eyelid *-plasty:* surgical repair	Cosmetic surgery that removes fatty tissue above and below the eyes that commonly form as a result of the aging process or excessive exposure to the sun
cochlear implant KŎK-lē-ăr ĬM-plănt *cochle:* cochlea *-ar:* pertaining to	Artificial hearing device that produces useful hearing sensations by electrically stimulating nerves inside the inner ear; also called *bionic ear*
cyclodialysis sī-klō-dī-ĂL-ĭ-sĭs *cycl/o:* ciliary body of eye; circular, cycle *dia:* through, across *-lysis:* separation; destruction; loosening	Formation of an opening between the anterior chamber and the suprachoroidal space for the draining of aqueous humor in glaucoma
enucleation ē-nū-klē-Ā-shŭn	Removal of the eyeball from the orbit *Enucleation is performed to treat cancer of the eye when the tumor is large and fills most of the structure.*
evisceration ē-vĭs-ĕr-Ā-shŭn	Removal of the contents of the eye while leaving the sclera and cornea intact *Evisceration is performed when the blind eye is painful or unsightly. The eye muscles are left intact, and a thin prosthesis called a **cover shell** is fitted over the sclera and cornea.*
mastoid antrotomy MĂS-toyd ăn-TRŎT-ō-mē	Surgical opening of a cavity within the mastoid process
otoplasty Ō-tō-plăs-tē *ot/o:* ear *-plasty:* surgical repair	Corrective surgery for a deformed or excessively large or small pinna *Otoplasty is also performed to rebuild new ears for those who lost them through burns or other trauma or were born without them.*
phacoemulsification fā-kō-ē-mŭl-sĭ-fĭ- KĀ-shŭn	Method of treating cataracts by using ultrasonic waves to disintegrate a cloudy lens, which is then aspirated and removed

(continued)

Diagnostic and Therapeutic Procedures—cont'd

Procedure	Description
radial keratotomy (RK) kĕr-ă-TŎT-ō-mē *kerat/o:* horny tissue; hard; cornea *-tomy:* incision	Incision of the cornea for treatment of nearsightedness or astigmatism. *In RK, hairline radial incisions are made on the outer portion of the cornea that allow the cornea to be flatten, to correct nearsightedness, or to reshape an irregular curvature of the cornea in astigmatism.*

sclerostomy
sklĕ-RŎS-tō-mē
scler/o: hardening; sclera (white
        of eye)
-stomy: forming an opening
        (mouth)
	Surgical formation of an opening in the sclera
	Sclerostomy is commonly performed in conjunction with surgery for glaucoma.

tuning fork test	Method use to evaluate sound conduction using a vibrating tuning fork
Rinne	Tuning fork test that evaluates bone conduction (BC) versus air conduction (AC) of sound *In the Rinne test, the base of a vibrating fork is placed against the mastoid bone (bone conduction) and in front of the auditory meatus (air conduction). If the sound is louder when the tuning fork is next to the ear, hearing in that ear is normal. If the sound is louder when the tuning fork touches the mastoid process, it is an indication of conductive hearing loss.*
Weber	Tuning fork test that evaluates bone conduction of sound in both ears at the same time *In the Weber test, the vibrating tuning fork is placed on the center of the forehead. If sound perception is equal in both ears, hearing is normal.*
tympanoplasty tĭm-păn-ō-PLĂS-tē *tympan/o:* tympanic membrane (eardrum) *-plasty:* surgical repair	Reconstruction of the eardrum, commonly due to perforation; also called *myringoplasty*

Pharmacology

Disorders of the eyes and ears are commonly treated with instillation of drops onto the surface of the eye or into the cavity of the ear. The eyes and ears are typically irrigated with liquid solution to remove foreign objects and to provide topical application of medications. Pharmacological agents used to treat eye disorders include antibiotics for bacterial eye infections, beta blockers and carbonic anhydrase inhibitors for glaucoma, and ophthalmic decongestants and moisturizers for irritated eyes. Mydriatics and miotics are used not only to treat eye disorders but also to dilate (mydriatics) and contract (miotics) the pupil during eye examinations. Ear medications include antiemetics to relieve nausea associated with inner ear infections, products to loosen and remove wax buildup in the ear canal, and local anesthetics to relieve pain associated with ear infections. (See Table 15–1.)

Table 15-1	**Drugs Used to Treat Sensory Disorders**

This table lists common drug classifications used to treat eye and ear disorders, their therapeutic actions, and selected generic and trade names.

Classification	Therapeutic Action	Generic and Trade Names
Eye **antibiotics,** **ophthalmic**	Inhibit growth of microorganisms that infect the eye. *Ophthalmic antibiotics are dispensed as topical ointments and solutions to treat various bacterial eye infections such as conjunctivitis (pinkeye).*	**erythromycin base** ĕ-rĭth-rō-MĪ-sĭn
antiglaucoma agents	Decrease aqueous humor production by constricting the pupil to open the angle between the iris and cornea.	**timolol** TĪ-mō-lŏl Betimol **acetazolamide** ăs-ĕt-ă-ZŌL-ă-mīd Diamox
mydriatics	Drugs that disrupt parasympathetic nerve supply to the eye or stimulate the sympathetic nervous system, causing the pupil to dilate. *Mydriatics are commonly used to dilate the pupil to treat inflammatory conditions or in preparation for internal examinations of the eye.*	**atropine sulfate** ĂT-rō-pēn SŬL-fāt
ophthalmic decongestants	Constrict the small arterioles of the eye, decreasing redness and relieving conjunctival congestion. *Ophthalmic decongestants are over-the-counter products that temporarily relieve the itching and minor irritation commonly associated with allergy.*	**tetrahydrozoline** tĕt-ră-hī-DRŎZ-ō-lēn Murine, Visine
ophthalmic moisturizers	Soothe dry eyes due to environmental irritants and allergens *Ophthalmic moisturizers are administered topically and may also be used to facilitate ophthalmoscopic examination in gonioscopy and ophthalmoscopy.*	**buffered isotonic solutions** BŬ-fĕrd ī-sō-TŎN-ĭk sō-LŪ-shŭnz Akwa Tears, Moisture Eyes
Ear **antiemetics**	Treat and prevent nausea, vomiting, dizziness, and vertigo by reducing the sensitivity of the inner ear to motion or inhibiting stimuli from reaching the part of the brain that triggers nausea and vomiting *Antiemetics are commonly used to treat vertigo.*	**meclizine** MĚK-lĭ-zēn Antrizine, Bonine, Meni-D

(continued)

Table 15-1	**Drugs Used to Treat Sensory Disorders—cont'd**	
Classification	**Therapeutic Action**	**Generic and Trade Names**
otic analgesics	Provide temporary relief from pain and inflammation associated with otic disorders *Otic analgesics may be prescribed for otitis media, otitis externa, and swimmer's ear. Some otic analgesics are also wax emulsifiers.*	**antipyrine and benzocaine** ăn-tĭ-PĪ-rēn, BĔN-zō-kān Allergan Ear Drops, A/B Otic
wax emulsifiers	Loosen and help remove impacted cerumen (ear wax) *Excessive wax may be washed out, vacuumed out, or removed using special instruments.*	**carbamide peroxide** KĂR-bă-mīd pĕr-ŎK-sīd Debrox Drops, Murine Ear Drops

Abbreviations

This section introduces abbreviations related to the eye and ear along with their meanings.

Abbreviation	Meaning	Abbreviation	Meaning
Eye			
Acc	accommodation	**OD**	right eye
ARMD, AMD	age-related macular degeneration	**O.D.**	Doctor of Optometry
Ast	astigmatism	**OS**	left eye
CK	conductive keratoplasty; creatine kinase (cardiac enzyme)	**OU**	both eyes
CT	computed tomography	**PERRLA**	pupils equal, round, and reactive to light and accommodation
D	diopter (lens strength)	**RK**	radial keratotomy
Em	emmetropia	**SICS**	small incision cataract surgery
EOM	extraocular movement	**SLE**	slit lamp examination; systemic lupus erythematosus
IOL	intraocular lens	**ST**	esotropia
IOP	intraocular pressure	**VA**	visual acuity
LASIK	laser-assisted *in situ* keratomileusis	**VF**	visual field
mix astig	mixed astigmatism	**XT**	exotropia
Myop	myopia (nearsightedness)		
Ear			
AC	air conduction	**AS**	left ear
AD	right ear	**AU**	both ears

Abbreviations—cont'd

Abbreviation	Meaning	Abbreviation	Meaning
BC	bone conduction	OM	otitis media
ENT	ears, nose, and throat	PE	physical examination; pulmonary embolism; pressure-equalizing (tube)
NIHL	noise-induced hearing loss	URI	upper respiratory infection

It is time to review procedures, pharmacology, and abbreviations by completing Learning Activity 15–5.

LEARNING ACTIVITIES

The following activities provide review of the eye and ear terms introduced in this chapter. Complete each activity and review your answers to evaluate your understanding of the chapter.

Learning Activity 15-1
Identifying Eye Structures

Label the following illustration using the terms listed below.

anterior chamber	conjunctiva	lens	pupil	suspensory ligaments
canal of Schlemm	cornea	optic disc	retina	vitreous chamber
choroid	fovea	optic nerve	sclera	
ciliary body	iris	posterior chamber		

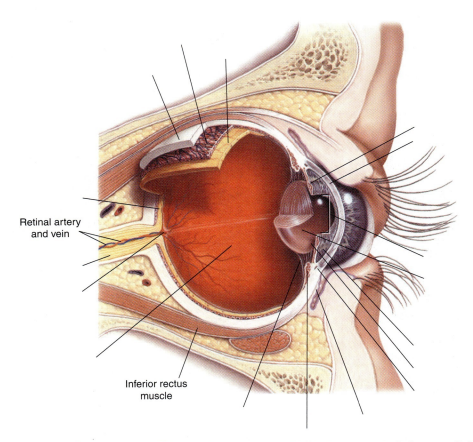

Retinal artery and vein

Inferior rectus muscle

 Check your answers by referring to Figure 15–1 on page 467. Review material that you did not answer correctly.

Identifying Ear Structures

Label the following illustration using the terms listed below.

auricle	*incus*	*stapes*
cochlea	*malleus*	*tympanic membrane*
eustachian tube	*oval window*	*vestibule*
external auditory canal	*semicircular canals*	

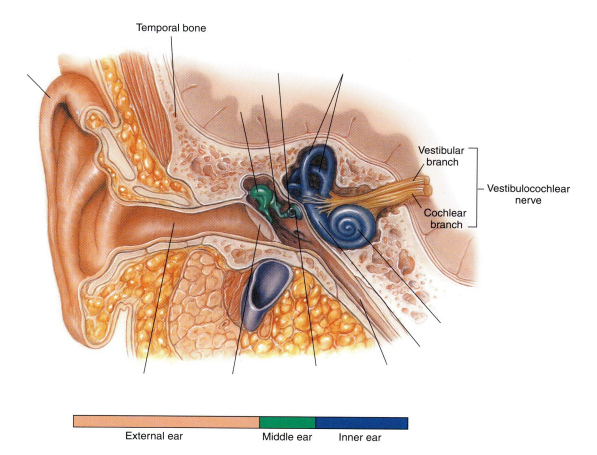

Temporal bone

Vestibular branch

Vestibulocochlear nerve

Cochlear branch

| External ear | Middle ear | Inner ear |

 Check your answers by referring to Figure 15–3 on page 469. Review material that you did not answer correctly.

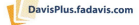 **DavisPlus.fadavis.com**

Enhance your study and reinforcement of word elements with the power of DavisPlus. Visit www.davisplus.fadavis.com/gylys/systems *for this chapter's flash-card activity. We recommend you complete the flash-card activity before completing Activity 15–3 below.*

Learning Activity 15-3
Building Medical Words

Use *ophthalm/o* (eye) to build words that mean:

1. paralysis of the eye _____
2. study of the eye _____

Use *pupill/o* (pupil) to build a word that means:

3. examination of the pupil _____

Use *kerat/o* (cornea) to build words that mean:

4. softening of the cornea _____
5. instrument for measuring the cornea _____

Use *scler/o* (sclera) to build words that mean:

6. inflammation of the sclera _____
7. softening of the sclera _____

Use *irid/o* (iris) to build words that mean:

8. paralysis of the iris _____
9. herniation of the iris _____

Use *retin/o* (retina) to build words that mean:

10. disease of the retina _____
11. inflammation of the retina _____

Use *blephar/o* (eyelid) to build words that mean:

12. paralysis of the eyelid _____
13. prolapse of the eyelid _____

Use *ot/o* (ear) to build a word that means:

14. flow of pus from the ear _____

Use *audi/o* (hearing) to build a word that means:

15. instrument for measuring hearing _____

Use *myring/o* (tympanic membrane [eardrum]) to build a word that means:

16. instrument for cutting the eardrum _____

Use the suffix *-opia* (vision) to build words that mean:

17. dim or dull vision _____
18. excessive (far-sighted) vision _____

Use the suffix -*acusis* (hearing) to build words that mean:

19. without hearing _____

20. excessive (sensitivity to) hearing _____

Build surgical words that mean:

21. removal of the stapes _____

22. incision of the labyrinth _____

23. removal of the mastoid process _____

24. surgical repair of the eardrum _____

25. incision of the cornea _____

Check your answers in Appendix A. Review material that you did not answer correctly.

Correct Answers _____ ✕ 4 = _____ % Score

Learning Activity 15-4
Matching Pathological, Diagnostic, Symptomatic, and Related Terms

Match the following terms with the definitions in the numbered list.

achromatopsia	chalazion	exotropia	nyctalopia	tinnitus
amblyopia	diopter	gonioscope	otitis externa	tonometer
anacusis	enucleation	Mènìëre disease	retinoblastoma	vertigo
cataract	epiphora	neovascular	strabismus	visual field

1. _____ opacity that forms on the lens and impairs vision
2. _____ complete color blindness
3. _____ inability to see well in dim light
4. _____ instrument for examining the angle of the anterior chamber of the eye
5. _____ complete deafness
6. _____ infection of the external auditory canal
7. _____ measurement of refractive errors
8. _____ instrument that measures the internal pressure of the eye
9. _____ area in which objects are seen when the eye is in a fixed position
10. _____ abnormal overflow of tears
11. _____ a condition in which one eye is misaligned with the other eye; also called heterotropia
12. _____ disorder of the labyrinth that leads to progressive hearing loss
13. _____ refers to the wet form of macular degeneration
14. _____ feeling of dizziness or spinning
15. _____ outward deviation of the eye
16. _____ removal of the eye
17. _____ tumor of the eyelid
18. _____ "lazy-eye" syndrome
19. _____ neoplastic disease of the eye found primarily in children
20. _____ perception of ringing in the ears with no external stimuli

Check your answers in Appendix A. Review any material that you did not answer correctly.

Correct Answers _____ × 5 = _____ % Score

Learning Activity 15-5
Matching Procedures, Pharmacology, and Abbreviations

Match the following terms with the definitions in the numbered list.

antiemetics	evisceration	ophthalmoscopy	ST
audiometry	fluorescein angiography	otic analgesics	tonometry
caloric stimulation test	gonioscopy	otoplasty	visual acuity test
cochlear implant	mydriatics	otoscopy	wax emulsifiers
enucleation	ophthalmic decongestants	radial keratotomy	XT

1. _____ test that uses different temperatures to assess the vestibular portion of the nerve

2. _____ visual examination of the interior of the eye

3. _____ artificial device that produces hearing sensations by electrically stimulating nerves inside the inner ear

4. _____ assesses blood vessels and retinal circulation using a colored dye while photographs are taken

5. _____ corrective surgery for large, small, or deformed ears

6. _____ agents that dilate the pupils and paralyze the eye muscles of accommodation

7. _____ measurement of the intraocular pressure for detecting glaucoma

8. _____ determines the smallest letters that can be read on a standardized chart

9. _____ removal of the contents of the eyeball, leaving the sclera and cornea

10. _____ treat and prevent nausea, vomiting, dizziness, and vertigo

11. _____ loosen and help remove impacted cerumen

12. _____ removal of the entire eyeball from its orbit

13. _____ esotropia

14. _____ constrict small arterioles of the eye to decrease redness and conjunctival congestion

15. _____ exotropia

16. _____ visual examination of the angle of the anterior chamber of the eye

17. _____ visual examination of the external auditory canal

18. _____ measurement of hearing acuity at various frequencies

19. _____ surgical treatment for nearsightedness that uses small incisions to flatten the cornea

20. _____ provide temporary relief from earache

✓ *Check your answers in Appendix A. Review any material that you did not answer correctly.*

Correct Answers _____ × 5 = _____ % Score

MEDICAL RECORD ACTIVITIES

The two medical records included in the following activities use common clinical scenarios to show how medical terminology is used to document patient care. Complete the terminology and analysis sections for each activity to help you recognize and understand terms related to the special senses.

Medical Record Activity 15-1
Operative Report: Retained Foreign Bodies

Terminology

Terms listed below come from the *Operative Report: Retained Foreign Bodies* that follows. Use a medical dictionary such as *Taber's Cyclopedic Medical Dictionary*, the appendices of this book, or other resources to define each term. Then review the pronunciations for each term and practice by reading the medical record aloud.

Term	Definition
bilateral bī-LĂT-ĕr-ăl	
cerumen sĕ-ROO-mĕn	
perforation pĕr-fō-RĀ-shŭn	
supine sū-PĪN	
tympanostomy tĭm-pă-NŎS-tō-mē	

Listen and Learn Online! *will help you master the pronunciation of selected medical words from this medical record activity. Visit* www.davisplus.com/gylys/systems *to find instructions on completing the* Listen and Learn Online! *exercise for this section and to practice pronunciations.*

OPERATIVE REPORT: RETAINED FOREIGN BO

Physicians Day Surgery

1514 Ninth Avenue ■■ **Sun City, USA 12345** ■■ **(555) 936-1933**

OPERATIVE REPORT

Date: 5/13/xx   Surgeon: Richard Roake, MD
Patient: Hirsch, Annie   Patient ID#:   33328

PREOPERATIVE DIAGNOSIS: Foreign body, ears.

POSTOPERATIVE DIAGNOSIS: Foreign body, ears.

OPERATIVE INDICATIONS: Patient is a 9-year-old girl who presents with bilateral retained tympanostomy tubes. The tubes had been placed for more than 2-1/2 years.

ANESTHESIA: General.

COMPLICATIONS: None.

OPERATIVE FINDINGS: Retained tympanostomy tubes, bilateral.

PROCEDURE: Removal of foreign bodies from ears with placement of paper patches.

INFORMED CONSENT: The risks and alternatives were explained to the mother, and she consented to the surgery.

In the supine position under satisfactory general anesthesia via mask, the patient was draped in a routine fashion.

The operating microscope was used to inspect the right ear. A previously placed tympanostomy tube was found to be in position and was surrounded with hard cerumen. The cerumen and the tube were removed, resulting in a very large perforation. The edges of the perforation were freshened sharply with a pick, and a paper patch was applied.

Patient tolerated the surgery very well, and was sent to recovery in stable condition.

Richard Roake, MD
Richard Roake, MD

rk:bg

D: 5-14-20xx
T: 5-14-20xx

Analysis

Review the medical record *Operative Report: Retained Foreign Bodies* to answer the following questions.

1. Did the surgery involve one or both ears?

   _____

2. What was the nature of the foreign body in the patient's ears?

   _____

3. What ear structure was involved?

   _____

4. What instrument was used to locate the tubes?

   _____

5. What was the material in which the tubes were embedded?

   _____

6. What occurred when the cerumen and tubes were removed?

   _____

7. How was the perforation treated?

   _____

Medical Record Activity 15-2
Operative Report: Phacoemulsification and Lens Implant

Terminology

Terms listed below come from *Operative report: Phacoemulsification and lens implant* that follows. Use a medical dictionary such as *Taber's Cyclopedic Medical Dictionary*, the appendices of this book, or other resources to define each term. Then review the pronunciations for each term and practice by reading the medical record aloud.

Term	Definition
anesthesia ăn-ĕs-THĒ-zē-ă	
blepharostat BLĔF-ă-rō-stăt	
capsulorrhexis kăp-sū-lŏ-RĔK-sĭs	
cataract KĂT-ă-răkt	
conjunctival kŏn-jŭnk-TĪ-văl	
diopter dī-ŎP-tĕr	
intravenous ĭn-tră-VĒ-nŭs	
keratome KĔR-ă-tōm	
peritomy pĕr-ĬT-ō-mē	
phacoemulsification făk-ō-ē-mŭl-sĭ-fĭ-KĂ-shŭn	
posterior chamber pŏs-TĔR-ē-or CHĂM-bĕr	
retrobulbar block rĕt-rŏ-BŬL-băr	
sutures SŪ-chŭrz	
TobraDex TŌ-bră-dĕks	

 Listen and Learn Online! *will help you master the pronunciation of selected medical words from this medical record activity. Visit www.davisplus.com/gylys/systems to find instructions on completing the* Listen and Learn Online! *exercise for this section and to practice pronunciations.*

OPERATIVE REPORT: PHACOEMULSIFICATION AND LENS IMPLANT

Physicians Day Surgery

1514 Ninth Avenue ■■ **Sun City, USA 12345** ■■ **(555) 936-1933**

OPERATIVE REPORT

Date: 5/14/xx   Surgeon: Lewis Sloope, MD
Patient: Deetrick, Douglas   Patient ID#: 33422

PREOPERATIVE DIAGNOSIS: Right eye cataract.

POSTOPERATIVE DIAGNOSIS: Right eye cataract.

OPERATION: Phacoemulsification, right eye, with posterior chamber lens implantation.

COMPLICATIONS: None.

PROCEDURE: This 68-year-old male was brought to the operating suite on 8/4/xx as an outpatient. Intravenous anesthesia and retrobulbar block to the right eye were administered. The right eye was prepped in the usual manner. A blepharostat was inserted and a surgical microscope was positioned. Conjunctival peritomy was performed. Using a keratome, the anterior chamber was entered at the 12 o'clock position. A capsulorrhexis was performed. The cataract was removed by phacoemulsification.

After confirming the 20.5 diopters on the package, the implant was easily inserted into the capsular bag. The wound was observed and shown to be fluid tight. The incision required no sutures. TobraDex ointment was applied and a sterile patch was taped into place.

Patient was monitored until stable. Postoperative care was reviewed, and patient was released with instructions to return to the office the following day.

Lewis Sloope, MD
Lewis Sloope, MD

rk:bg

D: 5-14-20xx
T: 5-14-20xx

Analysis

Review the medical record *Operative Report: Phacoemulsification and Lens Implant* to answer the following questions.

1. What technique was used to destroy the cataract?

_____

2. In what portion of the eye was the implant placed?

_____

3. What anesthetics were used for surgery?

_____

4. What was the function of the blepharostat?

_____

5. What is a keratome?

_____

6. Where was the implant inserted?

_____

Answer Key

CHAPTER 1—Basic Elements of a Medical Word

Learning Activity 1-1
Understanding Medical Word Elements

Fill in the following blanks to complete the sentences correctly.

1. root, combining form, suffix, and prefix.

2. arthr

Identify the following statements as either true or false. If false, rewrite the statement correctly in the space provided.

3. False—A combining vowel is usually an "o."

4. False—A word root links a suffix that begins with a vowel.

5. True

6. True

7. False—To define a medical word, first define the suffix or the end of the word. Second, define the first part of the word. Third, define the middle of the word.

8. True

Underline the word root in each of following combining forms.

9. splen/o

10. hyster/o

11. enter/o

12. neur/o

13. ot/o

14. dermat/o

15. hydr/o

Learning Activity 1-2
Identifying Word Roots and Combining Forms

Underline the word roots in the following terms.

1. nephritis

2. arthrodesis

3. dermatitis

4. dentist

5. gastrectomy

6. chondritis

7. hepatoma

8. muscular

9. gastria

10. osteoma

Underline the following elements that are combining forms.

11. nephr

12. hepat/o

13. arthr

14. oste/o/arthr

15. cholangi/o

Learning Activity 1-3
Understanding Pronunciations

1. macron

2. breve

3. long

4. short

5. k

6. n

7. is

8. eye

9. second

10. separate

Learning Activity 1-4
Identifying Suffixes and Prefixes

Analyze each term and write the element from each that is a suffix.

1. -tomy
2. -scope
3. -itis
4. -oma
5. -ectomy

Analyze each term and write the element from each that is a prefix.

6. an-
7. hyper-
8. intra-
9. para-
10. poly-

Learning Activity 1-5
Defining and Building Medical Words

Use the three basic steps to define the following words.

Term	Definition
1. gastritis găs-TRĪ-tĭs	inflammation of the stomach
2. nephritis nĕf-RĪ-tĭs	inflammation of the kidney(s)
3. gastrectomy găs-TRĔK-tō-mē	excision of the stomach
4. osteoma ŏs-tē-Ō-mă	tumor of bone
5. hepatoma hĕp-ă-TŌ-mă	tumor of the liver
6. hepatitis hĕp-ă-TĪ-tĭs	inflammation of the liver

Write the number for the rule that applies to each listed term as well as a short summary of the rule.

Term	Rule	Summary of the Rule
7. arthr/itis ăr-THRĪ-tĭs	1	WR links a suffix that begins with a vowel.
8. scler/osis sklĕ-RŌ-sĭs	1	WR links a suffix that begins with a vowel.
9. arthr/o/centesis ăr-thrō-sĕn-TĒ-sĭs	2	CF links a suffix that begins with a consonant.
10. colon/o/scope kō-LŎN-ō-skōp	2	CF links a suffix that begins with a consonant.

Term	Rule	Summary of the Rule
11. chondr/itis kŏn-DRĪ-tĭs	1	WR links a suffix that begins with a vowel.
12. chondr/oma kŏn-DRŌ-mă	1	WR links a suffix that begins with a vowel.
13. oste/o/chondr/itis ŏs-tē-ō-kŏn-DRĪ-tĭs	3,1	CF links multiple roots to each other. This rule holds true even if the next word root begins with a vowel. WR links a suffix that begins with a vowel.
14. muscul/ar MŬS-kū-lăr	1	WR links a suffix that begins with a vowel.
15. oste/o/arthr/itis ŏs-tē-ō-ăr-THRĪ-tĭs	3,1	CF links multiple roots to each other. This rule holds true even if the next word root begins with a vowel. WR links a suffix that begins with a vowel.

Chapter 2—Suffixes

Learning Activity 2-1
Building Surgical Words

1. episiotomy
2. colectomy
3. arthrocentesis
4. splenectomy
5. colostomy
6. osteotome
7. tympanotomy
8. tracheostomy
9. mastectomy
10. lithotomy
11. hemorrhoidectomy
12. colostomy
13. colectomy
14. osteotome
15. arthrocentesis
16. lithotomy
17. mastectomy
18. tympanotomy
19. tracheostomy
20. splenectomy

Learning Activity 2-2
Building More Surgical Words

1. arthrodesis
2. rhinoplasty
3. tenoplasty
4. myorrhaphy
5. mastopexy
6. cystorrhaphy
7. osteoclasis
8. lithotripsy
9. enterolysis
10. neurotripsy
11. rhinoplasty
12. arthrodesis
13. myorrhaphy
14. mastopexy
15. cystorrhaphy
16. tenoplasty
17. osteoclasis
18. lithotripsy
19. enterolysis
20. neurotripsy

Learning Activity 2-3
Selecting a Surgical Suffix

1. lithotripsy
2. arthrocentesis
3. splenectomy
4. colostomy
5. dermatome
6. tracheostomy
7. lithotomy
8. mastectomy
9. hemorrhoidectomy
10. tracheotomy
11. mastopexy
12. colectomy
13. gastrorrhaphy
14. hysteropexy
15. rhinoplasty
16. arthrodesis
17. osteoclasis
18. neurolysis
19. myorrhaphy
20. tympanotomy

Learning Activity 2-4
Selecting Diagnostic, Pathological, and Related Suffixes

1. hepatoma
2. neuralgia
3. bronchiectasis
4. carcinogenesis
5. dermatosis
6. nephromegaly
7. otorrhea
8. hysterorrhexis
9. blepharospasm
10. cystocele
11. hemorrhage
12. lithiasis
13. hemiplegia
14. myopathy
15. dysphagia
16. osteomalacia
17. aphasia
18. leukemia
19. erythropenia
20. pelvimetry

Learning Activity 2-5
Building Pathological and Related Words

1. bronchiectasis
2. cholelith
3. carcinogenesis
4. osteomalacia
5. hepatomegaly
6. cholelithiasis
7. hepatocele
8. neuropathy
9. dermatosis
10. hemiplegia
11. dysphagia
12. aphasia
13. cephalalgia
14. blepharospasm
15. hyperplasia or hypertrophy

Selecting Adjective, Noun, and Diminutive Suffixes

1. thoracic
2. gastric, gastral
3. bacterial
4. aquatic
5. axillary
6. cardiac or cardial
7. spinal or spinous
8. membranous
9. internist
10. leukemia
11. sigmoidoscopy
12. alcoholism
13. podiatry
14. allergist or allergy
15. mania
16. arteriole
17. ventricle
18. venule

Forming Plural Words

Singular	Plural	Rule	Singular	Plural	Rule
1. diagnosis	diagnoses	Drop *is* and add *es*.	9. ganglion	ganglia	Drop *on* and add *a*.
2. fornix	fornices	Drop *ix* and add *ices*.	10. prognosis	prognoses	Drop *is* and add *es*.
3. vertebra	vertebrae	Retain *a* and add *e*.	11. thrombus	thrombi	Drop *us* and add *i*.
4. keratosis	keratoses	Drop *is* and add *es*.	12. appendix	appendices	Drop *ix* and add *ices*.
5. bronchus	bronchi	Drop *us* and add *i*.	13. bacterium	bacteria	Drop *um* and add *a*.
6. spermatozoon	spermatozoa	Drop *on* and add *a*.	14. testis	testes	Drop *is* and add *es*.
7. septum	septa	Drop *um* and add *a*.	15. nevus	nevi	Drop *us* and add *i*.
8. coccus	cocci	Drop *us* and add *i*.			

Chapter 3—Prefixes

Identifying and Defining Pefixes

Word	Definition of Prefix	Word	Definition of Prefix
1. inter/dental	between	13. tri/ceps	three
2. hypo/dermic	under, below, deficient	14. poly/dipsia	many, much
3. epi/dermis	above, upon	15. ab/duction	from, away from
4. retro/version	backward, behind	16. an/esthesia	without, not
5. sub/lingual	under, below	17. macro/cyte	large
6. trans/vaginal	through, across	18. intra/muscular	in, within
7. infra/costal	under, below	19. supra/pelvic	above, excessive, superior
8. post/natal	after, behind	20. dia/rrhea	through, across
9. quadri/plegia	four	21. circum/duction	around
10. hyper/calcemia	excessive, above normal	22. ad/duction	toward
11. primi/gravida	first	23. peri/odontal	around
12. micro/scope	small	24. brady/cardia	slow

Word	Definition of Prefix	Word	Definition of Prefix
25. tachy/pnea	rapid	28. hetero/graft	different
26. dys/tocia bad,	painful, difficult	29. mal/nutrition	bad
27. eu/pnea good,	normal	30. pseudo/cyesis	false

Learning Activity 3-2
Matching Prefixes of Position, Number and Measurement, and Direction

1. retroversion
2. hypodermic
3. prenatal
4. subnasal
5. postoperative

6. intercostal
7. pseudocyesis
8. periodontal
9. diarrhea
10. ectogenous
11. suprarenal
12. hemiplegia
13. quadriplegia
14. macrocyte
15. polyphobia

Learning Activity 3-3
Matching Other Prefixes

1. dyspepsia
2. heterograft
3. panarthritis
4. antibacterial
5. bradycardia
6. malnutrition

7. amastia
8. anesthesia
9. eupnea
10. syndactylism
11. tachycardia
12. contraception
13. homograft
14. dystocia
15. homeoplasia

Chapter 4—Body Structure

Learning Activity 4-3
Matching Body Cavity, Spine, and Directional Terms

1. h. ventral cavity that contains digestive, reproductive, and excretory structures
2. k. movement toward the median plane
3. j. part of the spine known as the neck
4. b. tailbone
5. m. away from the surface of the body (internal)

6. f. turning outward
7. l. away from the head; toward the tail or lower part of a structure
8. i. turning inward or inside out
9. n. part of the spine known as the loin
10. a. pertaining to the sole of the foot
11. o. near the back of the body
12. e. lying horizontal with face downward
13. g. nearer to the center (trunk of the body)
14. d. toward the surface of the body (external)
15. c. ventral cavity that contains heart, lungs, and associated structures

Learning Activity 4-4
Matching Word Elements

1. kary/o
2. dist/o
3. -graphy
4. -gnosis
5. leuk/o
6. viscer/o
7. jaund/o
8. hist/o
9. -genesis

10. infra-
11. ultra-
12. caud/o
13. dors/o
14. poli/o
15. eti/o
16. morph/o
17. xer/o
18. idi/o
19. ad-
20. somat/o

Learning Activity 4-5
Matching Diagnostic and Therapeutic Terms and Procedures

1. radiology
2. Doppler
3. ultrasonography
4. thoracoscopy
5. punch biopsy
6. endoscopy

7. nuclear scan
8. fluoroscopy
9. morbid
10. radionuclide
11. febrile
12. resection
13. suppurative
14. cauterize
15. ablation

Medical Record Activity 4-1
Radiological Consultation Letter: Cervical and Lumbar Spine

1. What was the presenting problem?

The patient had neck and lower back pain for more than 2 years' duration.

2. What were the three views of the radiologic examination of June 14, 20xx?

Anterior posterior (AP), lateral, and odontoid

3. Was there evidence of recent bony disease or injury?

There was no evidence of recent bony disease or injury.

4. Which cervical vertebrae form the atlantoaxial joint?

The first cervical vertebra (atlas) and the second cervical vertebra (axis)

5. Was the odontoid fractured?

No, the odontoid was intact.

6. What did the AP and lateral films of the lumbar spine demonstrate?

Apparent minimal spina bifida occulta of the first sacral segment.

Medical Record Activity 4-2
Radiology Report: Injury of Left Wrist, Elbow, and Humerus

1. Where are the fractures located?

Distal shafts of the radius and ulna

2. What caused the soft-tissue deformity?

A fracture caused deformity to surrounding soft tissue.

3. Did the radiologist take any side views of the left elbow?

A single view of the left elbow was obtained in the lateral projection.

4. In the AP view of the humerus, what structure was also visualized?

A portion of the elbow

5. What findings are causes for concern to the radiologist?

Lucency through the distal humerus on the AP view along its medial aspect and elevation of the anterior and posterior fat pads

Chapter 5— Integumentary System

Learning Activity 5-2
Building Medical Words

1. adipoma, lipoma
2. adipocele, lipocele
3. adipoid, lipoid
4. adipocyte, lipocyte
5. dermatitis
6. dermatotome
7. onychoma
8. onychomalacia
9. onychosis
10. onychomycosis
11. onychocryptosis
12. onychopathy
13. trichopathy
14. trichomycosis
15. dermatology
16. dermatologist
17. adipectomy, lipectomy
18. onychectomy
19. onychotomy
20. dermatoplasty, dermoplasty

Learning Activity 5-4
Matching Burn and Oncology Terms

1. i. redness of skin
2. e. no evidence of primary tumor
3. h. cancerous; may be life threatening
4. g. heals without scar formation
5. f. determines degree of abnormal cancer cells compared with normal cells
6. a. develops from keratinizing epidermal cells
7. b. noncancerous
8. j. primary tumor size, small with minimal invasion
9. c. no evidence of metastasis
10. d. extensive damage to underlying connective tissue

Learning Activity 5-5
Matching Diagnostic, Symptomatic, Procedural, and Pharmacological Terms

1. pediculosis
2. vitiligo
3. tinea
4. scabies
5. impetigo
6. urticaria
7. chloasma
8. ecchymosis
9. petechiae
10. alopecia
11. antifungals
12. fulguration
13. corticosteroids
14. dermabrasion
15. parasiticides
16. keratolytics
17. intradermal test
18. patch test
19. autograft
20. xenograft

Medical Record Activity 5-1
Pathology Report: Skin Lesion

1. In the specimen section, what does "skin on dorsum left wrist" mean?

Skin was obtained from the back, or posterior, surface of the left wrist.

2. What was the inflammatory infiltrate?

Lymphocytic inflammatory infiltrate in the papillary dermis

3. What was the pathologist's diagnosis for the left forearm?

Nodular and infiltrating basal cell carcinoma near the elbow

4. Provide a brief description of Bowen disease, the pathologist's diagnosis for the left wrist.

Bowen disease is a form of intraepidermal carcinoma (squamous cell) characterized by red-brown scaly or crusted lesions that resemble a patch of psoriasis or dermatitis.

Medical record Activity 5-2
Patient Referral Letter: Onychomycosis

1. What pertinent disorders were identified in the past medical history?

History of hypertension and breast cancer

2. What pertinent surgery was identified in the past surgical history?

Mastectomy

3. Did the doctor identify any problems in the vascular system or nervous system?

Vascular and neurological systems were intact.

4. What was the significant finding in the laboratory results?

Alkaline phosphatase was elevated.

5. What treatment did the doctor employ for the onychomycosis?

Debridement and medication or Sporanox PulsePak

6. What did the doctor recommend regarding the abnormal laboratory finding?

The doctor recommended a repeat of the liver enzymes in approximately 4 weeks.

Chapter 6—Digestive System

Building Medical Words

1. esophagodynia, esophagalgia
2. esophagospasm
3. esophagostenosis
4. gastritis
5. gastrodynia, gastralgia
6. gastropathy
7. jejunectomy
8. duodenal
9. ileitis
10. jejunoileal

11. enteritis
12. enteropathy
13. enterocolitis
14. colitis
15. colorectal
16. coloptosis
17. colopathy
18. proctostenosis, rectostenosis
19. rectocele, proctocele
20. proctoplegia, proctoparalysis
21. cholecystitis
22. cholelithiasis
23. hepatoma
24. hepatomegaly
25. pancreatitis

Building Surgical Words

1. gingivectomy
2. glossectomy
3. esophagoplasty
4. gastrectomy
5. gastrojejunostomy
6. esophagectomy

7. gastroenterocolostomy
8. enteroplasty
9. enteropexy
10. choledochorrhaphy
11. colostomy
12. hepatopexy
13. proctoplasty, rectoplasty
14. cholecystectomy
15. choledochoplasty

Matching Pathological, Diagnostic, Symptomatic, and Related Terms

1. hematemesis
2. dysphagia
3. fecalith

4. halitosis
5. anorexia
6. dyspepsia
7. cirrhosis
8. cachexia
9. obstipation
10. lesion

Matching Procedures, Pharmacology, and Abbreviations

1. PTHC
2. bilirubin
3. emetics

4. antispasmodics
5. choledochoplasty
6. lower GI series
7. gastroscopy
8. stomatoplasty
9. intubation

10. anastomosis

11. stool guaiac

12. endoscopy

13. laxatives

14. antacids

15. ultrasonography

16. liver function tests

17. bariatric

18. stat.

19. proctosigmoidoscopy

20. upper GI series

Medical Record Activity 6-1
Chart Note: GI Evaluation

1. While referring to Figure 6–3, describe the location of the gallbladder in relation to the liver.

Posterior and inferior portion of the right lobe of the liver

2. Why did the patient undergo the cholecystectomy?

To treat cholecystitis and cholelithiasis

3. List the patient's prior surgeries.

Tonsillectomy, appendectomy, and cholecystectomy

4. How does the patient's most recent postoperative episode of discomfort (pain) differ from the initial pain she described?

The continuous, deep right-sided pain took a crescendo pattern and then a decrescendo pattern. Initially, it was intermittent and sharp epigastric pain.

Medical Record Activity 6-2
Operative Report: Esophagogastroduodenoscopy with Biopsy

1. What caused the hematemesis?

Etiology was unknown. Inflammation of the stomach and duodenum was noted.

2. What procedures were carried out to determine the cause of bleeding?

During x-ray tomography using the videoendoscope, biopsies were taken of the stomach and duodenum. It was also noted that previously the patient had esophageal varices.

3. How much blood did the patient lose during the procedure?

None

4. Were there any ulcerations or erosions found during the exploratory procedure that might account for the bleeding?

No

5. What type of sedation was used during the procedure?

Demerol and Versed administered intravenously

6. What did the doctors find when they examined the stomach and duodenum?

Diffuse and punctate erythema

Chapter 7—Respiratory System

Learning Activity 7-2
Building Medical Words

1. rhinorrhea

2. rhinitis

3. laryngoscopy

4. laryngitis

5. laryngostenosis

6. bronchiectasis

7. bronchopathy

8. bronchospasm

9. pneumothorax

10. pneumonitis

11. pulmonologist

12. pulmonary, pulmonic

13. dyspnea

14. bradypnea

15. tachypnea

16. apnea

17. rhinoplasty

18. thoracocentesis, thoracentesis

Learning Activity 7-3
Matching Pathological, Diagnostic, Symptomatic, and Related Terms

1. atelectasis

2. empyema

3. surfactant

4. consolidation

5. auscultation

6. anosmia

7. hypoxemia

8. tubercles

Learning Activity 7-4
Matching Procedures, Pharmacology, and Abbreviations

1. lung scan

2. polysomnography

3. radiography

4. antral lavage

5. antihistamine

6. antitussive

7. sweat test

8. oximetry

Medical Record Activity 7-1
SOAP Note: Respiratory Evaluation

1. What symptom caused the patient to seek medical help?

Shortness of breath

2. What was the patient's previous history?

Difficult breathing, high blood pressure, chronic obstructive pulmonary disease, and peripheral vascular disease

3. What were the abnormal findings of the physical examination?

Bilateral wheezes and rhonchi heard anteriorly and posteriorly

19. pulmonectomy, pneumonectomy

20. tracheostomy

9. apnea

10. emphysema

11. compliance

12. epistaxis

13. pulmonary edema

14. crackle

15. deviated septum

16. coryza

17. pneumonoconiosis

18. pleurisy

19. stridor

20. pertussis

9. AFB

10. aerosol therapy

11. decongestant

12. Mantoux test

13. ABGs

14. expectorant

15. throat culture

16. pulmonary function tests

17. laryngoscopy

18. septoplasty

19. pneumectomy

20. rhinoplasty

4. What changes were noted from the previous film?

Interstitial vascular congestion with possible superimposed inflammatory change and some pleural reactive change

5. What are the present assessments?

Acute exacerbation of chronic obstructive pulmonary disease, heart failure, hypertension, peripheral vascular disease

6. What new diagnosis was made that did not appear in the previous medical history?

Heart failure

Medical Record Activity 7-2
SOAP Note: Chronic Interstitial Lung Disease

1. When did the patient notice dyspnea?

With activity

2. Other than the respiratory system, what other body systems are identified in the history of present illness?

Cardiovascular, urinary, and nervous system

3. What were the findings regarding the neck?

Supple and no evidence of thyromegaly or ade-nomegaly

4. What was the finding regarding the chest?

Basilar crackles without wheezing or rhonchi

5. What appears to be the likely cause of the chronic interstitial lung disease?

Combination of pulmonary fibrosis and heart failure

6. What did the cardiac examination reveal?

Trace of edema without clubbing or murmur

Chapter 8— Cardiovascular System

Learning Activity 8-2
Building Medical Words

1. atheroma
2. atherosclerosis
3. phlebitis
4. phlebothrombosis
5. venous
6. venospasm
7. cardiologist
8. cardiorrhexis
9. cardiotoxic
10. cardiomegaly
11. angiomalacia
12. angioma
13. thrombogen, thrombogenesis
14. thrombosis
15. aortostenosis
16. aortography
17. cardiocentesis
18. arteriorrhaphy
19. embolectomy
20. thrombolysis

Learning Activity 8-3
Matching Pathological, Diagnostic, Symptomatic, and Related Terms

1. infarct
2. angina
3. incompetent
4. vegetations
5. varices
6. bruit
7. catheter
8. palpitation
9. deep vein thrombosis
10. aneurysm
11. embolus
12. arrhythmia
13. arrest
14. diaphoresis
15. stent
16. hypertension
17. hyperlipidemia
18. coarctation
19. ischemia
20. perfusion

Matching Procedures, Pharmacology, and Abbreviations

1. Holter monitor test

2. echocardiography

3. coronary angiography

4. nitrates

5. statins

6. diuretics

7. cardiac enzyme studies

8. scintigraphy

9. stress test

10. ligation and stripping

11. commissurotomy

12. arterial biopsy

13. catheter ablation

14. embolization

15. angioplasty

16. PTCA

17. CABG

18. atherectomy

19. venipuncture

20. thrombolysis

Chart Note: Acute Myocardial Infarction

1. How long had the patient experienced chest pain before she was seen in the hospital?

Approximately 2 hours

2. Did the patient have a previous history of chest pain?

Yes

3. Initially, what medications were administered to stabilize the patient?

Streptokinase and heparin

4. What two laboratory tests will be used to evaluate the patient?

Partial thromboplastin time and cardiac enzymes

5. During the current admission, what part of the heart was damaged?

The lateral front side of the heart (anterior of heart)

6. Was the location of damage to the heart for this admission the same as for the initial MI?

No, in the earlier admission, the damage was to the lower part of the heart.

Operative Report: Right Temporal Artery Biopsy

1. Why was the right temporal artery biopsied?

Rule out arteritis

2. In what position was the patient placed?

Supine

3. What was the incision area?

Right preauricular area

4. How was the temporal artery located for administration of Xylocaine?

By palpation

5. How was the dissection carried out?

Down through the subcutaneous tissue and superficial fascia

6. What was the size of the specimen?

Approximately 1.5-cm segment

Chapter 9—Blood, Lymph, and Immune Systems

Learning Activity 9-2
Building Medical Words

1. erythrocytosis
2. leukocytosis
3. lymphocytosis
4. reticulocytosis
5. erythropenia
6. leukopenia
7. thrombocytopenia, thrombopenia
8. lymphocytopenia
9. hemopoiesis, hematopoiesis
10. leukopoiesis, leukocytopoiesis
11. thrombocytopoiesis
12. immunologist
13. immunology
14. splenocele
15. splenolysis
16. splenectomy
17. thymectomy
18. thymolysis
19. splenotomy
20. splenopexy

Learning Activity 9-3
Matching Pathological, Diagnostic, Symptomatic, and Related Terms

1. exacerbations
2. hemoglobinopathy
3. bacteremia
4. aplastic anemia
5. active
6. Kaposi sarcoma
7. normocytic
8. lymphadenopathy
9. immunocompromised
10. hemophilia
11. infectious mononucleosis
12. myelogenous
13. passive
14. artificial
15. hemolysis
16. hematoma
17. graft rejection
18. anisocytosis
19. opportunistic infection
20. septicemia

Learning Activity 9-4
Matching Procedures, Pharmacology, and Abbreviations

1. aspiration
2. hematocrit
3. Monospot
4. anticoagulants
5. WBC
6. homologous
7. lymphangiectomy
8. RBC indices
9. Shilling
10. lymphadenography
11. autologous
12. sentinel
13. RBC
14. thrombolytics
15. differential

Discharge Summary: Sickle Cell Crisis

1. What blood product was administered to the patient?

Two units of packed red blood cells

2. Why was this blood product given to the patient?

The patient was anemic due to sickle cell anemia.

Discharge Summary: PCP and HIV

1. How do you think the patient acquired the HIV infection?

From her husband, who died of HIV

2. What were the two diagnoses of the husband?

Multifocal leukoencephalopathy (PMN) and Kaposi sarcoma

3. Why was a CT scan performed on the patient?

To determine the cause of abdominal pain

4. What were the three findings of the CT scan?

Ileus in the small bowel, dilated small bowel loops, and abnormal enhancement pattern in the kidney

5. Why should the patient see his regular doctor?

To follow up on the renal abnormality

3. What four disorders in the medical history are significant for HIV?

Several episodes of diarrhea, sinusitis, thrush, and vaginal candidiasis

4. What was the x-ray finding?

Diffuse lower lobe infiltrates

5. What two procedures are going to be performed to confirm the diagnosis of PCP pneumonia?

Bronchoscopy and alveolar lavage

Chapter 10— Musculoskeletal System

Building Medical Words

1. osteocytes
2. ostealgia, osteodynia
3. osteoarthropathy
4. osteogenesis
5. cervical
6. cervicobrachial
7. cervicofacial
8. myeloma
9. myelosarcoma
10. myelocyte
11. myeloid
12. suprasternal
13. sternoid
14. chondroblast
15. arthritis
16. osteoarthritis
17. pelvimeter
18. myospasm
19. myopathy
20. myorrhexis
21. phalangectomy
22. thoracotomy
23. vertebrectomy
24. arthrodesis
25. myoplasty

Learning Activity 10-5
Matching Pathological, Diagnostic, Symptomatic, and Related Terms

1. subluxation
2. rickets
3. spondylolisthesis
4. claudication
5. muscular dystrophy
6. talipes
7. sequestrum
8. myasthenia gravis
9. prosthesis
10. ganglion cyst
11. hypotonia

12. Ewing sarcoma
13. greenstick fracture
14. kyphosis
15. osteoporosis
16. scoliosis
17. chondrosarcoma
18. comminuted fracture
19. spondylitis
20. gout
21. hematopoiesis
22. pyogenic
23. necrosis
24. ankylosis
25. phantom limb

Learning Activity 10-6
Matching Procedures, Pharmacology, and Abbreviations

1. myelography
2. open reduction
3. gold salts
4. CTS
5. laminectomy
6. arthrography

7. arthrodesis
8. amputation
9. HNP
10. salicylates
11. arthroscopy
12. sequestrectomy
13. ACL
14. relaxants
15. closed reduction

Medical Record Activity 10-1
Operative Report: Right Knee Arthroscopy and Medial Meniscectomy

1. Describe the meniscus and identify its location.

The meniscus is the curved, fibrous cartilage in the knees and other joints.

2. What is the probable cause of the tear in the patient's meniscus?

The continuous pressure on the knees from jogging on a hard surface, such as the pavement

3. What does normal ACL and PCL refer to in the report?

The anterior and posterior cruciate ligaments appeared to be normal.

4. Explain the McMurray sign test.

Rotation of the tibia on the femur is used to determine injury to meniscal structures. An audible click during manipulation of the tibia with the leg flexed is an indication that the meniscus has been injured.

5. Because Lachman and McMurray tests were negative (normal), why was the surgery performed?

The medial compartment of the knee showed an inferior surface posterior and mid medial meniscal tear that was flipped up on top of itself. The surgeon resected the tear, and the remaining meniscus was contoured back to a stable rim.

Medical Record Activity 10-2
Radiographic Consultation: Tibial Diaphysis Nuclear Scan

1. Where was the pain located?

Middle one third of the left tibia

2. What medication was the patient taking for pain and did it provide relief?

He finds no relief with NSAIDs.

3. How was the blood flow to the affected area described by the radiologist?

There is focal, increased blood flow and blood pooling.

4. How was the radiotracer accumulation described?

The radiotracer accumulated within the left mid posterior tibial diaphysis was delayed.

5. What will be the probable outcome with continued excessive repetitive stress?

The rate of resorption will exceed the rate of bone replacement.

6. What will happen if resorption continues to exceed replacement?

A stress fracture will occur.

Chapter 11— Genitourinary System

Learning Activity 11-3
Building Medical Words

1. nephrolith
2. nephropyosis, pyonephrosis
3. hydronephrosis, nephrohydrosis
4. pyelectasis, pyelectasia
5. pyelopathy
6. ureterectasis, ureterectasia
7. ureterolith
8. cystitis
9. cystoscope
10. vesicocele
11. vesicoprostatic
12. urethrostenosis
13. urethrotome
14. urography
15. uropathy
16. dysuria
17. oliguria
18. orchidopathy, orchiopathy
19. orchialgia, orchiodynia, orchidalgia
20. balanorrhea
21. orchidectomy, orchiectomy
22. balanoplasty
23. vasectomy
24. pyelotomy
25. cystopexy

Learning Activity 11-4
Matching Pathological, Diagnostic, Symptomatic, and Related Terms

1. urgency
2. fistula
3. anorchidism
4. anuria
5. azotemia
6. hydronephrosis
7. benign prostatic hypertrophy
8. hesitancy
9. oliguria
10. nephrotic syndrome
11. phimosis
12. sterility
13. epispadias
14. aspermia
15. pyuria
16. herniorrhaphy
17. nocturia
18. enuresis
19. hydrocele
20. balanitis

Learning Activity 11-5
Matching Procedures, Pharmacology, and Abbreviations

1. KUB
2. semen analysis
3. cystoscopy
4. antibiotics
5. C&S
6. diuretics
7. urethrotomy
8. ESWL
9. peritoneal dialysis
10. PSA
11. vasectomy
12. orchidectomy
13. circumcision
14. androgens
15. potassium supplements

Medical Record Activity 11-1
Operative Report: Ureterocele and Ureterocele Calculus

1. What were the findings from the resectoscopy?

The prostate and bladder appeared normal but there was a left ureterocele.

2. What was the name and size of the urethral sound used in the procedure?

#26 French Van Buren

3. What is the function of the urethral sound?

Dilate the urethra

4. In what direction was the ureterocele incised?

Longitudinally

5. Was fulguration required? Why or why not?

Fulguration was not required because there was no bleeding.

Medical Record Activity 11-2
Operative Report: Extracorporeal Shock-Wave Lithotripsy

1. What previous procedures were performed on the patient?

ESWL and double-J stent placement

2. Why is this current procedure being performed?

To fragment the remaining calculus and remove the double-J stent

3. What imaging technique was used for positioning the patient to ensure that the shock waves would strike the calculus?

Fluoroscopy

4. In what position was the patient placed in the cystoscopy suite?

Dorsal lithotomy

5. How was the double-J stent removed?

Using grasping forceps and removing it as the scope was withdrawn

Chapter 12—Female Reproductive System

Learning Activity 12-3
Building Medical Words

1. gynecopathy
2. gynecologist
3. cervicovaginitis
4. cervicovesical
5. colposcope
6. colposcopy
7. vaginitis
8. vaginocele
9. hysteromyoma
10. hysteropathy
11. hysterosalpingography
12. metrorrhagia
13. parametritis
14. uterocele
15. uterocervical

16. uterovesical

17. oophoritis

18. oophorosalpingitis

19. salpingocele

20. salpingography

21. oophoropexy, ovariopexy

22. hystero-oophorectomy

23. episiorrhaphy, perineorrhaphy

24. hysterosalpingo-oophorectomy

25. amniocentesis

Matching Pathological, Diagnostic, Symptomatic, and Related Terms

1. pyosalpinx

2. primipara

3. gestation

4. chancre

5. retroversion

6. congenital

7. dystocia

8. atresia

9. Down syndrome

10. pruritus vulvae

11. asymptomatic

12. metrorrhagia

13. menarche

14. leiomyoma

15. oligomenorrhea

16. parturition

17. eclampsia

18. viable

19. condylomas

20. primigravida

Matching Procedures, Pharmacology, and Abbreviations

1. Pap test

2. hysterosalpingography

3. amniocentesis

4. antifungals

5. colpocleisis

6. D&C

7. TAH

8. tubal ligation

9. OCPs

10. laparoscopy

11. episiotomy

12. ultrasonography

13. chorionic villus sampling

14. estrogens

15. oxytocins

16. cryocautery

17. IUD

18. cordocentesis

19. lumpectomy

20. prostaglandins

SOAP Note: Primary Herpes 1 Infection

1. Did the patient have any discharge? If so, describe it.

A brownish discharge

2. What type of discomfort did the patient experience around the vulvar area?

She was experiencing severe itching (pruritus), fever, and blisters.

3. Has the patient been taking her oral contraceptive pills regularly?

Yes

4. Where was the viral culture obtained?

Ulcerlike lesion on the right labia

Medical Record Activity 12-2
Postoperative Consultation: Menometrorrhagia

1. How many pregnancies did this woman have? How many viable infants did she deliver?

Two pregnancies and one viable birth

2. What is a therapeutic abortion?

An abortion performed when the pregnancy endangers the mother's mental or physical health or when the fetus has a known condition incompatible with life

3. Why did the physician propose to perform a hysterectomy?

Patient desires definitive treatment for menometrorrhagia and has declined palliative treatment

Chapter 13—Endocrine System

Learning Activity 13-2
Building Medical Words

1. hyperglycemia
2. hypoglycemia
3. glycogenesis

Learning Activity 13-3
Matching Pathological, Diagnostic, Symptomatic, and Related Terms

1. virile
2. myxedema
3. diuresis
4. hirsutism
5. cretinism
6. insulin

5. Even though her partner used a condom, how do you think the patient became infected with herpes?

She probably got infected from the cold sore when having oral-genital sex.

4. What is a vaginal hysterectomy?

Surgical removal of the uterus through the vagina

5. Does the surgeon plan to remove one or both ovaries and fallopian tubes?

The surgeon plans to perform a bilateral (relates to two sides) salpingo-oophorectomy.

6. Why do you think the physician will use the laparoscope to perform the hysterectomy?

To permit visualization of the abdominal cavity as the ovaries and fallopian tubes are removed through the vagina

4. pancreatitis
5. pancreatolysis
6. pancreatopathy
7. thyroiditis
8. thyromegaly
9. parathyroidectomy
10. adrenalectomy

7. Addison disease
8. exophthalmic goiter
9. hyperkalemia
10. pheochromocytoma
11. type 1 diabetes
12. hyponatremia
13. glycosuria
14. Cushing syndrome
15. type 2 diabetes

Matching Procedures, Pharmacology, and Abbreviations

1. FBS
2. RAIU
3. corticosteroids
4. growth hormone
5. thyroid scan
6. T_4

7. oral antidiabetics
8. GTT
9. antithyroids
10. protein-bound iodine
11. T3
12. MRI
13. exophthalmometry
14. CT scan
15. Humulin

Consultation Note: Hyperparathyroidism

1. What is an adenoma?

Benign tumor of a gland

2. What does the physician suspect caused the patient's hyperparathyroidism?

Possible parathyroid adenoma

3. What type of laboratory findings revealed parathyroid disease?

Elevated calcium level

4. What is hypercalciuria?

Excessive amount of calcium in the urine

5. If the patient smoked 548 packs of cigarettes per year, how many packs did she smoke in an average day?

Approximately 1.5 packs per day (365 days per yr/548 pks = 1.5)

SOAP Note: Diabetes Mellitus

1. How long has this patient been experiencing voracious eating?

For the past 10 days

2. Was the patient's obesity due to overeating or metabolic imbalance?

Overeating

3. Why did the doctor experience difficulty in examining the patient's abdomen?

Because she was so obese

4. Was the patient's blood glucose above or below normal on admission?

Above normal

5. What is the reference range for fasting blood glucose?

The range for fasting blood glucose is 70/110 mg/dL.

Chapter 14—Nervous System

Building Medical Words

1. encephalopathy
2. encephalocele
3. encephalography
4. cerebropathy
5. cerebritis

6. craniocele
7. craniometer
8. neuralgia, neurodynia
9. neurologist
10. neurotripsy
11. myelocele
12. myeloplegia
13. psychotic, psychic
14. psychosis
15. bradykinesia

16. dyskinesia

17. hemiplegia

18. quadriplegia

19. dysphasia

20. aphasia

21. neurolysis

22. craniotomy

23. cranioplasty

24. neurorrhaphy

25. encephalotomy

Learning Activity 14-3
Matching Pathological, Diagnostic, Symptomatic, and Related Terms

1. hemiparesis

2. aphasia

3. Alzheimer disease

4. bulimia nervosa

5. clonic phase

6. Guillain-Barrè syndrome

7. phobias

8. bipolar disorder

9. epilepsies

10. ischemic stroke

11. shingles

12. radiculopathy

13. paraplegia

14. poliomyelitis

15. lethargy

16. myelomeningocele

17. autism

18. Parkinson disease

19. multiple sclerosis

20. concussion

Learning Activity 14-4
Matching Procedures, Pharmacology, and Abbreviations

1. NCV

2. psychostimulants

3. antipsychotics

4. general anesthetics

5. echoencephalography

6. cryosurgery

7. myelography

8. cerebral angiography

9. CSF analysis

10. electromyography

11. lumbar puncture

12. PET

13. tractotomy

14. hypnotics

15. trephination

Medical Record Activity 14-1
Discharge Summary: Subarachnoid Hemorrhage

1. In what part of the head did the patient feel pain?

Occipital, the back part of the head

2. What imaging tests were performed, and what was the finding in each test?

CT scan showed blood in the cisterna subarachnoidalis and mild acute hydrocephalus. Cerebral angiogram and MRI showed no aneurysm.

3. What was the result of the lumbar puncture?

The results were consistent with recurrent subarachnoid hemorrhage.

4. What was the result of the repeat MRI?

It again showed no evidence of an aneurysm.

5. Regarding activity, what limitations were placed upon the patient?

Avoid activity that could raise the pressure in the head, and perform no activity more vigorous than walking.

Consultation Report: Acute Onset Paraplegia

1. What was the original cause of the patient's current problems and what treatments were provided?

Fall at work about 15 to 20 years ago and four subsequent lumbar surgeries

2. Why was the patient admitted to the hospital?

Pain management

3. What medications did the patient receive and why was each given?

Clonidine for hypertension and methadone for pain

4. What was the cause of bladder retention?

Administration of clonidine

5. What occurred after the catheter was removed?

Subacute onset of paresis, paresthesias, and pain in the legs, approximately 2.5 to 3.0 hours later

6. What three disorders were listed in the differential diagnosis?

Subarachnoid hemorrhage, epidural abscess, and transverse myelitis

7. How will lymphedema be controlled should physical therapy be undertaken?

Compression stockings

Chapter 15—Special Senses

Learning Activity 15-3
Building Medical Words

1. ophthalmoplegia, ophthalmoparalysis
2. ophthalmology
3. pupilloscopy
4. keratomalacia
5. keratometer
6. scleritis
7. scleromalacia
8. iridoplegia, iridoparalysis
9. iridocele
10. retinopathy

11. retinitis
12. blepharoplegia
13. blepharoptosis
14. otopyorrhea
15. audiometer
16. myringotome
17. amblyopia
18. hyperopia
19. anacusis
20. hyperacusis
21. stapedectomy
22. labyrinthotomy
23. mastoidectomy
24. myringoplasty, tympanoplasty
25. keratotomy

Learning Activity 15-4
Matching Pathological, Diagnostic, Symptomatic, and Related Terms

1. cataract
2. achromatopsia
3. nyctalopia
4. gonioscope
5. anacusis
6. otitis externa

7. diopter
8. tonometer
9. visual field
10. epiphora
11. strabismus
12. Mèniëre disease
13. neovascular
14. vertigo
15. exotropia
16. enucleation

17. chalazion

18. amblyopia

19. retinoblastoma

20. tinnitus

Learning Activity 15-5
Matching Procedures, Pharmacology, and Abbreviations

1. caloric stimulation test

2. ophthalmoscopy

3. cochlear implant

4. fluorescein angiography

5. otoplasty

6. mydriatics

7. tonometry

8. visual acuity test

9. evisceration

10. antiemetics

11. wax emulsifiers

12. enucleation

13. ST

14. ophthalmic decongestants

15. XT

16. gonioscopy

17. otoscopy

18. audiometry

19. radial keratotomy

20. otic analgesics

Medical Record Activity 15-1
Operative Report: Retained Foreign Bodies

1. Did the surgery involve one or both ears?

It was bilateral, involving both ears.

2. What was the nature of the foreign body in the patient's ears?

Retained tympanostomy tubes

3. What ear structure was involved?

Eardrum, or tympanum

4. What instrument was used to locate the tubes?

Operating microscope

5. What was the material in which the tubes were embedded?

Earwax, or cerumen

6. What occurred when the cerumen and tubes were removed?

It resulted in a large perforation.

7. How was the perforation treated?

The edges were freshened sharply with a pick, and a paper patch was applied.

Medical Record Activity 15-2
Operative Report: Phacoemulsification and Lens Implant

1. What technique was used to destroy the cataract?

Phacoemulsification, an ultrasound technique

2. In what portion of the eye was the implant placed?

Posterior chamber

3. What anesthetics were used for surgery?

Intravenous and retrobulbar block

4. What was the function of the blepharostat?

To separate the eyelids during surgery

5. What is a keratome?

A knife used to incise the cornea

6. Where was the implant inserted?

In the capsular bag

APPENDIX

B

Common Abbreviations and Symbols

Common Abbreviations

The table below lists common abbreviations used in health care and related fields along with their meanings.

Abbreviation	Meaning	Abbreviation	Meaning
A		**ARDS**	acute respiratory distress syndrome
		ARF	acute renal failure
AAA	abdominal aortic aneurysm	**ARMD, AMD**	age-related macular degeneration
A&P	auscultation and percussion	**AS**	aortic stenosis
A, B, AB, O	blood types in ABO blood group	**AS***	left ear
AB, Ab, ab	antibody; abortion	**ASD**	atrial septal defect
ABC	aspiration biopsy cytology	**ASHD**	arteriosclerotic heart disease
ABG	arterial blood gas(es)	**AST**	angiotensin sensitivity test; aspartate aminotransferase
AC	air conduction		
a.c.*	before meals	**Ast**	astigmatism
Acc	accommodation	**ATN**	acute tubular necrosis
ACE	angiotensin-converting enzyme (inhibitor)	**AU***	both ears
		AV	atrioventricular; arteriovenous
ACL	anterior cruciate ligament		
ACS	acute coronary syndrome	**B**	
ACTH	adrenocorticotropic hormone	**Ba**	barium
AD	Alzheimer disease	**baso**	basophil (type of white blood cell)
AD*	right ear	**BBB**	bundle branch block
ADH	antidiuretic hormone (vasopressin)	**BC**	bone conduction
ADHD	attention-deficit hyperactivity disorder	**BCC**	basal cell carcinoma
		BE	barium enema; below the elbow
ad lib.	as desired	**BEAM**	brain electrical activity mapping
ADLs	activities of daily living	**b.i.d.***	twice a day
AE	above the elbow	**BK**	below the knee
AED	automatic external defibrillator	**BKA**	below-knee amputation
AF	atrial fibrillation	**BM**	bowel movement
AFB	acid-fast bacillus (TB organism)	**BMI**	body mass index
AGN	acute glomerulonephritis	**BMR**	basal metabolic rate
AI	artificial insemination	**BNO**	bladder neck obstruction
AICD	automatic implantable cardioverter defibrillator	**BP, B/P**	blood pressure
		BPH	benign prostatic hyperplasia; benign prostatic hypertrophy
AIDS	acquired immune deficiency syndrome		
		BS	blood sugar
AK	above the knee	**BSE**	breast self-examination
alk phos	alkaline phosphatase	**BUN**	blood urea nitrogen
ALL	acute lymphocytic leukemia	**Bx, bx**	biopsy
ALS	amyotrophic lateral sclerosis; also called *Lou Gehrig disease*	**C**	
ALT	alanine aminotransferase	**c̄**	with
AM, a.m.	in the morning or before noon	**C&S**	culture and sensitivity
AML	acute myelogenous leukemia	**c/o**	complains of, complaints
ANS	autonomic nervous system	**C1, C2, and so on**	first cervical vertebra, second cervical vertebra, and so on
ant	anterior		
AOM	acute otitis media	**CA**	cancer; chronological age; cardiac arrest
AP	anteroposterior		
APC	antigen-presenting cell	**Ca**	calcium; cancer
APTT	activated partial thromboplastin time	**CABG**	coronary artery bypass graft
		CAD	coronary artery disease

Common Abbreviations—cont'd

Abbreviation	Meaning	Abbreviation	Meaning
CAH	chronic active hepatitis; congenital adrenal hyperplasia	**D**	
CAT	computed axial tomography	D	diopter (lens strength)
Cath	catheterization; catheter	D&C	dilatation (dilation) and curettage
CBC	complete blood count	dc, DC, D/C*	discharge; discontinue
CC	cardiac catheterization; chief complaint	Decub.	decubitus (lying down)
cc*	cubic centimeters; same as mL (1/1000 of a liter)	D.O.	Doctor of Osteopathy
		D.P.M.	Doctor of Podiatric Medicine
		Derm	dermatology
CCU	coronary care unit	DES	diffuse esophageal spasm; drug-eluting stent
CDH	congenital dislocation of the hip	DEXA, DXA	dual energy x-ray absorptiometry
CF	cystic fibrosis	DI	diabetes insipidus; diagnostic imaging
CHD	coronary heart disease		
chemo	chemotherapy	diff	differential count (white blood cells)
CHF	congestive heart failure		
Chol	cholesterol	DJD	degenerative joint disease
CIS	carcinoma in situ	DKA	diabetic ketoacidosis
CK	creatine kinase (cardiac enzyme); conductive keratoplasty	DM	diabetes mellitus
		DNA	deoxyribonucleic acid
CLL	chronic lymphocytic leukemia	DOE	dyspnea on exertion
cm	centimeter (1/100 of a meter)	DPI	dry powder inhaler
CML	chronic myelogenous leukemia	DPT	diphtheria, pertussis, tetanus
CNS	central nervous system	DO	Doctor of Osteopathy
CO	coccygeal nerves	DRE	digital rectal examination
c/o	complains of	DSA	digital subtraction angiography
CO₂	carbon dioxide	DUB	dysfunctional uterine bleeding
COLD	chronic obstructive lung disease	DVT	deep vein thrombosis; deep venous thrombosis
COPD	chronic obstructive pulmonary disease		
		Dx	diagnosis
CP	cerebral palsy	**E**	
CPAP	continuous positive airway pressure	EBR	external beam radiation
CPD	cephalopelvic disproportion	EBT	external beam therapy
CPK	creatine phosphokinase (enzyme released into bloodstream after a heart attack)	EBV	Epstein-Barr virus
		ECCE	extracapsular cataract extraction
		ECG, EKG	electrocardiogram; electrocardiography
CPR	cardiopulmonary resuscitation		
CRF	chronic renal failure	ECHO	echocardiogram; echocardiography; echoencephalogram; echoencephalography
CRRT	continuous renal replacement therapy		
CS, C-section	cesarean section	ECRB	extensor carpi radialis brevis (muscle or tendon)
CSF	cerebrospinal fluid		
CT	computed tomography	ED	erectile dysfunction; emergency department
	computed tomography		
CTS	carpal tunnel syndrome	EEG	electroencephalography
CV	cardiovascular	EENT	eyes, ears, nose, throat
CVA	cerebrovascular accident	EF	ejection fraction
CVD	cardiovascular disease	EGD	esophagogastroduodenoscopy
CVS	chorionic villus sampling	ELT	endovenous laser ablation; endolumina laser ablation
CWP	childbirth without pain		
CXR	chest x-ray, chest radiograph	Em	emmetropia
cysto	cystoscopy		

(continued)

Common Abbreviations—cont'd

Abbreviation	Meaning	Abbreviation	Meaning
EMG	electromyography	HCG	human chorionic gonadotropin
ENT	ears, nose, and throat	HCl	hydrochloric acid
EOM	extraocular movement	HCT, Hct	hematocrit
eos	eosinophil (type of white blood cell)	HCV	hepatitis C virus
ERCP	endoscopic retrograde cholangiopancreatography	HD	hemodialysis; hip disarticulation; hearing distance
ESR	erythrocyte sedimentation rate	HDL	high-density lipoprotein
ESRD	end-stage renal disease	HDN	hemolytic disease of the newborn
ESWL	extracorporeal shock-wave lithotripsy	HDV	hepatitis D virus
ETT	exercise tolerance test	HEV	hepatitis E virus
ETT-MIBI	exercise tolerance test combined with a radioactive tracer (sestamibi) scan	HF	heart failure
		HIV	human immunodeficiency virus
		H_2O	water
EU	excretory urography	HMD	hyaline membrane disease
		HNP	herniated nucleus pulposus (herniated disk)
F		HP	hemipelvectomy
FBS	fasting blood sugar	HPV	human papillomavirus
FECG, FEKG	fetal electrocardiogram	HRT	hormone replacement therapy
FH	family history	hs*	half strength
FHR	fetal heart rate	h.s.*	at bedtime
FHT	fetal heart tone	HSG	hysterosalpingography
FS	frozen section	HSV	herpes simplex virus
FSH	follicle-stimulating hormone	HTN	hypertension
FTND	full-term normal delivery	Hx	history
FVC	forced vital capacity		
Fx	fracture	**I, J**	
		IAS	interatrial septum
G		IBD	irritable bowel disease
G	gravida (pregnant)	I&D	incision and drainage
GB	gallbladder	IBS	irritable bowel syndrome
GBP	gastric bypass	ICD	implantable cardioverter-defibrillator
GBS	gallbladder series (x-ray studies)	ICP	intracranial pressure
GC	gonococcus (*Neisseria gonorrhoeae*)	ICU	intensive care unit
G-CSF	granulocyte-colony-stimulating factor	ID	intradermal
		IDDM	insulin-dependent diabetes mellitus
GER	gastroesophageal reflux	Igs	immunoglobulins
GERD	gastroesophageal reflux disease	IM	intramuscular; infectious mononucleosis
GH	growth hormone		
GI	gastrointestinal	IMP	impression (synonymous with diagnosis)
GTT	glucose tolerance test		
GU	genitourinary	INR	international normalized ratio
GVHD	graft-versus-host disease	IVP	instravenous pyelogram; intravenous pyelography
GVHR	graft-versus-host reaction		
GYN	gynecology	IOL	intraocular lens
		IOP	intraocular pressure
H		IPPB	intermittent positive-pressure breathing
HAV	hepatitis A virus		
Hb, Hgb	hemoglobin	IRDS	infant respiratory distress syndrome
HBV	hepatitis B virus		

Common Abbreviations—cont'd

Abbreviation	Meaning	Abbreviation	Meaning
IS	intracostal space	MCHC	mean cell hemoglobin concentration (average concentration of hemoglobin per red cell)
ITP	idiopathic thrombocytopenic purpura		
IU*	international unit	MCV	mean cell volume (average volume or size per red cell
IUD	intrauterine device		
IUGR	intrauterine growth rate; intrauterine growth retardation	MDI	metered-dose inhaler
		MEG	magnetoencephalography
IV	intravenous	MG	myasthenia gravis
IVC	intravenous cholangiogram; intravenous cholangiography	mg	milligram (1/1000 of a gram)
		mg/dl, mg/dL	milligram per deciliter
IVF	*in vitro* fertilization	MI	myocardial infarction
IVF-ET	*in vitro* fertilization and embryo transfer	mix astig	mixed astigmatism
		ml, mL	milliliters (1/1000 of a liter)
IVP	intravenous pyelogram; intravenous pyelography	mm	millimeter (1/1000 of a meter)
		mm Hg	millimeters of mercury
K		MR	mitral regurgitation
K	potassium (an electrolyte)	MRA	magnetic resonance angiogram; magnetic resonance angiography
KD	knee disarticulation		
KUB	kidney, ureter, bladder	MRI	magnetic resonance imaging
L		MS	mitral stenosis; musculoskeletal; multiple sclerosis; mental status; magnesium sulfate
L1, L2, and so on	first lumbar vertebra, second lumbar vertebra, and so on		
		MSH	melanocyte-stimulating hormone
LA	left atrium	MUGA	multiple-gated acquisition (scan)
LASIK	laser-assisted in situ keratomileusis	MVP	mitral valve prolapse
LAT, lat	lateral	MVR	mitral valve replacement; massive vitreous retraction (blade); microvitreoretinal
LBBB	left bundle branch block		
LBW	low birth weight		
LD	lactate dehydrogenase; lactic acid dehydrogenase (cardiac enzyme)	Myop	myopia (nearsightedness)
		N	
LDL	low-density lipoprotein	Na	sodium (an electrolyte)
LES	lower esophageal sphincter	NB	newborn
LFT	liver function test	NCV	nerve conduction velocity
LH	luteinizing hormone	NG	nasogastric
LLQ	left lower quadrant	NIDDM	non–insulin-dependent diabetes mellitus
LMP	last menstrual period		
LOC	loss of consciousness	NIHL	noise-induced hearing loss
LP	lumbar puncture	NK cell	natural killer cell
LPR	laryngopharyngeal reflux	NMT	nebulized mist treatment
LS	lumbosacral spine	NPH	neutral protamine Hagedorn (insulin)
LSO	left salpingo-oophorectomy		
lt	left	NPO, n.p.o.*	nothing by mouth
LUQ	left upper quadrant	NSAIDs	nonsteroidal anti-inflammatory drugs
LV	left ventricle		
lymphos	lymphocytes	NSR	normal sinus rhythm
M		**O**	
MCH	mean cell hemoglobin (average amount of hemoglobin per red cell)	O_2	oxygen
		OB	obstetrics
		OCPs	oral contraceptive pills
		OD	overdose

(continued)

Common Abbreviations—cont'd

Abbreviation	Meaning	Abbreviation	Meaning
O.D.	Doctor of Optometry	PO$_2$	partial pressure of oxygen
OD*	right eye	poly, PMN, PMNL	polymorphonuclear leukocyte
OM	otitis media		
OP	outpatient; operative procedure	post	posterior
ORTH, ortho	orthopedics	PPV	pars plana vitrectomy
OS*	left eye; by mouth (pharmacology)	PRL	prolactin
OU*	both eyes	p.r.n.*	as required
OSA	obstructive sleep apnea	PSA	prostate-specific antigen
		PT	prothrombin time, physical therapy
P		pt	patient
P	phosphorus; pulse	PTHC	percutaneous transhepatic cholan-
p̄	after		geography
PBI	protein-bound iodine	PTCA	percutaneous transluminal coro-
PCO$_2$	partial pressure of carbon dioxide		nary angioplasty
PID	pelvic inflammatory disease	PTH	parathyroid hormone; also called
PA	posteroanterior; pernicious ane-		*parathormone*
	mia; pulmonary artery	PTT	partial thromboplastin time
PAC	premature atrial contraction	PUD	peptic ulcer disease
Pap	Papanicolaou (test)	PVC	premature ventricular contraction
para 1, 2, 3 and so on	unipara, bipara, tripara and so on (number of viable births)		
		Q	
PAT	paroxysmal atrial tachycardia	qAM*	every morning
PBI	protein-bound iodine	q.2h.*	every 2 hours
pc, p.c.*	after meals	q.d.*	every day
PCL	posterior cruciate ligament	qEEG	quantitative electroencephalography
PCNL	percutaneous nephrolithotomy	q.h.*	every hour
PCO$_2$	partial pressure of carbon dioxide	q.i.d.*	four times a day
PCP	*Pneumocystis* pneumonia; primary	q.o.d.*	every other day
	care physician; phencyclidine	qPM*	every evening
	(hallucinogen)		
PCV	packed cell volume	**R**	
PE	physical examination; pulmonary	RA	right atrium; rheumatoid
	embolism; pressure-equalizing		arthritis
	(tube)	RAI	radioactive iodine
PERRLA	pupils equal, round, and reactive to	RAIU	radioactive iodine uptake
	light and accommodation	RBC, rbc	red blood cell
PET	positron emission tomography	RD	respiratory distress
PFT	pulmonary function tests	RDS	respiratory distress syndrome
PGH	pituitary growth hormone	RF	rheumatoid factor; radio
pH	symbol for degree of acidity or		frequency
	alkalinity	RGB	Roux-en-Y gastric bypass
PID	pelvic inflammatory disease	RK	radial keratotomy
PIH	pregnancy induced hypertension	RLQ	right lower quadrant
PKD	polycystic kidney disease	R/O	rule out
PMH	past medical history	ROM	range of motion
PMI	point of maximum impulse	RP	retrograde pyelogram; retrograde
PMP	previous menstrual period		pyelography
PMS	premenstrual syndrome	RSO	right salpingo-oophorectomy
PND	paroxysmal nocturnal dyspnea	rt	right
PNS	peripheral nervous system	RUQ	right upper quadrant
p.o.*	by mouth	RV	residual volume; right ventricle

Common Abbreviations—cont'd

Abbreviation	Meaning	Abbreviation	Meaning
S		**TKR**	total knee replacement
s̄	without	**TPPV**	trans pars plana vitretomy
S1, S2, and so on	first sacral vertebra, second sacral vertebra, and so on	**TPR**	temperature, pulse, and respiration
		TRAM	transverse rectus abdominis muscle
SA, S-A	sinoatrial	**TSE**	testicular self-examination
SaO₂	arterial oxygen saturation	**TSH**	thyroid-stimulating hormone
SD	shoulder disarticulation	**TURP**	transurethral resection of the prostate
segs	segmented neutrophils		
SIADH	syndrome of inappropriate antidiuretic hormone	**TVH**	total vaginal hysterectomy
		Tx	treatment
SICS	small incision cataract surgery	**U**	
SIDS	sudden infant death syndrome	**U***	unit
SLE	systemic lupus erythematosus; slit-lamp examination	**U&L, U/L**	upper and lower
		UA	urinalysis
SNS	sympathetic nervous system	**UC**	uterine contractions
SOB	shortness of breath	**UGI**	upper gastrointestinal
sono	sonogram	**UGIS**	upper gastrointestinal series
SPECT	single photon emission computed tomography	**ung**	ointment
		UPP	uvulopalatopharyngoplasty
sp. gr.	specific gravity	**URI**	upper respiratory infection
ST	esotropia	**US**	ultrasound; ultrasonography
stat., STAT	immediately	**UTI**	urinary tract infection
STD	sexually transmitted disease	**V**	
subcu*, Sub-Q, subQ	subcutaneous (injection)	**VA**	visual acuity
		VC	vital capacity
Sx	symptom	**VCUG**	voiding cystourethrography
T		**VD**	venereal disease
T&A	tonsillectomy and adenoidectomy	**VF**	visual field
T1, T2, and so on	first thoracic vertebra, second thoracic vertebra, and so on	**VSD**	ventricular septal defect
		VT	ventricular tachycardia
T₃	triiodothyronine (thyroid hormone)	**VUR**	vesicoureteral reflux
		W	
T₄	thyroxine (thyroid hormone)	**WBC, wbc**	white blood cell
TAH	total abdominal hysterectomy	**WD**	well-developed
TB	tuberculosis	**WN**	well-nourished
TFT	thyroid function test	**WNL**	within normal limits
THA	total hip arthroplasty	**X, Y, Z**	
THR	total hip replacement	**XP, XDP**	xeroderma pigmentosum
ther	therapy	**XT**	exotropia
TIA	transient ischemic attack		
t.i.d.*	three times a day		
TKA	total knee arthroplasty		

*Although these abbreviations are currently found in medical records and clinical notes, they are easily misinterpreted. Thus, the Joint Commission (formerly JCAHO) requires their discontinuance. Instead, they recommend to write out their meanings. For a summary of these abbreviations, see the table below.

Summary of Discontinued Abbreviations

As noted above, the Joint Commission has recommended the discontinuance of certain abbreviations that are easily misinterpreted in medical records. The table below lists these abbreviations along with their meanings.

Abbreviation	Meaning
Medication and Therapy Time Schedule	
a.c.	before meals
b.i.d.	twice a day
hs	half strength
h.s.	at bedtime
NPO, n.p.o.	nothing by mouth
p.c.	after meals
p.o.	by mouth
p.r.n.	as required
qAM	every morning
q.d.	every day
q.h.	every hour
q.2h.	every 2 hours
q.i.d.	four times a day
q.o.d.	every other day
qPM	every evening
t.i.d.	three times a day
Other Related Abbreviations	
AD	right ear
AS	left ear
AU	both ears
cc	cubic centimeters; same as mL, ml (1/1000 of a liter)
	Use ml *for milliliters or write out the meaning.*
dc, DC,	discharge; discontinue
OD	right eye
OS	left eye
OU	both eyes
subcu, Sub-Q, subQ	subcutaneous (injection)
U	unit

Common Symbols

Symbol	Meaning	Symbol	Meaning
@	at	−	minus, negative
aa	of each	±	plus or minus; either positive or negative; indefinite
'	foot	∅	no
"	inch	#	number; following a number; pounds
Δ	change; heat	÷	divided by
Rx	prescription, treatment, therapy	/	divided by
		×	multiplied by; magnification
→	to, in the direction of	=	equals
↑	increase(d), up	⊕	approximately equal
↓	decrease(d), down	°	degree
+	plus, positive	%	percent
		♀	female
		♂	male

Glossary of Medical Word Elements

Medical Word Elements

Element	Meaning	Element	Meaning
A		**-ary**	pertaining to
		asbest/o	asbestos
a-	without, not	**-asthenia**	weakness, debility
ab-	from, away from	**astr/o**	star
abdomin/o	abdomen	**-ate**	having the form of, possessing
abort/o	to miscarry	**atel/o**	incomplete; imperfect
-ac	pertaining to	**ather/o**	fatty plaque
acid/o	acid	**-ation**	process (of)
acous/o	hearing	**atri/o**	atrium
acr/o	extremity	**audi/o**	hearing
acromi/o	acromion (projection of scapula)	**audit/o**	hearing
-acusis	hearing	**aur/o**	ear
-ad	toward	**auricul/o**	ear
ad-	toward	**auto-**	self, own
aden/o	gland	**ax/o**	axis, axon
adenoid/o	adenoids	**azot/o**	nitrogenous compounds
adip/o	fat		
adren/o	adrenal glands	**B**	
adrenal/o	adrenal glands		
aer/o	air	**bacteri/o**	bacteria (singular, bacterium)
af-	toward	**balan/o**	glans penis
agglutin/o	clumping, gluing	**bas/o**	base (alkaline, opposite of acid)
agora-	marketplace	**bi-**	two
-al	pertaining to	**bil/i**	bile, gall
albin/o	white	**bi/o**	life
albumin/o	albumin (protein)	**-blast**	embryonic cell
-algesia	pain	**blast/o**	embryonic cell
-algia	pain	**blephar/o**	eyelid
allo-	other, differing from the normal	**brachi/o**	arm
alveol/o	alveolus; air sac	**brachy-**	short
ambly/o	dull, dim	**brady-**	slow
amni/o	amnion (amniotic sac)	**bronch/o**	bronchus (plural, bronchi)
an-	without, not	**bronchi/o**	bronchus (plural, bronchi)
an/o	anus	**bronchiol/o**	bronchiole
ana-	against; up; back	**bucc/o**	cheek
andr/o	male		
aneurysm/o	widened blood vessel	**C**	
angi/o	vessel (usually blood or lymph)		
aniso-	unequal, dissimilar	**calc/o**	calcium
ankyl/o	stiffness; bent, crooked	**calcane/o**	calcaneum (heel bone)
ante-	before, in front of	**-capnia**	carbon dioxide (CO_2)
anter/o	anterior, front	**carcin/o**	cancer
anthrac/o	coal, coal dust	**cardi/o**	heart
anti-	against	**-cardia**	heart condition
aort/o	aorta	**carp/o**	carpus (wrist bones)
append/o	appendix	**cata-**	down
appendic/o	appendix	**caud/o**	tail
aque/o	water	**cauter/o**	heat, burn
-ar	pertaining to	**cec/o**	cecum
-arche	beginning	**-cele**	hernia, swelling
arteri/o	artery	**-centesis**	surgical puncture
arteriol/o	arteriole	**cephal/o**	head
arthr/o	joint	**-ceps**	head
		-ception	conceiving
		cerebell/o	cerebellum

Element	Meaning
cerebr/o	cerebrum
cervic/o	neck; cervix uteri (neck of uterus)
chalic/o	limestone
cheil/o	lip
chem/o	chemical; drug
chlor/o	green
chol/e	bile, gall
cholangi/o	bile vessel
cholecyst/o	gallbladder
choledoch/o	bile duct
chondr/o	cartilage
chori/o	chorion
choroid/o	choroid
chrom/o	color
chromat/o	color
-cide	killing
cine-	movement
cinemat/o	things that move
circum-	around
cirrh/o	yellow
-cision	a cutting
-clasia	to break; surgical fracture
-clasis	to break; surgical fracture
-clast	to break
clavicul/o	clavicle (collar bone)
-cleisis	closure
clon/o	clonus (turmoil)
-clysis	irrigation, washing
coccyg/o	coccyx (tailbone)
cochle/o	cochlea
col/o	colon
colon/o	colon
colp/o	vagina
condyl/o	condyle
coni/o	dust
conjunctiv/o	conjunctiva
-continence	to hold back
contra-	against, opposite
cor/o	pupil
core/o	pupil
corne/o	cornea
coron/o	heart
corp/o	body
corpor/o	body
cortic/o	cortex
cost/o	ribs
crani/o	cranium (skull)
crin/o	secrete
-crine	secrete
cruci/o	cross
cry/o	cold
crypt/o	hidden

Element	Meaning
culd/o	cul-de-sac
-cusia	hearing
-cusis	hearing
cutane/o	skin
cyan/o	blue
cycl/o	ciliary body of eye; circular; cycle
-cyesis	pregnancy
cyst/o	bladder
cyt/o	cell
-cyte	cell

D

Element	Meaning
dacry/o	tear; lacrimal apparatus (duct, sac, or gland)
dacryocyst/o	lacrimal sac
dactyl/o	fingers; toes
de-	cessation
dendr/o	tree
dent/o	teeth
derm/o	skin
-derma	skin
dermat/o	skin
-desis	binding, fixation (of a bone or joint)
di-	double
dia-	through, across
dipl-	double
dipl/o	double
dips/o	thirst
-dipsia	thirst
dist/o	far, farthest
dors/o	back (of body)
duct/o	to lead; carry
-duction	act of leading, bringing, conducting
duoden/o	duodenum (first part of small intestine)
dur/o	dura mater; hard
-dynia	pain
dys-	bad; painful; difficult

E

Element	Meaning
-eal	pertaining to
ec-	out, out from
echo-	a repeated sound
-ectasis	dilation, expansion
ecto-	outside, outward
-ectomy	excision, removal
-edema	swelling
ef-	away from
electr/o	electricity
-ema	state of; condition
embol/o	embolus (plug)
-emesis	vomiting

(continued)

Element	Meaning	Element	Meaning
-emia	blood condition	glomerul/o	glomerulus
emphys/o	to inflate	gloss/o	tongue
en-	in, within	glott/o	glottis
encephal/o	brain	gluc/o	sugar, sweetness
end-	in, within	glucos/o	sugar, sweetness
endo-	in, within	glyc/o	sugar, sweetness
enter/o	intestine (usually small intestine)	glycos/o	sugar, sweetness
eosin/o	dawn (rose-colored)	gnos/o	knowing
epi-	above, upon	-gnosis	knowing
epididym/o	epididymis	gonad/o	gonads, sex glands
epiglott/o	epiglottis	goni/o	angle
episi/o	vulva	gon/o	seed (ovum or spermatozoon)
erythem/o	red	-grade	to go
erythemat/o	red	-graft	transplantation
erythr/o	red	-gram	record, writing
eschar/o	scab	granul/o	granule
-esis	condition	-graph	instrument for recording
eso-	inward	-graphy	process of recording
esophag/o	esophagus	-gravida	pregnant woman
esthes/o	feeling	gyn/o	woman, female
-esthesia	feeling	gynec/o	woman, female
eti/o	cause	**H**	
eu-	good, normal		
ex-	out, out from	hallucin/o	hallucination
exo-	outside, outward	hedon/o	pleasure
extra-	outside	hem/o	blood
F		hemangi/o	blood vessel
		hemat/o	blood
faci/o	face	hemi-	one half
fasci/o	band, fascia (fibrous membrane supporting and separating muscles)	hepat/o	liver
		hetero-	different
		hidr/o	sweat
femor/o	femur (thigh bone)	hist/o	tissue
-ferent	to carry	histi/o	tissue
fibr/o	fiber, fibrous tissue	home/o	same, alike
fibul/o	fibula (smaller bone of lower leg)	homeo-	same, alike
fluor/o	luminous, fluorescence	homo-	same
G		humer/o	humerus (upper arm bone)
		hydr/o	water
galact/o	milk	hyp-	under, below, deficient
gangli/o	ganglion (knot or knotlike mass)	hyper-	excessive, above normal
gastr/o	stomach	hyp/o	under, below, deficient
-gen	forming, producing, origin	hypn/o	sleep
gen/o	forming, producing, origin	hypo-	under, below, deficient
-genesis	forming, producing, origin	hyster/o	uterus (womb)
genit/o	genitalia	**I**	
gest/o	pregnancy		
gingiv/o	gum(s)	-ia	condition
glauc/o	gray	-iac	pertaining to
gli/o	glue; neuroglial tissue	-iasis	abnormal condition (produced by something specified)
-glia	glue; neuroglial tissue		
-globin	protein	iatr/o	physician; medicine; treatment

Element	Meaning
-iatry	medicine; treatment
-ic	pertaining to
-ical	pertaining to
-ice	noun ending
ichthy/o	dry, scaly
-ician	specialist
-icle	small, minute
-icterus	jaundice
idi/o	unknown, peculiar
-ile	pertaining to
ile/o	ileum (third part of small intestine)
ili/o	ilium (lateral, flaring portion of hip bone)
im-	not
immun/o	immune, immunity, safe
in-	in, not
-ine	pertaining to
infer/o	lower, below
infra-	below, under
inguin/o	groin
insulin/o	insulin
inter-	between
intra-	in, within
-ion	the act of
-ior	pertaining to
irid/o	iris
-is	noun ending
isch/o	to hold back; block
ischi/o	ischium (lower portion of hip bone)
-ism	condition
iso-	same, equal
-ist	specialist
-isy	state of; condition
-itic	pertaining to
-itis	inflammation
-ive	pertaining to
-ization	process (of)

J, K

Element	Meaning
jaund/o	yellow
jejun/o	jejunum (second part of small intestine)
kal/i	potassium (an electrolyte)
kary/o	nucleus
kerat/o	horny tissue; hard; cornea
kern/o	kernel (nucleus)
ket/o	ketone bodies (acids and acetones)
keton/o	ketone bodies (acids and acetones)
kinesi/o	movement
-kinesia	movement
kinet/o	movement

Element	Meaning
klept/o	to steal
kyph/o	humpback

L

Element	Meaning
labi/o	lip
labyrinth/o	labyrinth (inner ear)
lacrim/o	tear; lacrimal apparatus (duct, sac, or gland)
lact/o	milk
-lalia	speech, babble
lamin/o	lamina (part of vertebral arch)
lapar/o	abdomen
laryng/o	larynx (voice box)
later/o	side, to one side
lei/o	smooth
leiomy/o	smooth muscle (visceral)
-lepsy	seizure
lept/o	thin, slender
leuk/o	white
lex/o	word, phrase
lingu/o	tongue
lip/o	fat
lipid/o	fat
-listhesis	slipping
-lith	stone, calculus
lith/o	stone, calculus
lob/o	lobe
log/o	study of
-logist	specialist in the study of
-logy	study of
lord/o	curve, swayback
-lucent	to shine; clear
lumb/o	loins (lower back)
lymph/o	lymph
lymphaden/o	lymph gland (node)
lymphangi/o	lymph vessel
-lysis	separation; destruction; loosening

M

Element	Meaning
macro-	large
mal-	bad
-malacia	softening
mamm/o	breast
-mania	state of mental disorder, frenzy
mast/o	breast
mastoid/o	mastoid process
maxill/o	maxilla (upper jaw bone)
meat/o	opening, meatus
medi-	middle
medi/o	middle
mediastin/o	mediastinum
medull/o	medulla

(continued)

Element	Meaning
mega-	enlargement
megal/o	enlargement
-megaly	enlargement
melan/o	black
men/o	menses, menstruation
mening/o	meninges (membranes covering brain and spinal cord)
meningi/o	meninges (membranes covering brain and spinal cord)
ment/o	mind
meso-	middle
meta-	change, beyond
metacarp/o	metacarpus (hand bones)
metatars/o	metatarsus (foot bones)
-meter	instrument for measuring
metr/o	uterus (womb); measure
metri/o	uterus (womb)
-metry	act of measuring
mi/o	smaller, less
micr/o	small
micro-	small
mono-	one
morph/o	form, shape, structure
muc/o	mucus
multi-	many, much
muscul/o	muscle
mut/a	genetic change
my/o	muscle
myc/o	fungus (plural, fungi)
mydr/o	widen, enlarge
myel/o	bone marrow; spinal cord
myos/o	muscle
myring/o	tympanic membrane (eardrum)
myx/o	mucus

N

Element	Meaning
narc/o	stupor; numbness; sleep
nas/o	nose
nat/o	birth
natr/o	sodium (an electrolyte)
necr/o	death, necrosis
neo-	new
nephr/o	kidney
neur/o	nerve
neutr/o	neutral; neither
nid/o	nest
noct/o	night
nucle/o	nucleus
nulli-	none
nyctal/o	night

O

Element	Meaning
obstetr/o	midwife
ocul/o	eye
odont/o	teeth
-oid	resembling
-ole	small, minute
olig/o	scanty
-oma	tumor
omphal/o	navel (umbilicus)
onc/o	tumor
onych/o	nail
oophor/o	ovary
-opaque	obscure
ophthalm/o	eye
-opia	vision
-opsia	vision
-opsy	view of
opt/o	eye, vision
optic/o	eye, vision
or/o	mouth
orch/o	testis (plural, testes)
orchi/o	testis (plural, testes)
orchid/o	testis (plural, testes)
-orexia	appetite
orth/o	straight
-ory	pertaining to
-ose	pertaining to; sugar
-osis	abnormal condition; increase (used primarily with blood cells)
-osmia	smell
oste/o	bone
ot/o	ear
-ous	pertaining to
ovari/o	ovary
ox/i	oxygen
ox/o	oxygen
-oxia	oxygen
oxy-	quick, sharp

P

Element	Meaning
pachy-	thick
palat/o	palate (roof of mouth)
pan-	all
pancreat/o	pancreas
-para	to bear (offspring)
para-	near, beside; beyond
parathyroid/o	parathyroid glands
-paresis	partial paralysis
patell/o	patella (kneecap)
path/o	disease

Element	Meaning	Element	Meaning
-pathy	disease	-pnea	breathing
pector/o	chest	pneum/o	air; lung
ped/i	foot; child	pneumon/o	air; lung
ped/o	foot; child	pod/o	foot
pedicul/o	lice	-poiesis	formation, production
pelv/i	pelvis	poikil/o	varied, irregular
pelv/o	pelvis	poli/o	gray; gray matter (of brain or
pen/o	penis		spinal cord)
-penia	decrease, deficiency	poly-	many, much
-pepsia	digestion	polyp/o	small growth
per-	through	-porosis	porous
peri-	around	post-	after, behind
perine/o	perineum (area between scrotum	poster/o	back (of body), behind, posterior
	[or vulva in the female] and	-potence	power
	anus)	-prandial	meal
peritone/o	peritoneum	pre-	before, in front of
-pexy	fixation (of an organ)	presby/o	old age
phac/o	lens	primi-	first
phag/o	swallowing, eating	pro-	before, in front of
-phage	swallowing, eating	proct/o	anus, rectum
-phagia	swallowing, eating	prostat/o	prostate gland
phalang/o	phalanges (bones of fingers and	proxim/o	near, nearest
	toes)	pseudo-	false
pharmaceutic/o	drug, medicine	psych/o	mind
pharyng/o	pharynx (throat)	-ptosis	prolapse, downward displacement
-phasia	speech	ptyal/o	saliva
phe/o	dusky, dark	-ptysis	spitting
-phil	attraction for	pub/o	pelvis bone (anterior part of pelvic
phil/o	attraction for		bone)
-philia	attraction for	pulmon/o	lung
phim/o	muzzle	pupill/o	pupil
phleb/o	vein	py/o	pus
-phobia	fear	pyel/o	renal pelvis
-phonia	voice	pylor/o	pylorus
-phoresis	carrying, transmission	pyr/o	fire
-phoria	feeling (mental state)		
phot/o	light	*Q, R*	
phren/o	diaphragm; mind		
-phylaxis	protection	quadri-	four
-physis	growth	rachi/o	spine
pil/o	hair	radi/o	radiation, x-ray; radius (lower arm
pituitar/o	pituitary gland		bone on thumb side)
-plakia	plaque	radicul/o	nerve root
plas/o	formation, growth	rect/o	rectum
-plasia	formation, growth	ren/o	kidney
-plasm	formation, growth	reticul/o	net, mesh
-plasty	surgical repair	retin/o	retina
-plegia	paralysis	retro-	backward, behind
pleur/o	pleura	rhabd/o	rod-shaped (striated)
-plexy	stroke	rhabdomy/o	rod-shaped (striated) muscle
		rhin/o	nose

(continued)

Element	Meaning	Element	Meaning
rhytid/o	wrinkle	**spin/o**	spine
roentgen/o	x-rays	**spir/o**	breathe
-rrhage	bursting forth (of)	**splen/o**	spleen
-rrhagia	bursting forth (of)	**spondyl/o**	vertebrae (backbone)
-rrhaphy	suture	**squam/o**	scale
-rrhea	discharge, flow	**staped/o**	stapes
-rrhexis	rupture	**-stasis**	standing still
-rrhythm/o	rhythm	**steat/o**	fat
rube/o	red	**sten/o**	narrowing, stricture
		-stenosis	narrowing, stricture
S		**stern/o**	sternum (breastbone)
sacr/o	sacrum	**steth/o**	chest
salping/o	tube (usually fallopian or eustachian [auditory] tube)	**sthen/o**	strength
		stigmat/o	point, mark
-salpinx	tube (usually fallopian or eustachian [auditory] tube)	**stomat/o**	mouth
		-stomy	forming an opening (mouth)
sarc/o	flesh (connective tissue)	**sub-**	under, below
-sarcoma	malignant tumor of connective tissue	**sudor/o**	sweat
		super-	upper, above
scapul/o	scapula (shoulder blade)	**super/o**	upper, above
-schisis	a splitting	**supra-**	above; excessive; superior
schiz/o	split	**sym-**	union, together, joined
scler/o	hardening; sclera (white of eye)	**syn-**	union, together, joined
scoli/o	crooked, bent	**synapt/o**	synapsis, point of contact
-scope	instrument for examining	**synov/o**	synovial membrane, synovial fluid
-scopy	visual examination		
scot/o	darkness	**T**	
seb/o	sebum, sebaceous	**tachy-**	rapid
semi-	one half	**tax/o**	order, coordination
semin/o	semen; seed	**-taxia**	order, coordination
semin/i	semen; seed	**ten/o**	tendon
sept/o	septum	**tend/o**	tendon
sequestr/o	separation	**tendin/o**	tendon
ser/o	serum	**-tension**	to stretch
sial/o	saliva, salivary gland	**test/o**	testis (plural, testes)
sider/o	iron	**thalam/o**	thalamus
sigmoid/o	sigmoid colon	**thalass/o**	sea
silic/o	flint	**thec/o**	sheath (usually refers to meninges)
sin/o	sinus, cavity	**thel/o**	nipple
sinus/o	sinus, cavity	**therapeut/o**	treatment
-sis	state of; condition	**-therapy**	treatment
-social	society	**therm/o**	heat
somat/o	body	**thorac/o**	chest
somn/o	sleep	**-thorax**	chest
son/o	sound	**thromb/o**	blood clot
-spadias	slit, fissure	**thym/o**	thymus gland
-spasm	involuntary contraction, twitching	**-thymia**	mind; emotion
sperm/i	spermatozoa, sperm cells	**thyr/o**	thyroid gland
sperm/o	spermatozoa, sperm cells	**thyroid/o**	thyroid gland
spermat/o	spermatozoa, sperm cells	**tibi/o**	tibia (larger bone of lower leg)
sphygm/o	pulse	**-tic**	pertaining to,
-sphyxia	pulse	**ill/o**	to pull

Element	Meaning	Element	Meaning
-tocia	childbirth, labor	ureter/o	ureter
tom/o	to cut	urethr/o	urethra
-tome	instrument to cut	-uria	urine
-tomy	incision	urin/o	urine, urinary tract
ton/o	tension	-us	condition; structure
tonsill/o	tonsils	uter/o	uterus (womb)
tox/o	poison	uvul/o	uvula
-toxic	poison		
toxic/o	poison	**V, W**	
trabecul/o	trabecula (supporting bundles of fibers)	vagin/o	vagina
		valv/o	valve
trache/o	trachea (windpipe)	varic/o	dilated vein
trans-	across, through	vas/o	vessel; vas deferens; duct
tri-	three	vascul/o	vessel (usually blood or lymph)
trich/o	hair	ven/o	vein
trigon/o	trigone (triangular region at base of bladder)	ventr/o	belly, belly side
		ventricul/o	ventricle (of heart or brain)
-tripsy	crushing	-version	turning
-trophy	development, nourishment	vertebr/o	vertebrae (backbone)
-tropia	turning	vesic/o	bladder
-tropin	stimulate	vesicul/o	seminal vesicle
tubercul/o	a little swelling	vest/o	clothes
tympan/o	tympanic membrane (eardrum)	viscer/o	internal organs
		vitr/o	vitreous body (of eye)
U		vitre/o	glassy
		vol/o	volume
-ula	small, minute	voyeur/o	to see
-ule	small, minute	vulv/o	vulva
uln/o	ulna (lower arm bone on opposite side of thumb)		
		X, Y, Z	
ultra-	excess, beyond		
-um	structure, thing	xanth/o	yellow
umbilic/o	umbilicus, navel	xen/o	foreign, strange
ungu/o	nail	xer/o	dry
uni-	one	xiph/o	sword
ur/o	urine, urinary tract	-y	condition; process

English Terms

Meaning	Element	Meaning	Element
A		atrium	atri/o
abdomen	abdomin/o	attraction for	-phil
	lapar/o		phil/o
abnormal condition			-philia
(produced by		away from	ef-
something specified)	-iasis	away from, from	ab-
abnormal condition;		axis, axon	ax/o
increase (used		axon, axis	ax/o
primarily with blood cells)	-osis	**B**	
above normal, excessive	hyper-		
above, upon	epi-	babble, speech	-lalia
above, upper	super-	back (of body)	dors/o
above; excessive; superior	supra-	back (of body),	poster/o
acromion (projection	acromi/o	behind, posterior	
of scapula)		back; against; up	ana-
across, through	dia-	backward, behind	retro-
	trans-	bacteria (singular,	bacteri/o
the act of	-ion	bacterium)	
act of leading, bringing,	-duction	bad	mal-
conducting		bad; painful; difficult	dys-
act of measuring	-metry	band, fascia (fibrous	
adenoids	adenoid/o	membrane supporting	
adrenal glands	adren/o	and separating muscles)	fasci/o
	adrenal/o	base (alkaline, opposite	
after, behind	post-	of acid)	bas/o
against	anti-	to bear (offspring)	-para
against, opposite	contra-	before, in front of	ante-
against; up; back	ana-		pre-
air	aer/o		pro-
air; lung	pneum/o	beginning	-arche
	pneumon/o	behind, after	post-
air sac; alveolus	alveol/o	behind, backward	retro-
albumin (protein)	albumin/o	belly side, belly	ventr/o
alike, same	home/o	below, deficient, under	hyp-
	homeo-		hyp/o
all	pan-	below, lower	infer/o
alveolus; air sac	alveol/o	below, under	infra-
amnion (amniotic sac)	amni/o		sub-
angle	goni/o	bent, crooked	scoli/o
anterior, front	anter/o	bent, crooked; stiffness	ankyl/o
anus	an/o	beside, near; beyond	para-
anus, rectum	proct/o	between	inter-
aorta	aort/o	beyond, change	meta-
appendix	append/o	beyond, excess	ultra-
	appendic/o	beyond; near, beside	para-
appetite	-orexia	bile, gall	bil/i, chol/e
arm	brachi/o	bile duct	choledoch/o
around	circum-	bile vessel	cholangi/o
	peri-	binding, fixation	-desis
arteriole	arteriol/o	(of a bone or joint)	
artery	arteri/o	birth	nat/o
asbestos	asbest/o	black	melan/o

Meaning	Element	Meaning	Element
bladder	cyst/o	chemical; drug	chem/o
	vesic/o	chest	pector/o
blood	hem/o		steth/o
	hemat/o		thorac/o
blood clot	thromb/o		-thorax
blood condition	-emia	child; foot	ped/i
blood vessel	hemangi/o		ped/o
blue	cyan/o	childbirth, labor	-tocia
body	corp/o	chorion	chori/o
	corpor/o	choroid	choroid/o
	somat/o	ciliary body of eye; circular; cycle	cycl/o
bone	oste/o		
bone marrow; spinal cord	myel/o	clavicle (collar bone)	clavicul/o
brain	encephal/o	clear; to shine	-lucent
to break	-clast	clonus (turmoil)	clon/o
to break; surgical fracture	-clasia	closure	-cleisis
	-clasis	clothes	vest/o
breast	mamm/o	clumping, gluing	agglutin/o
	mast/o	coal dust, coal	anthrac/o
breathe	spir/o	coccyx (tailbone)	coccyg/o
breathing	-pnea	cochlea	cochle/o
bronchiole	bronchiol/o	cold	cry/o
bronchus (plural, bronchi)	bronch/o	colon	col/o
	bronchi/o		colon/o
burn, heat	cauter/o	color	chrom/o
bursting forth (of)	-rrhage		chromat/o
	-rrhagia	conceiving	-ception
		condition	-esis
C			-ia
			-ism
calcaneum (heel bone)	calcane/o	condition; process	-y
calcium	calc/o	condition; state of	-ema
calculus, stone	-lith		-isy
	lith/o		-sis
cancer	carcin/o	condition; structure	-us
carbon dioxide (CO_2)	-capnia	conducting, act of leading, bringing	-duction
carpus (wrist bones)	carp/o		
to carry	-ferent	condyle	condyl/o
carry; to lead	duct/o	conjunctiva	conjunctiv/o
carrying, transmission	-phoresis	coordination, order	tax/o
cartilage	chondr/o		-taxia
cause	eti/o	cornea	corne/o
cavity, sinus	sin/o	cornea; horny tissue; hard	kerat/o
	sinus/o	cortex	cortic/o
cecum	cec/o	cranium (skull)	crani/o
cell	cyt/o	crooked, bent	scoli/o
	-cyte	crooked, bent; stiffness	ankyl/o
cerebellum	cerebell/o	cross	cruci/o
cerebrum	cerebr/o	crushing	-tripsy
cervix uteri (neck of uterus); neck	cervic/o	cul-de-sac	culd/o
		curve, swayback	lord/o
cessation	de-	to cut	tom/o
change, beyond	meta-	cutting	-cision
cheek	bucc/o		

(continued)

Meaning	Element	Meaning	Element
cycle; ciliary body of eye; circular	cycl/o	eating, swallowing	phag/o
			-phage
D			-phagia
		electricity	electr/o
dark, dusky	phe/o	embolus (plug)	embol/o
darkness	scot/o	embryonic cell	-blast
dawn (rose-colored)	eosin/o		blast/o
death, necrosis	necr/o	emotion; mind	-thymia
debility, weakness	-asthenia	enlarge, widen	mydr/o
decrease, deficiency	-penia	enlargement	mega-
deficiency, decrease	-penia		megal/o
deficient, under, below	hyp-		-megaly
	hyp/o	epididymis	epididym/o
	hyp/o	epiglottis	epiglott/o
development; nourishment	-trophy	equal, same	iso-
diaphragm; mind	phren/o	esophagus	esophag/o
different	hetero-	excess, beyond	ultra-
differing from the normal, other	allo-	excessive, above normal	hyper-
		excision, removal	-ectomy
difficult; bad; painful	dys-	expansion, dilation	-ectasis
digestion	-pepsia	extremity	acr/o
dilated vein	varic/o	eye	ocul/o
dilation, expansion	-ectasis		ophthalm/o
dim, dull	ambly/o	eye, vision	opt/o
discharge, flow	-rrhea		optic/o
disease	path/o	eyelid	blephar/o
	-pathy		
dissimilar, unequal	aniso-	**F**	
double	di-		
	dipl-	face	faci/o
	dipl/o	false	pseudo-
down	cata-	far, farthest	dist/o
downward displacement, prolapse	-ptosis	fascia (fibrous membrane supporting and separating muscles), band	fasci/o
drug, medicine	pharmaceutic/o	fat	adip/o
drug; chemical	chem/o		lip/o
dry	xer/o		lipid/o
dry, scaly	ichthy/o		steat/o
duct; vessel; vas deferens	vas/o	fatty plaque	ather/o
dull, dim	ambly/o	fear	-phobia
duodenum (first part of small intestine)	duoden/o	feeling	esthes/o
			-esthesia
		feeling (mental state)	-phoria
dura mater; hard	dur/o	female, woman	gyn/o
dusky, dark	phe/o		gynec/o
dust	coni/o	femur (thigh bone)	femor/o
		fiber, fibrous tissue	fibr/o
E		fibula (smaller bone of lower leg)	fibul/o
ear	aur/o	fingers; toes	dactyl/o
	auricul/o	fire	pyr/o
	ot/o		

Meaning	Element	Meaning	Element
first	primi-	green	chlor/o
fissure, slit	-spadias	groin	inguin/o
fixation (of a bone or joint), binding	-desis	growth	-physis
		growth, formation	plas/o
fixation (of an organ)	-pexy		-plasia
flesh (connective tissue)	sarc/o		-plasm
flint	silic/o	gum(s)	gingiv/o
flow, discharge	-rrhea		
fluorescence, luminous	fluor/o	**H**	
foot	pod/o	hair	pil/o
foot; child	ped/i		trich/o
	ped/o	hallucination	hallucin/o
foreign, strange	xen/o	hard; dura mater	dur/o
form, shape, structure	morph/o	hardening; sclera (white of eye)	scler/o
formation, growth	plas/o	having the form of, possessing	-ate
	-plasia	head	cephal/o
	-plasm		-ceps
formation, production	-poiesis	hearing	acous/o
forming an opening (mouth)	-stomy		-acusis
forming, producing, origin	-gen		audi/o
	gen/o		audit/o
	-genesis		-cusia
four	quadri-		-cusis
frenzy, state of mental disorder	-mania	heart	cardi/o
from, away from	ab-	heart condition	-cardia
front, anterior	anter/o	heat	therm/o
fungus (plural, fungi)	myc/o	heat, burn	cauter/o
		hernia, swelling	-cele
G		hidden	crypt/o
gall, bile	chol/e	to hold back	-continence
gallbladder	cholecyst/o		isch/o
ganglion (knot or knotlike mass)	gangli/o	horny tissue; hard; cornea	kerat/o
		humerus (upper arm bone)	humer/o
genetic change	mut/a	humpback	kyph/o
gland	aden/o		
glans penis	balan/o	**I**	
glassy	vitre/o	ileum (third part of small intestine)	ile/o
glomerulus	glomerul/o		
glottis	glott/o	ilium (lateral, flaring portion of hip bone)	ili/o
glue; neuroglial tissue	gli/o	immune, immunity, safe	immun/o
	-glia	imperfect; incomplete	atel/o
gluing, clumping	agglutin/o	in, not	in-
gonads, sex glands	gonad/o	in, within	en-
good, normal	eu-		end-
granule	granul/o		endo-
gray	glauc/o		intra-
gray matter (of brain or spinal cord); gray	poli/o	in front of, before	ante-
gray; gray matter (of brain or spinal cord)	poli/o		pre-
			pro-

(continued)

Meaning	Element	Meaning	Element
incision	-tomy	larynx (voice box)	laryng/o
incomplete; imperfect	atel/o	to lead; carry	duct/o
increase (used primarily	-osis	lens	phac/o
with blood cells);		less, smaller	mi/o
abnormal condition		lice	pedicul/o
inflammation	-itis	life	bi/o
to inflate	emphys/o	light	phot/o
instrument for examining	-scope	limestone	chalic/o
instrument for measuring	-meter	lip	cheil/o
instrument for recording	-graph		labi/o
instrument to cut	-tome	liver	hepat/o
insulin	insulin/o	lobe	lob/o
internal organs	viscer/o	loins (lower back)	lumb/o
intestine (usually small	enter/o	loosening; separation;	-lysis
intestine)		destruction	
involuntary contraction,	-spasm	lower, below	infer/o
twitching		luminous, fluorescence	fluor/o
inward	eso-	lung	pulmon/o
iris	irid/o	lung; air	pneum/o
iron	sider/o		pneumon/o
irregular, varied	poikil/o	lymph	lymph/o
irrigation, washing	-clysis	lymph gland (node)	lymphaden/o
ischium (lower portion	ischi/o	lymph vessel	lymphangi/o
of hip bone)			

Meaning	Element	Meaning	Element
J		**M**	
jaundice	-icterus	male	andr/o
jejunum (second part of		malignant tumor of connective	-sarcoma
small intestine)	jejun/o	tissue	
joined, union, together	sym-	many, much	multi-
	syn-		poly-
joint	arthr/o	mark, point	stigmat/o
K		marketplace	agora-
		mastoid process	mastoid/o
kernel (nucleus)	kern/o	maxilla (upper jaw bone)	maxill/o
ketone bodies (acids	ket/o	meal	-prandial
and acetones)		measure; uterus (womb)	metr/o
	keton/o	meatus, opening	meat/o
kidney	nephr/o	mediastinum	mediastin/o
	ren/o	medicine, drug	pharmaceutic/o
killing	-cide	medicine; treatment	-iatry
knowing	gnos/o	medulla	medull/o
	-gnosis	meninges (membranes	mening/o
L		covering brain and	
		spinal cord)	
labor, childbirth	-tocia		meningi/o
labyrinth (inner ear)	labyrinth/o	menses, menstruation	men/o
lacrimal apparatus	dacry/o	mesh, net	reticul/o
(duct, sac, or gland); tear	lacrim/o	metacarpus (hand bones)	metacarp/o
lacrimal sac	dacryocyst/o	metatarsus (foot bones)	metatars/o
lamina (part of vertebral arch)	lamin/o	middle	medi-
large	macro-		medi/o
			meso-

Meaning	Element	Meaning	Element
midwife	obstetr/o	none	nulli-
milk	galact/o	normal, good	eu-
	lact/o	nose	nas/o
mind	ment/o		rhin/o
	psych/o	not	im-
mind; diaphragm	phren/o	not, in	in-
mind; emotion	-thymia	not, without	a-
minute, small	-icle		an-
	-ole	noun ending	-ice
	-ula		-is
	-ule	nourishment, development	-trophy
miscarry	abort/o	nucleus	kary/o
mouth	or/o		nucle/o
	stomat/o		
movement	cine-	**O**	
	kinesi/o	obscure	-opaque
	-kinesia	old age	presby/o
	kinet/o	one	mono-
much, many	multi-		uni-
	poly-	one half	hemi-
mucus	muc/o		semi-
	myx/o	opening, meatus	meat/o
muscle	muscul/o	opposite, against	contra-
	my/o	order, coordination	tax/o
	myos/o		-taxia
muzzle	phim/o	origin, forming, producing	-gen
N			gen/o
			-genesis
nail	onych/o	other, differing from the normal	allo-
	ungu/o		
narrowing, stricture	sten/o	out from, out	ec-
	-stenosis		ex-
navel, umbilicus	omphal/o	outside	extra-
	umbilic/o	outside, outward	ecto-
near, beside; beyond	para-		exo-
near, nearest	proxim/o	outward, outside	ecto-
neck; cervix uteri (neck of uterus)	cervic/o		exo-
		ovary	oophor/o
necrosis, death	necr/o		ovari/o
neither; neutral	neutr/o	own, self	auto-
nerve	neur/o	oxygen	ox/i
nerve root	radicul/o		ox/o
nest	nid/o		-oxia
net, mesh	reticul/o	**P, Q**	
neuroglial tissue; glue	gli/o		
	-glia	pain	-algesia
neutral; neither	neutr/o		-algia
new	neo-		-dynia
night	noct/o	palate (roof of mouth)	palat/o
	nyctal/o	pancreas	pancreat/o
nipple	thel/o	paralysis	-plegia
nitrogenous compounds	azot/o		

(continued)

Meaning	Element	Meaning	Element
parathyroid glands	parathyroid/o	process (of)	-ation
partial paralysis	-paresis		-ization
patella (kneecap)	patell/o	process; condition	-y
peculiar, unknown	idi/o	process of recording	-graphy
pelvis	pelv/i	production, formation	-poiesis
	pelv/o	prolapse, downward	-ptosis
pelvis bone (anterior part of	pub/o	displacement	
pelvic bone)		prostate gland	prostat/o
penis	pen/o	protection	-phylaxis
perineum (area between	perine/o	protein	-globin
scrotum [or vulva in		to pull	till/o
the female] and anus		pulse	sphygm/o
peritoneum	peritone/o		-sphyxia
pertaining to	-ac	pupil	cor/o
	-al		core/o
	-ar		pupill/o
	-ary		py/o
	-eal	pus	py/o
	-iac	pylorus	pylor/o
	-ic	quick, sharp	oxy-
	-ical		
	-ile	**R**	
	-ine		
	-ior	radiation, x-ray; radius (lower	radi/o
	-itic	arm bone on thumb side)	
	-ive	radius (lower arm bone on	radi/o
	-ory	humb side); radiation, x-ray	
	-ous	rapid	tachy-
	-tic	record, writing	-gram
pertaining to; sugar	-ose	rectum	rect/o
phalanges (bones of fingers	phalang/o	rectum, anus	proct/o
and toes)		red	erythem/o
pharynx (throat)	pharyng/o		erythemat/o
phrase, word	lex/o		erythr/o
physician; medicine; treatment	iatr/o		rube/o
pituitary gland	pituitar/o	removal, excision	-ectomy
plaque	-plakia	renal pelvis	pyel/o
pleasure	hedon/o	repeated sound	echo-
pleura	pleur/o	resembling	-oid
point, mark	stigmat/o	retina	retin/o
point of contact, synapse	synapt/o	ribs	cost/o
poison	tox/o	rod-shaped (striated)	rhabd/o
	-toxic	rod-shaped (striated) muscle	rhabdomy/o
	toxic/o	rupture	-rrhexis
porous	-porosis		
possessing, having the form of	-ate	**S**	
posterior, back (of body),	poster/o	sacrum	sacr/o
behind		safe, immune, immunity	immun/o
potassium (an electrolyte)	kal/i	saliva	ptyal/o
power	-potence	saliva, salivary gland	sial/o
pregnancy	-cyesis	salivary gland, saliva	sial/o
	gest/o	same	homo-
		same, alike	home/o
			homeo-
pregnant woman	-gravida	same, equal	iso-

Meaning	Element	Meaning	Element
scab	eschar/o	society	-social
scale	squam/o	sodium (an electrolyte)	natr/o
scaly, dry	ichthy/o	softening	-malacia
scanty	olig/o	sound	son/o
scapula (shoulder blade)	scapul/o	specialist	-ician
sclera (white of eye); hardening	scler/o		-ist
sea	thalass/o	specialist in the study of	-logist
sebaceous, sebum	seb/o	speech	-phasia
sebum, sebaceous	seb/o	speech, babble	-lalia
secrete	crin/o	sperm cells, spermatozoa	semin/o
	-crine		sperm/i
to see	voyeur/o		sperm/o
seizure	-lepsy		spermat/o
self, own	auto-	spinal cord; bone marrow	myel/o
seminal vesicle	vesicul/o	spine	rachi/o
separation	sequestr/o		spin/o
separation; destruction; loosening	-lysis	spitting	-ptysis
		spleen	splen/o
septum	sept/o	split	schiz/o
serum	ser/o	splitting	-schisis
sex glands, gonads	gonad/o	standing still	-stasis
sharp, quick	oxy-	stapes	staped/o
sheath (usually refers to meninges)	thec/o	star	astr/o
		state of mental disorder, frenzy	-mania
to shine; clear	-lucent	state of; condition	-ema
short	brachy-		-isy
side, to one side	later/o		-sis
sigmoid colon	sigmoid/o	to steal	klept/o
sinus, cavity	sin/o	sternum (breastbone)	stern/o
	sinus/o	stiffness; bent, crooked	ankyl/o
skin	cutane/o	stimulate	-tropin
	derm/o	stomach	gastr/o
	-derma	stone, calculus	-lith
	dermat/o		lith/o
sleep	hypn/o	straight	orth/o
	somn/o	strange, foreign	xen/o
sleep; stupor; numbness	narc/o	strength	sthen/o
slender, thin	lept/o	to stretch	-tension
slipping	-listhesis	stricture, narrowing	sten/o
slit, fissure	-spadias		-stenosis
slow	brady-	stroke	-plexy
small	micr/o	structure, form, shape	morph/o
	micro-	structure, thing	-um
small, minute	-icle	structure; condition	-us
	-ole	study of	log/o
	-ula		-logy
	-ule	stupor; numbness; sleep	narc/o
small growth	polyp/o	sugar, sweetness	gluc/o
smaller, less	mi/o		glucos/o
smell	-osmia		glyc/o
smooth	lei/o		glycos/o
smooth muscle (visceral)	leiomy/o		*(continued)*

Meaning	Element	Meaning	Element
sugar; pertaining to	-ose	thyroid gland	thyr/o
superior; above; excessive	supra-		thyroid/o
surgical fracture; to break	-clasia	tibia (larger bone of lower leg)	tibi/o
	-clasis	tissue	hist/o
surgical puncture	-centesis		histi/o
surgical repair	-plasty	to one side, side	later/o
suture	-rrhaphy	toes; fingers	dactyl/o
swallowing, eating	phag/o	tongue	gloss/o
	-phage		lingu/o
	-phagia	tonsils	tonsill/o
swayback, curve	lord/o	toward	-ad
sweat	hidr/o		ad-
	sudor/o		af-
sweetness, sugar	gluc/o	trabecula (supporting bundles of fibers)	trabecul/o
	glucos/o	trachea (windpipe)	trache/o
	glyc/o	transmission, carrying	-phoresis
	glycos/o	transplantation	-graft
swelling	-edema	treatment	therapeut/o
swelling (a little)	tubercul/o		-therapy
swelling, hernia	-cele	treatment; medicine	-iatry
sword	xiph/o	treatment; physician; medicine	iatr/o
synapsis, point of contact	synapt/o	tree	dendr/o
synovial fluid, synovial membrane	synov/o	trigone (triangular region at base of bladder)	trigon/o
T		tube (usually fallopian or eustachian [auditory] tubes)	salping/o
tail	caud/o		-salpinx
tear; lacrimal apparatus (duct, sac, or gland)	dacry/o	tumor	-oma
	lacrim/o		onc/o
teeth	dent/o	turning	-tropia
	odont/o		-version
tendon	ten/o		-spasm
	tend/o	twitching, involuntary contraction	
	tendin/o	two	bas/o
tension	ton/o	tympanic membrane (eardrum)	myring/o
testis (plural, testes)	orch/o		tympan/o
	orchi/o		
	orchid/o	**U**	
	test/o	ulna (lower arm bone on opposite side of thumb)	uln/o
thalamus	thalam/o		
thick	pachy-	umbilicus, navel	umbilic/o
thin, slender	lept/o	under, below	infra-
thing, structure	-um		sub-
things that move	cinemat/o	under, below, deficient	hyp-
thirst	dips/o		hyp/o
	-dipsia		hyp/o
three	tri-	unequal, dissimilar	aniso-
through	per-	union, together, joined	sym-
through, across	dia-		syn-
	trans-	unknown, peculiar	idi/o
thymus gland	thym/o		

Meaning	Element	Meaning	Element
upon, above	epi-	vomiting	-emesis
upper, above	super-	vulva	episi/o
ureter	ureter/o		vulv/o
urethra	urethr/o	**W**	
urine	ur/o	washing, irrigation	-clysis
	-uria	water	aque/o
	urin/o		hydr/o
uterus (womb)	hyster/o	weakness, debility	-asthenia
	metri/o	white	albin/o
	uter/o		leuk/o
uterus (womb); measure	metr/o	widen, enlarge	mydr/o
uvula	uvul/o	widened blood vessel,	aneurysm/o
V		a widening	
vagina	colp/o	within, in	en-
	vagin/o		end-
valve	valv/o		endo-
varied, irregular	poikil/o		intra-
vein	phleb/o	without, not	a-
	ven/o		an-
ventricle (of heart or brain)	ventricul/o	woman, female	gyn/o
vertebrae (backbone)	spondyl/o		gynec/o
	vertebr/o	word, phrase	lex/o
vessel (usually blood or lymph)	angi/o	wrinkle	rhytid/o
	vascul/o	writing, record	-gram
vessel; vas deferens; duct	vas/o	**X, Y, Z**	
view of	-opsy	x-ray, radiation; radius (lower	
vision	-opia	arm bone on thumb side),	
	-opsia	radiation	radi/o
vision, eye	opt/o	x-rays	roentgen/o
	optic/o	yellow	cirrh/o
visual examination	-scopy		jaund/o
vitreous body (of eye)	vitr/o		xanth/o
voice	-phonia		
volume	vol/o		

Index of Genetic Disorders

Index of Diagnostic Imaging Procedures

Index of Pharmacology

Index of Oncological Terms

Index